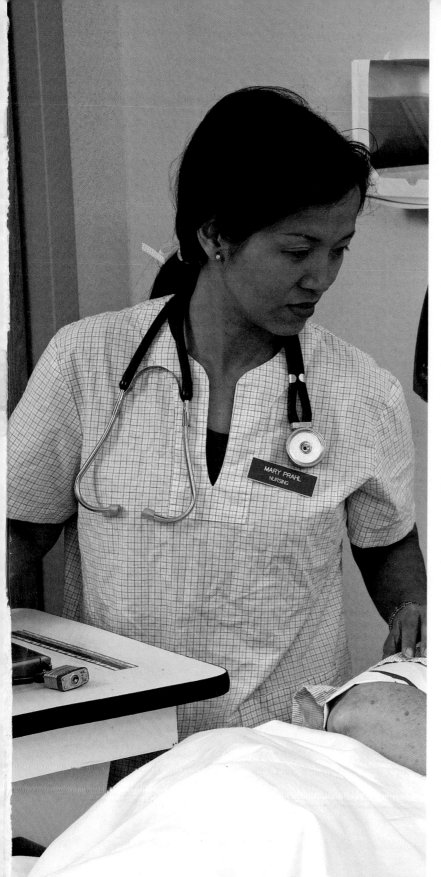

P9-CRU-899

Essentials of Medical Language

Second Edition

David M. Allan, MA, MD

Karen D. Lockyer, BS, RHIT, CPC

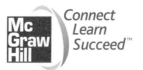
Connect
Learn
Succeed™

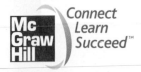
ESSENTIALS OF MEDICAL LANGUAGE, Second Edition

Published by McGraw-Hill, a business unit of The McGraw-Hill Companies, Inc., 1221 Avenue of the Americas, New York, NY, 10020. Copyright © 2012 by The McGraw-Hill Companies, Inc. All rights reserved. Previous edition © 2010. No part of this publication may be reproduced or distributed in any form or by any means, or stored in a database or retrieval system, without the prior written consent of The McGraw-Hill Companies, Inc., including, but not limited to, in any network or other electronic storage or transmission, or broadcast for distance learning.

Some ancillaries, including electronic and print components, may not be available to customers outside the United States.

✪ This book is printed on acid-free paper.

1 2 3 4 5 6 7 8 9 0 DOW/DOW 1 0 9 8 7 6 5 4 3 2 1

ISBN   978-0-07-337461-1
MHID   0-07-337461-X

Vice president/Editor in chief: *Elizabeth Haefele*
Vice president/Director of marketing: *John E. Biernat*
Publisher: *Kenneth S. Kasee, Jr.*
Senior sponsoring editor: *Natalie J. Ruffatto*
Director of development: *Sarah Wood*
Managing development editor: *Christine Scheid*
Marketing manager: *Mary B. Haran*
Lead digital product manager: *Damian Moshak*
Director, Editing/Design/Production: *Jess Ann Kosic*
Project manager: *Jean R. Starr*
Buyer: *Susan Culbertson*
Senior designer: *Srdjan Savanovic*
Lead photo research coordinator: *Carrie K. Burger*
Photo researcher: *Pam Carley*
Digital production coordinator: *Brent dela Cruz*
Outside development house: *Perrin Davis, Agate ProBooks*
Cover design: *Srdjan Savanovic*
Interior design: *Agate ProBooks*
Typeface: *10/11 Adobe Garamond Pro Regular*
Compositor: *Agate ProBooks*
Printer: *R. R. Donnelley*
Cover credit: © *Dr. David Phillips/Visuals Unlimited/Corbis*
Credits: The credits section for this book begins on page 567 and is considered an extension of the copyright page.

Library of Congress Cataloging in Publication Data

Library of Congress Control Number: 2010941605

The Internet addresses listed in the text were accurate at the time of publication. The inclusion of a Web site does not indicate an endorsement by the authors or McGraw-Hill, and McGraw-Hill does not guarantee the accuracy of the information presented at these sites.

www.mhhe.com

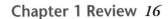
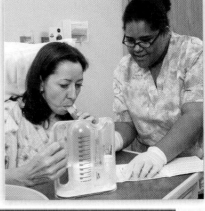
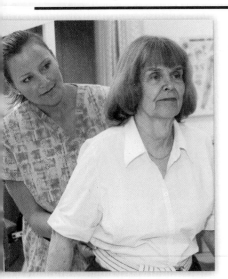
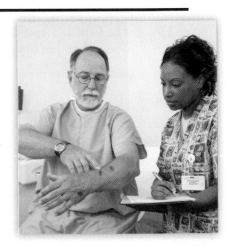

Chapter 4
The Skeletal System: *The Essentials of the Language of Orthopedics* 86

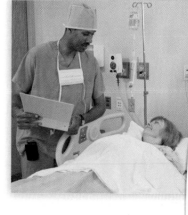

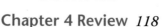

Chapter 5
Muscles and Tendons: *The Essentials of the Languages of Orthopedics and Rehabilitation* 130

Chapter 6
Cardiovascular and Circulatory Systems: *The Essentials of the Language of Cardiology* 152

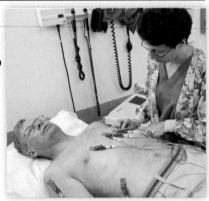

Chapter 7
The Blood, Lymphatic, and Immune Systems: *The Essentials of the Languages of Hematology and Immunology* 186

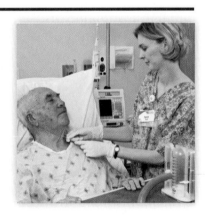

Chapter 8
Respiratory System: *The Essentials of the Language of Pulmonology* 226

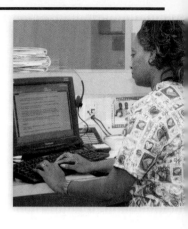

Chapter 9
The Digestive System: *The Essentials of the Language of Gastroenterology* 258

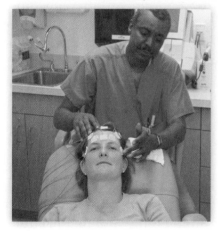

Chapter 10
The Nervous System and Mental Health: *The Essentials of the Languages of Neurology and Psychiatry* 300

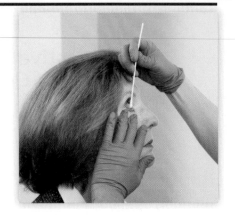
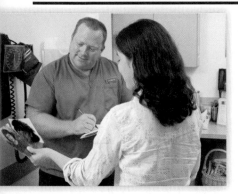
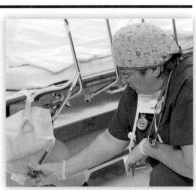

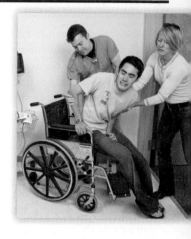
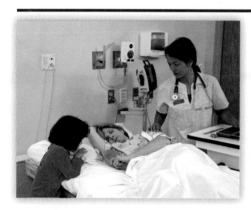

TO THE STUDENTS

Welcome to the second edition of *Essentials of Medical Language!* You may be asking yourself why taking Medical Terminology is so important. Considering you have chosen a major or a program that focuses on health care—whether it is nursing or medical assisting, medical coding or health information technology—understanding the language of medicine will be one of the most important skills you must master.

Right now, you are a student preparing for a career as a health professional. You may have already had a few health care-related courses, or this may be your very first course. Someday, you will be in a real medical office, hospital, or another health-care-related setting. *Essentials of Medical Language* is written using examples from **real-world health-care scenarios**—scenarios that you could actually encounter someday yourself. Just as one of the best ways to learn a foreign language is to be immersed in the language and culture of the country where it is spoken, one of the best ways to learn medical language is to be immersed within a vibrant, authentic, modern health care community.

To make sure your needs are addressed in this book, we asked both students and experienced medical terminology instructors, "What helps students learn medical terminology?" Overwhelmingly, the responses pointed to four common factors:

- motivation to learn
- retention of the material
- opportunities for application and practice
- readily available information

THIS TEXTBOOK INCORPORATES FEATURES DESIGNED TO ADDRESS THESE FOUR FACTORS:

Motivation to learn	→	In order for students to be motivated to learn, what they are learning must be meaningful and relevant. To ensure the chapters in *Essentials of Medical Language* fit these criteria, the student is asked to step into the role of an allied health professional in each chapter. Authentic patient cases are used to illustrate how medical language is used on the job.
Retention of the material	→	When students encounter new medical terms within the context of a patient case, they are able to remember it more effectively. In addition, each chapter presents medical terms from one body system or medical specialty, which further serves to "tie it all together" to help students retain the knowledge and skills.
Opportunities for application and practice	→	Practice makes perfect. This is especially true for learning medical terminology. This textbook provides many opportunities for students to apply what they are learning. Exercises are included in the lessons, as well as at the end of each chapter. Additional exercises are available on the student Online Learning Center (www.mhhe.com/AllanEss2e).
Readily available information	→	In this book, all the information needed for a specific topic is presented in self-contained two-page spreads. On the left-hand page, new medical terms are introduced. On the right-hand page, for each new term, the pronunciation, color-coded word elements, and definition are provided in a *Word Analysis and Definition (WAD) Table.*

Essentials of Medical Language will help you learn the terminology and language of modern health care in a way that bridges the gap between the classroom and a clinical setting.

RELEVANT MATERIALS – YOUR MOTIVATION TO LEARN!

Essentials of Medical Language 2e provides you with terminology, exercises, images and examples you can apply to other courses and within your career. You will step into the role of a health professional in every chapter and experience medical language illustrated through authentic patient cases.

BODY SYSTEMS AND MEDICAL SPECIALTIES – REMEMBER AND APPLY THE MATERIAL!

Encountering new medical terms within the context of each patient case will help you remember them more effectively. Every chapter presents medical terms from one body system or medical specialty, which helps tie it all together!

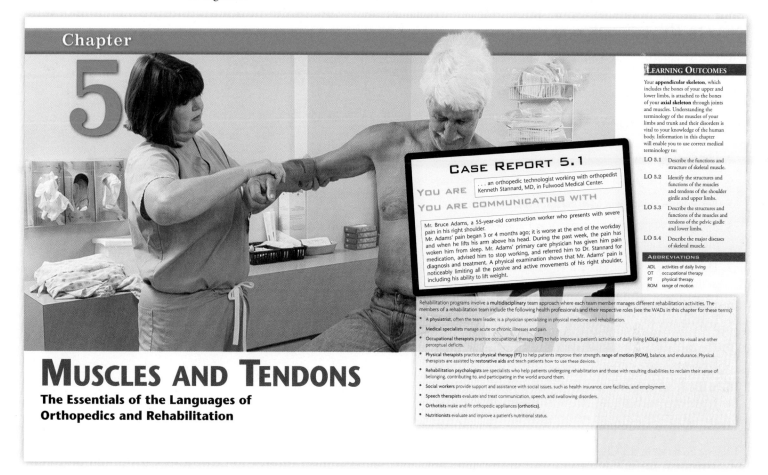

APPLICATION AND PRACTICE – YOUR KEY TO MASTERING MEDICAL TERMINOLOGY!

Practice makes perfect, especially when you are learning medical terminology. You will have plenty of opportunity to apply what you learn through exercises during the lessons and at the end of every chapter. Additional practice opportunities and exercises are available through LearnSmart Allied Health: Medical Terminology and Connect Plus (see pages xvi and xv).

To The Instructor

McGraw-Hill knows how much effort it takes to prepare for a new course. Through focus groups, symposia, reviews, and conversations with instructors like you, we have gathered information about what materials you need in order to facilitate successful courses. We are committed to providing you with high-quality, accurate instructor support.

Meeting Your Needs

New to This Edition!

1. The second edition contains 120 fewer text pages than the first edition. This has been achieved by reducing the anatomy and physiology; by focusing on essential terms, disorders and procedures; and by changing the layout of the text on each page.

2. The book's artwork has been enlarged and labeling has been reduced to allow greater focus on the terms covered within a spread.

3. The chapter sequence has been revised.

4. More word construction and deconstruction exercises have been added to the book.

5. The learning objectives have been revised and updated.

6. The lesson objectives have been tagged numerically and related to all questions in the Test Bank and to the exercises and activities in the Instructor Manual.

7. The learning objectives have been mapped to the content, with lessons in each chapter directly correlated to the learning objectives it satisfies.

8. The Word Analysis and Definition (WAD) tables and review exercises have been revamped and expanded and are now Bloom's taxonomy-progressive.

9. The contextual Case Reports have been emphasized within well-defined boxes. Each spread with a Case Report includes an exercise that reviews the Case Report.

10. In the opening spread of each chapter, we have included a list of health professionals involved in that particular specialty. The professions are also defined.

11. In each spread more questions and/or exercises have been added that are tied to the lesson objectives.

12. The exercises in the Chapter Reviews move from easy to more difficult based on Bloom's taxonomy.

13. The right page of each spread is now dedicated solely to WADs and exercises, and all content and art is confined to the left page of each spread.

14. The two musculoskeletal chapters have been segregated into one muscle chapter and one skeletal chapter.

15. The two female reproductive chapters have been combined into a single chapter.

16. The combined Urinary System and Male Reproductive System chapter has been split into a Urinary System chapter and a Male Reproductive System chapter.

17. The Life Span chapter can now be found in Create, McGraw-Hill's custom publishing alternative Web site (www.mcgrawhillcreate.com).

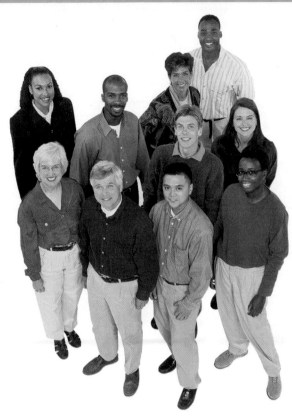

When you use *Essentials of Medical Language,* you will be supported at every point in the program. Each chapter in the book is broken down into lessons, and the Instructor's Manual provides lesson plans and additional materials for each lesson. Following are features of the textbook designed to address student needs:

Lesson-Based Approach

Each chapter of *Essentials of Medical Language* is divided into lessons covering different aspects of the overall chapter subject. Lessons within a chapter break down into topics. Each topic is designed so your students will not have to flip back and forth when completing exercises or looking at figures, tables, and boxes. All main concepts and ideas presented in topics begin and end within a two-page "spread." These spreads help learning flow smoothly by ensuring that valuable class and reading time is not wasted on flipping pages.

You Are . . . Your Patient Is . . . Case Scenarios

Each chapter and most lessons begin by immediately placing your students in the role of an allied health professional faced with a situation in which medical communication is necessary. Many different professional allied health and LPN-level nursing roles are utilized so your students can "experience" various specialties and positions. The patient cases introduced at the beginning of the chapters and lessons are referenced throughout the lessons to further unify the students' experience.

Chapter Outcomes and Lesson Objectives

The major learning outcomes for each chapter are previewed in the beginning so you and your students can focus on what they need to know and be able to do by the end of the chapter. Each lesson has outcome-based learning objectives. Accomplishing each lesson's objectives helps ensure students will be able to achieve the chapter outcomes and, ultimately, the goal of the textbook: to help them learn the essential terminology and language of modern health care.

Word Analysis and Definition Tables (WAD)

Each lesson contains tables listing important medical terms and their pronunciation, elements, and definition. Prefixes, suffixes, and combining forms are color-coded. These tables provide your students with an at-a-glance view of the terms covered. The tables are excellent for reference as well as for studying and reviewing.

End-of-Lesson and End-of-Chapter Exercises

At the end of each lesson is a series of exercises. The end-of-lesson exercises provide your students with immediate practice using the terms in the lesson. These exercises focus on basic understanding and ability to apply the terms. They are an excellent foundation for the end-of-chapter exercises, which are often based on authentic situations, such as interactions with patients, physicians, or medical documentation. The end-of-chapter exercises will require your students to understand, accurately apply, and think critically about the medical language they use. Throughout the text, frequent opportunities for application and reinforcement of medical language skills and concepts are provided to help your students build confidence and knowledge. A wide variety of exercises and activities are included to address different medical settings and levels of learning (including knowledge, comprehension, application, analysis, synthesis, and evaluation).

Introducing *Connect Plus™ Allied Health*: Medical Terminology

McGraw-Hill's new *Connect Plus Allied Health:* Medical Terminology is a revolutionary online assignment and assessment solution, providing instructors and students with tools and resources to maximize their success.

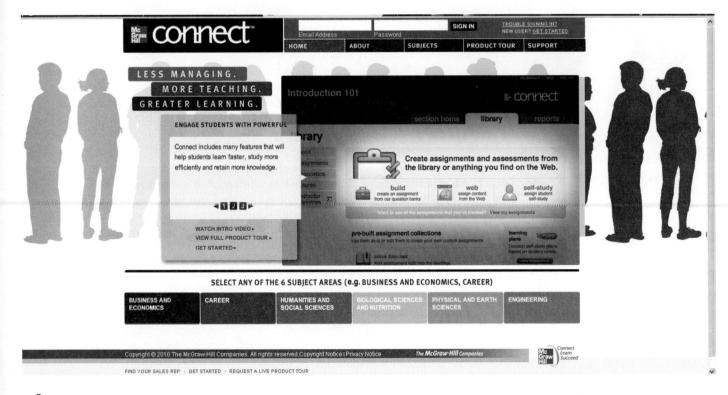

Simple assignment management

With *Connect Plus Allied Health:* Medical Terminology, creating assignments is easier than ever, so you can spend more time teaching and less time managing. The assignment management function enables you to:

- Create and deliver assignments easily with selectable Interactives, vocabulary exercises, end-of-chapter questions, and test bank items.

- Streamline lesson planning, student progress reporting, and assignment grading to make classroom management more efficient than ever.

- Go paperless with the eBook and online submission and grading of student assignments.

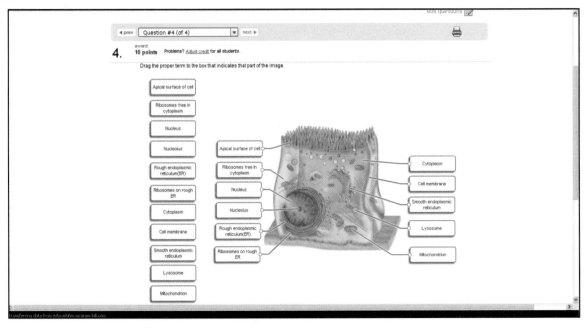

SMART GRADING

When it comes to studying, time is precious. *Connect Plus Allied Health:* Medical Terminology helps students learn more efficiently by providing feedback and practice material when they need it, where they need it. When it comes to teaching, your time also is precious. The grading function enables you to:

- Have assignments scored automatically, giving students immediate feedback on their work and side-by-side comparisons with correct answers.

- Access and review each response; manually change grades or leave comments for students to review.

- Reinforce classroom concepts with practice tests and instant quizzes.

INSTRUCTOR LIBRARY

The *Connect Plus Allied Health:* Medical Terminology Instructor Library is your repository for additional resources to improve student engagement in and out of class. You can select and use any asset that enhances your lecture. The *Connect Plus Allied Health:* Medical Terminology Instructor Library includes:

- *Instructor's Manual*

- *Testbank*

- *PowerPoint presentation*

- *Videos*

- *Animations (to come April 2011)*

- *eBook*
  - Fully integrated, allowing for anytime, anywhere access to the textbook.
  - Dynamic links between the exercises or questions you assign to your students and the location in the eBook where that exercise or question is covered.
  - A powerful search function to pinpoint and connect key concepts in a snap.

STUDENT PROGRESS TRACKING

Connect Plus Allied Health: Medical Terminology keeps instructors informed about how each student, section, and class is performing, allowing for more productive use of lecture and office hours. The progress-tracking function enables you to:

- View scored work immediately and track individual or group performance with assignment and grade reports.

- Access an instant view of student or class performance relative to learning objectives.

- Collect data and generate reports required by many accreditation organizations, such as CAAHEP or ABHES.

LECTURE CAPTURE

Increase the attention paid to lecture discussion by decreasing the attention paid to note taking. For an additional charge Lecture Capture offers new ways for students to focus on the in-class discussion, knowing they can revisit important topics later. Lecture Capture enables you to:

- Record and distribute your lecture with a click of a button.

- Record and index PowerPoint presentations and anything shown on your computer so they are easily searchable, frame by frame.

- Offer access to lectures anytime and anywhere by computer, iPod, or mobile device.

- Increase intent listening and class participation by easing students' concerns about note-taking. Lecture Capture will make it more likely you will see students' faces, not the tops of their heads.

McGraw-Hill's LearnSmart—Diagnostic and Adaptive Learning of Concepts

Students want to make the best use of their study time. The **LearnSmart** adaptive self-study technology within *Connect Plus Allied Health:* Medical Terminology provides students with a seamless combination of practice, assessment, and remediation of concepts found in their textbook. **LearnSmart's** intelligent software adapts to every student response and automatically delivers concepts that advance student understanding while reducing time devoted to the concepts already mastered. The result for every student is the fastest path to mastery of the chapter concepts. **LearnSmart:**

- Applies an intelligent concept engine to identify the relationships between concepts and to serve new concepts to each student only when he or she is ready.

- Adapts automatically to each student, so students spend less time on the topics they understand and practice more those they have yet to master.

- Provides continual reinforcement and remediation, but gives only as much guidance as students need.

- Integrates diagnostics as part of the learning experience.

- Enables you to assess which concepts students have efficiently learned on their own, thus freeing class time for more applications and discussion.

For more information about *Connect Plus Allied Health:* **Medical Terminology** or **LearnSmart,** go to **www. mcgrawhillconnect.com,** or contact your local McGraw-Hill sales representative.

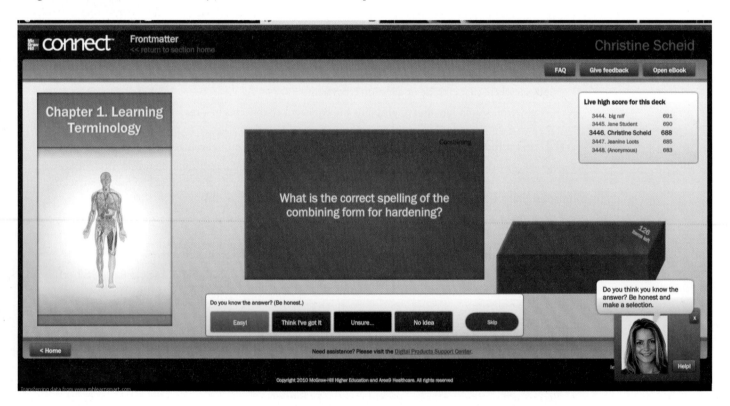

McGraw-Hill Higher Education and Blackboard have teamed up. What does this mean for you?

1. *Your life, simplified.* Now you and your students can access McGraw-Hill's Connect™ and Create™ right from within your Blackboard course—all with one single sign-on. Say goodbye to the days of logging in to multiple applications forever.

2. *Deep integration of content and tools.* Not only do you get single sign-on with Connect™ and Create™, you also get deep integration of McGraw-Hill content and content engines right in Blackboard. Whether you're choosing a book for your course or building Connect™ assignments, all the tools you need are right where you want them—inside of Blackboard.

3. *Seamless gradebooks.* Are you tired of keeping multiple gradebooks and manually synchronizing grades into Blackboard? We thought so. When a student completes an integrated Connect™ assignment, the grade for that assignment automatically (and instantly) feeds your Blackboard grade center.

4. *A solution for everyone.* Whether your institution is already using Blackboard or you just want to try Blackboard on your own, we have a solution for you. McGraw-Hill and Blackboard can now offer you easy access to industry leading technology and content—whether your campus hosts it, or we do. Be sure to ask your local McGraw-Hill representative for details.

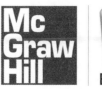

Do More

Instructors' Resources

Instructor Online Learning Center (OLC)

At www.mhhe.com/AllanEss2e, you will find the Instructor Online Learning Center. Your McGraw-Hill sales representative can provide you with the access you need to easily prepare for using *Essentials of Medical Language*, 2e. Our Online Learning Centers include:

- The Instructors' Manual, which contains valuable information that makes course prep a snap!

  - **Your Medical Terminology Course—An Introduction to Teaching Medical Terminology.** This valuable section includes information about student learning styles and instructor strategies; innovative learning activities; assessment techniques and strategies; classroom management tips; and techniques for teaching limited-English-proficiency students.

  - **Lesson Planning Guide.** Our Lesson Planning Guide comes complete with a customizable lesson plan for each of the lessons in this text. Each plan contains a step-by-step 50-minute teaching plan and master copies of handouts. Use these lessons alone or combined to accommodate different class schedules—you can even revise them to reflect your preferred topic or sequence. Each lesson plan is designed to be used with a corresponding PowerPoint® presentation that is also available on the OLC.

  - **PowerPoint® Lecture Outlines**. The PowerPoint lectures with speaking notes correlate to the Lesson Plans mentioned above and include the art and photos from the text. Covering the most important parts of every lesson, the slides are customizable to fit your course needs.

- **McGraw-Hill's EZ-Test Generator,** which makes creating tests easy!

  - This flexible electronic testing program allows instructors to create tests correlated to every chapter and learning outcome. Accommodating a variety of question types tied to Bloom's taxonomy, EZ-Test allows instructors to create multiple versions of the tests and then export to a course management system, such as Blackboard. EZ-Test Online gives you a place online to quickly and easily administer the exams you create.

How to Teach Medical Terminology

Online Course for Instructors to Support *Essentials of Medical Language* is found in the instructor resources section of the Online Learning Center at www.mhhe.com/AllanEss2e.

The **How to Teach Medical Terminology online course** provides instructors with the introductory knowledge and resources they need to begin effectively using the *Essentials of Medical Language* textbook and related materials. This course is designed to cover the "basics" of how to effectively teach medical terminology.

How to Teach Medical Terminology allows instructors to choose for themselves which module they wish to take, or they may opt to take a self-assessment survey that will recommend one of the three modules.

- **Module 1** is designed for the inexperienced instructor.
- **Module 2** is designed for the instructor who has previous classroom experience but who has never taught Medical Terminology.
- **Module 3** is designed for the experienced Medical Terminology instructor who has never taught using a contextualized approach.

Upon completion of a given module, instructors will take a final assessment designed to demonstrate their understanding and achievement of the learning objectives for that module. Those who score 70% or higher on the final assessment will receive a certificate that can be printed for professional development purposes.

MCGRAW-HILL CUSTOMER CARE CONTACT INFORMATION

At McGraw-Hill, we understand that getting the most from new technology can be challenging. That's why our services don't stop after you purchase our products. You can e-mail our Product Specialists 24 hours a day to get product training online. Or you can search our knowledge bank of Frequently Asked Questions on our support website. For Customer Support, call **800-331-5094,** e-mail **hmsupport@mcgraw-hill.com,** or visit **www.mhhe.com/support.** One of our Technical Support Analysts will be able to assist you in a timely fashion.

FOR THE STUDENT

Available at www.mhhe.com/AllanEss2e, the OLC offers an extensive array of learning and teaching tools. The site includes quizzes for each chapter, links to websites, and interactive activities. Students also will be able to access chapter-specific interactive exercises via McGraw-Hill Connect. These exercises provide multiple opportunities for practice and the mastery of core concepts. The exercises are designed to:

- Help students learn medical terms, including their definitions, roots, prefixes, and suffixes, plus accurate spelling.
- Help students understand the meaning and use of medical terms.
- Help students learn how and when to correctly apply medical terms in written and verbal communication.

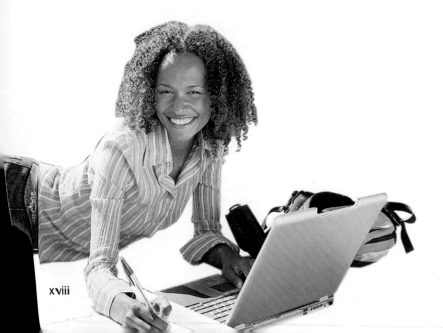

ACKNOWLEDGMENTS

For insightful reviews, constructive criticisms, helpful suggestions, and information, we would like to acknowledge the following:
Perrin Aikens Davis, Senior Vice President of Editorial Services at Agate Publishing in Evanston, Illinois, has been invaluable in the development of this second edition. She developed the original design and templates for execution of that design and supervised the complete production work of the book, including developmental editing, copyediting, proofreading, and art alteration. Most importantly we developed a collegial, cooperative relationship that enabled the process to keep on schedule and produce a creative outcome.

We would also like to thank our reviewers for the second edition for their helpful comments and feedback.

David Allan
Karen Lockyer

First Edition Reviewers

Kathryn G. Aguirre, MA
UEI College–El Monte Campus

Vanessa Austin, RMA, CAHI
Clarian Health Ed Sciences

Dr. Joseph H. Balabat, MD, RMA, RPT
Sanford-Brown Institute, New York

Dr. Seth Balogh, BS, MS, PhD
Brookline College

Sue Biedermann, MSHP, RHIA, FAHIMA
Texas State University–San Marcos

Bonnie Bonner, RDA, LVN
Franklin Career College

Quiana Bost, RMA
Bohecker College–Cincinnati

Dorisann Brandt, MSPT
Greenville Technical College

Bill Burke, BA
Madison Area Technical College; Blackhawk Technical College

Jennifer Campbell, BS, M.Ed
Tulsa Community College

Kim Carlson, M.Ed
Delta College of Arts and Technology

Marie Cissell, MN, RN, C
South Dakota State University

Ursula Cole, M.Ed, CMA, AAMA
Harrison College

Rosalind Collazo, CMA
ASA Institute of Business and Technology

Christina Rauberts Conklin, AA, RMA
Keiser University

Dr. Brian Conroy, MD
Lehigh Valley College

Kimberly Corsi, LRCP, CCS
Davenport University

Debra Mishoe Downs, LPN, AAS, RAM (AMT)
Okefenokee Technical College

Pat Dudek, RNM CHI, RMA
McCann School of Business and Technology

Tim Feltmeyer, MS
Erie Business Center

Jean Fennema, BA
Pima Medical Institute

Lance Followell, BS
Fremont College

Joanne Habenicht, MPA, RT, BS, ARRT
Manhattan College

Gregory Hartnett, BS, CPC
Sanford-Brown, Iselin, New Jersey

Diana Hollwedel, LPN
Career Institute of Florida

Susan Horn, AAS, CMA
Indiana Business College–Lafayette

Janet Hunter, MS, MBA
Northland Pioneer College

Judy Johnson, RN
Nashville State Community College

Tim Jones, BA, MA
Oklahoma City Community College; University of Oklahoma

Angela C. Jording, CMA
Fortis College

Judith Karls, RN, BSN, M.Ed
Madison Area Technical College

Shelli Lampi, PhD, RDH, NREMT
Dunwoody College of Technology

Sandra Lehrke, RN, LNC, RMA
Anoka Technical College

Nelly Mangarova, MD
Heald College

Pam McConnell, MA, AS
High Tech Institute

Jacqueline McNair, MA, RHIT
Baltimore City Community College

Cari McPherson, LP, N.II, AHI
Ross Medical Education Center

Susan Meeks, CPC-A
Milan Institute

Roxanna Montoya, M.Ed
Pima Medical Institute

Steve Moon, MS, CMI, FAMI
Ohio State University, College of Medicine

Cathleen Murphy, DC
Katherine Gibbs School

Sheila Newberry, M.Ed, RHIT
Remington College

Jennifer S. Painter,
Ohio Business College

Fred Pearson, PhD
Brigham Young University Idaho

Evie O'Nan, RMA
National College

Adrienne Reeves, BS, M.Ed
Westwood College

Becky Rodenbaugh, MBA, CMA
Baker College of Cadillac

Janette Rodriguez, RN, LNC RMA
Woot Tobe Coburn School, Manhattan New York

Shawn Marie Russell, BA, CPC
University of Alaska Fairbanks

Rebecca Schultz, PhD
University of Sioux Falls

Gene Simon, RHIA, RMD
Florida Career College

Susan Stockmaster, CMA (AAMA), MHS
Trident Technical College

Donna Slovensky, PhD, RHIA, FAHIMA
University of Alabama–Birmingham

Catherine A. Teel, AST, Health Care Technology, RMA
McCann School of Business and Technology

Margaret A. Tiemann, RN, BS
St. Charles Community College

Lenette Thompson, CST
Piedmont Technical College

Jonathan Thorsen, BS, RRT
Long Beach Community College

Lori A. Warren, MA, RN, CPC, CPC-I, CCP, CLNC
Spencerian College–Louisville KY

Kathryn Whitley, MSN, FNP
Patrick Henry Community College

Stacy Wilson, MT/PBT, CMA, MHA Program Chair
Cabarrus College of Health Sciences

Kathy Wishon, RN
North Metro Tech

Dr. Barbara Worley, DPM, BS, RMA, Program Manager, Medical Assisting
King's College

Carole A. Zeglin, MS, BS, RMA
Westmoreland County Community College

Daphne Zito, M.Ed, LPN
Katharine Gibbs School

Susan Zolvinski, BS, MBA
Brown Mackie College

Contextual Approach Promotes Active Learning

Chapters in the textbook are organized by body system in accordance with an overall anatomy and physiology (A & P) approach. Lessons introduce and define terminology through the context of A & P, pathology, and clinical and diagnostic procedures/tests. The organization of the body systems into chapters is based on an "outside to inside" sequence that reflects a physician's differential diagnosis method used during an examination.

To provide students with an authentic context, the medical specialty associated with each body area or system is introduced along with relevant anatomy and physiology. Students actually step into the role of an allied health professional associated with each specialty. Patient cases and documentation are used to illustrate the real-life application of medical terminology in modern health care: to care for and communicate with patients and to interact with other members of the health care team.

The A & P organizational approach, used in conjunction with an authentic medical setting and patient cases, encourages student motivation and facilitates active, engaged learning.

Innovative Pedagogical Aids Provide a Coherent Learning Program

Each chapter is structured around a consistent and unique framework of pedagogic devices. No matter what the subject matter of a chapter, the structure enables students to develop a consistent learning strategy, making *Essentials of Medical Language* a superior learning tool.

YOU ARE COMMUNICATING WITH . . .

Each chapter opens by placing the student in the role of an allied health professional related to the specialty and associated body systems/areas covered by the chapter. The student is also introduced to a patient and given information about the patient's case.

LEARNING OUTCOMES

At the same time, **Learning Outcomes** are presented to let students know what they will learn in the chapter. This technique immediately engages students, motivating them to read on to learn how this patient's case (and their role in the patient's care) relates to the medical terminology being introduced in the chapter.

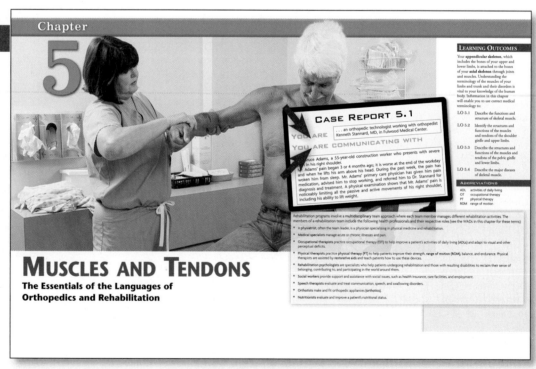

Lesson-Based Organization

The chapter content is broken down into chunks, or lessons, to help students digest new information and relate it to previously learned information. Rather than containing many various topics within a chapter, these lessons group the chapter material into logical, streamlined learning units designed to help students achieve the chapter outcomes. Lessons within a chapter build on one another to form a cohesive, coherent experience for the learner.

Each lesson is based on specific **Lesson Objectives** designed to support the students' achievement of the overall chapter outcomes.

Each lesson in a chapter contains an Introduction, Lesson Objectives, Lesson Topics, Word Analysis and Definition Tables, and Lesson Exercises. Within each lesson, all topics and information are presented in **self-contained two-page spreads.** This means students will no longer have to flip back and forth to see figures on one page that are described on another.

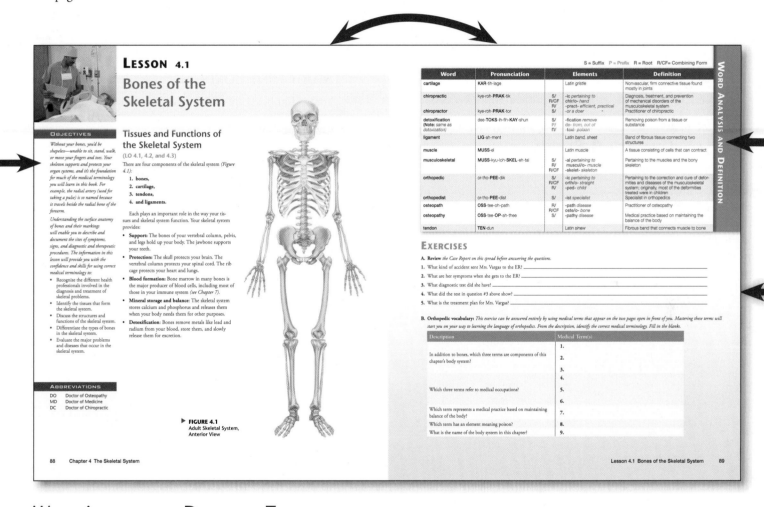

Word Analysis and Definition Tables

The medical terms covered in each lesson are introduced in context, either within a patient case or in the lesson topics. To facilitate easy reference and review, the terms are also listed in tables as a group. The **Word Analysis and Definition (WAD) Tables** list each term and its pronunciation, elements, and definition in a concise, color-coded, at-a-glance format.

LESSON AND CHAPTER-END EXERCISES

Each lesson within a chapter ends with exercises designed to allow students to check their basic understanding of the terms they just learned. These "checkpoints" can be used by instructors as assignments or for self-evaluation by students.

At the end of each chapter you will find 10–15 pages of exercises that ask students to apply what they learned in all lessons of a chapter. These chapter-end exercises reinforce learning and help students go beyond mere memorization to think critically about the medical language they use. In addition to reviewing and recalling the definitions of terms learned in the chapter, students are asked to use medical terms in new and different ways to ensure a thorough understanding.

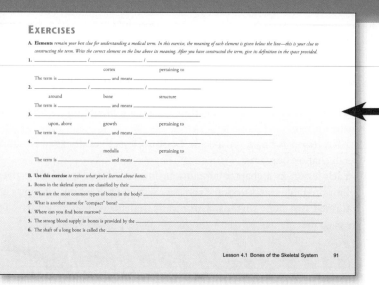

STUDY HINT BOXES

Study Hint boxes are found throughout the review exercises. They reinforce and remind students to use basic study skills.

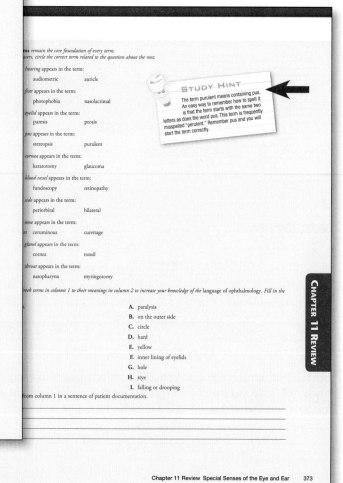

VIVID ILLUSTRATIONS AND PHOTOS

Colorful, precise anatomical illustrations and photos lend a realistic view of body structures and correlate to the clinical context of the lessons.

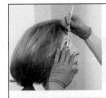

LESSON 11.2

The Eyeball and Seeing

The Eyeball (Globe)

(LO 11.1, 11.2, and 11.3)

The functions of your eyeball are to continuously:

1. **Adjust** the amount of light it lets in to reach the retina;
2. **Focus** on near and distant objects; and
3. **Produce** images of those objects and instantly transmit them to the brain.

As you learned earlier in this chapter, the front of the eyeball is covered by the conjunctiva. This thin layer of tissue lines the inside of the eyelids and curves over the eyeball to meet the **sclera** *(Figure 11.9)*, the tough, white outer layer of the eye.

At the center of the front of the eye is the **cornea**, a transparent, dome-shaped membrane. The cornea has no blood supply and obtains its nutrients from tears and from fluid in the anterior chamber behind it.

When light rays strike the eye, they pass through the cornea. Because of its dome curvature, those rays striking the edge of the cornea are bent toward its center. The light rays then go through the **pupil**, the black opening in the center of the colored area (the **iris**) in the front of the eye.

The iris controls the amount of light entering the eye. For example, when you're in the dark outside at night the iris opens (**dilates**) to allow more light into the eye. When you're in bright sunlight or in a well-lit room, the iris closes (**constricts**) to allow less light into the eye.

After traveling through the pupil, the light rays pass through the transparent **lens**. This lens can become thicker and thinner, enabling it to bend light rays and focus them on the **retina** at the back of the eye. Accommodation is the process of changing focus, and **refraction** is the process of bending light rays.

The lens does not contain blood vessels (**avascular**) or nerves, and with increasing age, it loses its elasticity. Because of this reduced elasticity, when you reach your forties, your eyes may have difficulty focusing on near objects, a condition called **presbyopia.**

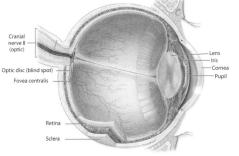

Cranial nerve II (optic)
Optic disc (blind spot)
Fovea centralis
Retina
Sclera
Lens
Iris
Cornea
Pupil

▲ **FIGURE 11.9** Anatomy of the Eyeball.

---

often irreversible side effects. These include with in adolescents, shrinking testes and rm counts, masculinization of women's bodies delusions, and paranoid jealousy. Long-term

Tenosynovitis is an inflammation of the sheath that surrounds a **tendon**, often in the wrist and hands. Repetitive use of these tendons can produce pain, tenderness in the tendon, and difficulty in related joint movement.

▼ **FIGURE 5.3**
RICE Treatment.

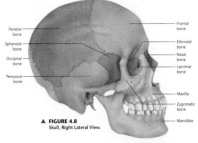

LESSON 4.2 Skull and Face

(LO 4.1, 4.2, and 4.3)

The Skull (LO 4.1, 4.2, and 4.3)

When you glance at your face in the mirror, chances are you're not thinking about what's behind your brown eyes or your slightly crooked smile. You see one image—not its layers, pieces, or parts. However, the human skull *(Figure 4.8)* is made up of 22 separate bones. Your **cranium**, the upper part of the skull that encloses the **cranial** cavity and protects the brain, contains 8 of these 22 bones; your facial skeleton contains the rest.

The bones of the cranium are joined together by sutures (joints that appear as seams), which are covered on the inside and outside by a thin layer of connective tissue. These bones have the following functions:

1. The **frontal** bone forms the forehead, roofs of the (eye) orbits, and part of the floor of the cranium, and contains a pair of right and left frontal sinuses above the orbits.
2. **Parietal** bones form the bulging sides and roof of the cranium.
3. The **occipital** bone forms the back of and part of the base of the cranium.
4. **Temporal** bones form the sides of and part of the base of the cranium.
5. The **sphenoid** bone forms part of the base of the cranium and the orbits.
6. The **ethmoid** bone is hollow and forms part of the nose, the orbits, and the ethmoid sinuses.

The lower part of the skull houses the bones of the facial skeleton *(Figure 4.9)*. These bones do the following:

1. **Maxillary** bones form the upper jaw (**maxilla**), hold the upper teeth, and are hollow, forming the maxillary sinuses.
2. **Palatine** bones are located behind the maxilla and cannot be seen on a lateral view of the skull.
3. **Zygomatic** bones are the prominences of the cheeks (cheekbones) below the eyes.
4. **Lacrimal** bones form the medial wall of each orbit.
5. **Nasal** bones form the sides and bridge of the nose.
6. The **mandible** is the lower jawbone, which holds the lower teeth. The mandible articulates (joins) with the temporal bone to form the **temporomandibular joint (TMJ).**

The third component of the axial skeleton, the rib cage, is discussed in Chapter 7, "Respiratory System."

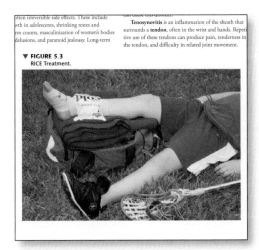

Parietal bone
Sphenoid bone
Occipital bone
Temporal bone
Frontal bone
Ethmoid bone
Nasal bone
Lacrimal bone
Maxilla
Zygomatic bone
Mandible

▲ **FIGURE 4.8**
Skull, Right Lateral View.

Nasal bone
Palatine bone
Maxilla
Mandible

▲ **FIGURE 4.9**
Facial Bones.

TABLES

Meaningful tables aid in summarizing concepts and lesson topics.

KEYNOTES AND ABBREVIATIONS

Keynotes and Abbreviations offer students additional information correlating to the lesson.

LESSON 4.1 Bone Fractures (FXS) (LO 4.1, 4.2, 4.3, and 4.4)

▼ **TABLE 4.1**
Classification and Definition of Bone Fractures

Name	Description	Reference
Closed (also called **simple** fracture)	A bone is broken, but the skin is not broken.	Figure 4.6g
Open (also called **compound** fracture)	A fragment of the fractured bone breaks the skin, or a wound extends to the site of the fracture.	Figure 4.6e
Displaced	The fractured bone parts are out of line.	Figure 4.6e
Complete	A bone is broken into at least two fragments.	Figure 4.6a
Incomplete	The fracture does not extend completely across the bone. It can be hairline, as in a stress fracture in the foot, when there is no separation of the two fragments.	Figure 4.6a
Comminuted	The bone breaks into several pieces, usually two major pieces and several smaller fragments.	Figure 4.6b
Transverse	The fracture is at right angles to the long axis of the bone.	Figure 4.6b
Impacted	The fracture consists of one bone fragment driven into another, resulting in shortening of a limb.	Figure 4.6c
Spiral	The fracture spirals around the long axis of the bone.	Figure 4.6d
Oblique	The fracture runs diagonally across the long axis of the bone.	Figure 4.6d
Linear	The fracture runs parallel to the long axis of the bone.	Figure 4.6f
Greenstick	This is a partial fracture. One side breaks, and the other bends.	Figure 4.6g
Pathologic	The fracture occurs in an area of bone weakened by disease, such as cancer.	—
Compression	The fracture occurs in a vertebra from trauma or pathology, leading to the vertebra being crushed.	—
Stress	This is a fatigue fracture caused by repetitive, local stress on a bone, as occurs in marching or running.	—

Healing of Fractures (LO 4.1, 4.2, 4.3, and 4.4)

When a bone is fractured, blood vessels bleed into the fracture site, forming a hematoma. After a few days, bone-forming cells called **osteoblasts** move in and start to produce new bone matrix, which develops into **osteocytes** (bone cells). Eventually the new bone fuses together the segments of the fracture.

Surgical Procedures for Fractures (LO 4.1, 4.2, 4.3, and 4.4)

The initial goal of fracture treatment is to bring the ends of the bone at the break back opposite each other so that they fit together as they did in the original bone. This is called **alignment.**

External manipulation is used frequently, sometimes with anesthesia. Here, the bone is pulled from the distal end (the farthest point from attachment) back into alignment through a process called **reduction**.

In **external fixation**, the alignment is maintained by immobilizing the bone via plaster casts, splints, traction, and/or **external fixators.** Traction involves applying gentle but continuous pulling force in order to align a fracture, reduce muscle spasms, and relieve pain. External fixators are implements, such as steel pins and rods, used to secure bone fragments together.

▲ **FIGURE 4.6**
Bone Fractures.

ABBREVIATIONS

Fx   fracture

94   Chapter 4 The Skeletal System

LESSON 4.1 Diseases of Bone
(LO 4.1, 4.2, 4.3, and 4.4)

KEYNOTE

- Osteomalacia occurs in some developing nations and occasionally in this country when children drink soft drinks instead of milk fortified with vitamin D.

One of the major bone diseases is **osteoporosis,** which results from a loss of bone density *(Figure 4.4).* More common in women than in men, the incidence of osteoporosis increases with age. In the United States alone, 10 million people are living with osteoporosis and 18 million more have low bone density (**osteopenia**). Osteopenia puts people at risk for developing osteoporosis.

In women, production of the hormone estrogen decreases after menopause, weakening the body's protection against bone loss and potentially resulting in fragile, brittle bones. In men, lower levels of testosterone have a similar but less noticeable effect.

Women at risk for osteoporosis should have a bone mineral density (**BMD**) screening using a **DEXA** scan, which is a measuring device that uses low-energy radiation beams. Men and women over 50 are often advised to follow a daily regimen of 1,200 milligrams (**mg**) of calcium, 400 to 600 international units (**IU**) of vitamin D, and 15 minutes of real sun exposure. In addition, there are several **FDA**-approved medications available for treating osteoporosis.

Other bone diseases that may not be as prevalent or publicized as osteoporosis are the following:

Osteomyelitis: an inflammation in a bone area caused by a bacterial infection, such as staphylococcus.

Osteomalacia: a disease (known as **rickets** in children) caused by vitamin D deficiency where the calcium-lacking bones become soft and flexible, lose their ability to bear weight, and become bowed.

Achondroplasia: a very rare condition where the long bones stop growing in childhood, but the axial skeleton bones are not affected *(Figure 4.5).* People with this condition are short in stature, with the average adult measuring about 4 feet tall. Although intelligence and life span are normal, the disease is caused by a spontaneous gene mutation that then becomes a dominant gene for succeeding generations.

Osteogenic sarcoma: the most common malignant bone tumor, which often occurs around the knee joint. Peak incidence is between the ages of 10 and 15 years.

Osteogenesis imperfecta: a rare genetic disorder producing very brittle bones that are easily fractured or broken, often **in utero** (while inside the uterus).

Normal bone   Osteoporotic bone

CASE REPORT 4.1 (CONTINUED)

On questioning, Amy Vargas demonstrated many of the risk factors for osteoporosis, including family history, lack of exercise, cigarette smoking, inadequate diet, postmenopause, and increasing age.

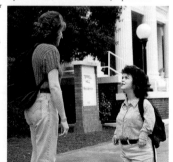

xxiv

David Allan

David Allan received his medical training at Cambridge University and Guy's Hospital in England. He was Chief Resident in Pediatrics at Bellevue Hospital in New York City before moving to San Diego, California.

Dr. Allan has worked as a family physician in England, a pediatrician in San Diego, and Associate Dean at the University of California, San Diego School of Medicine. He has designed, written, and produced more than 100 award-winning multimedia programs with virtual reality as their conceptual base. Dr. Allan resides happily in San Diego.

Karen Lockyer

Karen Lockyer holds a degree in Health Information (RHIT), a national coding certification (CPC), and a BS from Rutgers University. She is also a credentialed member of AHIMA (American Health Information Management Association) and AAPC (American Academy of Professional Coders).

Mrs. Lockyer has worked in medical practice administration and the Health Information Management fields for many years. She has taught medical terminology for high school, community college, and workforce development areas at the National Institutes of Health and the federal government's Office of Personnel Management. She has also taught coding and billing for undergraduate and certificate programs at the community college level.

Residing in Southlake, Texas, Karen enjoys the sights and flavors of the Southwest.

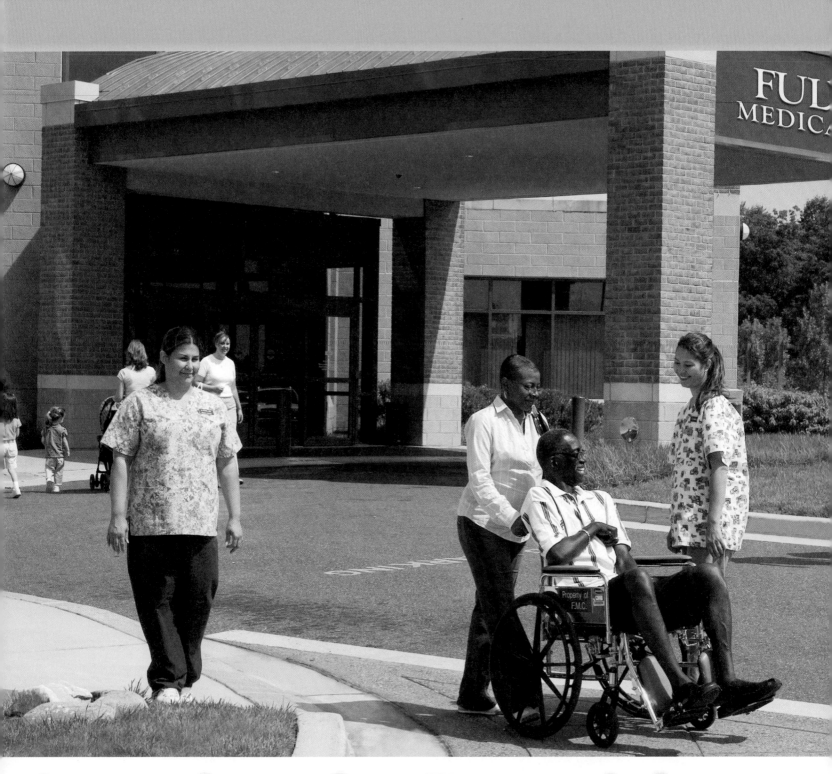

Learning the Essentials of Medical Language

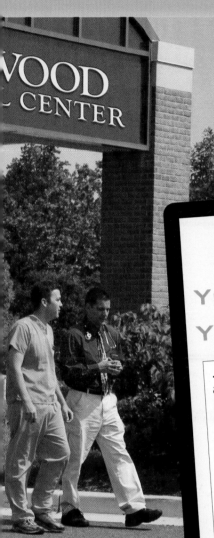

Welcome

LEARNING OUTCOMES

In order to get the most out of your learning experiences and this textbook, you need to:

W-1 Recognize the need to learn medical terminology.

W-2 Comprehend the value of learning medical terminology through the use of the realistic health care settings presented in this book.

W-3 Develop effective study habits and organizational strategies for learning and work.

W-4 Identify with the need for lifelong active learning as a health professional.

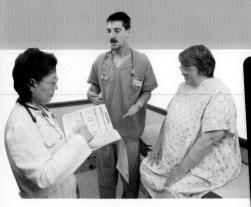

▲ **FIGURE W.1**
Direct Communication with Doctor and Patient.

THE HEALTH CARE TEAM

Fulwood Medical Center is a realistic health care setting that allows you to experience the use of medical language. Each chapter in this book focuses on the medical terminology used in a specific medical specialty and the body systems related to that specialty. A variety of health professionals make up the teams caring for patients in each medical specialty.

The team leader is a medical doctor, or physician, who can be an **MD** (doctor of medicine) or a **DO** (doctor of osteopathy). Most **managed care systems** require the patient to have a **primary care physician.** This physician can be a **family practitioner, internist,** or **pediatrician** (for children) and is responsible for the continuing overall care of the patient. In managed care, the primary care physician acts as the "gatekeeper" for the patient to enter the system, supervising all care the patient receives.

If needed medical care is beyond the expertise of the primary care physician, the patient is referred to a medical specialist whose expertise is based on a specific body system or even a part of a body system. For example, a **cardiologist** has expertise in diseases of the heart and vascular system, whereas a **dermatologist** specializes in diseases of the skin and an **orthopedist** in problems with the musculoskeletal system. A **gastroenterologist** is an expert in diseases of the whole digestive system, whereas a **colorectal surgeon** specializes only in diseases of the lower gastrointestinal tract.

Other health professionals work under the supervision of the physician and provide direct care to the patient. These can include a **physician assistant, nurse practitioner, medical assistant,** and, in specialty areas, different therapists, technologists, and technicians with expertise in the use of specific therapeutic and diagnostic tools.

Still other health professionals on the team provide indirect patient care. These include **administrative medical assistants, transcriptionists, health information technicians, medical insurance billers,** and **coders,** all of whom are essential to providing high-quality patient care.

As you study the language of each medical specialty at Fulwood Medical Center, you will also meet the members of each specialty's health care team and learn more about their roles in caring for the patient.

LISTENING, SPEAKING, READING, WRITING, AND CRITICAL THINKING

Daily in your practice as a health professional you will:

Listen to information from physicians about patient care, and carry out their instructions.

Listen to patients describing their symptoms, and translate their descriptions into medical terms.

Speak to physicians and other health professionals to report information and ask questions.

Speak to patients to translate and clarify information given to them by physicians and other health professionals.

Read physicians' comments and treatment plans in patient medical records and insurance reports.

Read the results of physical examinations, procedures, and laboratory and diagnostic tests.

Write to document actions taken by yourself and other members of the health care team *(Figure W.2)*.

Write to precisely record verbal orders, test results given over the phone, and other phone messages.

Think critically to evaluate medical documentation for accuracy.

Think critically to analyze and discover the meaning of unfamiliar medical terms using the strategies outlined in *Chapter 1* of this book.

IF YOU CANNOT SPEAK THE LANGUAGE, YOU CANNOT JOIN THE CLUB.

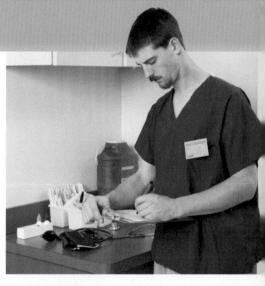

▲ **FIGURE W.2**
Accurate Documentation of Care Is Critical.

"WHY DO I NEED TO LEARN MEDICAL TERMINOLOGY?"

Communication Needs

Throughout your career as a health professional, you will need to communicate with other health professionals. This need is present whether you are providing direct patient care—for example, as a CMA like Luis Guitterez—or whether you are providing indirect patient care—for example, as a medical transcriptionist, biller, or coder. In this book, you will find all the medical terms necessary to equip yourself with the essential medical vocabulary needed for work and further study in any of the allied health professional careers.

As you can see in Case Report W.2, health professionals use specific terms and a different language to describe to each other situations they encounter each day. You need to be able to understand, spell, and pronounce the terms they use.

Modern medical terminology is an artificial language constructed over centuries using words and elements from Greek and Latin origins (where healing professions began). Some 15,000 or more words are formed from 1,200 Greek and Latin roots. New words are being added continually as new medical discoveries are made. Medical terminology enables health professionals from different fields, different specialties, and different countries to communicate clearly and precisely with each other. Every profession has its own language *(Figure W.3)*.

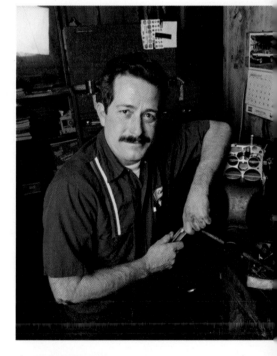

▲ **FIGURE W.3**
Every Profession Has Its Own Language
You may have difficulty understanding your auto mechanic when he tells you that the expansion valve, evaporator core, and orifice tubes in your air-conditioning system need replacing.

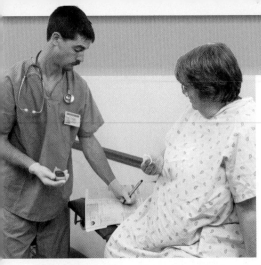

▲ FIGURE W.4
Every Patient Interaction Is an Opportunity for Learning.

"WHAT IS LIFELONG, ACTIVE LEARNING?"

Lifelong Learning

Your current training in medical terminology is necessary for you to be able to continue your education in your health care profession. But it is important to recognize that school is only one of the many places where you acquire knowledge.

You also acquire knowledge:

- Each time you ask a question about a patient or a report and receive an answer.

- Each time you analyze an unfamiliar medical term and discover its meaning.

- Each time you interact with a patient and see how that patient is coping with his or her problems *(Figure W.4)*.

All these are opportunities for learning to discover *your own* answers to *your own* problems or lack of knowledge.

This type of knowledge—discovered through your own experience and driven by your own needs and goals—is genuine, real, and trustworthy for you. It is not like what you learn in school, which is determined by some distant authority.

The authentic knowledge you gain from solving your own problems, whether by yourself or with the help of other people or resources, motivates you to acquire still more knowledge and helps you grow as a person and as a professional.

Throughout your working life, additional classroom training will be needed to keep your skills and professional knowledge up to date with new developments in medicine. You will also continue to learn through your own experience. Everything you do in life can result in learning.

Your own experience and judgment become your most valuable resources for making your life vibrant, strong, creative, and what *you* want *it* to be.

Your own experience and judgment maximize your professional and personal success.

ACTIVELY EXPERIENCING MEDICAL LANGUAGE

Medical terms were created to provide health care professionals a way to communicate with each other and document the care they provide. To provide effective patient care, all health care professionals must be fluent in medical language. One misused or misspelled medical term on a patient record can cause errors that can result in injury or death to patients, incorrect coding or billing of medical claims, and possible fraud charges.

When medical terms are separated from their intended context, as they are in other medical terminology textbooks, it is easy to lose sight of how important it is to use them accurately and precisely. Learning medical terminology in the context of the medical setting reinforces the importance of correct usage and precision in communication.

During your externship at Fulwood Medical Center, you will *experience* medical language. Just as in a real medical center, you will encounter and apply medical terminology in a variety of ways. Actively experiencing medical language will help ensure that you are truly learning, and not simply memorizing, the medical terms in each chapter. Memorizing a term allows you to use it in the same situation (e.g., repeating a definition) but doesn't help you apply it in new situations. Whether you are reading chart notes in a patient's medical record or a description of the treatment prescribed by a physician, you will see medical terms being used for the purpose they were intended.

ACTIVE LEARNING

It's no good sitting back and expecting someone else to pour knowledge into your head. You have to **actively work at learning.**

Get the Most Out of Lectures

- *Prepare* for your classroom experiences. Preview the book chapter before class, and the material will be much easier to understand.
- *Listen actively.* You cannot do this if you are looking at your cell phone, daydreaming, or worrying about what you have to get for dinner.
- *Ask* a question if you do not comprehend something the instructor is saying.
- *Write* good notes. Focus on the main points, and capture key ideas; review and edit your notes within 24 hours of the class.

Get the Most Out of Reading

- *Concentrate* on what you are reading. Review the titles, objectives, headings, and visuals for each lesson to identify what the lesson is all about.
- *Read* actively using the SQ3R method (see the Study Hint) to help you.
- *Write* down any questions you have.

Study with a Partner or Group

- *Find* a study partner. Schedule study dates, compare notes, talk through concepts and questions, and quiz each other.
- *Establish* a small study group, including your study partner. Again, compare notes and quiz each other.

Perform Well on Tests

- *Read* the directions carefully, and scan the entire test so that you know how long it is and what types of activities it contains.
- *Answer* the easy questions or sections first so that you finish as much as possible before doing the difficult questions, which might slow you down.
- *Use* any extra time, after you have finished the test, to check that you have answered all the questions and then to confirm your answers.

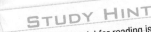

STUDY HINT

The SQ3R model for reading is a successful equation for studying:

Survey what you are going to read.

Question what you are going to learn after the preview.

Read the assignment.

Recite. Stop every once in a while, look up from the book, and put what you've just read into your own words.

Review. After you've finished, review the main points.

DIGITAL AIDS FOR ACTIVE LEARNING

Two powerful online digital tools are available for you and your instructors to extend the learning experience beyond the classroom so that you can engage with your coursework anytime, anywhere.

ConnectPlus™

ConnectPlus provides students with their textbook and homework assignments all in one easily accessible place. Students receive automatic scores for their assignments giving immediate feedback and side-by-side comparisons with correct answers. Because class materials are personalized and easily stored and accessed, ConnectPlus allows students to focus less on note-taking and more on class participation and interactions.

You can exeperience ConnectPlus at www.mcgrawhillconnect.com

LearnSmart™

LearnSmart is an insightful, intuitive learning system that diagnoses students' skill levels, delivers customized learning content based on their strengths and weaknesses, and predicts time and practice necessary to master content.

You can exeperience LearnSmart at www.mhlearnsmart.com.

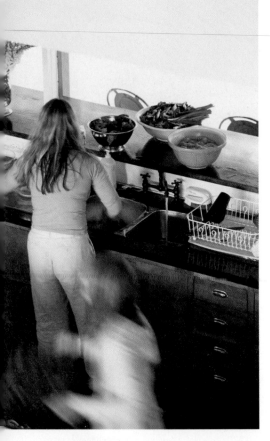

▲ FIGURE W.5 An Evening at Home.

CASE REPORT W.3

Your first day of externship at Fulwood Medical Center went well. You enjoyed being in the Primary Care Clinic with Dr. Lee and Luis Guitterez, CMA. You wonder if this could be a career choice for you. Now it's 6:15 p.m. at home, and you have yet to feed the kids, get them to bed, pay some bills, pick up around the house, and review a whole chapter in your medical terminology text to prepare for a test in class tomorrow. How are you going to do all this?

"HOW CAN I HELP MYSELF LEARN BETTER?"

You have a lot of time and money invested in your education. To succeed, you need to be able to focus and manage your time and your studies. To manage the difficulties described in Case Report W.3 *(Figure W.5)*, you need to:

- *Recognize* the stresses in your life at different times.
- *Prioritize* mentally, and handle each task in the order of importance. In this case, eat a healthy meal with your kids, enjoy putting them to bed, pay the bills, and then relax (or meditate) for 10 minutes. When you are relaxed, settle down to review the text, and go to bed at a reasonable hour. Picking up around the house will have to wait, since study and sleep are a higher priority. Sounds too easy? What other choices do you have to be able to study in an effective way?
- *Actively develop a support group.* Enlist the support of your spouse, parents, siblings, friends—any people you can trust and rely on. If you have a test every Thursday, get one of them to come over Wednesday night and put the kids to bed while you go over to his or her house or the library to study.
- *Find your own space.* Create a place where you keep everything for your courses at your fingertips, clutter-free.
- *Study when you are most productive.* Are you a night owl or an early bird? Set a daily study time for yourself.
- *Balance your life.* While studying should be a main focus, plan time for family, friends, leisure, exercise, and sleep.
- *Resist distractions.* Avoid the temptation to surf the Web, send instant messages, and make phone calls. Stick to your schedule.
- *Be realistic* when planning—know your limits and priorities.
- *Be prepared* for the unexpected (child's illness, your illness, inclement weather) that can turn your schedule into shambles.
- *Reprioritize* daily on the basis of schedule disruptions and other conflicts.
- *Identify* clear goals for what you need to get done today, this week, this month, before the end of the semester, and so on.

EXERCISES

Write out all of your activities for a typical week. On average, how many hours each week do you spend sleeping, grooming, eating, working, running errands, studying, attending your children's activities, and watching TV? Add all the hours up. There are 168 hours in the week. How many hours do you have left for studying? A sample time budget is shown below.

Activity	Number of Hours per Day	Number of Days per Week	Number of Hours per Week
Sleeping	8	7	56
Grooming	1	7	7
Meals: preparation, eating, cleanup	1	7	7
Cleaning, laundry	1	3	3
Commuting to and from school	1	5	5
In class	4	5	20
Doing errands	1	3	3
Family time	3	7	21
Church, workout, hobbies			5
Job			30
Friends, going out, TV, entertainment			6
TOTAL			163
TOTAL HOURS IN A WEEK			168
Hours remaining for study			5

• ARE 5 HOURS ENOUGH FOR STUDY?

• WHEN ARE THEY AVAILABLE?

• WHAT CAN YOU DO TO INCREASE THEM?

STUDY HOURS SHOULD BE SPENT IN A SETTING THAT ALLOWS YOU TO CONCENTRATE ON YOUR WORK AND NOT BE DISTRACTED. TURN OFF YOUR CELL PHONE AND TV. THE BIGGEST QUESTION TO ASK YOURSELF IS, "AM I INVESTING MY TIME WISELY?" IF NOT, HOW CAN YOU BUDGET YOUR TIME DIFFERENTLY SO THAT MORE TIME IS SPENT ON HIGHER-PRIORITY ACTIVITIES?

"What's New About This Book?"

Although the chapters in this book are organized by body system, as in many other textbooks on medical terminology, this book has many unique features that enhance learning, create interest, and provide a consistent learning strategy for you.

Each chapter is broken down into lessons; each lesson is broken down into self-contained topic areas so that there are smaller "chunks" of information to master.

You Are . . . You Are Communicating With . . .

At the beginning of each chapter and lesson, you are placed in the role of a health professional in a field related to the body system and medical specialty covered in the material. At the same time, learning objectives are presented for each chapter and lesson. These techniques immediately engage your attention, motivate you to read on to discover how this patient's diagnosis and care progress, and illustrate the medical terminology being introduced in the lessons.

Word Analysis And Definition

All the information needed for a topic area is presented in self-contained two-page spreads. On the left-hand page, the new medical terms are introduced. On the right-hand page, for each new medical term the pronunciation, color-coded word elements, and definition are provided in a **Word Analysis and Definition (WAD)** box. For example, in Case Report W.2 earlier in this chapter, the medical terms diabetic, retinopathy, neuropathy, tachycardia, tachypnea, hypotensive, ketoacidosis, glucometer, and pneumonia were used. On the right-hand page here, you can see an example of how these terms are analyzed. All these terms will appear again in the appropriate body-system chapter.

Also, below each WAD are exercises that test your understanding of key components of the terminology analyzed in the WAD.

Exercises

In addition to the exercises at the end of each topic area, there are several pages of exercises at the end of each chapter. More exercises are found on the Student Online Learning Center (www.mhhe.com/AllanEss2e).

The exercises are designed to help different styles of learners understand the logic of medical terminology. Exercises take comprehension beyond the basic level, and show you the practical application of the terminology you are learning in the classroom, and its use in the workplace. Constructing and deconstructing medical terms into their elements is the basic foundation on which this knowledge is built.

Attention is given to developing skills in pronunciation, spelling, forming plurals, using abbreviations, and writing medical language. The exercises take you beyond memorization and teach you to think critically about the realistic application of the medical language you are learning.

Additional Unique Features

Keynotes emphasize key points in the text or offer additional important information.

Study hints show you how to use basic study skills, and they provide ways by which to retain information.

Abbreviation boxes show common abbreviations accepted by The Joint Commission and AMA.

Illustrations and **photos** are vivid and colorful and are correlated precisely to the medical terminology of the lessons.

ABBREVIATIONS

AMA	American Medical Association
CMA	certified medical assistant

KEYNOTE

A few months of committed study now is a small sacrifice compared to the lifetime that awaits you.

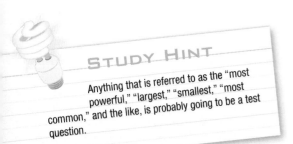

STUDY HINT

Anything that is referred to as the "most powerful," "largest," "smallest," "most common," and the like, is probably going to be a test question.

Word	Pronunciation		Elements	Definition
diabetes mellitus	dye-ah-**BEE**-teez **MEL**-ih-tus		diabetes, Greek *a siphon* mellitus, Latin *sweetened with honey*	Metabolic syndrome caused by absolute or relative insulin deficiency and/or insulin ineffectiveness
diabetic (adj)	dye-ah-**BET**-ik	S/ R/	-ic *pertaining to* diabet- *diabetes*	Pertaining to or suffering from diabetes
hypotension	**HIGH**-poh-**TEN**-shun	S/ P/ R/	-ion *action, condition* hypo- *below* -tens- *pressure*	Persistent low arterial blood pressure
hypotensive (adj)	**HIGH**-poh-**TEN**-siv	S/	-ive *pertaining to, quality of*	Pertaining to or suffering from hypotension
ketoacidosis	**KEY**-toe-ass-ih-**DOE**-sis	S/ R/CF R/CF	-sis *abnormal condition* ket/o- *ketone* -acid/o- *acid*	Excessive production of ketones, making the blood acidic
neuropathy	nyu-**ROP**-ah-thee	S/ R/CF	-pathy *disease* neur/o- *nerve*	Any disorder affecting the nervous system
pneumonia (Note: *The initial "p" is silent.*)	new-**MOH**-nee-ah	S/ R/	-ia *condition* pneumon- *air, lung*	Inflammation of the lung parenchyma
retinopathy	ret-ih-**NOP**-ah-thee	S/ R/CF	-pathy *disease* retin/o- *retina*	Any disease of the retina
tachycardia	tack-ih-**KAR**-dee-ah	S/ P/ R/	-ia *condition* tachy- *rapid* -card- *heart*	Rapid heart rate, above 100 beats per minute
tachypnea	tack-ip-**NEE**-ah	P/ R/	tachy- *rapid* -pnea *breathe*	Rapid breathing

The elements of a term are discussed in Chapter 1.

EXERCISES

Elements *are your best tool for understanding medical terms. In the chart below, the elements are listed in column 1. Identify the meaning of each element in column 2, and give an example of a term containing that element in column 3. Some terms will apply to more than one element. The first one is done for you.*

Element	Meaning of Elements	Medical Term Containing This Element
hypo	below	hypotension
tens		
ion		
neuro		
retino		
pathy		
ia		
pneumon		
pnea		
tachy		

1. Choose any term from column 3, and use it in a sentence of your choice:

_____

_____

_____

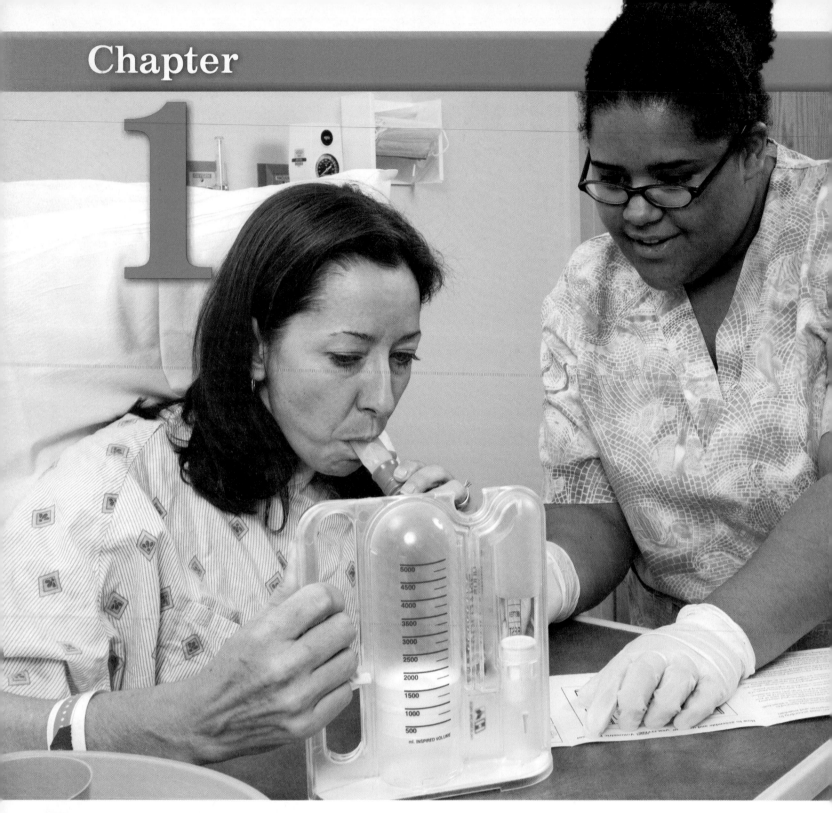

THE ANATOMY OF WORD CONSTRUCTION

The Essential Elements of the Language of Medicine

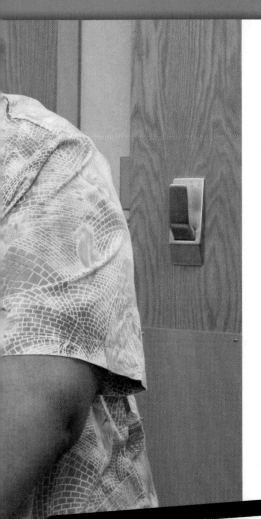

The technical language of medicine has been developed logically from Latin and Greek roots. In fact, the concept of treating patients was pioneered by ancient Greek culture. Medical terms are built from their individual parts, or **elements,** which form the **anatomy** of the word. The information in this chapter will enable you to:

LO 1.1   **Identify the roots, combining vowels, and combining forms of medical terms.**

LO 1.2   **Understand the importance of suffixes and prefixes in forming medical terms.**

LO 1.3   **Link word elements together to construct medical terms.**

LO 1.4   **Break down or deconstruct a medical term into its elements.**

LO 1.5   **Connect the singular and plural forms of medical terms.**

LO 1.6   **Verbalize the pronunciation of medical terms by employing the system used in the textbook and the Student Online Learning Center (www.mhhe.com/AllanEss2e).**

CASE REPORT 1.1

YOU ARE

. . . a respiratory therapist working with Tavis Senko, MD, a pulmonologist at Fulwood Medical Center.

YOU ARE COMMUNICATING WITH

. . . Mrs. Sandra Schwartz, a 43-year-old woman referred to Dr. Senko by her primary care physician, Dr. Andrew McDonald, an internist. Mrs. Schwartz has a persistent abnormality on her chest X-ray. You have been asked to determine her pulmonary function prior to a scheduled bronchoscopy.

THIS SUMMARY OF A CASE REPORT ILLUSTRATES FOR YOU THE USE OF SOME SIMPLE MEDICAL TERMS. MODERN HEALTH CARE AND MEDICINE HAS ITS OWN LANGUAGE. THE MEDICAL TERMS ALL HAVE PRECISE MEANINGS, WHICH ENABLE YOU, AS A HEALTH PROFESSIONAL, TO COMMUNICATE CLEARLY AND ACCURATELY WITH OTHER HEALTH PROFESSIONALS INVOLVED IN THE CARE OF A PATIENT. THIS COMMUNICATION IS CRITICAL FOR PATIENT SAFETY AND THE DELIVERY OF HIGH-QUALITY PATIENT CARE.

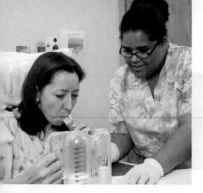

LESSON 1.1

The Construction of Medical Words

Your confidence in using and understanding the medical terms in this book will increase as you become familiar with the logic of how these terms are constructed. The information in this lesson will enable you to:

1.1.1 Build and construct medical terms using their elements.

1.1.2 Select and identify the meaning of essential medical term **roots.**

1.1.3 Define the elements **combining vowel** and **combining form.**

1.1.4 Identify the **combining vowel** and **combining form** of essential medical terms.

1.1.5 Define the elements **suffix** and prefix.

1.1.6 Select and identify the meaning of the **suffixes** and prefixes of essential medical terms.

ROOTS

- A **root** is the constant foundation and core of a medical term.

- **Roots** are usually of Greek or Latin origin.

- All medical terms have *one* or *more* **roots.**

- A **root** can appear anywhere in the term.

- More than one **root** can have the same meaning.

- A **root** plus a **combining vowel** creates a **combining form.**

Roots (LO 1.1)

Every medical term has a **root**—the element that provides the core meaning of the word. For example, in Case Report 1.1:

- The word *pneumonia* has the **root** *pneumon-*, taken from the Greek word meaning *lung* or *air*. The Greek **root** *pneum-* also means *lung* or *air*. *Pneumonia* is an infection of the lung tissue.

- Dr. Tavis Senko is a *pulmonologist*. The **root** *pulmon-* is taken from the Latin word meaning *lung*. A *pulmonologist* is a specialist who treats lung diseases.

> **CASE REPORT 1.1** (CONTINUED)
>
> From her medical records, you can see that 2 months ago Mrs. Schwartz developed a right upper lobe (RUL) pneumonia. After treatment with an antibiotic, a follow-up chest X-ray (CXR) showed some residual collapse in the right upper lobe and a small right pneumothorax. Mrs. Schwartz has smoked a pack a day since she was a teenager. Dr. Senko is concerned that she has lung cancer, and has scheduled her for a bronchoscopy.

Combining Forms (LO 1.1 and 1.2)

Roots are often joined to other elements in a medical term by adding a **combining vowel,** such as the letter **"o,"** to the end of the **root,** like *pneum-*, to form **pneum/o-.**

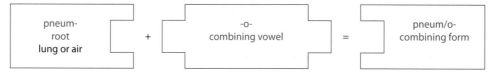

| pneum-
root
lung or air | + | -o-
combining vowel | = | pneum/o-
combining form |

Throughout this book, whenever a term is presented, a **slash** (/) will be used to separate the combining vowel from the **root.** Other examples of this approach are as follows:

- Adding the **combining vowel "o"** to the Latin **root** *pulmon-* makes the **combining form** *pulmon/o-.*

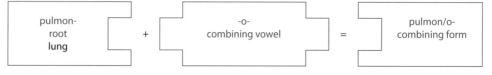

| pulmon-
root
lung | + | -o-
combining vowel | = | pulmon/o-
combining form |

Any vowel, "a," "e," "i," "o," or "u," can be used as a **combining vowel.**

- The **root** *respir-* means *to breathe*. Adding the **combining vowel "a"** makes the **combining form** *respir/a-.*

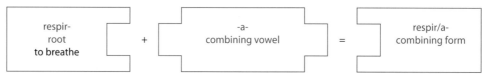

| respir-
root
to breathe | + | -a-
combining vowel | = | respir/a-
combining form |

Many medical terms contain more than one **root**; when two roots occur together, they are always joined by a **combining vowel**, as in the following example:

- The word **pneumothorax** has the **root** *pneum-,* from the Greek word meaning *air* or *lung,* and the **root** *-thorax,* from the Greek word meaning *chest.* The **combining vowel** "o" joins these two roots together to make the **combining form,** *pneum/o-.* A **pneumothorax** is the presence of air in the space that surrounds the lungs in the chest. As this amount of air increases, it causes pressure on the lung and forces the lung to collapse.

pneum- root lung or air	+	-o- combining vowel	+	-thorax root chest	=	pneumothorax air in the chest

COMBINING FORMS

- Combine a **root** and a **combining vowel**.
- Can be attached to another **root** or **combining form**.
- Can precede another word element called a **suffix**.
- Can follow a prefix.

KEYNOTES

- Throughout this book, look for the following patterns:

  Roots, combining forms, and combining vowels will be colored red.

  Prefixes will be colored green.

  Suffixes will be colored blue.

- Different roots can have the same meaning. *Pulmon-* and *pneumon-* both mean *lung*.

EXERCISES

Review *what you have just learned about the roots and combining forms on the two pages spread open in front of you. Fill in the blanks.*

1. Which element is the core or foundation of every medical term? _____

2. Give two examples of the element named in question #1 above: _____

3. If a **combining vowel** is added to the element in question #1, what is the name of the new element? _____

4. Give an example of a **root** that has become a **combining form**:

   _____ + _____ = _____

   Root   Combining vowel   Combining form (Don't forget the slash!)

5. More than one element can have the same meaning in medical terminology.
   Give an example from the elements on these two pages:

   _____ and _____

   both mean _____

6. Give an example of a term using each element in the above question:

   _____ means _____

   _____ means _____

STUDY HINT

Even though both these elements mean the same thing, they are not interchangeable. Only certain elements belong with certain terms, and you must know them.

7. The following terms have not been introduced yet, but the principle remains the same.
   The root/combining form will always carry the same meaning. Circle the roots/combining forms that you recognize, and provide the meaning of the root or combining form on the blank line.

7a. *Pneumonectomy, pneumonitis,* and *pneumococcal* all pertain to the _____.

7b. *Respirator* and *respiratory* both pertain to_____.

LESSON **1.1** Suffixes (LO 1.2 and 1.3)

SUFFIXES

- A **suffix** is a group of letters attached to the end of a **root** or **combining form.**
- A **suffix** changes the meaning of the word.
- If the **suffix** begins with a consonant, it must follow a **combining vowel.**
- If the **suffix** begins with a vowel, no **combining vowel** is needed.
- A few medical terms can have two **suffixes.**
- A **suffix** always appears at the end of a term.
- **Suffixes** that are different can have the same meaning.

A **suffix** is an element added to the end of a **root** or **combining form** to give it a new meaning. You can add different **suffixes** to the same **root** to build new words, all with different meanings. For example:

- Add the **suffix** -*ary* to the **root** *pulmon-* to create the term **pulmonary.** The **suffix** -*ary* means *pertaining to* or *relating to.* The adjective **pulmonary** means *pertaining to the lung.* **Pulmonary circulation** means the *passage of blood through the lungs.*

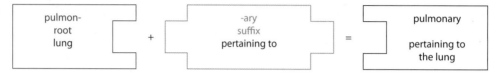

- Add the **suffix** -*logy* to the **combining form** *pulmon/o-* to make the term **pulmonology.** The **suffix** -*logy* means *study of.* **Pulmonology** is the study of the structure, functions, and diseases of the lungs.

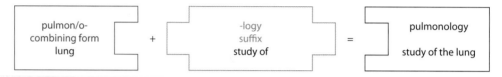

- Add the **suffix** -*ia* to the **root** *pneumon-* to make the term **pneumonia.** The **suffix** -*ia* means *a condition of.* **Pneumonia** is a condition of the lungs that involves an infection of the lung tissue.

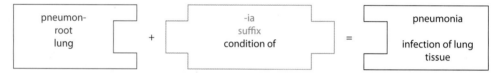

- Add the **suffix** -*ation* to the **root** *respir-* to make the term **respiration.** The **suffix** -*ation* means *a process.* Respiration is the process of breathing in and out.

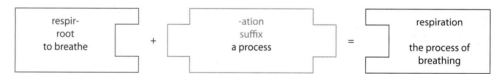

Although most **roots** are specific to body systems and medical specialties, **suffixes** are universal and can be applied to all body systems and specialties.

One user-friendly design concept of this book is that all the information you will need for any given topic is presented on the left-hand page of the two-page spread open in front of you. As part of this, you will find a Word Analysis and Definition (WAD) box on the right-hand side of each two-page spread. This section provides the elements, definition, and pronunciation of every new and repeated significant medical term that appears in the two-page spread.

Review all the terms in the WAD before you start any exercise.

Word	Pronunciation	Elements		Definition
pulmonary	PULL-moh-NAR-ee	S/ R/	-ary *pertaining to* pulmon- *lung*	Pertaining to the lungs
pulmonology	PULL-moh-NOL-oh-jee	S/ R/CF	-logy *study of* pulmon/o- *lung*	Study of the lungs, or the medical specialty of disorders of the lungs
pulmonologist	PULL-moh-NOL-oh-jist	S/	-logist *one who studies, specialist*	Specialist in treating disorders of the lungs
pneumonia	new-MOH-nee-ah	S/ R/	-ia *condition* pneumon- *lung, air*	Inflammation of the lung parenchyma (tissue)
pneumonitis (same as *pneumonia*)	new-moh-NI-tis	S/	-itis *inflammation*	
respiration	RES-pih-RAY-shun	S/ R/	-ation *process* respir- *to breathe*	Process of breathing; fundamental process of life used to exchange oxygen and carbon dioxide
respiratory (adj)	RES-pih-rah-tor-ee	S/	-atory *pertaining to*	Pertaining to respiration

EXERCISES

Elements: *It is important for you to recognize the identity of an element. Is it a root, combining form, or suffix? This will help you to determine its place in the term when you are building terms.*

A. Build the appropriate medical term *to match the definitions given. The placement of the elements is noted for you under the line; each different element is separated on the line. Write the correct elements on the line. The first one is done for you.*

1. Study of the lungs: _____ pulmon/o ___/___ logy _____

R/CF   S

2. Pertaining to the lung: _____ / _____

R/CF   S

3. The process of breathing: _____ / _____

R/CF   S

4. Condition of the lung: _____ / _____

R/CF   S

5. Use any one of the preceding terms in a sentence of your choice—one that is *not* a definition from above.

6. Choose another term from above and use it in patient documentation that you write below.

B. Answers *to all questions in this exercise can be found on the two-page spread open in front of you.*

1. What is another term for inflammation of the lung? _____

2. Which term is a body process? _____

3. Which suffix can be applied to a specialist? _____

LESSON 1.1 Prefixes (LO 1.2 and 1.3)

- A prefix always appears at the beginning of a term.
- A prefix precedes a root to change its meaning.
- Prefixes can have more than one meaning.
- Prefixes never require a **combining vowel.**
- An occasional medical term can have two prefixes.
- Not every term has a prefix.

PRACTICAL POINTS

- A **root** can start a term and does not become a prefix.
- A **root** can end a term and does not become a **suffix.**
- An example of both of these is **pneumothorax.**

A prefix is an element added to the beginning of a **root** or **combining form** to further expand the meaning of a medical term. Prefixes usually indicate time, number, color, or location. Examples of prefixes defining time are as follows:

- The term **mature** can refer to an infant born after a normal length of pregnancy, between 37 and 42 weeks.
- An infant born before 37 weeks is called **premature.** The prefix *pre-* means *before.* **Premature** means that the infant was born *before 37 weeks.*
- An infant born after 42 weeks is called **postmature.** The prefix *post-* means *after.* **Postmature** means that the *infant was born after 42 weeks.*

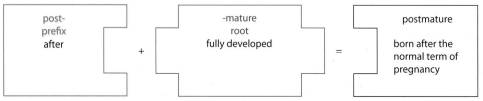

- The term **natal** contains the **root** *nat- (birth* or *born)* and the **suffix** *–al (pertaining to);* it means *pertaining to birth.*
- Add the prefix *pre- (before)* to form **prenatal,** which means *the time before birth.*
- Add the prefix *post- (after)* to form **postnatal,** which means *the time after birth.*
- Add the prefix *peri- (around)* to form **perinatal,** which means *around the time of birth.* This includes the time immediately *before, during,* and *directly after birth.*

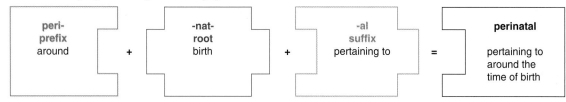

Examples of prefixes indicating number are as follows:

- The term **lateral** contains the **root** *later- (side)* and the **suffix** *–al (pertaining to).* **Lateral** means *pertaining to a side of the body.*
- Add the prefix *uni- (one)* to form **unilateral,** which means *pertaining to one side of the body only.*
- Add the prefix *bi- (two)* to form **bilateral,** which means *pertaining to both sides of the body.*

Examples of prefixes indicating location are as follows:

- The term **gastric** contains the **root** *gastr- (stomach)* and the **suffix** *–ic (pertaining to).* **Gastric** means *pertaining to the stomach.*
- Add the prefix *epi- (above)* to form **epigastric,** which means *pertaining to above the stomach.*
- Add the prefix *hypo- (below)* to form **hypogastric,** which means *pertaining to below the stomach.*

Examples of prefixes indicating size are as follows:

- The **root** *-cyte* means *cell.*
- Add the prefix *macro- (large)* to form **macrocyte,** which means *a large red blood cell.*
- Add the prefix *micro- (small)* to form **microcyte,** which means *a small red blood cell.*

Word	Pronunciation		Elements	Definition
gastric	GAS-trik	S/ R/	-ic *pertaining to* gastr- *stomach*	Pertaining to the stomach
epigastric hypogastric	ep-ih-GAS-trik high-poh-GAS-trik	P/ P/	epi- *above* hypo- *below*	Abdominal region above the stomach Abdominal region below the stomach
lateral	LAT-er-al	S/ R/	-al *pertaining to* later- *side*	Pertaining to one side of the body
bilateral unilateral	by-LAT-er-al you-nih-LAT-er-al	P/ P/	bi- *two* uni- *one*	Pertaining to both sides of the body Pertaining to one side of the body only
macrocyte	MACK-roh-site	P/ R/	macro- *large* -cyte *cell*	Large red blood cell
macrocytic (adj) (**Note:** *The "e" in* cyte *is deleted to allow the word to flow.*)	mack-roh-SIT-ik	S/	-ic *pertaining to*	Pertaining to a macrocyte
mature postmature	mah-TYUR post-mah-TYUR	P/ R/	*Latin* ready post- *after* -mature *fully developed*	Fully developed Infant born after 42 weeks of gestation
premature	pree-mah-TYUR	P/	pre- *before*	Occurring before the expected time; e.g., an infant born before 37 weeks of gestation.
microcyte	MY-kroh-site	P/ R/	micro- *small* -cyte *cell*	Small red blood cell
microcytic (adj) (**Note:** *The "e" in* cyte *is deleted to allow the word to flow.*)	my-kroh-SIT-ik	S/	-ic *pertaining to*	Pertaining to a small red blood cell
natal	NAY tal	S/ R/	-al *pertaining to* nat- *birth, born*	Pertaining to birth
perinatal postnatal prenatal	per-ih-NAY-tal post-NAY-tal pree-NAY-tal	P/ P/ P/	peri- *around* post- *after* pre- *before*	Around the time of birth After the birth Before the birth
pneumothorax	new-moh-THOR-ax	R/CF R/	pneum/o- *air, lung* -thorax *chest*	Air in the pleural cavity

EXERCISES

Prefixes: *Solid knowledge of prefixes will quickly help increase your medical vocabulary. A good example is the Word Analysis and Definition (WAD) entry for* natal. *The addition of three different prefixes builds three new medical terms.*

A. *To begin this exercise, underline every prefix in the bolded terms below. Answer the first question, and then build the correct term on the line next to the definitions in 2 through 4. Follow the instructions for question 5.*

natal   **prenatal**   **postnatal**   **perinatal**

1. The term *natal* means _____ .

2. Pertaining to around the time of birth: _____ / _____ / _____
                               P   R/CF   S

3. Pertaining to after the birth: _____ / _____ / _____
                               P   R/CF   S

4. Pertaining to before the birth: _____ / _____ / _____
                               P   R/CF   S

5. In 2 through 4 above, circle the word in the definition that is the clue to the correct prefix to use in the term.

B. Review *the prefixes for number, location and size. Check (✓) the correct box for the category, and write the meaning for every prefix in the chart.*

Prefix	Number	Location	Size	Prefix Means
1. hypo				
2. uni				

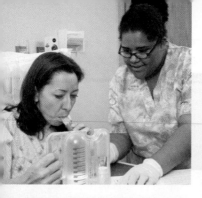

LESSON 1.2

Word Analysis and Deconstruction

OBJECTIVES

When you see an unfamiliar medical term, you can learn its meaning by **deconstructing** *it—reducing it to its basic elements. In this lesson you will learn to:*

1.2.1 Break down or deconstruct a medical term into its elements.

1.2.2 Use word analysis to help ensure the precise use of medical terms.

1.2.3 Use the word elements to analyze and determine the meaning of the term.

1.2.4 Apply the correct pronunciation to medical terms.

KEYNOTE

• Always begin deconstructing a medical term by identifying its suffix.

ABBREVIATIONS

AMI	acute myocardial infarction
CXR	chest x-ray
ECG/ EKG	electrocardiogram
IV	intravenous

CASE REPORT 1.2

YOU ARE: . . . a medical assistant working in the office of Lokesh Bannerjee, MD, a cardiologist in Fulwood Medical Center.

YOU ARE COMMUNICATING WITH:

. . . the 70-year-old wife and the 45-year-old son of James Donovan, a 75-year-old man who will be admitted to the hospital's acute care **cardiology** unit.

Dr. Bannerjee has diagnosed Mr. Donovan with an acute myocardial infarction (**AMI**), confirmed by changes in his **electrocardiogram (ECG/EKG)**. One of your tasks is to explain Mr. Donovan's diagnosis and reasons for admission to the hospital to Mrs. Donovan and her son. While Mr. Donovan is waiting to be admitted, he is receiving oxygen through nasal prongs. He is hypotensive, and an intravenous (**IV**) infusion of normal saline has been started. His medical record indicates that he is being seen in the neurology clinic for early dementia.

THE BOLD TERMS IN THE CASE REPORT ARE USED AS EXAMPLES IN THE TEXT AND/OR ARE DECONSTRUCTED IN THE WORD ANALYSIS AND DEFINITION BOX (OPPOSITE PAGE).

Word Deconstruction (LO 1.4)

When you see an unfamiliar medical term, first identify the **suffix.** Take the term **cardiologist.** Here, the **suffix** at the end of the word is *-logist,* which means *one who studies and is a specialist in.* This leaves the element *cardi/o-,* which is the **combining form** for *heart.* The term **cardiologist** means *a specialist in the heart and its diseases.* It has a **combining form** and a **suffix.**

In the term **myocardial,** the **suffix** at the end of the word is **-al,** which means pertaining to, as you learned earlier in this chapter. The **combining form** *my/o-,* which means *muscle,* is at the beginning of the word. The **root** *-cardi-,* which means *heart,* is in the middle of the word. So, the term **myocardial** means *pertaining to the heart muscle.* It has a **combining form,** a **root,** and a **suffix.**

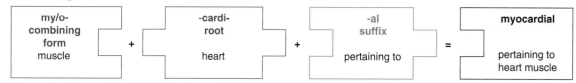

my/o- combining form muscle	+	-cardi- root heart	+	-al suffix pertaining to	=	**myocardial** pertaining to heart muscle

Changing the **suffix** to *-um,* meaning *a structure,* results in the term **myocardium,** *the structure called the heart muscle.*

The term **cardiomyopathy** contains the **suffix -pathy,** meaning *a disease,* the **combining form** *cardi/o-,* meaning the *heart,* and the **combining form** *my/o-,* meaning *muscle.* When you put this all together, the term **cardiomyopathy** means *a disease of the heart muscle.*

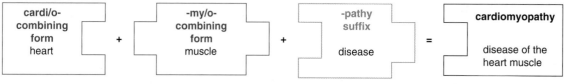

cardi/o- combining form heart	+	-my/o- combining form muscle	+	-pathy suffix disease	=	**cardiomyopathy** disease of the heart muscle

The term **ischemia** has the **suffix** *-emia,* which means *a blood condition.* The **root** *isch-* means *to block.* **Ischemia** means *a blockage of blood flow.* The term **myocardial ischemia** means *a blockage of blood flow to the heart muscle*—better known as a heart attack.

Changing the **suffix** *-emia* to *-emic,* which means *pertaining to a condition of the blood,* creates a new term, **ischemic,** that is an adjective. It means *pertaining to a blockage of blood flow.* It has a **root** and a **suffix.**

To help you learn, abbreviations are listed and defined in **Abbreviations boxes** throughout this book.

Word	Pronunciation	Elements		Definition
cardiologist	kar-dee-**OL**-oh-jist	S/ R/CF	-logist *one who studies and is a specialist in* cardi/o- *heart*	A medical specialist in the diagnosis and treatment of disorders of the heart
cardiology	kar-dee-**OL**-oh-jee	S/	-logy *study of*	Medical specialty of diseases of the heart
cardiomyopathy	KAR-dee-oh-my-**OP**-ah-thee	S/ R/CF R/CF	-pathy *disease* cardi/o- *heart* -my/o- *muscle*	Disease of the heart muscle, the myocardium
diagnosis (noun)	die-ag-**NO**-sis	P/ R/	dia- *complete* -gnosis *knowledge of an abnormal condition*	The determination of the cause of a disease
diagnoses (pl) diagnostic (adj) (Note: *The "is" in* -gnosis *is deleted to allow the word to flow.*)	die-ag-**NO**-sees die-ag-**NOS**-tik	S/	-tic *pertaining to*	Pertaining to or establishing a diagnosis
diagnose (verb)	die-ag-**NOSE**	R/	-gnose *recognize an abnormal condition*	To make a diagnosis
prognosis (noun)	prog-**NO**-sis	P/ R/	pro- *before, project forward* -gnosis *knowledge of an abnormal condition*	A forecast of the probable course and outcome of a disease
electrocardiogram	ee-lek-troh-**KAR**-dee-oh-gram	S/ R/CF R/CF	-gram *record* electr/o- *electricity* -cardi/o- *heart*	Record of the heart's electrical signals
infarct	in-**FARKT**	P/ R/	in- *in* -farct *area of dead tissue*	An area of cell death resulting from blockage of its blood supply
infarction	in-**FARK**-shun	S/	-ion *action, condition*	Sudden blockage of an artery
ischemia	is-**KEY**-me-ah	S/ R/	-emia *a blood condition* isch- *to block*	Lack of blood supply to tissue
ischemic (adj)	is-**KEY**-mik	S/	-emic *pertaining to a condition of the blood*	Pertaining to the lack of blood supply to tissue
myocardial (adj)	MY-oh-**KAR**-dee-al	S/ R/CF R/	-al *pertaining to* my/o- *muscle* -cardi- *heart*	Pertaining to heart muscle
myocardium	MY-oh-**KAR**-dee-um	S/	-um *structure*	All the heart muscle

EXERCISES

Precision in communication: *In addition to using the precise medical terms and speaking and spelling them correctly, you must use the appropriate form of the term as well.*

A. Reread the WAD entry for diagnosis. *Note that there are singular and plural forms of the term, as well as the noun, adjective, and verb forms. Insert the correct form of the term in the documentation below.*

> **Note:** A noun is a person, place, or thing. Singular: One
> A verb denotes action. Plural: More than one
> An adjective usually describes something.

1. The primary _____ for this patient is myocardial ischemia.

2. Dr. Bannerjee is unable to _____ this patient until he receives the lab results.

3. The _____ tests have been ordered for this patient first thing in the morning.

4. It is possible for this patient to have multiple _____ if there is more than one condition present.

B. Challenge your new knowledge *used in questions 1-4 above.*

1. Which sentence contains the verb form of the term? _____

2. Which sentence contains the plural form of the term? _____

3. Which sentence contains the singular noun? _____

4. Which sentence contains an adjective form? _____

LESSON 1.2 Plurals (LO 1.5)

Some medical terms are pronounced the same but spelled differently. For example:

- Both *ilium* and *ileum* are pronounced **ILL**-ee-um. *Ilium* is a bone in the pelvis; *ileum* is a segment of the small intestine.

- Both *mucus* and *mucous* are pronounced **MYU**-kus. *Mucus* is a noun and is the name of a fluid secreted by *mucous* (adjective) membranes that line body cavities.

A medical term may relate to more than one anatomical structure.

- The term cervical means relating to a neck in any sense.

- It can pertain to the neck that joins the head to the trunk with the cervical vertebrae.

- It can also pertain to the cervix of the uterus, with its cervical canal.

Some words, when incorrectly pronounced, sound the same. For example:

- The term *prostate,* pronounced **PROS**-tate, refers to the gland at the base of the male bladder. The term *prostrate* means to be physically weak or exhausted, or to lie flat on the ground.

- Train your ear to hear the differences—*reflex* is not *reflux.*

Many medical terms form a verb, a noun, a plural, and an adjective, and you have to know them all, as in diagnose, diagnosis, diagnoses, and diagnostic (see the WAD on the previous spread).

Many words in the English language allow you to change them from singular to plural by adding an "s." For medical terms, this rarely happens, as these plurals are formed in ways that were once logical to Greeks and Romans, but now have to be learned by memory in English. Examples of medical terms with Greek and Latin plurals are shown in *Table 1.1.*

Throughout this book, the Greek and Latin plurals of medical terms appear in the Word Analysis and Definition box with the singular medical term, as with the term **diagnosis** in the previous spread.

▼ TABLE 1.1
Singular and Plural Forms

Singular Ending	Plural Ending	Examples
-a	-ae	axilla axillae
-is	-es	diagnosis diagnoses
-on	-a	ganglion ganglia
-um	-a	septum septa

Adapted from Kenneth S. Saladin, Anatomy and Physiology, 3rd ed., fig. 1.2, p. 21. Copyright ©2004 The McGraw-Hill Companies, Inc. Reprinted with permission.

Pronunciation (LO 1.6)

Being able to pronounce words correctly is essential to effective communication. In the medical world, this concept is especially important. As a health professional, you will routinely use medical terms and your colleagues must be able to understand what you are saying. Correct pronunciation is crucial to patient safety and your ability to provide high-quality patient care.

Throughout this book, the pronunciation of medical terms is spelled out phonetically using modern English forms to show you exactly how the terms are pronounced. The word part to be emphasized is shown in bold, uppercase letters.

For example, **pulmonary** is phonetically written **PUL**-moh-nar-ee, and **pulmonology** is written **PUL**-moh-**NOL**-oh-jee. This illustrates that words derived from the same **root** can have their emphasis placed on different parts of the word, and that the emphasized part can be from different elements. The emphasized syllable **NOL** comes partly from the **combining form** *pulmon/o-* and partly from the **suffix** *-logy.* You can hear glossary terms pronounced correctly by visiting the Student Online Learning Center (www.mhhe.com/AllanEss2e).

Word	Pronunciation		Elements	Definition
axilla axillae (pl) axillary (adj)	AK-sill-ah AK-sill-ee AK-sill-air-ee	S/ R/	Latin *armpit* -ary *pertaining to* axill- *armpit*	Medical term for the armpit Pertaining to the armpit
dementia	dee-**MEN**-she-ah	S/ P/ R/	-ia *condition* de- *without* -ment- *mind*	Chronic, progressive, irreversible loss of intel-lectual and mental functions
ganglion ganglia (pl)	**GANG**-lee-on **GANG**-lee-ah		Greek *a swelling* or *knot*	A fluid-filled cyst or a collection of nerve cells outside the brain and spinal cord
ileum ilium ilia (pl)	**ILL**-ee-um **ILL**-ee-um **ILL**-ee-ah		Latin *to twist* or *roll up* Latin *groin*	Third portion of the small intestine. Large wing-shaped bone at the upper and posterior part of the pelvis
mucus (noun) mucous (adj) mucosa	**MYU**-kus **MYU**-kus myu-**KOH**-sah	 S/ R/ S/	Greek *slime* -ous *pertaining to* muc- *mucus* -osa *full of; like*	Sticky secretion of cells in mucous membranes Pertaining to mucus or the mucosa Lining of a tubular structure that secretes mucus
prostate prostrate prostration (noun)	**PROS**-tate pros-**TRAYT** pros-**TRAY**-shun		Greek *one who stands before* Latin *to stretch out*	Organ surrounding the urethra at the base of the male urinary bladder To lay flat or to be overcome by physical weakness and exhaustion
reflex reflux	**REE**-fleks **REE**-fluks		Latin *bend back* Latin *backward flow*	An involuntary response to a stimulus Backward flow
septum septa (pl)	**SEP**-tum **SEP**-tah		Latin *a partition*	A thin wall separating two cavities or two tis-sue masses

EXERCISES

A. Medical language: *Many terms in medicine sound and/or look very similar. The difference of only one letter can make a new term. Train your eye and ear to know the difference. Circle the correct choice of terms in the following documentation.*

1. The patient's nasal (mucus/mucous) membrane is severely infected.

2. Schedule this patient for a (prostrate/prostate) exam at his next annual physical.

3. The doctor checked the (reflex/reflux) in the patient's knee.

4. The patient's (ilium/ileum) was severely fractured in the motor vehicle accident.

B. Plurals: *Circle the correct form of the plural in the following sentences.*

1. Because of additional medical problems needing treatment, this patient's insurance claim form will have multiple (diagnoses/diagnosis).

2. Check both (axilla/axillae) for any evidence of enlarged lymph nodes.

3. Several (septa/septum) exist in the body—e.g., in the heart and in the nose.

4. A cluster of (ganglia/ganglion) has formed on her left wrist.

C. Terminology challenge. *Use your knowledge of the new medical terms you have learned in this chapter and answer the following questions.*

1. The term *cervical* can apply to two different places in the body. Where are they?

_____

_____

2. The term *ileum* and *ilium* are pronounced the same but are in two different body systems. Where are they?

_____

_____

LESSON 1.2 Precision in Communication (LO 1.5)

KEYNOTES

• Many words, when they are written or pronounced, have an element that if misspelled or mispronounced gives the intended word an entirely different meaning. A treatment response to the different meaning could cause a medical error or even the death of a patient.

• Precision in written and verbal communication is essential to prevent errors in patient care.

• The medical record in which you document a patient's care and your actions is a legal document. It can be used in court as evidence in professional medical liability cases.

It's important for you to note that being accurate and precise in both your written and verbal communication with your health care team can save someone's life. Each year in the United States, more than 400,000 people die because of drug reactions and medical errors, many of which are the result of poor communication. On the next page, you will find some specific examples of how certain medical terms could be seriously miscommunicated and misinterpreted.

In the above Case Report involving Mr. Donovan, if **hypotension** (low blood pressure) were confused with **hypertension** (high blood pressure), incorrect and dangerous treatment could be prescribed.

> ### CASE REPORT 1.2 (CONTINUED)
>
> Mr. Donovan is waiting to be admitted to the hospital and is receiving oxygen through nasal prongs. He is **hypotensive**, and an **intravenous (IV) infusion** of normal saline has been started. According to his medical record, he is being seen in the **neurology** clinic for early dementia.

• In the word **hypotension,** the **suffix** *-ion* means *a condition.* The prefix *hypo-* means *below or less than normal.* The **root** *-tens-* is from the Latin word for *pressure.* **Hypotension** is a condition of below-normal pressure, or low blood pressure.

• In the word **hypertension,** the prefix *hyper-* means *above or more than normal.* **Hypertension** is a condition of above-normal pressure, or high blood pressure.

Also in the above Case Report, the term **neurology,** the specialty of the nervous system *(see Chapter 10),* can sound very similar to **urology,** the study of the urinary system *(see Chapter 13).* In the urinary system, if a patient's **ureter** (the tube from the kidney to the bladder) were confused with the **urethra** (the tube from the bladder to the outside), the consequences could be serious.

As you can see from the above examples, your ability to correctly identify, spell, and pronounce different medical terms is essential. Being a health professional requires the utmost attention to detail, as a patient's life could be in your hands. Incorrect spelling and poor pronunciation does not only reflect badly on you and your health team—it could also be a matter of life and death.

ABBREVIATIONS

IV   intravenous

Word	Pronunciation	Elements		Definition
cervical (adj)	SER-vih-kal	S/ R/	-al *pertaining to* cervic- *neck*	Pertaining to the cervix or to the neck region
cervix	SER-viks		Latin *neck*	Lower part of the uterus
hypertension	HIGH-per-TEN-shun	S/ P/ R/	-ion *condition, action* hyper- *above normal* -tens- *pressure*	Persistent high arterial blood pressure
hypertensive (adj) hypotension hypotensive (adj)	HIGH-per-TEN-siv HIGH-poh-TEN-shun HIGH-poh-TEN-siv	S/ P/	-ive *pertaining to* hypo- *below normal*	Pertaining to or suffering from high blood pressure Persistent low arterial blood pressure Pertaining to or suffering from low blood pressure
infusion	in-FYU-zhun	P/ R/	in- *in* -fusion *to pour*	Introduction of a substance other than blood intravenously
transfusion	trans-FYU-zhun	P/	trans- *across, through*	Transfer of blood or a blood component from a donor to a recipient
intravenous	IN-trah-VEE-nus	S/ P/ R/	-ous *pertaining to* intra- *within, inside* -ven- *vein*	Inside a vein
neurology	nyu-ROL-oh-jee	S/ R/CF	-logy *study of* neur/o- *nerve*	Medical specialty of disorders of the nervous system
neurologist	nyu-ROL-oh-jist	S/	-logist *one who studies and is a specialist in*	Medical specialist in disorders of the nervous system
protocol	PRO-toe-kol		Latin *contents page of a book*	Detailed plan; in this case, for a regimen of therapy
ureter	you-REE-ter		Greek *urinary canal*	Tube that connects a kidney to the urinary bladder
urethra urology	you-REE-thrah you-ROL-oh-jee	S/ R/CF	Greek *passage for urine* -logy *study of* ur/o- *urine*	Canal leading from the bladder to the outside Medical specialty of disorders of the urinary system
uterus	YOU-ter-us		Latin *womb*	Organ in which an egg develops into a fetus
vertebra vertebrae (pl)	VER-teh-brah VER-teh-bree		Latin *bone in the spine*	One of the bones of the spinal column

EXERCISES

A. Patient documentation: *Read the following excerpts from patient charts, and insert the correct medical term from the above Word Analysis and Definition (WAD) box. Always review the WAD before you start the exercise.*

1. This patient has several badly fractured _____ in his spinal column.

2. This patient has nerve damage. Refer him to the department of _____.

3. Schedule this patient for an _____ of chemotherapy drugs today.

4. This patient has low blood pressure—he is _____ and anemic.

5. I am ordering an immediate _____ of 2 units of whole blood for this patient.

6. Send this patient for _____ x-rays of his neck immediately.

B. Brain teaser: *Challenge yourself to analyze the question and insert the correct answers.*

1. If a medical specialist in the study of disorders of the nervous system is a neurologist, what is a medical specialist in the study of disorders of the urinary system called?

   (Hint: Use your knowledge of suffixes and roots to help you.)

2. What element is the difference between high blood pressure and low blood pressure? _____

3. What substances go through an infusion? _____

4. What substances go through a transfusion that do not go through an infusion? _____

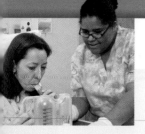

CHALLENGE YOUR KNOWLEDGE

A. Prefixes: *Prefixes can have more than one meaning, and always appear at the beginning of a medical term. Match the prefix in column 1 to its correct meaning or meanings in column 2.*

1.	peri	_____	**A.**	after
2.	de	_____	**B.**	within, inside
3.	epi	_____	**C.**	one
4.	hyper	_____	**D.**	below normal
5.	post	_____	**E.**	around
6.	trans	_____	**F.**	in
7.	uni	_____	**G.**	above
8.	intra	_____	**H.**	large
9.	dia	_____	**I.**	above normal
10.	pro	_____	**J.**	before
11.	hypo	_____	**K.**	two
12.	in	_____	**L.**	across, through
13.	macro	_____	**M.**	without
14.	pre	_____	**N.**	small
15.	bi	_____	**O.**	before, project forward
16.	micro	_____	**P.**	complete

B. Grouping opposites: *Fill in the chart, and then answer the questions that follow. After you have completed this exercise, use it for study review. Grouping opposite elements or terms into pairs will make them easier to remember.*

Element	Meaning of Element	Medical Term Containing This Element	Meaning of the Medical Term
pre	1.	2.	3.
post	4.	5.	6.
epi	7.	8.	9.
hypo	10.	11.	12.
macro	13.	14.	15.
micro	16.	17.	18.
hyper	19.	20.	21.

22. These elements are all (P, R, CF, S) _____.

The meaning of the above elements will help you determine the correct answers to the following questions, even though you have never seen these terms before! Finish this exercise by circling the word or words in questions 9 through 12 that led you to choose the correct element.

23. If a complication occurs after surgery, is it pre or post operative?

_____ operative

24. Which would be the topmost layer of skin (the one above everything else)—the epidermis or the hypodermis?

_____ dermis

25. Organisms that are too small to be seen with the naked eye are called _____ scopic.

26. Would too much sugar in the blood be hyperglycemia or hypoglycemia?

_____ glycemia.

C. Elements *will always remain your best clue to understandingπ a medical term. The following terms have one element underlined and bolded—define that element and define the term. Fill in the blanks.*

1. cardio**myo**pathy   element defined: _____

term defined: _____

2. **isch**emia   element defined: _____

term defined: _____

3. myocard**ium**   element defined: _____

term defined: _____

4. **cervic**al   element defined: _____

term defined: _____

5. hyperten**sion**   element defined: _____

term defined: _____

6. **trans**fusion   element defined: _____

term defined: _____

7. **neuro**logist   element defined: _____

term defined: _____

8. **bi**lateral   element defined: _____

term defined: _____

9. **gastr**ic   element defined: _____

term defined: _____

10. **intra**venous   element defined: _____

term defined: _____

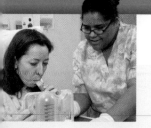

D. Identify and define *the elements in this chart. Then give an example of these elements in a medical term from this chapter. Fill in the chart.*

Element	Identify as P, R, CF, or S	Define Element	Medical Term Containing This Element
uro	1.	2.	3.
tens	4.	5.	6.
later	7.	8.	9.
nat	10.	11.	12.
cervic	13.	14.	15.
gram	16.	17.	18.

E. Roots/Combining Forms: *The meaning of the R/CF is given in column 1. Match the meaning to the correct term containing that R/CF in column 2.*

_____ 1. chest

_____ 2. armpit

_____ 3. heart

_____ 4. nerve

_____ 5. birth

_____ 6. pressure

_____ 7. knowledge

_____ 8. mind

_____ 9. area of dead tissue

_____ 10. cell

A. dementia

B. microcyte

C. hypertension

D. prognosis

E. neurologist

F. pneumothorax

G. infarct

H. myocardial

I. axillary

J. perinatal

Use any two terms from column 2 in patient documentation of your choice.

11. _____

_____

12. _____

_____

F. Suffixes: *A suffix always appears at the end of a term. Fill in the correct definition of all the suffixes that have appeared in this chapter, and answer the question.*

Suffix	Meaning of Suffix
ic	1.
al	2.
logist	3.
logy	4.
pathy	5.
tic	6.
gram	7.
ion	8.
emia	9.
emic	10.
um	11.
ary	12.
ia	13.
ous	14.
ive	15.

16. What is the most frequent meaning that appears in this list of suffixes? _____

Remember: More than one element can have the same meaning.

G. Difference between: *If you really understand a term, you can explain it to someone else. Briefly explain these terms to a patient, in language he or she can understand.*

1. transfusion: _____

_____

2. infusion: _____

_____

3. diagnosis: _____

_____

4. prognosis: _____

_____

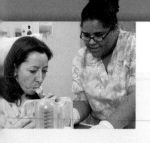

H. Spelling demons: *The following terms from this chapter are particularly difficult to spell and pronounce. Correct pronunciation and spelling of medical terms is the mark of an educated professional. Circle the correct spelling, and then check (✓) that you have practiced the pronunciation. Remember that pronunciations are on the Student Online Learning Center* (www.mhhe.com/AllanEss2e).

Pronunciation ✓

1. diagnosis   diagnossis   diagnosiss   _____

2. infart   infarct   infarrct   _____

3. isscemia   iskchemia   ischemia   _____

4. miocardium   myocardeum   myocardium   _____

5. axila   axilla   axeila   _____

6. septtum   siptum   septum   _____

7. dementia   dimentia   dementea   _____

8. intraveinous   intravenous   intravinous   _____

9. vertebrae   verteebrae   vertebray   _____

10. pnumothorax   pneumothorax   pneumonthorax   _____

I. Latin and Greek terms *do not deconstruct into the elements of* prefix, **root, combining form,** *and* **suffix** *the way most medical terms do. You just have to know them for what they are. Test yourself by matching the literal or defined meaning in column 1 with the correct Latin or Greek term in column 2.*

_____ **1.** armpit   A. ganglion

_____ **2.** one who stands before   B. mature

_____ **3.** bend back   C. prostrate

_____ **4.** neck   D. reflex

_____ **5.** backward flow   E. mucus

_____ **6.** slime   F. ileum

_____ **7.** wing-shaped bone in pelvis   G. axilla

_____ **8.** fluid-filled cyst   H. reflux

_____ **9.** ripe   I. cervical

_____ **10.** third portion of small intestine   J. ilium

J. Terminology challenge.

1. Write the precise medical language for what, in layperson's terms, is called a "heart attack":

_____

K. Keynotes *contain useful information and will often be the source of test questions. All the answers for this exercise on medical term elements can be found in Keynotes earlier in this chapter. For each statement, circle T (true) or (F) false. If the statement is false, rewrite the statement so that it is true on the lines below.*

1. A suffix changes the meaning of a term.   T   F

2. Different suffixes can have the same meaning.   T   F

3. The core foundation of every term is a root or combining form.   T   F

4. Every term must have a prefix.   T   F

5. If the suffix begins with a consonant, it must follow a root.   T   F

6. A root plus a combining vowel equals a combining form.   T   F

7. A medical term will never have more than one suffix.   T   F

8. A prefix always comes at the beginning of the term.   T   F

9. Combining forms can precede a suffix.   T   F

10. Always begin deconstructing a term by identifying the root.   T   F

Corrected statements: _____

_____

_____

_____

L. Build medical terms *in this exercise. The first column in the chart below presents statements relating to the terms you will build. Look for clues in the statement words that will help you select the elements from the list. Build the term by inserting the correct elements in the appropriate columns (some elements you will use more than once, and some you will not use at all). The first term has been built, and the elements highlighted, to help you understand.*

To complete the exercise, use any one of the terms in a brief sentence that is not a definition.

pneum/o-	-cyte	-logy	trans-	-ic	-thorax	-um	macro-	gastr-	-tension
-emia	isch-	-logy	cardio-	-mature	bi-	peri-	-ation	-al	respir-
-my/o-	-pathy	intra-	-later-	-nat-	post-	hypo-	pulmon/o-	epi-	card/i-
neur/o-	cervic-								

Statement	Prefix	Root/CF	Suffix
air in the chest		pneum/o-, -thorax	
1. the heart muscle			
2. pertaining to around the time of birth			
3. large red blood cell			
4. pertaining to both sides of the body			
5. study of the lung			

6. Sentence: _____

_____

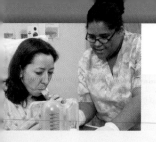
M. Layperson's language: *Patients may request that you "translate" medical language into language they can more easily understand. Practice communicating the correct information with this exercise. If there are abbreviations in the sentence, "translate" them as well.*

1. The pulmonologist read the patient's CXR and diagnosed a cancer in her RUL.

_____

_____

_____

2. The patient's past medical history includes pneumonia and pneumothorax, as well as problems with her ileum.

_____

_____

_____

3. Because of her diabetes, this patient must be seen for closely supervised prenatal and postnatal care.

_____

_____

_____

N. Plurals: *Because many medical terms are directly from Greek or Latin, they do not form their plurals just by adding "s" as happens in English. In this exercise, you are given the singular form of five terms. Choose one of the endings to form the correct plural of each term (some endings you will use more than once, and some you will not use at all).*

ae	es	ides	ges	ies	era	a

Singular	Plural
1. diagnosis	_____
2. axilla	_____
3. ganglion	_____
4. septum	_____
5. vertebra	_____

O. Partner exercise: *Ask your study partner to close his or her text. Dictate the following sentences to your partner, and then ask him or her to write the sentences and show them to you. Check your partner's sentences against the text below. The sentence is not correct unless every word is present and everything is spelled correctly. When you have finished checking your partner's answers, close your book and ask your partner to dictate the sentences to you and you write them down.*

1. Mr. Donovan's chest pain is caused by myocardial ischemia, and an intravenous infusion has been started.

2. In addition to his hypotension, the record notes that Mr. Donovan is also being seen in the neurology clinic for dementia.

3. Mr. Donovan's physician has diagnosed an acute myocardial infarction based on a diagnostic electrocardiogram.

P. Proofread *the following sentences for errors in fact or spelling. Underline any misspelled terms or errors in fact in a sentence; then rewrite the incorrect sentences correctly on the lines below. There is only one sentence that is entirely correct.*

1. An acute myocardial infraction can be confirmed by an EGK.

2. Patients with chest pain could possibly have myocardeal ischemic.

3. An electrocardiogram is a diagnostic tool to check for possible heart attack.

4. The pulmonalogist ordered an IV transfusion of saline and nasal oxygen.

5. Mr. Donovan's dimentia may be a complicating factor in the treatment for his heart attack.

Rewrites: _____

_____

_____

_____

_____

Q. Chapter challenge: *Read all the possible choices before you circle the correct answer.*

1. Which answer best describes *pulmono* and *pneumo?*

    a. They are both roots and mean *chest.*

    b. They are both combining forms but have different meanings.

    c. One is a root, and the other is a combining form.

    d. They are both combining forms and mean lung.

    e. One is a suffix, and the other is a prefix.

2. Based on their *elements,* pick the pair of terms that logically belong together:

    a. reflex and urology   **d.** ganglia and ganglion

    b. pulmonology and pulmonologist   **e.** multilateral and epigastric

    c. prostate and prostrate

3. Which two sets of terms have prefixes denoting numbers?

    a. hypotension and hypertension   **d.** pericardial and perinatal

    b. premature and postmature   **e.** epigastric and hypogastric

    c. bilateral and unilateral

4. The body system concerned with air or breathing is the _____, and an organ in that system is the _____.

    a. urinary   ureter

    b. musculoskeletal   ilium

    c. respiratory   lung

    d. cardiovascular   heart

    e. digestive   stomach

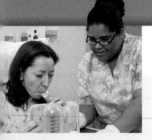

R. Chapter challenge: *Read all the possible choices before you circle the correct answer.*

1. The terms *myocardial* and *myocardium* both refer to the:

   a. lung   **d.** heart

   b. hip   **e.** blood

   c. pelvis

2. The prefix in *intravenous* means:

   a. across   **d.** two

   b. around   **e.** before

   c. within

3. Which pair of terms do not deconstruct into word elements?

   a. axillary and axilla   **d.** respiration and pulmonary

   b. pulmonologist and pulmonology   **e.** cervix and cervical

   c. ileum and ilium

4. Circle the only choice that does not contain a combining form:

   a. pneumothorax   **d.** myocardial

   b. pulmonology   **e.** cardiomyopathy

   c. pneumonia

5. The medical term for "armpit" is:

   a. septum   **d.** ganglion

   b. mucosa   **e.** ilium

   c. axilla

6. Brain teaser: Circle the terms used to describe newborn babies' development.

   a. unilateral and bilateral   **d.** perigastric and perinatal

   b. epigastric and hypogastric   **e.** prenatal and postnatal

   c. premature and postmature

5. The term *cardiomyopathy* has a suffix meaning:

   a. condition   **d.** structure

   b. disease   **e.** pertaining to

   c. action

6. Which pair contains terms that are both diagnoses?

   a. pneumothorax and pulmonologist   **d.** reflux and reflex

   b. cervix and ureter   **e.** pneumonia and pneumothorax

   c. pulmonology and pneumonia

7. Which word element appears at the beginning of the term?

   a. root

   b. combining vowel

   c. combining form

   d. suffix

   e. prefix

S. **Case Report challenge:** *Now that you are more comfortable with the terms in this chapter, you can apply that knowledge and briefly answer the questions about the case report.*

CASE REPORT 1.1

YOU ARE

a respiratory therapist working with Tavis Senko, MD, a pulmonologist at Fulwood Medical Center.

YOU ARE COMMUNICATING WITH

Mrs. Sandra Schwartz, a 43-year-old woman referred to Dr. Senko by her primary care physician, an internist. She has a persistent abnormality on her chest x-ray. You have been asked to determine her pulmonary function prior to a scheduled bronchoscopy.

From her medical records, you see that 2 months ago Mrs. Schwartz developed a right upper lobe (RUL) pneumonia. After treatment with an antibiotic, a follow-up chest x-ray (CXR) showed some residual collapse in the right upper lobe and a small right pneumothorax. Mrs. Schwartz has smoked a pack a day for many years. Concerned that she has lung cancer, Dr. Senko has scheduled her for bronchoscopy.

1. What type of specialist is Dr. Senko? _____

2. What sign did Mrs. Schwartz have that meant she needed to see a specialist?

_____

3. What disease or condition is in Mrs. Schwartz's past medical history?

_____

4. Give a brief definition of the condition in question 3 above: _____

5. What diagnostic test did Mrs. Schwartz have done? _____

6. What part of Mrs. Schwartz's lung shows residual collapse? _____

7. What procedure has Dr. Senko scheduled for Mrs. Schwartz? _____

8. Based on her past medical history, history of smoking, and current diagnostic findings, what is a probable diagnosis for

   Mrs. Schwartz? _____

Congratulations! You are on your way to learning medical terminology.

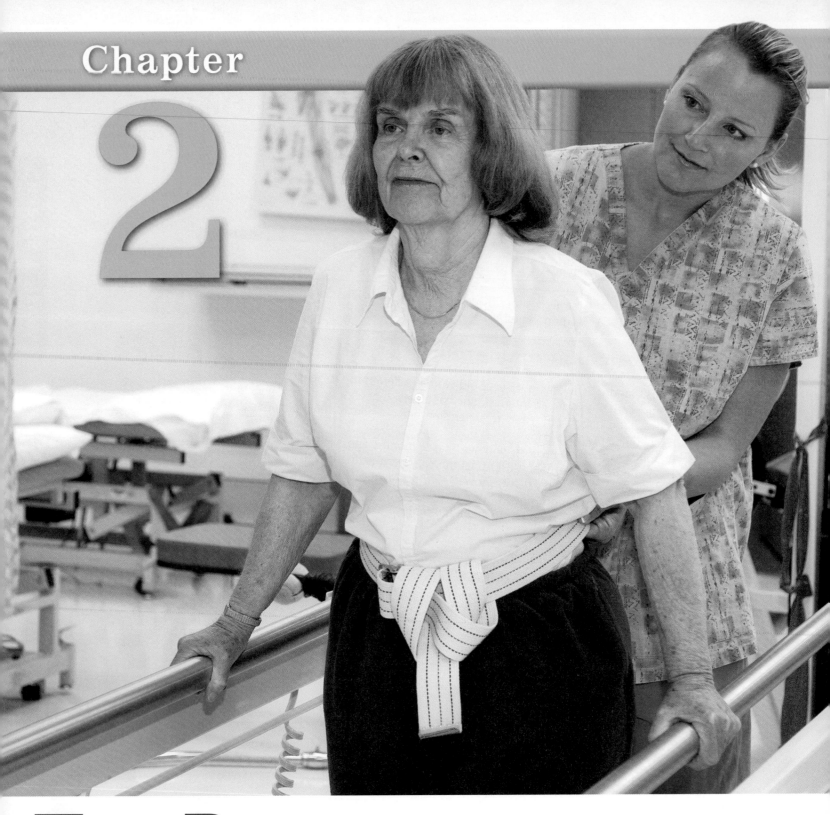

THE BODY AS A WHOLE

The Essentials of the Language of Anatomy

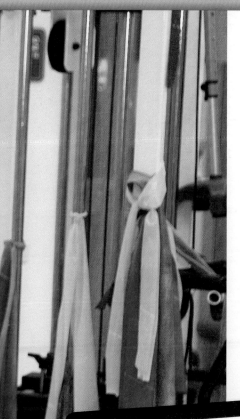

LEARNING OUTCOMES

Effective medical treatment recognizes that each organ, tissue, and cell in your body, no matter where it's located, is connected to and functions in harmony with every other organ, tissue, and cell. To understand these concepts, you need to be able to:

LO 2.1   Describe the medical terms of the different anatomical planes, directions, and body regions.

LO 2.2   Integrate individual body systems into the organization and function of the body as a whole.

LO 2.3   Comprehend, spell, and write medical terms pertaining to the body as a whole so that you communicate and document these terms accurately and precisely.

LO 2.4   Recognize and pronounce medical terms pertaining to the body as a whole so that you communicate verbally with accuracy and precision.

CASE REPORT 2.1

YOU ARE

. . . a physical therapy assistant (PTA) employed in the Rehabilitation Unit at Fulwood Medical Center.

YOU ARE COMMUNICATING WITH

. . . Mrs. Amy Vargas, a 70-year-old housewife, who is 2 weeks postop following an emergency right hip replacement for a hip fracture. Your task is to help Mrs. Vargas increase her walking ability and improve the strength and mobility in her hip joint and upper arms.

You know that in order to prevent her hip replacement from dislocating, she has been instructed to avoid:

- Bringing the right leg or knee **medially** across the **sagittal** plane, meaning not to cross the right leg over the left leg.
- Lifting the right knee so that it is superior to the right hip.
- Bending the trunk anteriorly beyond a 90-degree angle in relation to the thigh.

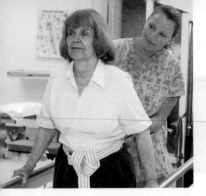

LESSON 2.1

Anatomical Positions, Planes, and Directions

OBJECTIVES

Medical terms have been developed over the past several thousand years to help you describe clearly the location of different anatomical structures and lesions and their relation to each other in the human body. To do this, you need to be able to:

2.1.1 Define the fundamental anatomical position on which all descriptions of anatomical locations are based.

2.1.2 Describe the medical terminology of the different anatomical planes and directions.

2.1.3 Relate these terms to physical sites on the body.

2.1.4 Locate the body cavities.

2.1.5 Identify the medical terminology of the four abdominal quadrants and the nine main regions.

KEYNOTE

• The transverse plane is the only horizontal body plane.

Fundamental Anatomical Position

(LO 2.1, 2.2, 2.3, and 2.4)

When all anatomical descriptions are used, it's assumed that the body is in the "anatomical position" *(Figure 2.1)*. Here is how this position looks if you're standing in front of a full-length mirror: your body is standing erect, your feet are flat on the floor, your face and eyes are facing forward, and your arms are at your sides with your palms facing forward.

When you lie down flat on your back with your palms upward, you are **supine.** When you lie down flat on your belly with your palms facing the floor, you are **prone.**

Anatomical Directional Terms

(LO 2.1, 2.2, 2.3, and 2.4)

Directional terms describe the position of one body structure or part relative to another body structure or part. These directional terms are shown in *Figures 2.1* and *2.2*.

Anatomical Planes (LO 2.1, 2.2, 2.3, and 2.4)

Different views of your body are based on imaginary "slices," which produce flat surfaces called **planes** that pass through your body *(Figure 2.3)*. The **three major anatomical planes** are the following:

▼ **FIGURE 2.1**
Anatomical Position, with Directional Terms.

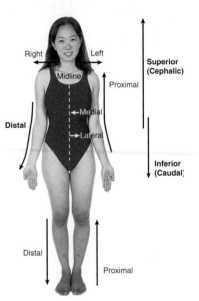

▼ **FIGURE 2.2**
Other Directional Terms.

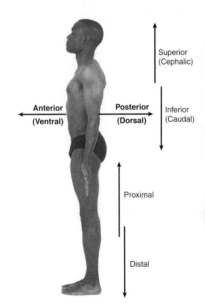

▼ **FIGURE 2.3**
Anatomical Planes.

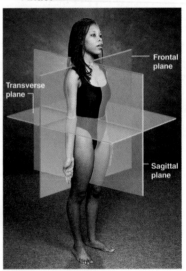

• **Transverse or horizontal:** a plane passing across the body parallel to the floor and perpendicular to the body's long axis. It divides the body into an upper/superior portion and a lower/inferior portion.

• **Sagittal:** a vertical plane that divides the body into right and left portions.

• **Frontal (coronal):** a vertical plane that divides the body into front (**anterior**) and back (**posterior**) portions.

ABBREVIATIONS

PTA   physical therapy assistant

Word	Pronunciation	Elements		Definition
abdomen abdominal (adj)	**AB**-doh-men ab-**DOM**-in-al	 S/ R/	Latin *abdomen* -al *pertaining to* abdomin- *abdomen*	Part of the trunk between thorax and pelvis Pertaining to the abdomen
anatomy anatomical (adj)	ah-**NAT**-oh-mee an-ah-**TOM**-ik-al	S/ R/ S/	-tomy *process of separating* ana- *apart from* -ical *pertaining to*	Study of the structures of the human body Pertaining to anatomy
anterior *(opposite of posterior)*	an-**TEER**-ee-or	S/ R/	-ior *pertaining to* anter- *before, front part*	The front surface of the body; situated in front
caudal *(opposite of cephalic, same as inferior)*	**KAW**-dal	S/ R/	-al *pertaining to* caud- *tail*	Portaining to or nearer to the tailbone
cephalic *(opposite of caudal, same as superior)*	seh-**FAL**-ik	S/ R/	-ic *pertaining to* cephal- *head*	Pertaining to or nearer to the head
coronal *(same as frontal)*	**KOR**-oh-nal	S/ R/	-al *pertaining to* coron- *crown*	Pertaining to the vertical plane dividing the body into anterior and posterior portions
distal *(opposite of proximal)*	**DISS**-tal	S/ R/	-al *pertaining to* dist- *away from the center*	Situated away from the center of the body
dorsal *(same as posterior)*	**DOOR**-sal	S/ R/	-al *pertaining to* dors- *back*	Pertaining to the back or situated behind
lateral *(opposite of medial)*	**LAT**-er-al	S/ R/	-al *pertaining to* later- *side*	Situated at the side of a structure
medial *(opposite of lateral)*	**ME**-dee-al	S/ R/	-al *pertaining to* medi- *middle*	Nearer to the middle of the body
posterior *(opposite of anterior)*	pohs-**TEER**-ee-or	S/ R/	-ior *pertaining to* poster- *back part*	Pertaining to the back surface of the body; situated behind
prone *(opposite of supine)*	**PROHN**		Latin *bending forward*	Lying face down, flat on your belly
proximal *(opposite of distal)*	**PROK**-sih-mal	S/ R/	-al *pertaining to* proxim- *nearest to the center*	Situated nearest to the center of the body
sagittal	**SAJ**-ih-tal	S/ R/	-al *pertaining to* sagitt- *arrow*	Vertical plane through the body dividing it into right and left portions
supine *(opposite of prone)*	soo-**PINE**		Latin *lying on the back*	Lying face up, flat on your spine
transverse	trans-**VERS**		Latin *crosswise*	Horizontal plane dividing the body into upper and lower portions
ventral *(same as anterior)*	**VEN**-tral	S/ R/	-al *pertaining to* ventr- *belly*	Pertaining to the belly or situated nearer the surface of the belly

EXERCISES

A. Review *the Case Report on the chapter opening spread before answering the questions.*

1. What emergency surgery was necessary for Mrs. Vargas? _____

2. Why is Mrs. Vargas in the rehabilitation unit following her surgery?

_____

3. What two specific tasks does Mrs. Vargas' treatment plan focus on?

_____ and _____

4. Name one thing Mrs. Vargas has been instructed to avoid: _____

5. What does a PTA assist with? _____

STUDY HINT

Help your memory with little tricks of association for medical terms. Example: The medical term *supine* has the word up in it. The meaning of *supine* is lying with the face and the anterior part of the body UP. Associate UP with sUPine, and you will have no trouble remembering its definition. Then associate the opposite term, and you will know the meaning of *prone* as well.

B. Some of the terms *in the WADs are opposites, and some are synonyms. Identify the following pairs of terms as either opposites or synonyms.*

1. anterior/posterior _____

4. coronal/frontal _____

2. ventral/anterior _____

5. cephalic/caudal _____

3. prone/supine _____

6. cephalic/superior _____

LESSON 2.1 Abdominal Quadrants

(LO 2.1, 2.2, 2.3, and 2.4)

To simplify your job of locating and identifying abdominal structures and sites of abdominal pain and other abnormalities, you can mentally divide the abdomen into **quadrants,** as shown in *Figure 2.5a.* This approach allows you to separate these locations into manageable parts. So, here you have the right upper quadrant **(RUQ),** left upper quadrant **(LUQ),** right lower quadrant **(RLQ),** and left lower quadrant **(LLQ).**

In addition, there are three main regions of your abdomen—the epigastric, umbilical, and hypogastric regions, as shown in *Figure 2.5b.*

Body Cavities

(LO 2.1, 2.2, 2.3, and 2.4)

Your body contains many **cavities** or hollow spaces. Some, like the nasal cavity, open to the outside of your body. Five cavities that do not open to the outside are shown in *Figure 2.4* and listed below.

1. The **cranial cavity** contains the brain within the skull.
2. The **thoracic cavity** contains the heart, lungs, thymus gland, trachea and esophagus, and numerous blood vessels and nerves.
3. The **abdominal cavity,** separated from the thoracic cavity by the **diaphragm,** contains the stomach, intestines, liver, spleen, pancreas, and kidneys. There are nine regions in the abdomen, as shown in *Figure 2.5b.*
4. The **pelvic cavity,** surrounded by the pelvic bones, contains the urinary bladder, part of the large intestine, the rectum and anus, and the internal reproductive organs.
5. The **spinal cavity** contains the spinal cord.

The abdominal cavity and pelvic cavity can be combined as the **abdominopelvic cavity.**

▶ **FIGURE 2.4**
Major Body Cavities.

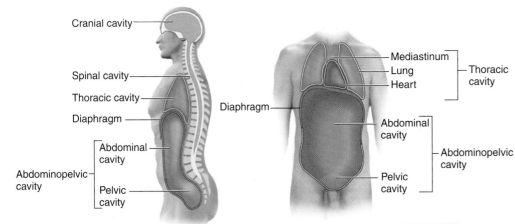

▶ **FIGURE 2.5**
Regional Anatomy.

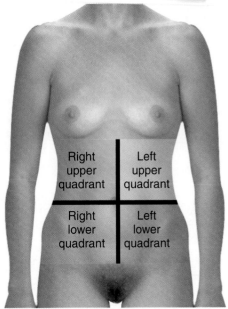

(a) Abdominal quadrants

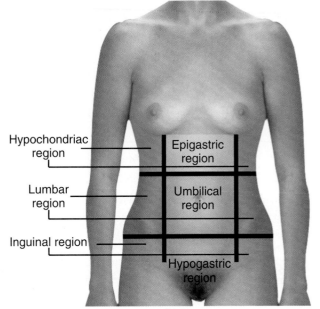

(b) Abdominal regions

Word	Pronunciation		Elements	Definition
abdominopelvic	ab-**DOM**-ih-no-PEL-vik	S/ R/CF R/	-ic *pertaining to* abdomin/o- *abdomen* -pelv- *pelvis*	Pertaining to the abdomen and pelvis
cavity cavities (pl)	KAV-ih-tee KAV-ih-tees	S/ R/	-ity *state, condition* cav- *hollow space*	A hollow space or body compartment
cranial (adj) cranium	KRAY-nee-al KRAY-nee-um	S/ R/ S/	-al *pertaining to* crani- *skull* -um *structure*	Pertaining to the cranium The skull
diaphragm diaphragmatic (adj)	DIE-ah-fram DIE-ah-frag-**MAT**-ik	 S/ R/	Greek *diaphragm, fence* -ic *pertaining to* diaphragmat- *diaphragm*	Muscular sheet separating the abdominal and thoracic cavities Pertaining to the diaphragm
quadrant	KWAD-rant		Latin *one quarter*	One quarter of a circle; one of four regions of the surface of the abdomen
spine spinal (adj)	SPYN SPY-nal	 S/ R/	Latin *spine* -al *pertaining to* spin- *spine*	The vertebral column or a short bony projection Pertaining to the spine
thoracic (adj) thorax	THOR-ass-ik THOR-acks	S/ R/	-ic *pertaining to* thorac- *chest* Greek *chest*	Pertaining to the chest (thorax) The part of the trunk between the abdomen and neck
umbilical (adj) umbilicus	um-**BILL**-ih-kal um-**BILL**-ih-kuss	S/ R/ R/	-al *pertaining to* umbilic- *navel (belly button)* umbilicus *navel (belly button)*	Pertaining to the umbilicus or the center of the abdomen Pit in the abdomen where the umbilical cord entered the fetus

EXERCISES

A. Deconstruct the following terms *into their basic elements. Note that not every type of element will appear in every term. The only element every term needs is a root or a combining form. Fill in the blanks.*

1. diaphragmatic _____/_____/_____
                P   R/CF   S

2. abdominopelvic _____/_____/_____
                P   R/CF   S

3. umbilical _____/_____/_____
                P   R/CF   S

4. cranial _____/_____/_____
                P   R/CF   S

5. thoracic _____/_____/_____
                P   R/CF   S

6. cavity _____/_____/_____
                P   R/CF   S

B. Analyze the elements *in the terms in Exercise A to get the correct answers.*

1. Which term contains a root and a combining vowel? _____

2. Which term is a muscle that separates body cavities? _____

3. The term "quadrant" represents what number? _____

4. The term "spine" also means _____.

5. What term in the WAD is a dentist likely to use? _____

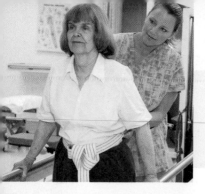

LESSON 2.2

Organization of the Body

Composition of the Body
(LO 2.1, 2.2, 2.3, and 2.4)

* The whole body or organism is composed of **organ systems.**
  * Organ systems are composed of **organs.**
    * Organs are composed of **tissues.**
      * Tissues are composed of **cells.**
        * Cells are composed in part of **organelles.**
          * Organelles are composed of **molecules.**
            * Molecules are composed of **atoms.**

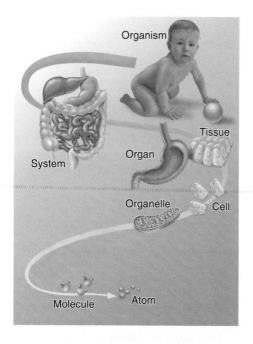

The Cell (LO 2.1, 2.2, 2.3, and 2.4)

The result of the **fertilization** of an egg by a sperm is a single fertilized cell called a **zygote** *(Figure 2.6).* This process is also called **conception.** This zygote is the origin of every cell in your body. It divides and multiplies into trillions of cells which become the basic unit of every tissue and organ. These cells are responsible for the structure and all the functions of your tissues and organs. **Cytology** is the study of cell structure and function.

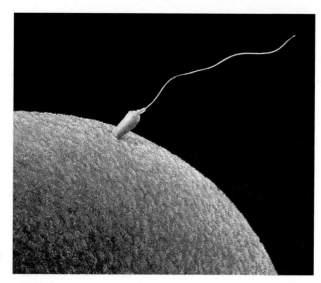

▶ **FIGURE 2.6**
Fertilization of Egg by Single Sperm.

S = Suffix   P = Prefix   R = Root   R/CF= Combining Form

Word	Pronunciation		Elements	Definition
cell	**SELL**		Latin a *storeroom*	The smallest unit of the body capable of independent existence
conception	kon-**SEP**-shun		Latin *something received*	Fertilization of the egg by sperm to form a zygote
cytology	**SIGH**-tol-oh-jee	S/ R/CF	-logy *study of* cyt/o- *cell*	Study of the cell
cytologist	**SIGH**-tol-oh-jist	S/	-logist *one who studies, a specialist*	Specialist in the structure, chemistry, and pathology of the cell
fertilization (noun)	**FER**-til-eye-**ZAY**-shun	S/ R/	-ation *process* fertiliz- *to make fruitful*	Union of a male sperm and a female egg
fertilize (verb)	**FER**-til-ize		Greek *to bear*	Penetration of the egg by sperm
organ	**OR**-gan		Latin *instrument, tool*	Structure with specific functions in a body system
organelle	**OR**-gah-nell	S/ R/	-elle *small* organ- *organ*	Part of a cell having specialized function(s).
organism	**OR**-gan-izm	S/	-ism *condition, process*	Any whole living, individual plant or animal
tissue	**TISH**-you		Latin *to weave*	Collection of similar cells
zygote	**ZYE**-goat		Greek *yolk*	Cell resulting from the union of sperm and egg

EXERCISES

A. Review *the terms in the WAD box above and the text on the opposite page before answering the questions. Pay careful attention to word elements and meanings. Fill in the blanks.*

1. Put the following terms in the ascending order of their size:

organism	cells	molecules	organs
organ systems	organelles	atoms	tissues

a. _____

b. _____

c. _____

d. _____

e. _____

f. _____

g. _____

h. _____

B. Review the WAD *before answering the questions.*

1. The suffix _____ means *study of*. The suffix that means *specialist (in the study of)* is _____ .

2. What part of *cyt/o* makes it a combining form rather than a root? _____

3. What is the medical term for *union of a male sperm and a female egg?* _____

4. What suffix in the WAD describes the size of something? _____

5. What does a cytologist study? _____

LESSON 2.2 Structure and Function of Cells (LO 2.1, 2.2, 2.3, and 2.4)

As the zygote divides, every cell it creates becomes a complex little factory that carries out these basic life functions:

• **Manufacture** of **proteins** and **lipids;**

• **Production** and use of energy;

• **Communication** with other cells;

• **Replication** of **deoxyribonucleic acid (DNA);** and

• **Reproduction** of itself.

All your cells contain a fluid called **cytoplasm** (intracellular fluid) surrounded by a cell **membrane** *(Figure 2.7).* Your cell membrane—made of **proteins** and **lipids**—allows water, oxygen, glucose, **electrolytes, steroids,** and alcohol to pass through it. On the outside of the cell membrane, you have receptors that bind to chemical messengers like **hormones** sent by other cells. These are the chemical signals by which your cells communicate with each other.

Organelles are small structures in the cytoplasm of the cell that carry out special **metabolic** tasks (the chemical processes that occur in the cell). These organelles and their respective jobs include the following:

Organelles (LO 2.1, 2.2, 2.3, and 2.4)

The **nucleus** is the largest organelle *(Figure 2.7).* It is surrounded by its own membrane and directs all the cell's activities. The 46 molecules of DNA in the nucleus form 46 **chromosomes.**

A **nucleolus** is a small, dense body composed of **ribonucleic acid (RNA)** and protein found in the nucleus. It is involved in the manufacture of proteins from simple materials—a process called **anabolism.**

Mitochondria are the cell's powerhouses. They produce energy by breaking down compounds like glucose and fat in a process called **catabolism.**

• **Metabolism** is the sum of the constructive processes of anabolism and the destructive processes of catabolism within a cell **(intracellular).**

ABBREVIATIONS

DNA deoxyribonucleic acid
RNA ribonucleic acid

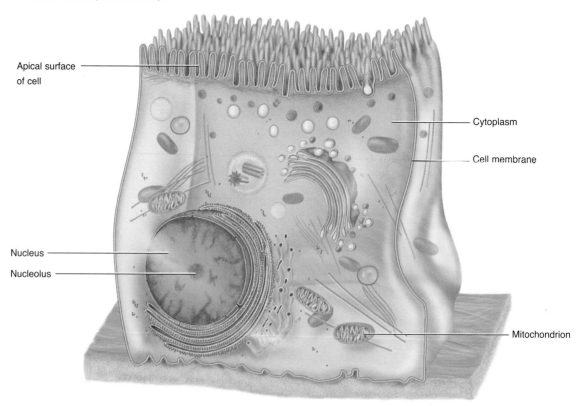

Apical surface of cell

Cytoplasm

Cell membrane

Nucleus

Nucleolus

Mitochondrion

▲ **FIGURE 2.7**
Structure of a Representative Cell.

Word	Pronunciation	Elements		Definition
anabolism	an-**AB**-oh-lizm	S/ R/	-ism *process, condition* anabol- *build up*	The buildup of complex substances in the cell from simpler ones as a part of metabolism
catabolism	kah-**TAB**-oh-lizm	S/ R/	-ism *process, condition* catabol- *break down*	The breakdown of complex substances into simpler ones as a part of metabolism
chromosome	**KROH**-moh-sohm	S/ R/CF	-some *body* chrom/o- *color*	Body in the nucleus that contains DNA and genes
cytoplasm	**SIGH**-toh-plazm	S/ R/CF	-plasm *something formed* cyt/o- *cell*	Clear, gelatinous substance that forms the substance of a cell, except for the nucleus
deoxyribonucleic acid (DNA)	dee-**OCK**-see-rye-boh-noo-**KLEE**-ik **ASS**-id		deoxyribose *a sugar* nucleic acid *a protein*	Source of hereditary characteristics found in chromosomes
electrolyte	ee-**LEK**-troh-lite	S/ R/CF	-lyte *soluble* electr/o- *electricity*	Substance that, when dissolved in a suitable medium, forms electrically charged particles
hormone	**HOR**-mohn		Greek *set in motion*	Chemical formed in one tissue or organ and carried by the blood to stimulate or inhibit a function of another tissue or organ
hormonal (adj)	hor-**MOHN**-al	S/ R/	-al *pertaining to* hormon- *hormone*	Pertaining to a hormone
intracellular	in-trah-**SELL**-you-lar	S/ P/ R/	-ar *pertaining to* intra- *within* -cellul- *small cell*	Within the cell
lipid	**LIP**-id		Greek *fat*	General term for all types of fatty compounds; for example, cholesterol, triglycerides and fatty acids
membrane	**MEM**-brain		Latin *parchment*	Thin layer of tissue covering a structure or cavity
membranous (adj)	**MEM**-brah-nus	S/ R/	-ous *pertaining to* membran- *cover, skin*	Pertaining to a membrane
metabolism	meh-**TAB**-oh-lizm	S/ R/	-ism *condition, process* metabol- *change*	The constantly changing physical and chemical processes occurring in the cell that are the sum of anabolism and catabolism
metabolic (adj)	met-ah-**BOL**-ik	S/	-ic *pertaining to*	Pertaining to metabolism
mitochondria (pl)	my-toe-**KON**-dree-ah	S/ R/CF R/	-ia *condition* mit/o- *thread* -chondr- *granule*	Organelles that generate, store, and release energy for cell activities
mitochondrion (singular)	my-toe-**KON**-dree-on	S/	-ion *condition*	
nucleolus	nyu-**KLEE**-oh-lus	S/ R/CF	-lus *small* nucle/o- *nucleus*	Small mass within the nucleus
nucleus	**NYU**-klee-us	R/	Latin *command center* nucle- *nucleus*	Functional center of a cell or structure
nuclear (adj)	**NYU**-klee-ar	S/	-ar *pertaining to*	Pertaining to a nucleus
protein	**PRO**-teen		Greek *protein*	Class of food substances based on amino acids
ribonucleic acid (RNA)	**RYE**-boh-nyu-**KLEE**-ik **ASS**-id	S/ P/ R/	-ic *pertaining to* ribo- *from ribose, a sugar* -nucle- *nucleus*	The information carrier from DNA in the nucleus to an organelle to produce protein molecules
steroid	**STER**-oyd	S/ R/	-oid *resembling* ster- *solid*	Large family of chemical substances found in many drugs, hormones, and body components

EXERCISE

A. Elements: *Knowledge of elements is your best clue to determining the meaning of medical terminology. Analyze the elements in these questions to find your answers. Review the WAD before attempting to answer the questions. Circle the BEST ANSWER to the question.*

1. Which term relates to electrically charged particles?

   protein   hormonal   electrolyte

2. Which term relates to change?

   steroid   metabolic   lipid

3. Which term is a condition?

   metabolism   cytoplasm   hormone

4. What is a thin layer of tissue that covers a structure or cavity?

   lipid   membrane   hormone

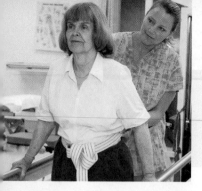

LESSON 2.3

Tissues, Organs, and Organ Systems

OBJECTIVES

Your tissues, organs, and organ systems must continually adapt and adjust in order to work in sync with each other. The information in this lesson will enable you to:

2.3.1 Define the four primary tissue groups.

2.3.2 Discuss the medical terminology for the structure and functions of each tissue group.

2.3.3 Name the organ systems.

2.3.4 Describe the medical terminology for the functions of each organ system.

Tissues (LO 2.1, 2.2, 2.3, and 2.4)

Tissues hold your body together. Each tissue is different but made of similar cells with unique materials around them manufactured by the cells. The many tissues of your body have different structures that enable them to perform specialized functions.

Histology is the study of the structure and function of tissues. The four primary tissue groups are outlined in *Table 2.1.*

CASE REPORT 2.2

YOU ARE

. . . a physical therapy assistant employed in the Rehabilitation Unit in Fulwood Medical Center.

YOU ARE COMMUNICATING WITH

. . . Mr. Richard Josen, a 22-year-old man who injured tissues in his left knee while playing football *(Figure 2.8)*. Using **arthroscopy,** the orthopedic surgeon removed his torn **anterior cruciate ligament (ACL)** and replaced it with a graft from his patellar tendon. The torn medial collateral ligament was sutured together. The tear in his medial **meniscus** was repaired. Rehabilitation is focused on strengthening the **muscles** around his knee joint and regaining joint mobility and stability.

▼ **TABLE 2.1**
THE FOUR PRIMARY TISSUE GROUPS

Type	Function	Location
Connective	Bind, support, protect, fill spaces, store fat	Widely distributed throughout the body, e.g., in blood, bone cartilage, and fat
Epithelial	Protect, secrete, absorb, excrete	Cover body surface, cover and line internal organs, compose glands
Muscle	Movement	Attached to bones; found in the walls of hollow tubes, organs, and the heart
Nervous	Transmit impulses for coordination, sensory reception, motor actions	Brain, spinal cord, nerves

Adapted from Shier, Butler, and Lewis, *Hole's Human Anatomy and Physiology*, 10th ed. Copyright © 2004 The McGraw-Hill Companies, Inc. Adapted with permission.

▶ **FIGURE 2.8**
Knee Anatomy.
(a) Injury to left knee.
(b) Normal knee.

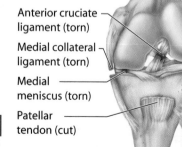

Anterior cruciate ligament (torn)

Medial collateral ligament (torn)

Medial meniscus (torn)

Patellar tendon (cut)

(a)

Femur

Cartilage

Tibia

Quadriceps muscle

Patella

Synovial fluid

Synovial membrane

Patellar tendon

(b)

Word	Pronunciation	Elements		Definition
arthroscopy	ar-**THROS**-koh-pee	S/ R/CF	-scopy *to examine, to view* arthr/o- *joint*	Visual examination of the interior of a joint
connective tissue	koh-**NECK**-tiv **TISH**-you	S/ R/	-ive *pertaining to* connect- *join together* tissue Latin *to weave*	The supporting tissue of the body
cruciate	**KRU**-she-ate		Latin *cross*	Shaped like a cross
graft	**GRAFT**		French *transplant*	Transplantation of living tissue
histology	his-**TOL**-oh-jee	S/ R/CF	-logy *study of* hist/o- *tissue*	Study of the structure and function of cells, tissues, and organs
histologist	his-**TOL**-oh-jist	S/	-logist *one who studies, specialist*	Specialist in histology
ligament	**LIG**-ah-ment		Latin *band*	Band of fibrous tissue connecting two structures
meniscus	meh-**NISS**-kuss		Greek *crescent*	Disc of cartilage between the bones of a joint
muscle	**MUSS**-el		Latin *muscle*	A tissue consisting of contractile cells
patella (singular) patellae (pl)	pah-**TELL**-ah pah-**TELL**-ee		Latin *small plate*	Thin, circular bone embedded in the patellar tendon in front of the knee joint; also called the kneecap
patellar (adj)	pah-**TELL**-ar	S/ R/	-ar *pertaining to* patell- *patella*	Pertaining to the patella
therapy	**THAIR**-ah-pee	 S/	Greek *medical treatment* -ic *pertaining to*	Systematic treatment of a disease, dysfunction, or disorder
therapeutic	**THAIR**-ah-**PYU**-tik	R/ S/	therapeut- *treatment* -ist *specialist*	Relating to the treatment of a disease or disorder
therapist	**THAIR**-ah-pist	R/	therap- *treatment*	Professional trained in the practice of a particular therapy

EXERCISES

A. Review *the Case Report on this two-page spread before answering the questions.*

1. How was Mr. Josen injured? _____

2. What type of procedure is an arthroscopy? _____

3. Where is the patellar tendon located? _____

4. What two specific knee components were repaired? _____

5. What other component could not be repaired and required replacement? _____

B. Dictionary exercise: *When you are working in the medical field, you will be exposed to medical terms you may not recognize. Learn to use the glossary or a good medical dictionary, or practice going online to find the definitions you need. The Case Report on the opposite page contains some terms that are not defined in the WAD above.*

Use the glossary or a dictionary (or go online) to define each of the following terms and identify it as noun, verb, or adjective.

1. orthopedic   (noun, verb, adjective) _____

   Definition: _____

2. collateral   (noun, verb, adjective) _____

   Definition: _____

3. sutured   (noun, verb, adjective) _____

   Definition: _____

Connective Tissues

(LO 2.1, 2.2, 2.3, and 2.4)

The relation of structure to function in your body tissues is key. To help you understand this important connection, this lesson uses the knee joint to illustrate the structures and functions of the different tissues found in this joint.

Connective Tissues in the Knee Joint (LO 2.1, 2.2, 2.3, and 2.4)

The connective tissues in your knee joint make it possible for you to enjoy your daily life—from standing, sitting, walking, bending, and running. These tissues and their roles are listed below:

- The **bones** of the knee joint are the **femur, tibia,** and **patella** *(see Chapter 4).* Bone is the hardest connective tissue in your body because it contains calcium mineral salts (mainly calcium phosphate). Bones have a good blood supply so they can heal well after a fracture. Bones in general are covered with a thick fibrous tissue called the **periosteum.**

- **Cartilage** has a flexible, rubbery **matrix** (in the knee as a **meniscus**) that allows it to function as a shock absorber and a gliding surface where two bones meet to form a joint. Cartilage has very few blood vessels and heals poorly—sometimes not at all. When it is injured or torn, surgery is often needed. Cartilage also forms the shape of your ear, the tip of your nose, and your larynx.

- **Ligaments** are strips or bands of fibrous connective tissue made of **collagen** fibers. The

knee joint has a complex array of 11 ligaments that hold it together. The blood supply to these ligaments is poor, so they do not heal well without surgery *(Figure 2.9).*

- **Tendons** are thick, strong ligaments that attach muscles to bone.

- The **joint capsule** of the knee joint encloses the joint cavity. It's made of thin, fibrous connective tissue and strengthened by fibers that extend over it from the surrounding ligaments and muscles. These features are common to most joints.

- The **synovial membrane** lines many joint capsules and secretes **synovial fluid**—a slippery lubricant stored in the joint cavity. This fluid makes joint movement almost friction-free. It distributes **nutrients** to the cartilage on the joint surfaces of bone.

- **Muscle tissue** stabilizes the joint. Extensions of the large muscle tendons in the front and the rear of the thigh are major stabilizers of the knee joint. The muscles alone extend and flex the knee joint *(see Chapter 4).*

- **Nervous tissue** carries messages between the brain and the knee structures. All the knee structures are packed with nerves, which is why a knee injury is excruciatingly painful.

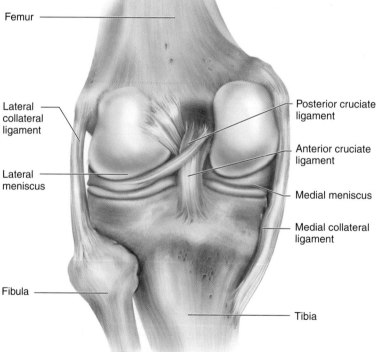

Femur

Lateral collateral ligament

Lateral meniscus

Fibula

Posterior cruciate ligament

Anterior cruciate ligament

Medial meniscus

Medial collateral ligament

Tibia

Anterior view

▶ **FIGURE 2.9**
Ligaments of Knee Joint, with the Patellar Tendon Removed.

Word	Pronunciation		Elements	Definition
capsule	**KAP**-syul		Latin *little box*	Fibrous tissue layer surrounding a joint or other structure
capsular (adj)	**KAP**-syu-lar	S/ R/	-ar *pertaining to* capsul- *box*	Pertaining to a capsule
cartilage	**KAR**-tih-lage		Latin *gristle*	Nonvascular, firm connective tissue found mostly in joints
collagen	**KOLL**-ah-jen	S/ R/CF	-gen *produce, form* coll/a- *glue*	Major protein of connective tissue, cartilage, and bone
matrix	**MAY**-triks		Latin mater *mother*	Substance that surrounds and protects cells, is manufactured by the cells, and holds them together
nutrient	**NYU**-tree-ent	S/ R/	-ent *end result* nutri- *nourish*	A substance in food required for normal physiologic function
periosteum	**PER**-ee-**OSS**-tee-um	S/ P/ R/	-um *tissue* peri- *around* -oste- *bone*	Fibrous membrane covering a bone
synovial	si-**NOH**-vee-al	S/ P/ R/CF	-al *pertaining to* syn- *together* -ov/i- *egg*	Pertaining to the synovial membrane or fluid
tendon	**TEN**-dun		Latin *sinew*	Fibrous band that connects muscle to bone

EXERCISES

A. Construct *the medical term given by the definition.*

1. Fibrous membrane covering a bone: _____/_____/_____
   P R/CF S

2. Major protein of connective tissue: _____/_____/_____
   P R/CF S

3. Pertaining to the synovial membrane _____/_____/_____
   P R/CF S

4. Substance in food _____/_____/_____
   P R/CF S

B. Construct *the medical term that correctly answers the question.*

1. What is the only term in the WAD that
   contains a prefix, root, and suffix? _____/_____/_____
   P R/CF S

2. Which term contains an element
   that means *glue*? _____/_____/_____
   P R/CF S

3. What is the only term in the WAD
   that contains a prefix, combining form, and suffix? _____/_____/_____
   P R/CF S

4. What is the term for nonvascular,
   firm connective tissue found mostly in joints? _____/_____/_____
   P R/CF S

5. What terms in this WAD do not deconstruct into elements? _____

LESSON **2.3** Organs and Organ Systems (LO 2.1, 2.2, 2.3, and 2.4)

An **organ** is a structure composed of several tissues that work together to carry out specific functions. For example, your skin is an organ that has different tissues in it, such as epithelial cells, hair, nails, and glands *(see Chapter 3).*

An **organ system** is a group of organs with a specific collective function, like digestion, circulation, or respiration. For example, your nose, pharynx, larynx, trachea, bronchi, and lungs all work together to achieve the total function of respiration *(see Chapter 8).*

The different organs in an organ system are usually interconnected. For example, in the **urinary** organ system *(Figure 2.10),* the organs are the kidneys, ureters, bladder, and urethra, and they are all connected *(see Chapter 13).*

All your organ systems work together to ensure that your body's internal environment remains relatively constant. This process is called **homeostasis.** It ensures that cells receive adequate nutrients and oxygen. It also ensures that cell waste products are removed so your cells can function normally. Disease affecting an organ or organ system disrupts the homeostasis game plan.

Your body has 11 organ systems, as shown in *Table 2.2.* Muscular and **skeletal** are considered one organ system called the musculoskeletal system *(see Chapters 4 and 5).* Each body system has a chapter in this book where the terms associated with it are defined.

▼ **TABLE 2.2**
ORGAN SYSTEMS

Organ System	Major Organs	Major Functions
Integumentary	Skin, hair, nails, sweat glands, sebaceous glands	Protect tissues, regulate body temperature, support sensory receptors
Skeletal	Bones, ligaments, cartilages	Provide framework, protect soft tissues, provide attachments for muscles, produce blood cells, store inorganic salts
Muscular	Muscles	Cause movements, maintain posture, produce body heat
Nervous	Brain, spinal cord, nerves, sense organs	Receive and interpret sensory information, and in response, stimulate muscles, glands, and other organ systems
Endocrine	Glands that secrete hormones: pituitary, thyroid, parathyroid, adrenal, pancreas, ovaries, testes, pineal, thymus	Control metabolic activities of organs
Cardiovascular	Heart, blood vessels	Move blood and transport substances throughout body
Lymphatic	Lymph vessels and nodes, thymus, spleen	Defend body against infection, return tissue fluid to blood, carry certain absorbed food molecules
Digestive	Mouth, tongue, teeth, salivary glands, pharynx, esophagus, stomach, liver, gallbladder, pancreas, small and large intestines	Receive, break down, and absorb food; eliminate unabsorbed material
Respiratory	Nasal cavity, pharynx, larynx, trachea, bronchi, lungs	Intake and output air, exchange gases between air and blood
Urinary	Kidneys, ureters, urinary bladder, and urethra	Remove wastes from blood, maintain water and electrolyte balance, store and transport urine
Reproductive	Male: scrotum, testes, epididymides, vasa deferentia, seminal vesicles, prostate, bulbourethral glands, urethra, penis	Produce and maintain sperm cells, transfer sperm cells into female reproductive tract
	Female: ovaries, fallopian tubes, uterus, vagina, vulva	Produce and maintain egg cells, receive sperm cells, support development of an embryo, function in birth process

Adapted from Shier, Butler, and Lewis, *Hole's Human Anatomy and Physiology, 10th ed.* Copyright © 2004 The McGraw-Hill Companies, Inc. Adapted with permission.

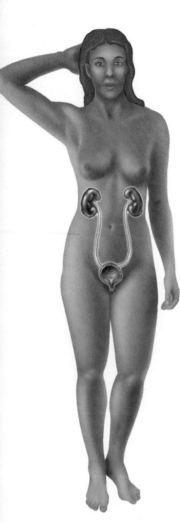

▲ **FIGURE 2.10**
The Urinary System.

Word	Pronunciation	Elements		Definition
cardiovascular	KAR-dee-oh-VAS-kyu-lar	S/ R/CF R/	-ar *pertaining to* cardi/o- *heart* -vascul- *blood vessel*	Pertaining to the heart and blood vessels
digestion	die-**JEST**-shun	S/ R/	-ion *action* digest- *break down food*	Breakdown of food into elements suitable for cell metabolism
digestive (adj)	die-**JEST**-iv	S/	-ive *pertaining to*	Pertaining to digestion
endocrine	**EN**-doh-krin	P/ R/	endo- *within* -crine *to secrete*	A gland that produces an internal or hormonal substance
homeostasis (Note: *Hemostasis is the arrest of bleeding.*)	hoh-mee-oh-**STAY**-sis	S/ R/CF	-stasis *standstill, control* home/o- *the same*	Maintaining the stability of a system or the body's internal environment
integument	in-**TEG**-you-ment		Latin *a covering*	Organ system that covers the body, the skin being the main organ within the system
integumentary (adj)	in-**TEG**-you-**MENT**-ah-ree	S/ R/	-ary *pertaining to* integument- *covering of the body*	Pertaining to the covering of the body
lymph	LIMF		Latin *clear spring water*	Clear fluid collected from body tissues and transported by lymph vessels to the venous circulation
lymphatic (adj)	lim-**FAT**-ic	S/ R/	-atic *pertaining to* lymph- *lymph, lymphatic system*	Pertaining to lymph or the lymphatic system
nervous	**NER**-vus	S/ R/	-ous *pertaining to* nerv- *nerve*	Pertaining to a nerve or the nervous system; or easily excited or agitated
nervous system	**NER**-vus **SIS**-tem		system Greek *an organized whole*	The whole, integrated nerve apparatus
respiration	**RES**-pih-**RAY**-shun	S/ R/	-ation *process* respir- *to breathe*	Process of breathing; fundamental process of life used to exchange oxygen and carbon dioxide
respiratory (adj)	**RES**-pih-rah-tor-ee	S/	-atory *pertaining to*	Pertaining to respiration
skeleton skeletal (adj)	**SKEL**-eh-ton **SKEL**-eh-tal	S/ R/	Greek *skeleton or mummy* -al *pertaining to* skelet- *skeleton*	The bony framework of the body Pertaining to the skeleton
urinary (adj)	**YUR**-in-ary	S/ R/	-ary *pertaining to* urin- *urine*	Pertaining to urine

EXERCISES

A. Build *the correct medical terms by working with the literal meanings of the elements in the WAD above. Write the correct elements on the line to complete the term.*

1. _____ /_____ /_____

                       lymph   pertaining to

2. _____ /_____ /_____

        heart and blood vessels   pertaining to

3. _____ /_____ /_____

            skeleton   pertaining to

4. _____ /_____ /_____

              skin   pertaining to

5. _____ /_____ /

           digestion   pertaining to

B. Continue *working with the medical terms in the above WAD.*

1. List all the terms in the WAD that refer to names of body systems: _____

2. What is the difference between the terms *homeostasis* and *hemostasis*? _____

3. What is the main organ in the integumentary system? _____

4. What is the bony framework of the body called? _____

5. What term refers to clear fluid? _____

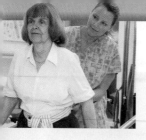

CHAPTER 2 REVIEW THE BODY AS A WHOLE

CHALLENGE YOUR KNOWLEDGE

A. Construct the following medical terminology, using the elements as your guide. *The word in capitals will be your clue to the missing element. Fill in the blanks.*

1. resembling a SOLID _____/_____ /oid

2. small ORGAN _____/_____ /elle

3. pertaining to CHANGE _____/_____/ic

4. process of BREAKING DOWN _____/_____ /ism

5. use of an instrument to examine a JOINT _____/_____/scopy

6. one who studies TISSUE _____/_____ /logist

7. tissue AROUND bone _____/_____ /oste/ um

8. standing THE SAME _____/_____ / stasis

9. pertaining to THE BACK _____/_____/al

10. pertaining to a NERVE _____/_____ /ous

B. Word attack exercise: *This exercise will help you develop a method of analyzing medical terminology questions to determine the correct answer. Work the exercise step-by-step.*

Question: *Which of the following terms means fibrous membrane covering a bone?*

a. collagen

b. synovial

c. integumentary

d. endocrine

e. periosteum

1. The question concerns a "fibrous membrane covering a bone." Do you recognize in any of the above words an element that matches an answer?

Write them here:

_____

2. Read the answer choices again, and cross off any that you know are not correct.

The incorrect ones are _____.

3. Of the remaining answer choices, look for one that contains any element that matches any of the words in the question.

(See answer 1 above.) _____.

4. The correct answer to this question is _____

because it contains the element(s) _____.

C. Spelling correctly is always important *and is the mark of an educated professional. Choose the correct spelling to complete the patient's documentation. Circle the best choice.*

1. This patient's (electrolite/electrolyte) balance should be checked once a day.

2. Mr. Josen has torn his anterior (cruxiate/cruciate) ligament and will require a surgical repair.

3. The medial (meniscus/menniscus) will be repaired at the same time.

4. The patient has worn away the (cartiledge/cartilage) in his kneecap.

5. This injectable drug should help replace the loss of (sinovial/synovial) fluid in the patient's knee.

6. Mr. Rose's (umbilical/umbellical) hernia surgery should be scheduled as soon as possible.

7. The patient's broken ribs have punctured his lung in his (thoracic/thorascic) cavity.

8. The doctor has ordered an x-ray of the patient's left (patella/patela).

9. Because she is bedridden, the patient's (integementary/integumentary) system is severely compromised.

10. Her (resperation/respiration) is shallow and labored.

D. Roots/combining forms *are the foundation of every medical term. List here the 10 roots/combining forms in this chapter that you have the most difficulty remembering. Be sure to include their meanings, and provide an example of each in a medical term.*

Root/Combining Form	Meaning of R/CF	Example of a Medical Term
1.	2.	3.
4.	5.	6.
7.	8.	9.
10.	11.	12.
13.	14.	15.
16.	17.	18.
19.	20.	21.
22.	23.	24.
25.	26.	27.
28.	29.	30.

E. Difference between: *If you know the meaning of the term, you can briefly explain it to someone else. Write your explanations below.*

1. organ _____

   _____

2. organelle _____

   _____

3. The difference in these two terms is the element _____,

   which means _____.

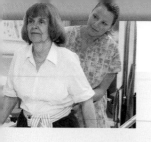

F. Partner exercise: *Ask your study partner to close his or her text. Dictate the following sentences to your partner, and then ask him or her to spell the sentences back to you. Check your partner's sentences against the text below. The sentence is not correct unless every word is present and everything is spelled correctly. When you have finished checking your partner's answers, close your book. Ask your partner to dictate the sentences to you. You should write them down, and then have your partner check them.*

1. In order to prevent her hip replacement from dislocating, she has been instructed to not bring the right leg or knee medially across the sagittal plane.

2. The transverse, or horizontal, plane divides the body into an upper or superior portion and a lower or inferior portion.

3. The abdominal cavity is separated from the thoracic cavity by the diaphragm and contains the stomach, intestines, liver, spleen, pancreas, and kidneys.

G. Layperson's language: *Translate the following sentences into language your patient can understand. Be brief, but be sure you are conveying the complete information. Rewrite the sentences on the lines below.*

1. The doctor has told the patient her knee joint lacks synovial fluid and this is the cause of her severe pain.

_____

_____

_____

_____

2. The orthopedic surgeon has recommended an arthroscopy to repair the torn ACL ligament and the torn medial meniscus.

_____

_____

_____

H. Brain teaser: *From the description given, can you determine what the medical term is?*

1. "The body is standing erect with feet flat on the floor, face and eyes are facing forward, and the arms are at the side with the palms facing forward."

Medical term: _____

2. "Opposite of *caudal,* same as *superior:*

Medical term: _____

3. "Contains the heart, lungs, thymus gland, trachea, esophagus, and numerous blood vessels and nerves."

Medical term: _____

I. Group the elements to make studying easier. *Fill in the chart below with the meaning of the given element, and list a medical term containing that element. Remember to answer the question at the end of the exercise.*

Element	Meaning of Element	Medical Term with This Element
al	1.	2.
ar	3.	4.
ation	5.	6.
elle	7.	8.
ia	9.	10.
ic	11.	12.
ior	13.	14.
ity	15.	16.
logist	17.	18.
logy	19.	20.
lus	21.	22.
oid	23.	24.
um	25.	26.

27. These elements are all _____ .

J. What am I? *A brief clue is given as to the identity of the term. Can you name them all? Fill in the blanks.*

1. largest organelle _____

2. part of the trunk between abdomen and neck _____

3. powerhouse of the cell _____

4. stable internal environment of the body _____

5. the skin _____

6. belly button (navel) _____

7. fertilized egg _____

8. smallest unit of the body capable of independent existence _____

9. clear fluid collected from body tissues _____

10. chemical messenger _____

K. Terminology challenge: *More than one element can have the same meaning. For example, there are many elements that all mean pertaining to. Find more pairs of elements in this chapter that both mean the same thing. Do not use any examples of pertaining to.*

1. _____ and _____ both mean _____

2. _____ and _____ both mean

3. _____ and _____ both mean _____

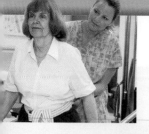

L. Recall and review: *There is a large volume of medical terminology to learn. This exercise reviews terms that appear in this chapter and the previous one. S-t-r-e-t-c-h your memory—try to answer the questions without turning back in your book. Your knowledge of roots and two different suffixes will help you fill in the blanks and the chart.*

Suffix for study of = _____

Suffix for specialist = _____

Base of Term	Medical Term for the *Study of* This Field	Medical Term for a *Specialist* in This Field
the lungs	1.	2.
the heart	3.	4.
the nervous system	5.	6.
cells	7.	8.
the urinary system	9.	10.
tissues	11.	12.

M. Latin and Greek terms *cannot be further deconstructed into prefix, root, or suffix. You must know them for what they are. Test your knowledge of these terms with this exercise. Match the meaning in column l with the correct medical term in column 2.*

Meaning

_____ **1.** union of egg and sperm

_____ **2.** sinew

_____ **3.** band

_____ **4.** separating muscle

_____ **5.** fat

_____ **6.** flat on your belly

_____ **7.** small plate

_____ **8.** parchment

_____ **9.** lying on the back

_____ **10.** middle

Medical Term

A. lipid

B. supine

C. patella

D. membrane

E. prone

F. zygote

G. tendon

II. medial

I. diaphragm

J. ligament

N. Identification *of elements, and knowledge of their meaning, will aid your understanding of the meaning of a term. Know your elements to increase your medical vocabulary! Fill in the chart.*

Element	Meaning of Element	Medical Term Example	Meaning of Medical Term
caud	1.	2.	3.
cephal	4.	5.	6.
colla	7.	8.	9.
electro	10.	11.	12.
endo	13.	14.	15.
metabol	16.	17.	18.
oste	19.	20.	21.
poster	22.	23.	24.
scopy	25.	26.	27.
vascul	28.	29.	30.

O. Build the correct medical term *using the appropriate combination of elements. There are more elements than you need. Some elements you may use twice. Fill in the blanks.*

caud	cav	homeo	cyto	ism	cyt	cellul
arthro	ity	stasis	logist	syn	lyte	endo
intra	ar	catabol	logy	anabol	al	proxim
scopy	histo	ovi	ic	hemo	cephal	ia

1. pertaining to, or near, the head _____ / _____ / _____
   P   R/CF   S

2. nearest to the center of the body _____ / _____ / _____
   P   R/CF   S

3. hollow space _____ / _____ / _____
   P   R/CF   S

4. study of the cell _____ / _____ / _____
   P   R/CF   S

5. within the cell _____ / _____ / _____
   P   R/CF   S

6. buildup process in metabolism _____ / _____ / _____
   P   R/CF   S

7. visual examination of a joint _____ / _____ / _____
   P   R/CF   S

8. one who studies tissue _____ / _____ / _____
   P   R/CF   S

9. fluid that lubricates a joint _____ / _____ / _____
   P   R/CF   S

10. maintaining body's internal environment _____ / _____ / _____
    P   R/CF   S

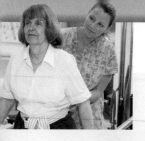

P. Precision in communication: *The terminology for positions, planes, and directions includes very important terms you will hear often in medical practice, and you need to use them precisely. Some of the following statements are incorrect; rewrite them correctly on the lines below.*

1. Inferior pertains to being situated above something.

2. Directional terms describe the position of one structure or part of the body relative to another structure or part of the body.

3. The heart is superior to the abdominopelvic cavity.

4. Saggital is a horizontal plane that divides the body into right and left portions.

5. Another name for a coronal plane is frontal plane.

6. Distal is opposite to dorsal.

7. Posterior is the opposite of cephalic.

8. When you lie flat on your back, you are prone.

9. Ventral is the same as posterior.

10. The transverse plane is the only one that is not vertical.

11. A flat surface that passes through the body is a plane.

Rewrite the incorrect statements: _____

_____

_____

_____

_____

_____

_____

_____

Q. Chapter challenge: *Circle the correct answer.*

1. Circle the pair of terms that relate to the knee joint:

   a. skeleton   lymphatic

   b. integumentary   ligament

   c. coronal   quadrant

   d. diaphragm   zygote

   e. cruciate   meniscus

2. The suffix *stasis* means:

   a. breaking down   d. something formed

   b. stand still, control   e. producing

   c. to secrete

3. Choose the term that has a root meaning *blood vessel*:

   a. integument   d. lymph

   b. cardiovascular   e. dorsal

   c. respiratory

4. **Brain teaser:** Which term functions as a "shock absorber"?

   a. ligament   d. meniscus

   b. membrane   e. muscle

   c. tendon

R. Chapter challenge: *Circle the correct answer.*

1. Which statement is most correct?

   a. Another name for cytoplasm is *intracellular fluid.*   **d.** The nucleus, nucleolus, and electrolytes are organelles.

   b. Organelles have no specific functions.   **e.** The cell membrane does not allow alcohol to pass through.

   c. The cell membrane is made of cartilage and lipids.

2. *Patella* is the correct medical term for:

   a. the thigh   **d.** the membrane covering a bone

   b. the muscle between two body cavities   **e.** the disc of connective tissue in the knee

   c. the kneecap

3. In the abbreviation *LLQ,* the first "L" stands for:

   a. lower   **d.** ligament

   b. left   **e.** lateral

   c. long

4. Circle the pair of correct opposites:

   a. superior and lateral   **d.** distal and inferior

   b. transverse and horizontal   **e.** cephalic and proximal

   c. coronal and frontal

5. The diaphragm separates:

   a. the pelvic cavity and the spinal cavity   **d.** the stomach and the intestines

   b. the lungs and the heart   **e.** the thoracic cavity and the abdominopelvic cavity

   c. the cranial cavity and the thoracic cavity

6. Choose the correct body system and the organ it contains:

   a. integumentary/patella

   b. endocrine/pineal

   c. urinary/pancreas

   d. digestive/uterus

   e. reproductive/urethra

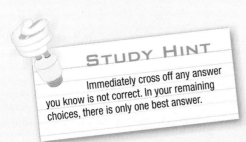

STUDY HINT

Immediately cross off any answer you know is not correct. In your remaining choices, there is only one best answer.

7. Circle the term with a combining form meaning *egg:*

   a. synovial   **d.** urinary

   b. metabolism   **e.** cranial

   c. homeostasis

8. Maintaining the body's internal environment is:

   a. hemostasis   **d.** homeostasis

   b. metabolism   **e.** catabolism

   c. anabolism

9. *Epigastric, hypogastric,* and *umbilical* describe:

   a. body planes   **d.** anatomical positions

   b. directional terms   **e.** body regions

   c. body cavities

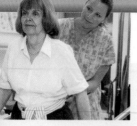

10. Which term is the opposite of *caudal* and the same as *superior:*

    a. anterior   **d.** distal

    b. cephalic   **e.** sagittal

    c. coronal

11. Circle the term that has a root that means *chest:*

    a. umbilicus   **d.** nucleolus

    b. cranial   **e.** collagen

    c. thoracic

12. What does a histologist specialize in studying?

    a. blood   **d.** heart

    b. cells   **e.** skin

    c. tissues

13. "A chemical formed in one tissue or organ and carried by the blood to stimulate or inhibit a function of another tissue or organ" is the definition of:

    a. lipid   **d.** hormone

    b. electrolyte   **e.** steroid

    c. protein

14. Which term has an element that means *color?*

    a. metabolism   **d.** collagen

    b. chromosome   **e.** endocrine

    c. intracellular

15. Which of the following is the only horizontal plane?

    a. posterior   **d.** transverse

    b. anterior   **e.** coronal

    c. superior

16. Find the only pair of incorrectly spelled medical terms:

    a. mitochondria   organelle

    b. membraneous   chromosone

    c. muscle   cruciate

    d. patellar   cartilage

    e. synovial   cytology

S. Case Report challenge: *Now that you are more comfortable with the terms in this chapter, you can apply that knowledge and briefly answer the questions about the case report **in your own words**. If you read the report through once and then go back and underline all the medical terminology, this will make it easier to answer the questions. Fill in the blanks.*

1. What type of procedure is an *arthroscopy?*

   _____

   _____

   _____

   _____

2. What is the function of a *ligament?*

   _____

   _____

3. A *cruciate* ligament forms what shape?

   _____

4. What was removed from this patient? _____

5. What is *transplanted,* and where did it come from?

   _____

   _____

6. Describe the location of *medial:*

   _____

   _____

7. What two parts of this patient's knee were repaired?

   _____

   _____

8. What is the function of a *meniscus?*

   _____

   _____

9. What is the meaning of the term *rehabilitation?*

   _____

   _____

10. Describe "joint mobility and stability":

    _____

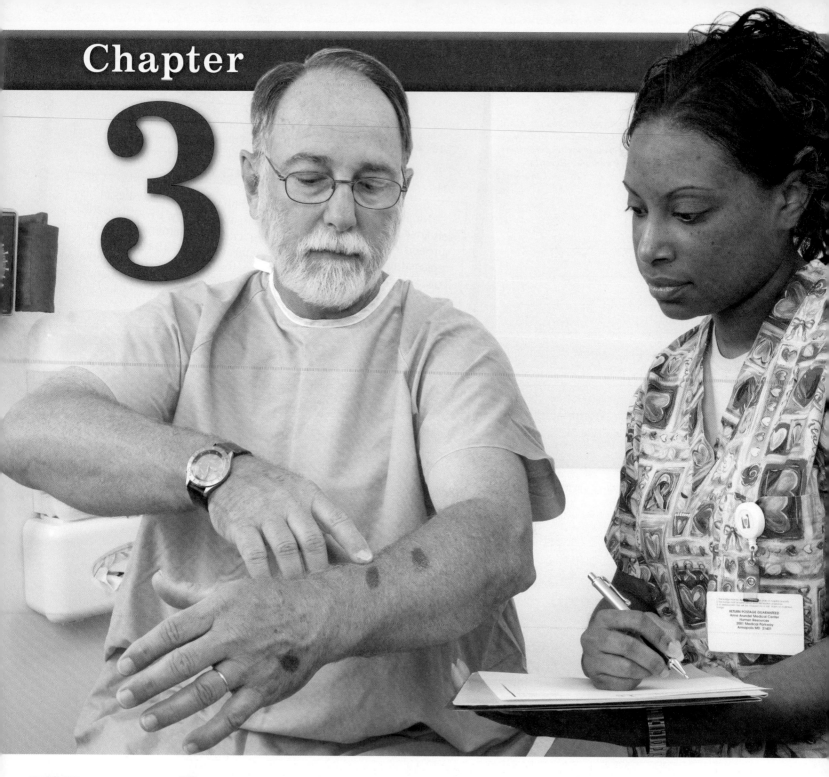

THE INTEGUMENTARY SYSTEM

The Essentials of the Language of Dermatology

In addition to anticipating Dr. Echols' needs for equipment to **biopsy,** diagnose, and treat the lesions, you also have to be able to communicate clearly with her in medical terms and understand her language as she communicates with you and the patient about the **etiology** (cause) and structure of the lesions. You will then need to document the medical history and treatment and communicate clearly with Mr. Andrews about the treatment of his lesions and their **prognosis.**

To perform these tasks, you must be able to:

LO 3.1   Apply the language of dermatology to the skin and its associated organs.

LO 3.2   Comprehend, analyze, spell, and write the medical terms of dermatology.

LO 3.3   Recognize and pronounce the medical terms of dermatology.

LO 3.4   Describe the etiology, treatment, and prognosis of common dermatologic conditions.

CASE REPORT 3.1

YOU ARE

. . . a dermatology technologist working with dermatologist Laura Echols, MD, a member of the Fulwood Medical Group.

YOU ARE COMMUNICATING WITH

. . . Mr. Rod Andrews, a 60-year-old man, who shows you three skin lesions—two on his left forearm and one on the back of his left hand. You learn that he has been living in Arizona for the past 10 years but has recently returned to this area in order to live near his daughter and young grandchildren. You find no other skin lesions on his body.

The health professionals involved in the diagnosis and treatment of problems with the integumentary system include the following:

- **Dermatologists** are medical doctors who are specialists in skin disorders.
- **Dermatology technologists** are nurses or medical assistants who have an additional year of training in dermatology.

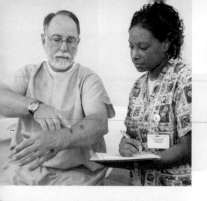

LESSON 3.1

Structure and Function of the Skin

OBJECTIVES

*Your skin is your largest organ—it covers your entire body. The three lesions on Mr. Andrews' arm and hand developed in the outer layer of the skin, the **epidermis**. This lesson looks at the structure and function of the skin so that you will be able to use correct medical terminology to:*

3.1.1 Describe the functions of the skin.

3.1.2 Name the tissues in the different layers of the skin.

3.1.3 Specify the functions of the different layers of the skin.

Your skin's nerves allow you to feel heat, cold, pain, and comfort. Your skin wards off infections and protects your body from harmful environmental elements. Your skin is constantly shedding old cells in order to make room for new skin growth.

The **integumentary system** consists of your skin and its associated organs. **Dermatology** is the study and treatment of the integumentary system. A **dermatologist** is a medical specialist in the disorders of the skin.

CASE REPORT 3.1 (CONTINUED)

When Dr. Echols examined Mr. Andrews, she determined that two of his lesions were basal cell **carcinomas** and treated them with **cryosurgery,** an approach that involves freezing cancerous tissue. She believed that the third lesion was a **squamous cell** carcinoma and performed a biopsy removal of the **cutaneous** (skin) lesion. You sent this to the laboratory with a request for a pathologic diagnosis and determination of whether the lesion had been completely removed.

Functions of the Skin

(LO 3.1, 3.2, and 3.3)

Your skin functions in several ways to keep you healthy and safe. These important functions include the following:

- **Protection:** Your skin is a physical barrier against injury, chemicals, ultraviolet rays, microbes, and toxins, and is not easily breached *(Figure 3.1)*. Bacteria and other pathogens, called normal **flora,** populate your skin's surface.

- **Water resistance:** You don't swell up every time you take a bath because your skin is water resistant. It also prevents water from leaking out of body tissues.

- **Temperature regulation:** A network of capillaries in your skin opens up or dilates (**vasodilation**) when your body is too hot. When your body is cold, this capillary network narrows (**vasoconstriction**),

blood flow decreases, and your body retains heat *(see Chapter 6)*.

- **Vitamin D synthesis:** As little as 15 to 30 minutes of sunlight each day allows your skin cells to initiate the metabolism of vitamin D, which is essential for bone growth and maintenance.

- **Sensation:** Nerve endings that detect touch, pressure, heat, cold, pain, vibration, and tissue injury are particularly numerous in the skin of your face, fingers, palms, soles, nipples, and genitals.

- **Excretion and secretion:** Water and small amounts of waste products from cell metabolism are lost through your skin by **excretion** and **secretion** from your sweat glands.

- **Social functions:** The skin reflects your emotions: it blushes when you are self-conscious, goes pale when you are frightened, and wrinkles when you register disgust.

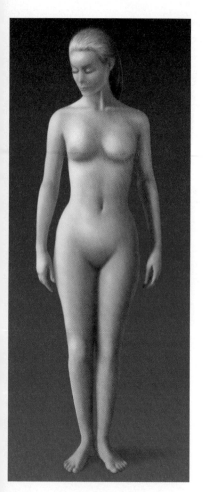

◀ **FIGURE 3.1**
Integumentary System.
The skin provides protection, contains sensory organs, and helps control body temperature.

Word	Pronunciation	Elements		Definition
biopsy	**BI**-op-see	S/ R/	-opsy *to view* bi- *life*	Removing tissue from a living person for laboratory examination
carcinoma	kar-sih-**NOH**-mah	S/ R/	-oma *tumor, mass* carcin- *cancer*	A malignant and invasive epithelial tumor
cryosurgery	cry-oh-**SUR**-jer-ee	S/ R/ R/	-ery *process of* cryo- *icy cold* -surg- *operate*	Use of liquid nitrogen or argon gas in a probe to freeze and kill abnormal tissue
cutaneous	kyu-**TAY**-nee-us	S/ R/CF	-ous *pertaining to* cutan/e- *skin*	Pertaining to the skin
dermatology	der-mah-**TOL**-oh-jee	S/ R/CF	-logy *study of* dermat/o- *skin*	Medical specialty concerned with disorders of the skin
dermatologist	der-mah-**TOL**-oh-jist	S/	-logist *one who studies, specialist*	Medical specialist in diseases of the skin
dermatologic (adj)	der-mah-toh-**LOJ**-ik	S/	-ic *pertaining to*	Pertaining to the skin and dermatology
etiology	ee-tee-**OL**-oh-jee	S/ R/CF	-logy *study of* eti/o- *cause*	The study of the causes of a disease
excrete (verb)	eks-**KREET**	P/ R	ex- *out of, away from* -crete *separate*	To pass waste products of metabolism out of the body
excretion (noun)	eks-**KREE**-shun	S/	-ion *action*	Removal of waste products of metabolism out of the body
flora	**FLO**-rah		Latin *flower*	The population of microorganisms covering the exterior and interior surfaces of healthy animals
integument	in-**TEG**-you-ment		Latin *a covering*	Organ system that covers the body, the skin being the main organ within the system
integumentary (adj)	in-**TEG**-you-MENT-ah-ree	S/ R/	-ary *pertaining to* integument- *covering of the body*	Pertaining to the covering of the body
prognosis	prog-**NO**-sis	P/ R/	pro- *projecting forward* -gnosis *knowledge*	Forecast of the probable future course and outcome of a disease
squamous cell	**SKWAY**-mus **SELL**		squamous Latin *scaly*	Flat, scale-like epithelial cell
secrete (verb) secretion (noun)	seh-**KREET** seh-**KREE**-shun	R/ S/	secret- *produce* -ion *action*	To produce a chemical substance in a cell and release it from the cell
synthesis	**SIN**-the-sis	P/ R/	syn- *together* -thesis *to organize, arrange*	The process of building a compound from different elements
synthetic (adj)	sin-**THET**-ik	S/ R/	-ic *pertaining to* -thet- *arrange, organize*	Built up or put together from simpler compounds
vasoconstriction	VAY-soh-con-**STRIK**-shun	S/ R/CF R/	-ion *action* vas/o- *blood vessel* -constrict- *narrow*	Reduction in diameter of a blood vessel
vasodilation	VAY-soh-dih-**LAY**-shun	R/	-dilat- *widen, open up*	Increase in diameter of a blood vessel

EXERCISE

A. Review *the Case Report on this spread before answering the questions.*

1. Mr. Andrews' skin lesions were two different types. What were they? _____

2. What different types of treatment did Dr. Echols use to remove these lesions? _____

3. What two questions does Dr. Echols need the pathologist to answer?

_____ and _____

4. What treatment approach involves freezing cancerous tissue? _____

5 . *Cutaneous* means: _____

LESSON 3.1 Structure of the Skin
(LO 3.1, 3.2, and 3.3)

Epidermis (LO 3.1, 3.2, and 3.3)

Mr. Andrews' three lesions were present in his **epidermis,** the most superficial layer of his skin.

The outer layer of your epidermis *(Figure 3.2)* is a keratin-packed cover of compact, dead cells that you continually shed. **Keratin**—a tough, scaly protein that is also the basis for your hair and nails—shields your body from harmful elements like chemicals and bacteria. **Dandruff** is essentially clumps of these dead keratin cells stuck together with **sebum** (oil) from **sebaceous glands.**

In the lower layers of your epidermis, cells are filled with a protein that becomes keratin. Other cells produce a brown/black pigment called **melanin,** which determines the color of your skin and protects it from **ultraviolet (UV)** light damage.

Dermis (LO 3.1, 3.2, and 3.3)

Figure 3.3 shows that the **dermis** is a much thicker connective tissue layer than the epidermis. Your dermis is the middle layer of your skin between your epidermis and **hypodermis.** It consists mostly of collagen fibers. Your dermis is well supplied with blood vessels and nerves. It contains your other skin organs: sweat glands, sebaceous glands, hair **follicles,** and nail roots.

ABBREVIATIONS

IM	intramuscular
SC	subcutaneous
TB	tuberculosis
UV	ultraviolet

Hypodermis or Subcutaneous Tissue Layer (LO 3.1, 3.2, and 3.3)

This layer beneath your dermis is the site of **subcutaneous** fat (**adipose** tissue), nerves, and blood vessels. Also called the subcutaneous tissue layer, it regulates your body's temperature and helps to protect your vital organs. When this layer becomes thinner or deteriorates, as with the aging process, your skin begins to sag.

Clinical Applications
(LO 3.1, 3.2, and 3.3)

Injections are given into the three areas of the skin using the following approaches:

- **Intradermal,** in which a short, thin needle is introduced into the epidermis, raising a small **wheal** on the skin. This site is used for allergy testing or a tuberculosis (**TB**) test.

- **Subcutaneous (SC),** in which a longer needle pierces the epidermis and dermis to reach the hypodermis (subcutaneous) layer. This site is used for insulin injections and immunizations.

- **Intramuscular (IM),** in which a long needle penetrates the epidermis, dermis, and hypodermis to reach into the muscles underneath. Some antibiotics and immunizations are given this way.

In addition, there are **transdermal** applications. Here, medications are administered through the skin by an adhesive transdermal patch applied to the skin. The medication diffuses across the epidermis and enters the blood vessels in the dermis. Contraceptive hormones, **analgesics,** and antinausea/antiseasickness medications are examples of transdermal applications.

▼ **FIGURE 3.2**
Epidermis.

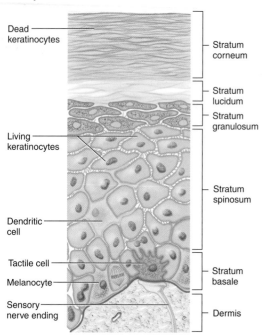

▼ **FIGURE 3.3**
Dermis and Its Organs.

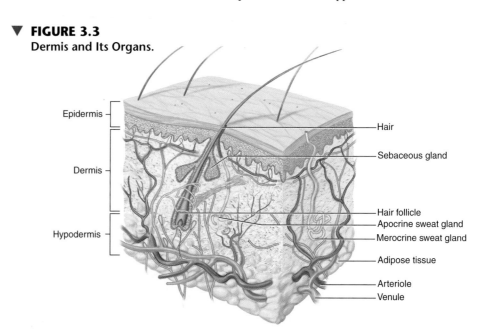

Word	Pronunciation	Elements		Definition
adipose	ADD-ih-pose	S/ R/	-ose *full of* adip- *fat*	Containing fat
analgesic (adj) analgesia	an-al-**JEE**-sic an-al-**JEE**-zee-ah	S/ P/ R/ S/	-ic *pertaining to* an- *without* -alges- *sensation of pain* -ia *condition*	Substance that reduces or relieves the response to pain without producing loss of consciousness State in which pain is reduced or relieved
dandruff	DAN-druff		Source unknown	Scales in hair from shedding of the epidermis
dermis dermal	DER-miss DER-mal	S/ R/	Greek *skin* -al *pertaining to* derm- *skin*	Connective tissue layer of the skin beneath the epidermis Pertaining to the skin
epidermis epidermal (adj)	ep-ih-**DER**-miss ep-ih-**DER**-mal	P/ R/ S/ R/	epi- *above, upon* -dermis *skin* -al *pertaining to* -derm- *skin*	Top layer of the skin Pertaining to the epidermis
follicle	FOLL-ih-kull		Latin *small sac*	Spherical mass of cells containing a cavity or a small cul-de-sac, such as a hair follicle
hypodermis hypodermic (adj) (same as subcutaneous)	high-poh-**DER**-miss high-poh-**DER**-mik	P/ R/ S/ R/	hypo- *below* -dermis *skin* -ic *pertaining to* -derm- *skin*	Loose connective tissue layer of skin below the dermis Pertaining to the hypodermis
intradermal	in-trah-**DER**-mal	S/ P/ R/	-al *pertaining to* intra- *within* -derm- *skin*	Within the epidermis
intramuscular	in-trah-**MUSS**-kew-lar	S/ P/ R/	-ar *pertaining to* intra- *within* -muscul- *muscle*	Within the muscle
keratin	KER-ah-tin	S/ R/	-in *substance* kerat- *hard protein*	Protein present in skin, hair, and nails
melanin	MEL-ah-nin	S/ R/	-in *substance* melan- *black pigment*	Black pigment found in skin, hair, and the retina
sebaceous glands sebum	seh-**BAY**-shus **GLANZ** SEE-bum	S/ R/CF	-ous *pertaining to* sebac/e- *wax* Latin *tallow*	Glands in the dermis that open into hair follicles and secrete a waxy fluid called sebum Waxy secretion of the sebaceous glands
subcutaneous (same as hypodermic)	sub-kew-**TAY**-nee-us	S/ P/ R/CF	-ous *pertaining to* sub- *below* -cutan/e- *skin*	Below the skin
transdermal	trans-**DER**-mal	S/ P/ R/	-al *pertaining to* trans- *across, through* -derm- *skin*	Going across or through the skin
ultraviolet	ul-trah-**VIE**-oh-let	P/ R/	ultra- *beyond* -violet *violet, bluish purple*	Light rays at a higher frequency than the violet end of the spectrum
wheal (same as hives)	WHEEL		Old English *wheal*	Small, itchy swelling of the skin. (Wheals raised by an injection do not itch)

EXERCISES

A. Review *the Case Report on the previous two-page spread before answering the questions.*

1. What role did sunlight play in Mr. Andrews' skin cancer? _____

2. What treatments were given for Mr. Andrews' skin cancer? _____

3. What future precautions should Mr. Andrews take? _____

B. Practice *using your medical terminology in the following exercise. When possible, be sure to deconstruct the term using the slashes provided. Fill in the blanks.*

1. This pigment is responsible for skin color: _____ / _____ / _____
P   R/CF   S

2. Skin needs protection from this type of light: _____ / _____ / _____
P   R/CF   S

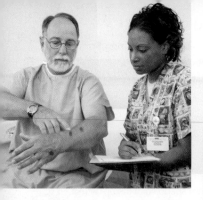

LESSON 3.2

Disorders of the Skin

OBJECTIVES

*Your skin provides your body's first line of defense against injury, disease, **allergens,** and pollutants. Because your skin is continually exposed to the elements, it's susceptible to various problems and disorders. The skin shows the same types of disease as most organs—infections, tumors, cancers—but because of its protective covering, it's the first responder to many irritant and **allergenic** agents. The information in this lesson will enable you to use correct medical terminology to:*

3.2.1 Name common disorders of the skin.

3.2.2 Describe the effects of these disorders on health.

CASE REPORT 3.2

YOU ARE

. . . a medical assistant working with dermatologist Dr. Lenore Echols in Fulwood Medical Center.

YOU ARE COMMUNICATING WITH

. . . Ms. Cheryl Fox, a 37-year-old nursing assistant working in a surgical unit in Fulwood Medical Center.

Recently, Ms. Fox's fingers have become red and itchy, with occasional **vesicles.** She has also noticed irritation and swelling of her earlobes and **pruritus.** Over the weekends, both the itching and the **rash** on her hands worsen. A patch test by Dr. Echols showed that Ms. Fox is **allergic** to nickel, which is present in the rings she wears on both hands and in her earrings. She only wears this jewelry on the weekends, not during her workdays.

Dermatitis (LO 3.1, 3.2, 3.3, and 3.4)

Dermatitis, also called **eczema,** is an inflammation that produces swollen, red, itchy skin. Ms. Fox has a dermatitis *(Figure 3.4)* resulting from direct exposure to an irritating agent.

The different types of dermatitis and their related causes are as follows:

- **Contact dermatitis** results from direct contact with irritants or allergens, including soaps, detergents, cleaning products, and solvents.

- **Atopic** or **allergic dermatitis** is due to allergens that include nickel in jewelry (as with Ms. Fox), perfume, cosmetics, poison ivy, and latex.

- **Eczema** is a general term used for inflamed and itchy skin conditions. When the itchy skin is scratched, it becomes **excoriated** and produces the dry, red, scaly patches characteristic of eczema. The atopic dermatitis that Ms. Fox developed is a common form of eczema.

- **Seborrheic dermatitis** produces a red rash overlaid with a yellow, oily scale and is common in people with oily skin or hair.

- **Stasis dermatitis** occurs in the lower leg when varicose veins slow the return of blood and the accumulation of fluid interferes with the nourishment of the skin.

CASE REPORT 3.2 (CONTINUED)

For Ms. Fox, the **allergy** is not just a local reaction to an irritant. Her form of **atopic** or allergic dermatitis develops when the whole body becomes sensitive to an allergen. This whole-body involvement is shown by her systemic symptoms of pruritus distant from the local irritant site. Ms. Fox has stopped wearing rings and earrings that contain nickel.

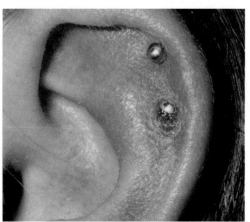

▲ **FIGURE 3.4**
Dermatitis of the Ear.

Word	Pronunciation	Elements		Definition
allergen *(The duplicate "g" is deleted.)*	AL-er-jen	S/ R/ R/	-gen- *produce* all- *strange, other* -erg- *work, activity*	Substance producing a hypersensitivity (allergic) reaction
allergenic (adj)	al-er-JEN-ik	S/	-ic *pertaining to*	Pertaining to the capacity to produce an allergic reaction
allergy	AL-er-jee			Hypersensitivity to an allergen
allergic (adj)	ah-LER-jik			Pertaining to being hypersensitive
atopy	AT-oh-pee		Greek *strangeness*	State of hypersensitivity to an allergen—allergic
atopic (adj)	ay-TOP-ik			
dermatitis	der-mah-TYE-tis	S/ R/	-itis *inflammation* dermat- *skin*	Inflammation of the skin
eczema	EK-zeh-mah		Greek *to boil* or *ferment*	Inflammatory skin disease, often with a serous discharge
eczematous (adj)	EK-zem-ah-tus	S/ R/CF	-tous *pertaining to* eczem/a- *eczema*	Pertaining to or marked by eczema
excoriate (verb)	eks-KOR-ee-ate	S/ P/ R/	-ate *pertaining to* ex- *away from* -cori- *skin*	To scratch
excoriation (noun)	eks-KOR-ee-AY-shun	S/	-ation *process*	Scratch mark
pruritus	proo-RYE-tus		Latin *to itch*	Itching
pruritic (adj)	proo-RIT-ik	S/ R/	-ic *pertaining to* prurit- *itch*	Itchy
antipruritic	AN-tee-proo-RIT-ik	P/	anti- *against*	Medication against itching
rash	RASH		French *skin eruption*	Skin eruption
seborrhea	seb-oh-REE-ah	S/ R/CF	-rrhea *flow* seb/o- *sebum*	Excessive amount of sebum
seborrheic (adj) *(The "a" is deleted to enable the word to flow.)*	seb-oh-REE-ik	S/	-ic *pertaining to*	Pertaining to seborrhea
stasis	STAY-sis		Greek *staying in one place*	Stagnation in the flow of any body fluid
vesicle	VES-ih-kull		Latin *blister*	Small sac containing liquid; e.g., a blister

EXERCISES

A. Review *the Case Report on this two-page spread before answering the questions.*

1. What two parts of Ms. Fox's body were exhibiting symptoms? _____

2. What were the symptoms? _____

3. Why are the symptoms confined to those two areas? _____

4. What is Ms. Fox allergic to? _____

5. Why do her symptoms worsen on the weekends? _____

B. Medical documentation *should always be neat, legible, and spelled correctly for patient safety. Also remember that the patient record is a legal document. The WAD above contains some medical terms that are difficult to spell and pronounce. After you finish this exercise listen to the pronunciation of these terms on the Student Online Learning Center (www.mhhe.com/AllanEss2e) and practice them yourself. Below, insert the correct spelling of the term on the line.*

1. Medication has been prescribed for this patient's case of _____ dermatitis.
   seborheic   seborrheic

2. The _____ rash on the patient's face is slowly clearing after she tried the new medication.
   eczematous   exzematous

3. Ms. Fox's _____ is an allergic reaction to her jewelry, which contains nickel.
   purritis   pruritus

LESSON 3.2 Disorders of the Skin *(continued)*

Skin Cancers

(LO 3.1, 3.2, 3.3, and 3.4)

The two basal cell carcinomas *(Figure 3.5)* on Mr. Andrews' arm arose from the basal (bottom) layer of his epidermis. This is the most common and the least dangerous form of skin cancer because it does not **metastasize** (spread).

The squamous cell carcinoma on Mr. Andrews' hand arose from cells in the middle layers of the epidermis. This skin cancer responds well to surgical removal but can metastasize to lymph glands if neglected.

Malignant melanoma *(Figure 3.6)* is the least common but most dangerous skin cancer. It arises in melanin-producing cells in the basal layer of the epidermis and metastasizes quickly. If neglected, this cancer is fatal.

Excess **sunlight** can also be an irritant to the skin. Too much sun can burn the skin and may lead to cancer, as it did for Mr. Andrews.

Any *congenital* (present at birth) lesion of the skin, including various types of birthmarks and all moles, is referred to as a **nevus.**

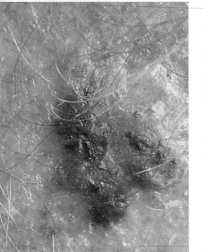

▲ **FIGURE 3.5**
Basal Cell Carcinoma.

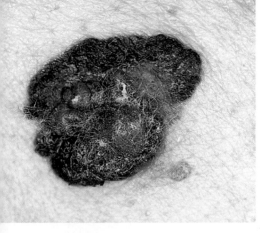

▲ **FIGURE 3.6**
Malignant Melanoma.

Pressure Ulcers

(LO 3.1, 3.2, 3.3, and 3.4)

When a patient lies in one position for a long period, the pressure between the bed and the body's bony projections, such as the lower spine or heel, cuts off the blood supply to the skin. Under these circumstances, **pressure** or **decubitus ulcers** can appear *(Figure 3.7)*. When this happens, the skin's protective function is compromised, making it easy for germs to enter the body. The elderly are often at risk for pressure ulcers because their skin is usually thin and dry. In addition, poor nutritional status can deplete the fatty protective layer in the hypodermis under the skin, making the body more susceptible to pressure ulcers.

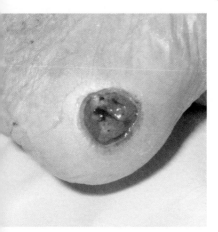

◀ **FIGURE 3.7**
Decubitus (Pressure)
Ulcer on the Heel.

Infections of the Skin

(LO 3.1, 3.2, 3.3, and 3.4)

The skin can be susceptible to many different types of infections, including viral, fungal, parasitic, and bacterial infections.

Viral Infections

(LO 3.1, 3.2, 3.3, and 3.4)

Warts (verrucas) are skin growths caused by the human **papillomavirus** invading the epidermis *(Figure 3.8)*.

Varicella-zoster virus causes chickenpox in unvaccinated people. Here, **macules** (small, flat spots different in color from the surrounding skin), **papules** (small, solid elevations), and **vesicles** (small sacs containing fluid) form. The virus can then remain dormant in the peripheral nerves (near the skin's surface) for decades before erupting as the painful vesicles of **herpes zoster,** also called **shingles** *(Figure 3.9)*.

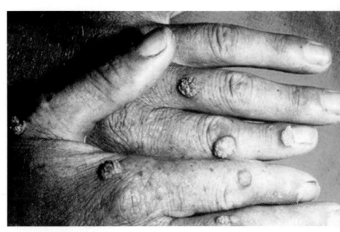

▲ **FIGURE 3.8**
Warts on Hands.

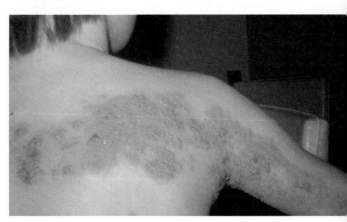

▲ **FIGURE 3.9**
Shingles.

Word	Pronunciation	Elements		Definition
decubitus ulcer (pressure ulcer)	deh-**KYU**-bit-us **UL**-ser	P/ R/ R/	de- *from* -cubitus *lying down* ulcer *sore*	Sore caused by lying down for long periods of time
herpes zoster (shingles)	**HER**-pees **ZOS**-ter		herpes Greek *to creep or spread* zoster Greek *belt, girdle*	Painful eruption of vesicles that follows a nerve root on one side of the body
macule	**MACK**-yul		Latin *spot*	Small, flat spot or patch on the skin
malignant	mah-**LIG**-nant	S/ R/	-ant *forming, pertaining to* malign- *harmful, bad*	Tumor that invades surrounding tissues and metastasizes to distant organs
malignancy	mah-**LIG**-nan-see	S/	-ancy *state of*	State of being malignant
melanin melanoma	**MEL**-ah-nin mel-ah-**NO**-mah	S/ R/	Greek *black* -oma *tumor, mass* melan- *black pigment*	Black pigment found in skin, hair, and retina Malignant neoplasm formed from cells that produce melanin
metastasis (noun)	meh-**TAS**-tah-sis	R/ P/	-stasis *stagnate, stay in one place* meta- *beyond, subsequent to*	Spread of a disease from one part of the body to another
metastasize (verb)	meh-**TAS**-tah-size	S/ R/	-ize *affect in a specific way* -stat- *stationary*	To spread to distant parts
metastatic (adj)	meh-tah-**STAT**-ik	S/	-ic *pertaining to*	Pertaining to the character of cells that can metastasize
nevus nevi (pl)	**NEE**-vus **NEE**-veye		Latin *mole, birthmark*	Congenital lesion of the skin
papillomavirus	pap-ih-**LOH**-mah-vi-rus	S/ R/CF	-oma *mass, tumor* papill/o- *papilla, pimple* virus Latin *poison*	Virus that causes warts and is associated with cancer
papule	**PAP**-yul		Latin *pimple*	Small, circumscribed elevation on the skin
verruca (wart)	ver-**ROO**-cah		Latin *wart*	Wart caused by a virus

EXERCISES

A. **Identify** *the italicized element in the first column of the chart, define it, and use it to determine the meaning of the medical term.*

Medical Term	Identity of Element (P, S, R, or CF)	Meaning of Element	Meaning of Medical Term
metastasis	1.	2.	3.
malignant	4.	5.	6.
melanoma	7.	8.	9.
decubitus	10.	11.	12.

B. **Use any two terms** *from the chart above in sentences of your choice that are* not *definitions.*

Sentence:

1. _____

_____

_____

_____

2. _____

_____

_____

_____

_____

Fungal Infections

(LO 3.1, 3.2, 3.3, and 3.4)

Tinea is a general term for a group of related skin infections caused by different species of **fungi.**

Tinea pedis, or athlete's foot, causes itching, redness, and peeling of the skin of the foot, particularly between the toes *(Figure 3.10)*. **Tinea capitis** describes an infection of the scalp (ringworm). **Tinea corporis** refers to ringworm infections of the body's skin and hands. **Tinea cruris,** or jock itch, is the name for infections of the groin. The fungus spreads from animals, from the soil, and by direct contact with infected individuals.

A yeast-like fungus, ***Candida albicans,*** can produce recurrent infections of the skin, nails, and mucous membranes. The first sign can be a frequent diaper rash or oral **thrush** in infants. Older children can show repeated or persistent lesions on the scalp. In adults, chronic **mucocutaneous candidiasis** can affect the mouth (thrush) *(Figure 3.11)*, vagina, and skin. It can also occur with diseases of the immune system *(see Chapter 7)*, as those with a compromised immune system are more susceptible to chronic infections, including fungal infections.

Parasitic Infestations

(LO 3.1, 3.2, 3.3, and 3.4)

A **parasite** is an organism that lives in contact with and feeds off another organism or host. This process is called an **infestation** and is different from an **infection.**

Lice *(Figure 3.12)* are small, wingless, blood-sucking parasites that produce the disease **pediculosis** by attaching their nits (eggs) to hair and clothing.

Itch mites *(Figure 3.13)* produce an intense, itching rash called **scabies,** which generally occurs in the genital area or near the waist, breasts, and armpits. These mites lay eggs under the skin.

Bacterial Infections

(LO 3.1, 3.2, 3.3, and 3.4)

Staphylococcus aureus (commonly called "staph") is the most common bacterium to invade the skin. Staph causes pimples, boils, **carbuncles,** and **impetigo** *(Figure 3.14)*. It can also produce a **cellulitis** of the epidermis and dermis. *Group A Streptococcus* (strep) can also cause cellulitis.

Occasionally, some strains of both staph and strep can be extremely **toxic,** especially when their enzymes digest the connective tissues and spread into the muscle layers. This condition is called **necrotizing fasciitis** and it requires highly aggressive surgical and antibiotic treatment.

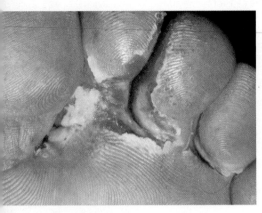

▲ **FIGURE 3.10**
Tinea Pedis Between the Toes.

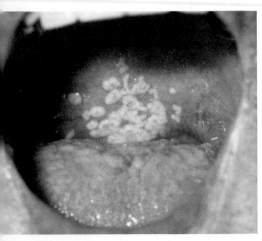

▲ **FIGURE 3.11**
Thrush.

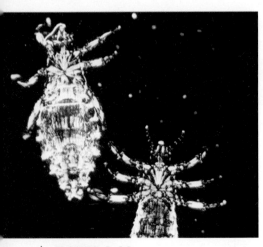

▲ **FIGURE 3.12**
Body Lice.

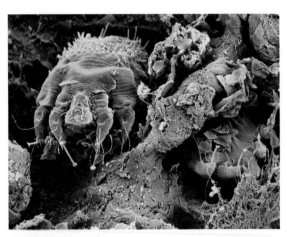

▲ **FIGURE 3.13**
The Itch Mite of Scabies.

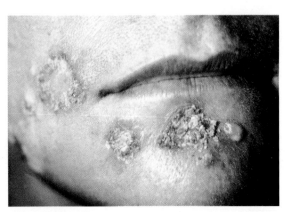

▲ **FIGURE 3.14**
Impetigo.

Word	Pronunciation		Elements	Definition
Candida candidiasis	KAN-did-ah kan-dih-**DIE**-ah-sis	 S/ R/	Latin *dazzling white* -iasis *state of, condition* candid- *Candida*	A yeastlike fungus Infection with the yeastlike fungus
Candida albicans thrush	KAN-did-ah **AL**-bih-kanz **THRUSH**		albicans *white*	The most common form of *Candida* Another name for infection with *Candida*
carbuncle	KAR-bunk-ul		Latin *carbuncle*	Infection of many hair follicles in a small area, often on the back of the neck
cellulitis	sell-you-**LIE**-tis	S/ R/	-itis *inflammation* cellul- *cell*	Infection of subcutaneous connective tissue
fungus fungi (pl)	FUN-gus FUN-jee or FUN-gee		Latin *mushroom*	General term used to describe yeasts and molds
impetigo	im-peh-**TIE**-go		Latin *scabby eruption*	Infection of the skin producing thick, yellow crusts
infection infectious (adj)	in-**FECK**-shun in-**FECK**-shus	S/ R/ S/	-ion *action* infect- *internal invasion, infection* -ious *pertaining to*	Invasion of the body by disease-producing microorganisms Capable of being transmitted, or a disease caused by the action of a microorganism
infestation	in-fes-**TAY**-shun	S/ R/	-ation *process* infest- *invade*	Act of being invaded on the skin by a troublesome other species, such as a parasite
louse lice (pl)	LOWSE LISE		Old English *louse*	Parasitic insect
mucocutaneous	MYU-koh-kyu-**TAY**-nee-us	S/ R/CF R/CF	-ous *pertaining to* muc/o- *mucous membrane* -cutan/e- *skin*	Junction of skin and mucous membrane; e.g., the lips
necrotizing fasciitis (Note the spelling.)	NEH-kroh-**TIZE**-ing fash-eh -**EYE**-tis	S/ R/CF S/ S/ R/CF	-ing *quality of* necr/o- *death* -tiz- *pertaining to* -itis *inflammation* fasc/i *fascia*	Inflammation of fascia producing death of the tissue
parasite parasitic (adj)	PAR-ah-site par-ah-**SIT**-ik	 S/ R/	Greek *guest* -ic *pertaining to* parasit- *parasite*	An organism that attaches itself to, lives on or in, and derives its nutrition from another species Pertaining to a parasite
pediculosis	peh-dick-you-**LOH**-sis	S/ R/	-osis *condition* pedicul- *louse*	An infestation with lice
scabies	SKAY-bees		Latin *to scratch*	Skin disease produced by mites
tinea	TIN-ee-ah		Latin *worm*	General term for a group of related skin infections caused by different species of fungi
toxin toxic (adj) toxicity *(contains two suffixes)*	TOK-sin TOK-sick toks-**ISS**-ih-tee	 S/ R/ S/	Greek *poison* -ic *pertaining to* tox- *poison* -ity *state, condition*	Poisonous substance formed by a cell or organism Pertaining to a toxin The state of being poisonous

EXERCISES

A. Terminology challenge. *Employ the language of dermatology to answer the following questions.*

1. Demonstrate your understanding of the terms *infection* and *infestation* by explaining how they are different.

   Infection: _____

   Infestation: _____

2. What are lice eggs called? _____

B. Proofread your documentation. *The following sentence has either an error in fact or an error in spelling. Correct the sentence.*

1. An infection of lice can be troublesome to eliminate. _____

Collagen Diseases (LO 3.1, 3.2, 3.3, and 3.4)

Collagen, a fibrous protein, comprises 30% of your total body protein. Because your body contains so much of this protein, collagen diseases can have a dramatic effect throughout the body and in the skin.

Systemic lupus erythematosus (SLE) is an **autoimmune** disease that occurs most commonly in women. It produces characteristic skin lesions like a butterfly-shaped, red rash on both cheeks that is joined across the bridge of the nose *(Figure 3.15)*. This disease also affects multiple organs, including the kidneys, brain, heart, and joints.

Rosacea produces a similar facial rash to that of SLE, but there are no systemic complications.

Scleroderma is a chronic, persistent autoimmune disease that also occurs more often in women. It's characterized by a hardening and shrinking of the skin that makes it feel leathery *(Figure 3.16)*. Joints show swelling, pain, and stiffness. Internal organs, including the heart, lungs, kidneys, and digestive tract, are involved in a similar process. The etiology is unknown, and there is no effective treatment.

Other Skin Diseases (LO 3.1, 3.2, 3.3, and 3.4)

Psoriasis *(Figure 3.17)* is marked by itchy, flaky, red patches of skin of various sizes covered with white or silvery scales. It appears most commonly on the scalp, elbows, and knees, and its cause is unknown.

Skin Manifestations of Internal Disease

(LO 3.1, 3.2, 3.3, and 3.4)

The presence of cancer inside the body is often shown by skin lesions visible on the body's surface, even before the cancer or other disease has produced **symptoms** or been diagnosed.

Dermatomyositis *(Figure 3.18)* is often associated with ovarian cancer, which can appear within 4 to 5 years after the skin disease is diagnosed. This skin disease presents with a reddish-purple rash around the eyes. Muscle weakness commonly follows weeks or months after the appearance of the rash.

Kaposi sarcoma mostly develops in association with **HIV** infection. Raised red or brown blotches or bumps in tissues occur below the skin's surface and eventually spread throughout the body.

Herpes zoster, referred to earlier in this chapter, is common in immunocompromised patients, including the elderly, individuals with HIV, and patients on chemotherapy *(see Chapter 7)*.

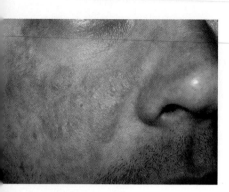

▲ **FIGURE 3.15**
Systemic Lupus
Erythematosus.

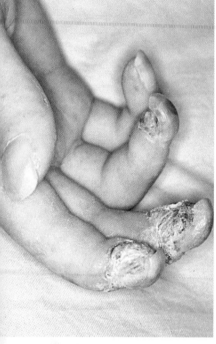

▲ **FIGURE 3.16**
Scleroderma.

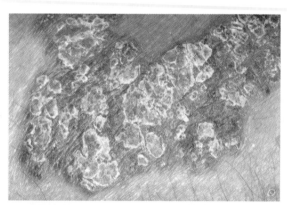

▲ **FIGURE 3.17**
Psoriasis.

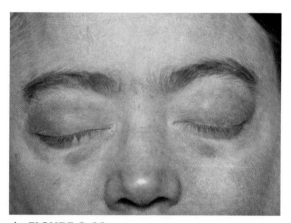

▲ **FIGURE 3.18**
Periorbital Rash of Dermatomyositis.

ABBREVIATIONS

HIV	human immunodeficiency virus
SLE	systemic lupus erythematosus

S = Suffix   P = Prefix   R = Root   R/CF= Combining Form

Word	Pronunciation	Elements		Definition
autoimmune	awe-toe-im-**YUNE**	P/ R/	auto- *self* -immune *protected from*	Diseases in which the body makes antibodies directed against its own tissues
dermatomyositis	**DER**-mah-toe-**MY**-oh-site-is	S/ R/CF R/	-itis *inflammation* dermat/o- *skin* -myos- *muscle*	Inflammation of the skin and muscles
Kaposi sarcoma	kah-**POH**-see sar-**KOH**-mah		Moritz Kaposi, Hungarian dermatologist, 1837–1902	A form of skin cancer seen in AIDS patients
psoriasis	so-**RYE**-ah-sis		Greek *the itch*	Rash characterized by reddish, silver-scaled patches
rosacea	roh-**ZAY**-she-ah		Latin *rosy*	Persistent erythematous rash of the central face
scleroderma	sklair-oh-**DERM**-ah	S/ R/CF	-derma *skin* scler/o- *hard*	Thickening and hardening of the skin due to new collagen formation
symptom *(subjective)*	**SIMP**-tum		Greek *event or feeling that has happened to someone*	Departure from normal health experienced by the patient
symptomatic *(adj)*	simp-toe-**MAT**-ik	S/ R/	-atic *pertaining to* symptom *symptoms*	Pertaining to the symptoms of a disease
sign *(objective)*	SINE		Latin *mark*	Physical evidence of a disease process
systemic lupus erythematosus	sis-**TEM**-ik **LOO**-pus er-ih-**THEE**-mah-toe-sus	S/ R/ S/ R/	-ic *pertaining to* system- *the body as a whole* lupus *Latin wolf* -osus *condition* erythemat- *redness*	Inflammatory connective tissue disease affecting the whole body

EXERCISES

A. Document *using the language of dermatology by inserting the correct term in the space provided. Always review the above WAD before you start any exercise.*

1. According to the patient's symptoms, the physician diagnosed (body attacks its own tissues) _____ disease.

2. What we thought was originally a localized problem has now spread, and the patient's final diagnosis is (inflammatory connective tissue disease affecting the whole body) _____ .

3. Because of this patient's past history of HIV, his new skin lesions have been diagnosed by the pathologist as (a form of skin cancer seen in AIDS patients) _____ .

4. Patients with (rash with reddish, silver-scaled patches) _____ often wear long sleeves to hide their elbows.

B. Critical thinking *and the language of dermatology will help you answer the following questions. Using the two medical terms* symptom *and* sign *from the WAD, explain which term is objective, and which term is subjective, and what that means to the patient.*

1. _____
_____
_____
_____

2. Briefly describe an immunocompromised patient. _____
_____

3. What is the role of skin lesions as a precursor to cancer? _____
_____

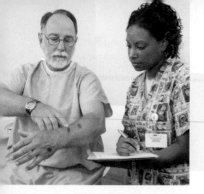

LESSON 3.3

Accessory Skin Organs

OBJECTIVES

Hair follicles, sebaceous glands, sweat glands, and nails are accessory organs located in your skin. Each of these skin organs has specific anatomical and physiological characteristics. This lesson will enable you to use correct medical terminology to:

3.3.1 Distinguish the different accessory skin organs.

3.3.2 Identify the structure and functions of the accessory skin organs.

3.3.3 Describe certain disorders affecting the accessory skin organs.

CASE REPORT 3.3

YOU ARE . . . a pharmacist working in the pharmacy at Fulwood Medical Center.

YOU ARE COMMUNICATING WITH

. . . Mr. Wayne Winter, an 18-year-old man who will be starting college in a few months.

Mr. Winter has had **acne** since the age of 15. He has tried several over-the-counter products, all of which have been unsuccessful in treating his acne. He's even tried retinoic acid. He has numerous **comedones**, papules, **pustules**, and **scars** on his face and forehead, and has severe **cystic** lesions and scars on his back. His social life is nonexistent, and his peers frequently tease him. He wishes to change all this before he gets to college.

Your role is to explain to him how to use the medications Dr. Echols, a dermatologist, has prescribed, what their effects will be, and what possible complications may occur.

Hair Follicles and Sebaceous Glands

(LO 3.1, 3.2, 3.3, and 3.4)

Each hair follicle on your face has a sebaceous gland opening into it *(Figure 3.19)*. This gland secretes into the follicle oily, acidic sebum, which mixes with broken-down keratin cells from the base of the follicle.

Around puberty, **androgens,** male sex hormones, are thought to trigger an excessive production of sebum from the sebaceous glands. Sebum brings with it excessive numbers of broken-down keratin cells. This blocks the hair follicle, forming a **comedo** (whitehead or blackhead). Comedones can stay closed, leading to papules, or can rupture, allowing bacteria to get in and produce **pustules.** These are the classic signs of **acne.** Acne affects about 85% of people between the ages of 12 and 25 years *(Figure 3.20).*

Another skin problem involving the sebaceous glands is seborrheic dermatitis. Here, the glands are thought to be inflamed and to produce a different sebum. The skin around the face and scalp is reddened and covered with yellow, greasy scales. In infants, this condition is called "cradle cap." Seborrheic dermatitis of the scalp produces dandruff.

Hair shaft

Apocrine sweat gland

Sebaceous gland

Hair matrix

Hair root

Hair bulb

Blood capillaries

▲ **FIGURE 3.19**
Hair Follicle and Sebaceous Gland.

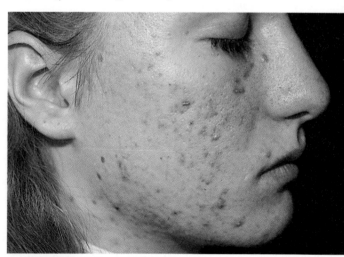

▲ **FIGURE 3.20**
Acne.

Word	Pronunciation		Elements	Definition
acne	AK-nee		Greek *point*	Inflammatory disease of sebaceous glands and hair follicles
androgen	AN-droh-jen	S/ R/CF	-gen *to produce, create* andr/o- *male*	Hormone that promotes masculine characteristics
comedo *(whitehead or blackhead)* comedones (pl)	KOM-ee-doh Kom-ee-**DOH**-nz		Latin *eat up*	Too much sebum and too many keratin cells block the hair follicle to produce the comedo
cyst cystic (adj)	SIST SIS-tik		Greek *sac, bladder*	Abnormal fluid-filled sac surrounded by a membrane
pustule	PUS-tyul		Latin *pustule*	Small protuberance on the skin containing pus
scar	SKAR		Greek *scab*	Fibrotic seam that forms when a wound heals

EXERCISES

A. Review *the Case Report on this spread before answering the questions.*

1. What does it mean if a medication is "over the counter" (OTC) in a pharmacy? _____
_____

2. Name one medication you can buy OTC in a pharmacy: _____

3. What types of skin eruptions does Mr. Winter have on his face? _____

4. What type of eruption does he have on his back that he does not have on his face? _____

5. Why does severe acne make it difficult for Mr. Winter to have an active social life? _____

6. What type of specialist did Mr. Winter consult? _____

B. Patient communication: *Rewrite the following sentences from the above Case Report and text in language Mr. Winter can understand. Substitute layperson's language for medical terms.*

1. "He has numerous comedones, papules, pustules, and scars on his face and forehead and has severe cystic lesions and scars on his back."

_____

_____

2. "Around puberty, androgens are thought to trigger excessive production of sebum from the sebaceous glands, and sebum brings with it excessive numbers of broken-down cells."

_____

_____

3. "Comedones can stay closed, leading to papules, or can rupture, allowing bacteria to get in and produce pustules."

_____

_____

LESSON 3.3 Accessory Skin Organs (LO 3.1, 3.2, 3.3, and 3.4)

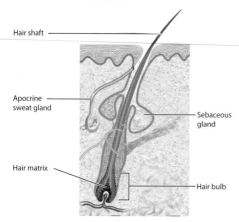

▲ **FIGURE 3.21**
Hair Follicle.

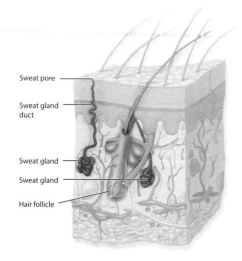

▲ **FIGURE 3.22**
Sweat Glands.

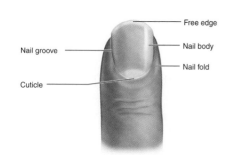

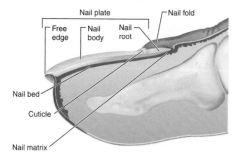

◄ **FIGURE 3.23**
Anatomy of a Fingernail.

Hair (LO 3.1, 3.2, 3.3, and 3.4)

Every hair on your body or scalp originates from epidermal cells at the base (**matrix**) of a hair follicle. As these cells divide and grow, they push older cells upward, away from the source of nutrition in the hair papilla (*Figure 3.21*). The older cells become keratinized and die.

In most people, aging causes **alopecia,** thinning of the hair, and baldness as the follicles shrink and produce thin, wispy hairs.

Sweat Glands (LO 3.1, 3.2, 3.3, and 3.4)

You have 3 million to 4 million sweat glands scattered all over your skin, with clusters on your palms, soles, and forehead (*Figure 3.22*). Their main function is to produce the watery perspiration (sweat) that cools your body. Some sweat glands open directly onto the surface of your skin. Others open into your hair follicles (*Figure 3.22*).

In the dermis, the sweat gland is a coiled tube lined with epithelial, sweat-secreting cells. In your armpits (axillae), around your nipples, in your groin, and around your anus, different sweat glands produce a thick, cloudy secretion. This interacts with your normal skin bacteria to produce a distinct, noticeable smell. The ducts of these glands lead directly into your hair follicles (*see Figure 3.21*).

Nails (LO 3.1, 3.2, 3.3, and 3.4)

Your nails consist of closely packed, thin, dead skin cells that are filled with parallel fibers of hard keratin. On the average, your fingernails grow about 1 millimeter (mm) per week. New cells are added by cell division in the nail matrix, which is protected by the nail fold of skin and the **cuticle** at the base of your nail (*Figure 3.23*).

Diseases of Nails (LO 3.1, 3.2, 3.3, and 3.4)

Fifty percent of all nail disorders are caused by fungal infections and are called **onychomycosis** (*Figure 3.24*). With these infections, the fungus grows under the nail and leads to yellow, brittle, cracked nails that separate from the underlying nail bed.

Paronychia (*Figure 3.25*) is a bacterial infection, usually staphylococcal, of the nail base. The nail fold and cuticle become swollen, red, and painful, and pus forms under the nail.

With an **ingrown toenail,** the nail grows into the skin at the side of the nail, particularly if pressured by tight, narrow shoes. An infection can then grow underneath this ingrown toenail.

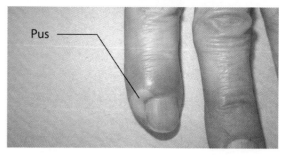

▲ **FIGURE 3.24**
Onychomycosis (Fungal Infection).

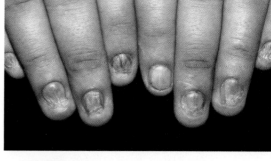

▲ **FIGURE 3.25**
Paronychia.

S = Suffix P = Prefix R = Root R/CF= Combining Form

Word	Pronunciation	Elements		Definition
alopecia	al-oh-**PEE**-shah		Greek *mange*	Partial or complete loss of hair, naturally or from medication
cuticle	**KEW**-tih-cul		Diminutive of cutis *skin*	Nonliving epidermis at base of fingernails and toenails
matrix	**MAY**-tricks		Latin mater *mother*	The formative portion of a hair, nail, or tooth
onychomycosis	oh-nih-koh-my-**KOH**-sis	S/ R/CF R/	-osis *condition* onych/o-*nail* -myc- *fungus*	Condition of a fungus infection in a nail
paronychia **(Note:** *The vowel "a" at the end of* para *is dropped to make the composite word flow more easily.)*	par-oh-**NICK**-ee-ah	S/ P/ R/	-ia *condition* para- *alongside* -onych- *nail*	Infection alongside the nail

WORD ANALYSIS AND DEFINITION

Exercises

A. Elements *are clues to the meaning of a medical term. Identify each given element in the following chart, and list its meaning. Then answer the questions below.*

Element	Identity of Element (P, R, CF, or S)	Meaning of Element
para	1.	2.
ia	3.	4.
myc	5.	6.
onycho	7.	8.
osis	9.	10.
onych	11.	12.

B. Construct terms *from the elements in the WAD.*

1. The elements in the chart above form which two terms in the WAD?

_______________ and _______________

2. Use the two medical terms from question 1 in different sentences that would appear in patient documentation.

Sentence:

a. _______________

____

____

b. _______________

____

____

3. The root form of the element meaning *nail* is _______________

4. Make the root form in question 3 above into a combining form: _______________

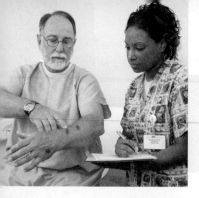

LESSON 3.4

Burns and Injuries to the Skin

CASE REPORT 3.4

YOU ARE . . . a burn technologist employed in the Burn Unit at Fulwood Medical Center.

YOU ARE COMMUNICATING WITH

. . . the son and daughter of Mr. Steven Hapgood, a 52-year-old man. Mr. Hapgood has been admitted to the Fulwood Burn Unit with severe burns over his face, chest, and abdomen. After an evening of drinking, he began smoking in bed and fell asleep. His next-door neighbors smelled smoke and called 911. In the Burn Unit, his initial treatment included large volumes of intravenous fluids to prevent **shock.**

Burns (LO 3.1, 3.2, 3.3, and 3.4)

Burns are the leading cause of accidental death. The immediate threats to life are from fluid loss, infection, and the systemic effects of burned dead tissue. Burn injury to the lungs through damage from heat or smoke inhalation is responsible for 60% or more of burn-related fatalities.

Burns are classified according to the depth of burnt tissue involved *(Figure 3.26):*

First-degree (superficial) burns involve only the epidermis and produce superficial **inflammation,** with redness, pain, and slight edema. Healing takes 3 to 5 days without scarring.

Second-degree (partial-thickness) burns involve the epidermis and dermis but leave some of the dermis intact. They produce redness, blisters, and more severe pain. Healing takes 2 to 3 weeks, with minimal scarring.

Third-degree (full-thickness) burns involve the epidermis, dermis, and subcutaneous tissues, which are often completely destroyed. Healing takes a long time and involves skin **grafts.**

Fourth-degree burns destroy all layers of the skin and involve underlying tendons, muscles, and, sometimes, bones.

▼ **FIGURE 3.26**
Partial- and Full-Thickness Burns.
(a) First degree (superficial thickness).
(b) Second degree (partial thickness).
(c) Third degree (full thickness).

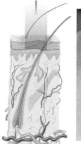 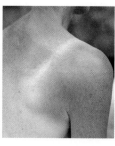 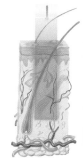 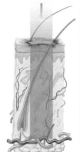 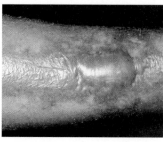 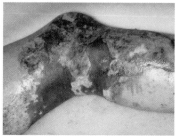

(a)   (b)   (c)

S = Suffix   P = Prefix   R = Root   R/CF= Combining Form

Word	Pronunciation	Elements		Definition
inflammation	in-flah-**MAY**-shun	S/ P/ R/	-ion *action, condition* in- *in* -flammat- *flame*	A complex of cell and chemical reactions occurring in response to an injury or chemical or biologic agent
inflammatory (adj)	in-**FLAM**-ah-tor-ee	S/	-ory *having the function of*	Causing or affected by inflammation
scald	**SKAWLD**		Latin *wash in hot water*	Burn from contact with hot liquid or steam
shock	**SHOCK**		German *to clash*	Sudden physical or mental collapse or circulatory collapse

EXERCISES

A. Review *the Case Report on this spread before answering the questions.*

1. Why is Mr. Hapgood in the Burn Unit and not on a regular surgical unit in the hospital?

_____

2. What areas of his body have the most severe burns? _____

3. How did Mr. Hapgood sustain these burns? _____

4. How do intravenous fluids get into the body? _____

5. What is the fluid treatment designed to prevent in Mr. Hapgood's case? _____

B. Lesson objectives: *Meet the lesson objectives with this exercise on burns. Employ your knowledge of medical terms from the integumentary system. Fill in the blanks.*

1. Hit by lightning:

    Degree of burn: _____   Symptoms: _____

    Layers of skin involved: _____

    What other specific type of injury/accident could produce this burn? _____

2. Scald:

    Degree of burn: _____   Symptoms: _____

    Layers of skin involved: _____

    What is a scald? _____

    How quickly does this heal? _____

3. Prolonged flame contact in a house fire:

    Degree of burn: _____   Symptoms: _____

    Layers of skin involved: _____

    What specific surgical procedure is used to promote healing for this type of burn? _____

4. Sunburn:

    Degree of burn: _____   Symptoms: _____

    Layers of skin involved: _____

    Why is this burn only superficial? _____

LESSON 3.4 Burns and Injuries to the Skin

(LO 3.1, 3.2, 3.3, and 3.4)

CASE REPORT 3.4 (CONTINUED)

Mr. Hapgood's burns were mostly third-degree. The burned, dead tissue formed an **eschar** that can have toxic effects on the digestive, respiratory, and cardiovascular systems. The eschar was surgically removed by **debridement**.

In full-thickness burns, because there is no dermal tissue left for **regeneration,** skin grafts are necessary. The ideal graft is an **autograft,** taken from another location on the patient's body, because it is not rejected by the immune system. Mr. Hapgood had autografts taken from his unburned legs and back.

If the patient's burns are too extensive, **allografts**—grafts from another person—are used. **Homograft** is another name for allograft. These grafts are provided by skin banks, which acquire them from deceased people **(cadavers).** A **xenograft** or **heterograft** is a graft from another species, such as a pig for heart valves.

In addition, artificial skin is being developed commercially and can stimulate the growth of new connective tissues from the patient's underlying tissue.

The treatment and prognosis for a burn patient also depend on how much of the body surface is affected. This is estimated by subdividing the skin's surface into regions, each one of which is a fraction of or multiple of 9% of the total surface area *(Figure 3.27)*. To give you a clearer idea of how these numbers come into play, the body's surface areas are assigned the following percentages:

- Head and neck = 9% (4½% anterior and posterior).
- Each arm = 9% (4½% anterior and 4½% posterior).
- Each leg = 18% (9% anterior and 9% posterior).
- The anterior trunk = 18%.
- The posterior trunk = 18%.
- Genitalia = 1%.

KEYNOTE

- In third- and fourth-degree burns, there is no dermal tissue left for regeneration, and skin grafts are necessary.

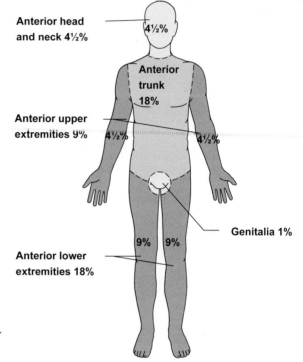

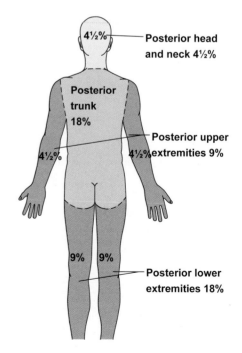

▶ **FIGURE 3.27**
Rule of Nines.

Word	Pronunciation	Elements		Definition
allograft	**AL**-oh-graft	P/ R/	allo- *other* -graft *transplant*	Skin graft from another person or a cadaver
autograft	**AWE**-toe-graft	P/ R/	auto- *self, same* -graft *transplant*	A graft removed from the patient's own skin
cadaver	kah-**DAV**-er		Latin *dead body*	A dead body or corpse
debridement	day-**BREED**-mon (French pronun- ciation of -ment)	S/ P/ R/	-ment *resulting state* de- *take away* -bride- *rubbish*	The removal of injured or necrotic tissue
eschar	**ESS**-kar		Greek *scab of a burn*	The burnt, dead tissue lying on top of third- degree burns
heterograft *(same as xenograft)*	**HET**-er-oh-graft	P/ R/	hetero- *different* -graft *transplant*	A graft from another species (not human)
homograft *(same as allograft)*	**HOH**-moh-graft	P/ R/	homo- *same, alike* -graft *transplant*	Skin graft from another person or a cadaver
regenerate (verb)	ree-**JEN**-eh-rate	S/ P/ R/	-ate *composed of* re- *again* -gener- *produce*	Reconstitution of a lost part
regeneration (noun)	ree-**JEN**-eh-**RAY**-shun	S/	-ation *process*	The process of reconstitution
xenograft *(same as heterograft)*	**ZEN**-oh-graft **HET**-er-oh-graft	P/ R/	xeno- *foreign* -graft *transplant*	A graft from another species (not human)

EXERCISES

A. Review *the Case Report on this spread before answering the questions.*

1. What is *dermal tissue?* _____

2. What degree of burns did Mr. Hapgood suffer? _____

3. The burned, dead tissue is referred to as: _____

4. What is the surgical procedure called that removes burned, dead tissue? _____

5. Why are grafts necessary for Mr. Hapgood _____

6. What is the ideal type of graft for Mr. Hapgood? _____

7. Why? _____

B. Employ *medical language in written communication. Insert the correct term from the spread on the appropriate blank; then proofread your paragraph for spelling errors.*

1. If the burn is deep enough, the tissue cannot _____ itself, and a skin graft is needed. This graft can come from the patient, _____, or from another person, _____, or even from another species _____. Grafts may also come from skin banks or _____

2. An _____ is taken from the patient; an _____ can come from another person. Donor skin comes from skin banks, which acquire skin from _____. A _____ is from a different species, not human. An example of this would be a _____ for the heart.

3. Two of the terms in question 2 are also known by another name. Write them below.

   _____ is the same as _____

   _____ is the same as _____

4. What other body systems can be affected by severe burns? _____

LESSON 3.4 Wounds and Tissue Repair (LO 3.1, 3.2, 3.3, and 3.4)

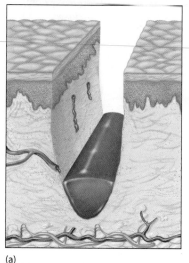

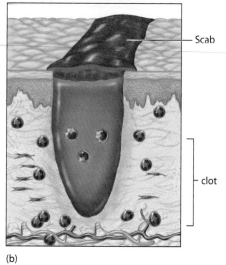

(a)

(b)

▲ **FIGURE 3.28**
Wound Healing.
(a) Bleeding into the wound. (b) Scab formation.

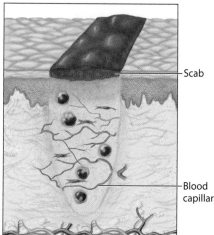

▲ **FIGURE 3.29**
Formation of Granulation Tissue.

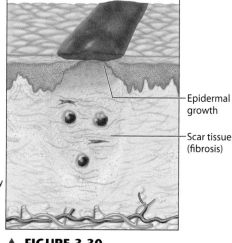

▲ **FIGURE 3.30**
Scar Formation.

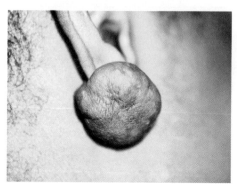

▲ **FIGURE 3.31**
A Keloid of the Earlobe.
This scar resulted from piercing the ear for earrings.

If you cut yourself when shaving and produce a superficial **laceration** in the epidermis, the epithelial (surface tissue) cells along the laceration's edges will split rapidly and fill in the gap to heal it.

If you cut yourself more deeply, creating a **wound** in the dermis or hypodermis, blood vessels in the dermis break and blood escapes into the wound *(Figure 3.28a).* The same happens when a surgeon makes an **incision.** On the other hand, a surgeon would perform an **excision** if he or she removed a lesion from the skin or any other tissue.

Escaped blood from a wound or surgical procedure forms a **clot** in the wound. The clot consists of the protein fibrin together with platelets, blood cells, and dried tissue fluids trapped in the fibers. Cells that digest and clean up the tissue debris enter the wound *(see Chapter 7).* The surface of the clot dries and hardens in the air to form a **scab.** The scab seals and protects the wound from becoming infected *(Figure 3.28b).*

New capillaries from the surrounding dermis then invade the clot. Three or four days after the injury, other cells migrate into the wound. These cells form new collagen fibers that pull the wound together. This soft tissue in the wound is called **granulation** tissue *(Figure 3.29),* which is later replaced by a scar *(Figure 3.30).*

Suturing brings together the edges of the wound to enhance tissue healing.

In some patients, there is excessive fibrosis and scar tissue, producing raised, irregular, lumpy, shiny scars called **keloids** *(Figure 3.31).* Keloids, most commonly found on the upper body and earlobes, can extend beyond the edges of the original wound and often return if they are surgically removed.

A superficial scraping of the skin, a mucous membrane, or the cornea *(Chapter 3)* is called an **abrasion.**

Surgery on the skin is now being performed using focused light beams called lasers. These lasers remove lesions like birthmarks and tattoos, and create a fresh surface over which new skin can grow.

Cosmetic Procedures (LO 3.1, 3.2, 3.3, and 3.4)

Surgical procedures that cosmetically alter or improve the appearance of your face or body are becoming more and more common. These cosmetic procedures include:

Abdominoplasty: a "tummy tuck."
Blepharoplasty: the correction of defects in the eyelids.
Dermabrasion: the removal of upper layers of skin using a high-powered rotating brush.
Lipectomy: the surgical removal of fatty tissue by excision.
Liposuction: the surgical removal of fatty tissue using suction.
Mammoplasty: the surgical procedure to alter the size or shape of the breasts.
Rhinoplasty: the surgical procedure to alter the size or shape of the nose.

Word	Pronunciation		Elements	Definition
abdominoplasty (tummy tuck)	ab-**DOM**-ih-noh-plas-tee	S/ R/CF	-plasty *surgical repair* abdomin/o- *abdomen*	Surgical removal of excess subcutaneous fat from abdominal wall
abrasion	ah-**BRAY**-shun		Latin *to scrape*	Area of skin or mucous membrane that has been scraped off
blepharoplasty	**BLEF**-ah-roh-plas-tee	S/ R/CF	-plasty *surgical repair* blephar/o- *eyelid*	Surgical repair of an eyelid
clot	**KLOT**		German *to block*	The mass of fibrin and cells that is produced in a wound
dermabrasion	der-mah-**BRAY**-shun	S/ R/ R/	-ion *action* derm- *skin* -abras- *scrape off*	Removal of upper layers of skin by rotary brush
granulation	gran-you-**LAY**-shun	S/ R/	-ation *process* granul- *small grain*	New fibrous tissue formed during wound healing
incision	in-**SIZH**-un	S/ R/	-ion *action, condition* incis- *cut into*	A cut or surgical wound
excision	ek-**SIZH**-un	R/	excis- *cut out*	Surgical removal of part or all of a structure
keloid	**KEY**-loyd		Greek *stain*	Raised, irregular, lumpy scar due to excess collagen fiber production during healing of a wound
laceration	lass-eh-**RAY**-shun	S/ R/	-ation *process* lacer- *to tear*	A tear or jagged wound of the skin caused by blunt trauma; not a cut
lipectomy	lip-**ECK**-toe-me	S/ R/	-ectomy *surgical excision* lip- *lipid, fat*	Surgical removal of adipose tissue
liposuction	**LIP**-oh-suck-shun	S/ R/CF R/	-ion *action* lip/o- *fat* -suct- *suck*	Surgical removal of adipose tissue using suction
mammoplasty	**MAM**-oh-plas-tee	S/ R/CF	-plasty *surgical repair* mamm/o- *breast*	Surgical procedure to change the size or shape of the breast
rhinoplasty	**RYE**-no-plas-tee	S/ R/CF	-plasty *surgical repair* rhin/o- *nose*	Surgical procedure to change the size or shape of the nose
scab	**SKAB**		Old English *crust*	Crust that forms over a wound or sore during healing
suture (noun) suture (verb)	**SOO**-chur		Latin *seam*	Stitch to hold the edges of a wound together To stitch the edges of a wound together
wound	**WOOND**		Old English *wound*	Any injury that interrupts the continuity of skin or a mucous membrane

EXERCISES

A. Wounds: *Use your knowledge of the meaning of the following medical terms to put them in the correct order of their appearance and give a brief description of each term. Fill in the chart.*

keloid   scab   clot   laceration   wound   granulation

Medical Term	Brief Description
1.	2.
3.	4.
5.	6.
7.	8.
9.	10.
11.	12.

B. Terminology challenge: *Precision in communication is using the correct medical term for the appropriate meaning.*

1. What is the difference between *abrasion* and *dermabrasion*? _____

2. Which term in the WAD is an accepted treatment for acne? _____

3. Consider the terms *clot* and *scab*. Which is inside the wound, and which is outside the wound? Inside: _____ Outside: _____

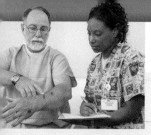

CHAPTER **3** REVIEW THE ANATOMY OF WORD CONSTRUCTION

CHALLENGE YOUR KNOWLEDGE

A. Prefixes *can work across all body systems and still have the same meaning. Hypo***dermic** *means pertaining to below the* **skin,** *while* hypo**gastr**ic *means pertaining to below the* **stomach.** *Prefix and suffix remain the same; only the body system root (derm and gastr) changes. Increase your medical vocabulary with a working knowledge of the following prefixes. Fill in the blanks.*

Prefix	Meaning of refix	Medical Term with this Prefix	Meaning of Medical Term
allo	1.	2.	3.
pro	4.	5.	6.
auto	7.	8.	9.
cryo	10.	11.	12.
de	13.	14.	15.
epi	16.	17.	18.
ex	19.	20.	21.
hetero	22.	23.	24.
homo	25.	26.	27.
hypo	28.	29.	30.
an	31.	32.	33.
syn	34.	35.	36.

B. Roots/Combining Forms *are the core foundations of every medical term. You are given a brief definition of a term. Construct the complete term by adding the correct R/CF. Fill in the blanks.*

1. inflammation of the skin _____ /itis

2. to scratch ex/ _____ /ate

3. medication against itching anti/ _____ /ic

4. infestation with lice _____ /osis

5. pertaining to poison _____ /ic

6. thickening of the skin due to excess collagen _____ /derma

7. infection alongside a nail para/ _____ /ia

8. surgical removal of injured or necrotic tissue de/ _____ /ment

9. skin graft from a cadaver homo/ _____

10. a tear of the skin _____ /ation

Remember: A root or combining form can begin or end a medical term, and it does not become a prefix or suffix. Its identity always remains a root, and every term needs at least one root.

C. Prefixes: *Continue working with the important prefixes in this chapter. These prefixes will appear again in succeeding chapters and terminology for other body systems. Knowing them will greatly increase your medical vocabulary. Fill in the blanks.*

Prefix	Meaning of Prefix	Medical Term with this Prefix	Meaning of Medical Term
in	1.	2.	3.
intra	4.	5.	6.
para	7.	8.	9.
re	10.	11.	12.
sub	13.	14.	15.
trans	16.	17.	18.
ultra	19.	20.	21.
xeno	22.	23.	24.

D. Train your eye and ear *to hear and see the slight differences in medical terms. System is not symptom, and a macule is not a papule. Briefly explain to your patient the differences in the following terms.*

1. system:

_____

symptom:

_____

2. macule:

_____

papule:

_____

E. Some Latin and Greek *terms cannot be further deconstructed into prefix, root, or suffix. You must know them for what they are. Test your knowledge of these terms with this exercise. There are more answer choices than you need.*

parasite	rosacea	tinea	impetigo
armpit	vesicle	cyst	fungus
psoriasis	toxin	verruca	macule

1. small sac containing liquid _____

2. organism living off another species _____

3. scabby eruption _____

4. wart _____

5. worm _____

6. poison _____

7. axilla _____

8. spot _____

9. sac, bladder _____

10. rosy _____

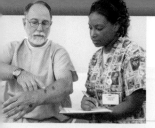

F. Spelling demons: *Every chapter contains some very difficult spelling demons. Challenge your ability to spell all these terms correctly. Circle the best choice below; then listen to the pronunciations on the Student Online Learning Center* (www.mhhe.com/AllanEss2e) *to be sure you can pronounce them correctly.*

1. allopecia   alopecia   allopechia

2. onchomycosis   onychomycosis   onycomycosis

3. zenograft   xenograft   zennograft

4. mamoplasty   manoplasty   mammoplasty

5. syntethis   synthetis   synthesis

6. sebaceous   sebeceous   sebacious

7. puritis   pruritis   pruritus

8. subcutaneous   subcutenious   subcutanous

9. sebborheic   seborrheic   seborheic

10. blefaroplasty   belpharoplasty   blepharoplasty

G. Review and recall, *from Chapters l through 3, all the suffixes that mean* pertaining to. *List them here.*

Pertaining to	Pertaining to	Pertaining to	Pertaining to
1.	2.	3.	4.
5.	6.	7.	8.
9.	10.	11.	12.
13.	14.	15.	16.

H. Partner exercise: *Ask your study partner to close his or her text. Dictate the following sentences to your partner, so that he or she can write them down on a separate piece of paper and then hand them back to you. Check your partner's sentences against the text below. The sentence is not correct unless every word is present and every word is spelled correctly. When you have finished checking your partner's answers, review them with him or her. Then close your book and ask your partner to dictate the sentences to you. Write them down on a separate piece of paper and have him or her check them and review them with you.*

1. Suturing brings together the edges of the wound to enhance tissue healing. In some people there is excessive fibrosis and scar tissue formation, which may produce a keloid.

2. A subcutaneous injection consists of using a longer needle to pierce the epidermis and dermis to reach the hypodermis or subcutaneous layer of skin.

3. The varicella-zoster virus causes chickenpox in unvaccinated people and can remain dormant in the peripheral nerves for decades before erupting as the painful vesicles of shingles.

Brain teaser: In the preceding sentence, what is the meaning of the word ***dormant?*** (Use your glossary or your dictionary, or go online to find out.) Define it on the lines below.

Dormant: _____

_____

I. **Seek and find:** *Some terms in this book are defined in context and do not appear in a WAD. These terms could also appear on a test, so pay attention to them! Here is a sample of terms that have appeared in this chapter. Challenge yourself to answer without turning back to check in the book. Fill in the blanks, and then check your spelling!*

What is another name for:

subcutaneous fat	1.
hives	2.
pressure ulcer	3.
allergic dermatitis	4.
shingles	5.
lice eggs	6.
itch mites	7.
cradle cap	8.
blackhead/whitehead	9.
thrush	10.
subcutaneous	11.
dead body	12.
allergic reaction	13.
warts	14.
armpits	15.
bottom	16.
cause	17.
athlete's foot	18.
base	19.
ringworm	20.

J. **Terminology challenge:** *Express yourself in medical vocabulary. Briefly explain how the terms diagnosis, prognosis, and etiology are related in the disease process.*

_____

_____

_____

_____

_____

_____

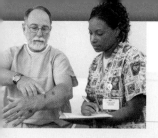

K. Make the connection: *In this exercise, each set of terms has something in common. Use the elements to help you determine what that is. Fill in the blanks.*

Medical   **Terms All Relate To:**

1. cuticle, paronychia, onychomycosis   _____

2. cadavers, skin banks, homograft   _____

3. mammoplasty, abdominoplasty, blepharoplasty   _____

4. integumentary, dermatitis, subcutaneous   _____

5. comedo, papule, vesicle   _____ _____

STUDY HINT

Equate it to an animal in English.

L. Create your own study hint *for the medical term rhinoplasty.*

_____

_____

_____

_____

M. Demonstrate your knowledge *of the language of dermatology by indicating whether the following medical terms are a diagnosis or a procedure. Place a check mark (✔) in the appropriate column.*

Medical Term	Diagnosis	Procedure
1. pruritus		
2. pediculosis		
3. biopsy		
4. debridement		
5. laceration		
6. abdominoplasty		
7. carcinoma		
8. autograft		
9. verruca		
10. stasis dermatitis		
11. rhinoplasty		
12. SLE		
13. lipectomy		

N. Difference between: *If you know the meaning of a term, you will be able to explain it to someone else. Briefly write how you would explain to a fellow student the difference between:*

1. vasoconstriction:

_____

_____

vasodilation:

_____

_____

2. incision:

_____

_____

excision:

_____

_____

3. infection:

_____

_____

infestation:

_____

_____

O. Chapter challenge: *Circle the correct answer.*

1. A *transdermal patch* can be used to administer:

   a. contraceptive hormones

   b. analgesics

   c. antinausea medications

   d. a, b, and c

   e. only a and c

2. The abbreviations **SC** and **IM** relate to:

   a. lobes of the lung

   b. body regions

   c. injection sites

   d. layers of a wound

   e. accessory skin organs

3. Tummy tuck, breast alteration, and nose alteration are:

   a. abdominoplasty, mammoplasty, and rhinoplasty

   b. liposuction, lipectomy, and blepharoplasty

   c. abdominoplasty, liposuction, and blepharoplasty

   d. dermabrasion, mammoplasty, and lipectomy

   e. abdominoplasty, dermabrasion, and blepharoplasty

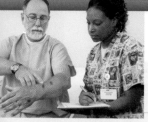

4. Burnt, dead tissue lying on top of third-degree burns is called:

   a. granulation

   b. keloid

   c. necrotizing

   d. eschar

   e. keratin

5. *Tinea pedis, capitis, corporis,* and *cruris* are all:

   a. bacterial infections

   b. viral infections

   c. fungal infections

   d. systemic infections

   e. parasitic infestations

6. Which three terms represent a process?

   a. abdominoplasty, biopsy, liposuction

   b. host, parasite, infestation

   c. cellulitis, pediculosis, dermatitis

   d. sebaceous glands, sweat glands, hair follicles

   e. intradermal, hypodermic, subcutaneous

7. *Comedones, papules, pustules*—if these three signs are present, what is the condition?

   a. necrotizing fasciitis

   b. acne

   c. onychomycosis

   d. scleroderma

   e. squamous cell carcinoma

8. A synonym for *subcutaneous* is:

   a. epidermal

   b. dermal

   c. intradermal

   d. hypodermic

   e. transdermal

9. Which medical term contains an element meaning *self?*

   a. allograft

   b. autograft

   c. homograft

   d. xenograft

   e. heterograft

10. The most common skin cancer and the least dangerous is:

   a. Kaposi sarcoma

   b. basal cell carcinoma

   c. melanoma

   d. squamous cell carcinoma

   e. herpes zoster

11. "Can extend beyond the edges of the original wound and often return if they are surgically removed." This describes:

   a. papules

   b. macules

   c. pustules

   d. scars

   e. keloids

12. Circle the pair of terms that have roots or combining forms meaning skin:

    a. seborrheic allergenic   **d.** nevus hypodermic

    b. dermatitis subcutaneous   **e.** integumentary shingles

    c. metastasize decubitus

13. Which pair of terms is spelled correctly?

    a. fascitis pediculosis   **d.** dermatomyositis alopecia

    b. staphylococus aureus   **e.** onycomycosis paronchia

    c. scleroderma soriasis

14. *Pimples, boils, carbuncles,* and *impetigo* can be caused by:

    a. papillomavirus   **d.** varicella

    b. herpes zoster   **e.** *Candida*

    c. staph

P. Case Report challenge: *Now that you are more comfortable with the terms in this chapter, you can apply that knowledge and briefly answer the questions about the Case Report. If you read the report through and underline all the medical terminology, this will make it easier to answer the questions.*

YOU ARE

. . . a burn technologist employed in the Burn Unit at Fulwood Medical Center.

YOU ARE COMMUNICATING WITH

. . . the son and daughter of Mr. Steven Hapgood, a 52-year-old man admitted to the Fulwood Burn Unit with severe burns over his face, chest, and abdomen. After an evening of drinking, he had been smoking in bed and fell asleep. His next-door neighbors in the apartment building smelled smoke and called 911. In the Burn Unit, his initial treatment included large volumes of intravenous fluids to prevent shock.

Mr. Hapgood's burns were mostly third-degree. The burned, dead tissue formed an eschar that can have toxic effects on the digestive, respiratory, and cardiovascular systems. The eschar was surgically removed by debridement.

1. Explain to Mr. Hapgood's son and daughter exactly which layers of skin are affected by his third-degree burn.

Use nonmedical language they can understand.

_____

_____

_____

_____

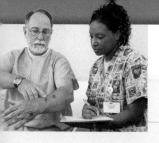

2. Explain to them also the surgical procedure their father is about to undergo.

_____

_____

_____

_____

3. Why does this procedure need to be performed?

_____

_____

_____

_____

4. What is meant by _toxic effects?_

_____

_____

_____

_____

5. Define *shock:*

_____

_____

_____

_____

6. Describe *eschar:*

_____

_____

_____

_____

7. Why do you think burn patients are kept in a separate unit and not mixed in with other medical/surgical patients?

_____

_____

_____

_____

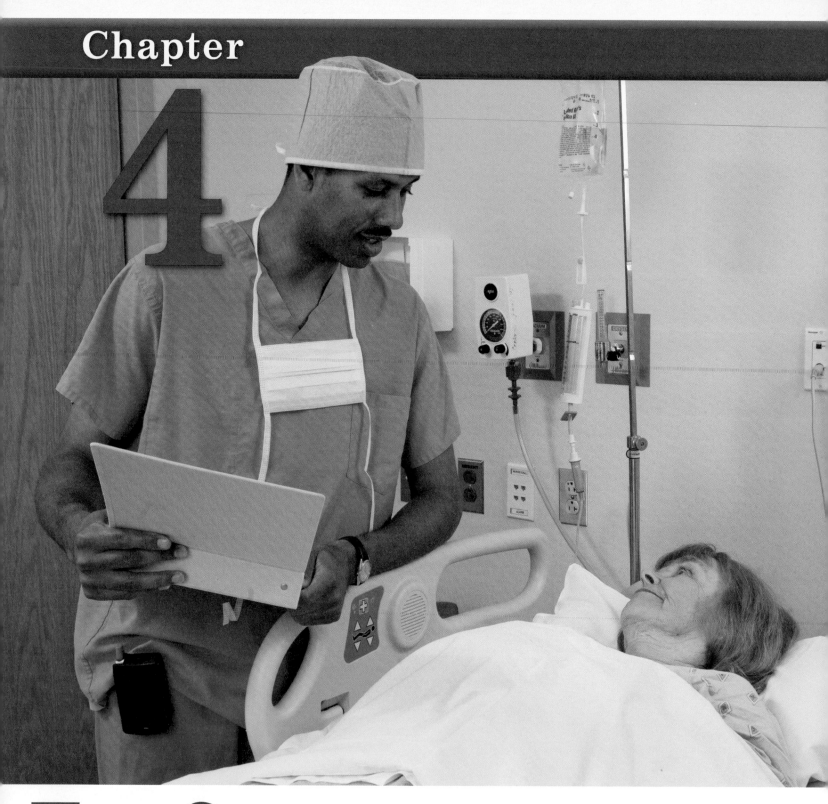

THE SKELETAL SYSTEM

The Essentials of the Language of Orthopedics

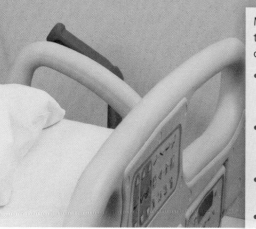

CASE REPORT 4.1

YOU ARE

. . . an orthopedic technologist working for Kenneth Stannard, MD, an orthopedist in the Fulwood Medical Group.

YOU ARE COMMUNICATING WITH

. . . Mrs. Amy Vargas, a 70-year-old housewife, who tripped while walking down the front steps of her house. She has severe pain in her right hip and is unable to stand. An X-ray shows a hip fracture and marked osteoporosis. Dr. Stannard examined her in the Emergency Department, and Mrs. Vargas is being admitted for a hip replacement.

Many health professionals are involved in the diagnosis and treatment of problems in the skeletal system. You may work directly and/or indirectly with one or more of the following:

- **Orthopedic surgeons (orthopedists)** are medical doctors **(MDs)** who deal with the prevention and correction of injuries of the skeletal system and associated **muscles**, joints, and ligaments.

- **Osteopathic physicians** have earned a doctor of osteopathy **(DO)** degree and receive additional training in the **musculoskeletal system** and how it affects the whole body.

- **Chiropractors (DC)** focus on the manual adjustment of joints—particularly the spine—in order to maintain and restore health.

- **Physical therapists** evaluate and treat pain, disease, or injury by physical therapeutic measures, as opposed to medical or surgical measures.

- **Physical therapist assistants** work under the direction of a physical therapist to assist patients with their physical therapy.

- **Orthopedic technologists** and **technicians** assist orthopedic surgeons in treating patients.

- **Podiatrists** are practitioners in the diagnosis and treatment of disorders and injuries of the foot.

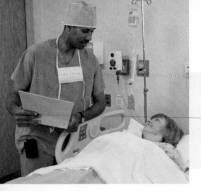

LESSON 4.1

Bones of the Skeletal System

OBJECTIVES

Without your bones, you'd be shapeless—unable to sit, stand, walk, or move your fingers and toes. Your skeleton supports and protects your organ systems, and it's the foundation for much of the medical terminology you will learn in this book. For example, the radial artery (used for taking a pulse) is so named because it travels beside the radial bone of the forearm.

Understanding the surface anatomy of bones and their markings will enable you to describe and document the sites of symptoms, signs, and diagnostic and therapeutic procedures. The information in this lesson will provide you with the confidence and skills for using correct medical terminology to:

4.1.1 Recognize the different health professionals involved in the diagnosis and treatment of skeletal problems.

4.1.2 Identify the tissues that form the skeletal system.

4.1.3 Discuss the structures and functions of the skeletal system.

4.1.4 Differentiate the types of bones in the skeletal system.

4.1.5 Evaluate the major problems and diseases that occur in the skeletal system.

ABBREVIATIONS

DO   Doctor of Osteopathy
MD   Doctor of Medicine
DC   Doctor of Chiropractic

Tissues and Functions of the Skeletal System

(LO 4.1, 4.2, and 4.3)

There are four components of the skeletal system *(Figure 4.1):*

1. **bones,**
2. **cartilage,**
3. **tendons,**
4. **and ligaments.**

Each plays an important role in the way your tissues and skeletal system function. Your skeletal system provides:

- **Support:** The bones of your vertebral column, pelvis, and legs hold up your body. The jawbone supports your teeth.

- **Protection:** The skull protects your brain. The vertebral column protects your spinal cord. The rib cage protects your heart and lungs.

- **Blood formation:** Bone marrow in many bones is the major producer of blood cells, including most of those in your immune system *(see Chapter 7).*

- **Mineral storage and balance**: The skeletal system stores calcium and phosphorus and releases them when your body needs them for other purposes.

- **Detoxification**: Bones remove metals like lead and radium from your blood, store them, and slowly release them for excretion.

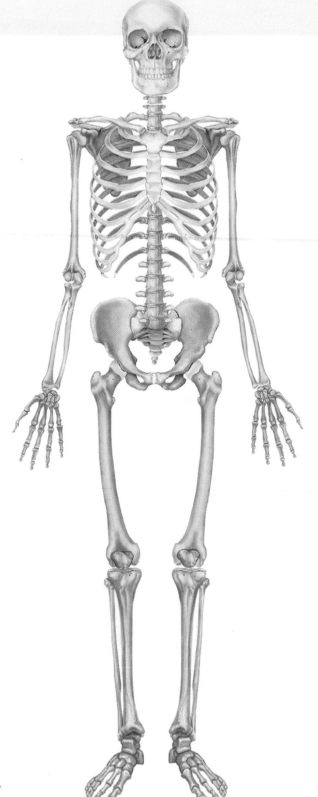

▶ **FIGURE 4.1**
Adult Skeletal System, Anterior View

Word	Pronunciation		Elements	Definition
cartilage	KAR-tih-lage		Latin *gristle*	Nonvascular, firm connective tissue found mostly in joints
chiropractic	kye-roh-**PRAK**-tik	S/ R/CF R/	-ic *pertaining to* chir/o- *hand* -pract- *efficient, practical*	Diagnosis, treatment, and prevention of mechanical disorders of the musculoskeletal system
chiropractor	kye-roh-**PRAK**-tor	S/	-or *a doer*	Practitioner of chiropractic
detoxification (Note: *same as detoxication*)	dee-**TOKS**-ih-fih-**KAY**-shun	S/ P/ R/	-fication *remove* de- *from, out of* -toxi- *poison*	Removing poison from a tissue or substance
ligament	**LIG**-ah-ment		Latin *band, sheet*	Band of fibrous tissue connecting two structures
muscle	**MUSS**-el		Latin *muscle*	A tissue consisting of cells that can contract
musculoskeletal	**MUSS**-kyu-loh-**SKEL**-eh-tal	S/ R/ R/CF	-al *pertaining to* muscul/o- *muscle* -skelet- *skeleton*	Pertaining to the muscles and the bony skeleton
orthopedic	or-tho-**PEE**-dik	S/ R/CF R/	-ic *pertaining to* orth/o- *straight* -ped- *child*	Pertaining to the correction and cure of deformities and diseases of the musculoskeletal system; originally, most of the deformities treated were in children
orthopedist	or-tho-**PEE**-dist	S/	-ist *specialist*	Specialist in orthopedics
osteopath	**OSS**-tee-oh-path	R/ R/CF	-path *disease* oste/o- *bone*	Practitioner of osteopathy
osteopathy	**OSS**-tee-**OP**-ah-thee	S/	-pathy *disease*	Medical practice based on maintaining the balance of the body
tendon	**TEN**-dun		Latin *sinew*	Fibrous band that connects muscle to bone

EXERCISES

A. Review *the Case Report on this spread before answering the questions.*

1. What kind of accident sent Mrs. Vargas to the ER? _____

2. What are her symptoms when she gets to the ER? _____

3. What diagnostic test did she have? _____

4. What did the test in question #3 above show? _____

5. What is the treatment plan for Mrs. Vargas? _____

B. Orthopedic vocabulary: *This exercise can be answered entirely by using medical terms that appear on the two pages open in front of you. Mastering these terms will start you on your way to learning the language of orthopedics. From the description, identify the correct medical terminology. Fill in the blanks.*

Description	Medical Term(s)
In addition to bones, which three terms are components of this chapter's body system?	1. 2. 3. 4
Which three terms refer to medical occupations?	5. 6.
Which term represents a medical practice based on maintaining balance of the body?	7.
Which term has an element meaning poison?	8.
What is the name of the body system in this chapter?	9.

► **FIGURE 4.2**
Femur: Long Bone of the Thigh.
(a) Anterior view. (b) Interior view.

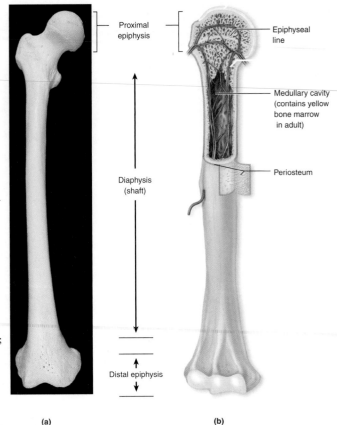

Proximal epiphysis

Epiphyseal line

Medullary cavity (contains yellow bone marrow in adult)

Periosteum

Diaphysis (shaft)

Distal epiphysis

(a)　　　(b)

Bones

(LO 4.1, 4.2, and 4.3)

Classification of Bones

(LO 4.1, 4.2, and 4.3)

The bones of your skeletal system are classified by their shape. Each falls into one of the following four shape categories:

- **Long** (considerably longer than they are wide), like the main bones of the limbs, palms, soles, fingers, and toes;

- **Short** (nearly as long as they are wide), like the bones of the wrists, ankles, and the patella (kneecap);

- **Flat,** like the bones of the skull and the ribs; or

- **Irregular,** like the vertebrae.

Structure of Bones

(LO 4.1, 4.2, and 4.3)

Think about how long your arms and legs are, and then consider how few bones make up all that length. In that context, it's likely no surprise that **long bones** are the most common bones in your body *(Figure 4.2)*. The shaft **(diaphysis)** of a long bone contains compact bone (also called **cortical** bone), while each end of the bone (the **epiphysis)** is composed of spongy bone. Sandwiched between the diaphysis and epiphysis are thin layers of cartilage cells in the **epiphysial plate** or **line** that allow your bones to grow longer.

A tough, connective tissue sheath called **periosteum** covers the outer surface of all bones; it protects the bone and anchors blood vessels and nerves to the bone's surface. Strong collagen fibers attach the periosteum to the cortical bone.

Inside the diaphysis is a hollow cylinder called the **medulla** *(Figure 4.2b)*, which contains bone **marrow,** a fatty tissue in adults. Red bone marrow with blood cells in varying stages of development can be found in the epiphyseal ends of the bone, the flat bones of the skull, the sternum, and the hip bones. Because red bone marrow is normally concentrated here, the medulla of the sternum and hip bone is the ideal source for bone marrow aspiration, a procedure where a needle is inserted into the bone to withdraw a sample of bone marrow fluid and cells to be checked for abnormalities.

Most bones have a strong blood supply *(Figure 4.3)* because of the blood vessels that travel through them in a system of small **Haversian canals.** The good supply of blood through your bones promotes healing.

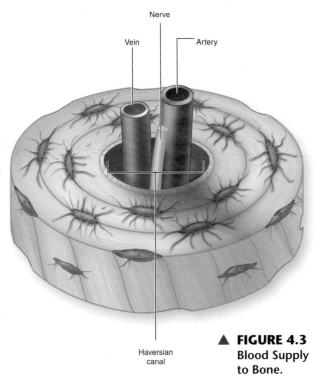

Nerve

Vein

Artery

Haversian canal

▲ **FIGURE 4.3**
Blood Supply to Bone.

Word	Pronunciation		Elements	Definition
cortex cortical (adj)	KOR-teks KOR-tih-cal	S/ R/	Latin *bark* -al *pertaining to* cortic- *cortex*	Outer portion of an organ, such as bone Pertaining to a cortex
diaphysis	die-AF-ih-sis		Greek *growing between*	The shaft of a long bone
epiphysis	eh-PIF-ih-sis	P/ R/	epi- *upon, above* -physis *growth*	Expanded area at the proximal and distal ends of a long bone to provide increased surface area for attachment of ligaments and tendons
epiphysial (adj) (Note: *The part "is" is deleted to enable the word to flow.*)	eh-PIF-ih-see-al	S/	-ial *pertaining to*	Pertaining to an epiphysis
Haversian canals	hah-VER-shan ka-NALS		Clopton Havers, English physician, 1655–1702	Vascular canals in bone
marrow	MAH-roe		Old English *marrow*	Fatty, blood-forming tissue in the cavities of long bones
medulla	meh-DULL-ah		Latin *marrow*	Central portion of a structure surrounded by cortex
medullary (adj)	meh-DULL-ah-ree	S/ R/	-ary *pertaining to* medulla- *medulla*	Pertaining to a medulla
periosteum	PER-ee-OSS-tee-um	S/ P/ R/	-um *structure* peri- *around* -oste- *bone*	Strong membrane surrounding a bone
periosteal (adj)	PER-ee-OSS-tee-al	S/	-al *pertaining to*	Pertaining to the periosteum

EXERCISES

A. Elements *remain your best clue for understanding a medical term. In this exercise, the meaning of each element is given below the line—this is your clue to constructing the term. Write the correct element on the line above its meaning. After you have constructed the term, give its definition in the space provided.*

1. _____ / _____ / _____
                           cortex   pertaining to

    The term is _____ and means _____.

2. _____ / _____ / _____
       around   bone   structure

    The term is _____ and means _____.

3. _____ / _____ / _____
      upon, above   growth   pertaining to

    The term is _____ and means _____.

4. _____ / _____ / _____
                       medulla   pertaining to

    The term is _____ and means _____.

B. Use this exercise *to review what you've learned about bones.*

1. Bones in the skeletal system are classified by their _____.

2. What are the most common types of bones in the body? _____.

3. What is another name for "compact" bone? _____.

4. Where can you find bone marrow? _____.

5. The strong blood supply in bones is provided by the _____.

6. The shaft of a long bone is called the _____.

LESSON 4.1 Diseases of Bone
(LO 4.1, 4.2, 4.3, and 4.4)

- Osteomalacia occurs in some developing nations and occasionally in this country when children drink soft drinks instead of milk fortified with vitamin D.

One of the major bone diseases is **osteoporosis,** which results from a loss of bone density *(Figure 4.4).* More common in women than in men, the incidence of osteoporosis increases with age. In the United States alone, 10 million people are living with osteoporosis and 18 million more have low bone density **(osteopenia).** Osteopenia puts people at risk for developing osteoporosis.

In women, production of the hormone estrogen decreases after menopause, weakening the body's protection against bone loss and potentially resulting in fragile, brittle bones. In men, lower levels of testosterone have a similar but less noticeable effect.

Women at risk for osteoporosis should have a bone mineral density **(BMD)** screening using a **DEXA** scan, which is a measuring device that uses low-energy radiation beams. Men and women over 50 are often advised to follow a daily regimen of 1,200 milligrams **(mg)** of calcium, 400 to 600 international units **(IU)** of vitamin D, and 15 minutes of real sun exposure. In addition, there are several **FDA**-approved medications available for treating osteoporosis.

Other bone diseases that may not be as prevalent or publicized as osteoporosis are the following:

Osteomyelitis: an inflammation in a bone area caused by a bacterial infection, such as staphylococcus.

Osteomalacia: a disease (known as **rickets** in children) caused by vitamin D deficiency where the calcium-lacking bones become soft and flexible, lose their ability to bear weight, and become bowed.

Achondroplasia: a very rare condition where the long bones stop growing in childhood, but the axial skeleton bones are not affected *(Figure 4.5).* People with this condition are short in stature, with the average adult measuring about 4 feet tall. Although intelligence and life span are normal, the disease is caused by a spontaneous gene mutation that then becomes a dominant gene for succeeding generations.

Osteogenic sarcoma: the most common malignant bone tumor, which often occurs around the knee joint. Peak incidence is between the ages of 10 and 15 years.

Osteogenesis imperfecta: a rare genetic disorder producing very brittle bones that are easily fractured or broken, often **in utero** (while inside the uterus).

CASE REPORT 4.1 (CONTINUED)

On questioning, Amy Vargas demonstrated many of the risk factors for osteoporosis, including family history, lack of exercise, cigarette smoking, inadequate diet, postmenopause, and increasing age.

ABBREVIATIONS

BMD	bone mineral density
DEXA	dual energy x-ray absorptiometry
FDA	Food and Drug Administration
IU	international unit(s)
mg	milligram

Normal bone   Osteoporotic bone

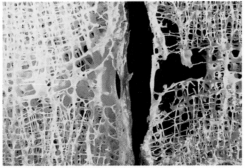

LM 5×

▲ **FIGURE 4.4**
Normal Bone and Osteoporotic Bone.

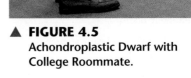

▲ **FIGURE 4.5**
Achondroplastic Dwarf with College Roommate.

S = Suffix   P = Prefix   R = Root   R/CF= Combining Form

Word	Pronunciation	Elements		Definition
achondroplasia	a-kon-droh-**PLAY**-zee-ah	S/ P/ R/CF	-plasia *formation* a- *without* -chondr/o- *cartilage*	Condition with abnormal, early conversion of cartilage into bone, leading to dwarfism
osteogenesis imperfecta	**OSS**-tee-oh-**JEN**-eh sis im-per-**FEK**-tah	S/ R/CF	-genesis *creation, formation* oste/o- *bone* imperfecta, Latin *unfinished*	Inherited condition when bone formation is incomplete, leading to fragile, easily broken bones
osteomalacia	**OSS**-tee-oh-mah-**LAY**-she-ah	S/ R/CF	-malacia *abnormal softness* oste/o- *bone*	Soft, flexible bones lacking in calcium (rickets)
osteomyclitis	**OSS**-tee-oh-my-eh-**LIE**-tis	S/ R/CF R/	-itis *inflammation* oste/o- *bone* -myel- *bone marrow*	Inflammation of bone tissue
osteopenia	**OSS**-tee-oh-**PEE**-nee-ah	S/ R/CF	-penia *deficient* oste/o- *bone*	Decreased calcification of bone
osteoporosis	**OSS**-tee-oh-poh-**ROE**-sis	S/ R/CF R/CF	-sis *condition* oste/o- *bone* -por/o- *opening*	Condition in which the bones become more porous, brittle, and fragile and more likely to fracture
rickets	**RICK**-ets		Old English *to twist*	Disease due to vitamin D deficiency, producing soft, flexible bones
sarcoma	sar-**KOH**-mah	S/ R/	-oma *tumor, mass* sarc- *flesh*	Malignant tumor originating in connective tissue
osteogenic sarcoma	**OSS**-tee-oh-**JEN**-ik sar-**KOH**-mah	S/ R/ R/CF	-ic *pertaining to* -gen- *creation* oste/o- *bone*	Malignant tumor originating in bone-producing cells

EXERCISES

A. Review *the Case Report on this spread before answering the questions.*

1. What is a *risk factor?* _____

2. What does *post menopause* mean? _____

3. What bone disease is Mrs. Vargas at risk to develop? _____

4. What does it mean if this diagnosis is *in her family history?* _____

5. How can Mrs. Vargas alter her lifestyle to improve her health? _____

6. Name the disease that puts people at risk to develop osteoporosis. _____

B. Suffixes: *The combining form oste/o means bone, and it is the main element in each of the following terms. You choose the correct suffix to complete the term. Fill in the blanks.*

genesis   genic   sarcoma   penia   malacia   porosis   myclitis

1. Disease caused by vitamin D deficiency   osteo/ _____

2. Low bone density   osteo/ _____

3. Porous, brittle, fragile bones   osteo/ _____

4. Most common malignant bone tumor   osteo/ _____

5. Rare genetic disorder producing easily fractured bones, often in utero   osteo/ _____

6. Inflammation of bone tissue   osteo/ _____

Note: *The meaning of the combining form never changes. The addition of six different suffixes has helped you learn six new terms in orthopedic vocabulary!*

LESSON 4.1 Bone Fractures (FXS) (LO 4.1, 4.2, 4.3, and 4.4)

▼ **TABLE 4.1**
Classification and Definition of Bone Fractures

Name	Description	Reference
Closed (also called **simple** fracture)	A bone is broken, but the skin is not broken.	Figure 4.6g
Open (also called **compound** fracture)	A fragment of the fractured bone breaks the skin, or a wound extends to the site of the fracture.	Figure 4.6e
Displaced	The fractured bone parts are out of line.	Figure 4.6e
Complete	A bone is broken into at least two fragments.	Figure 4.6a
Incomplete	The fracture does not extend completely across the bone. It can be hairline, as in a stress fracture in the foot, when there is no separation of the two fragments.	Figure 4.6a
Comminuted	The bone breaks into several pieces, usually two major pieces and several smaller fragments.	Figure 4.6b
Transverse	The fracture is at right angles to the long axis of the bone.	Figure 4.6b
Impacted	The fracture consists of one bone fragment driven into another, resulting in shortening of a limb.	Figure 4.6c
Spiral	The fracture spirals around the long axis of the bone.	Figure 4.6d
Oblique	The fracture runs diagonally across the long axis of the bone.	Figure 4.6d
Linear	The fracture runs parallel to the long axis of the bone.	Figure 4.6f
Greenstick	This is a partial fracture. One side breaks, and the other bends.	Figure 4.6g
Pathologic	The fracture occurs in an area of bone weakened by disease, such as cancer.	—
Compression	The fracture occurs in a vertebra from trauma or pathology, leading to the vertebra being crushed.	—
Stress	This is a fatigue fracture caused by repetitive, local stress on a bone, as occurs in marching or running.	—

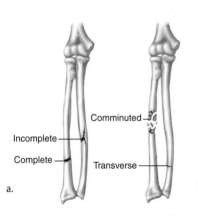

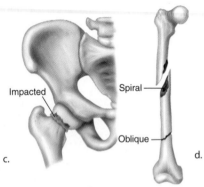

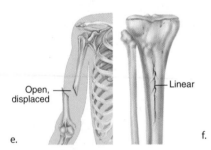

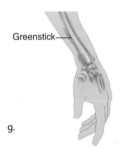

▲ **FIGURE 4.6**
Bone Fractures.

Healing of Fractures (LO 4.1, 4.2, 4.3, and 4.4)

When a bone is fractured, blood vessels bleed into the fracture site, forming a hematoma. After a few days, bone-forming cells called **osteoblasts** move in and start to produce new bone matrix, which develops into **osteocytes** (bone cells). Eventually the new bone fuses together the segments of the fracture.

Surgical Procedures for Fractures (LO 4.1, 4.2, 4.3, and 4.4)

The initial goal of fracture treatment is to bring the ends of the bone at the break back opposite each other so that they fit together as they did in the original bone. This is called **alignment.**

External manipulation is used frequently, sometimes with anesthesia. Here, the bone is pulled from the distal end (the farthest point from attachment) back into alignment through a process called **reduction.**

In **external fixation,** the alignment is maintained by immobilizing the bone via plaster casts, splints, traction, and/or **external fixators.** Traction involves applying gentle but continuous pulling force in order to align a fracture, reduce muscle spasms, and relieve pain. External fixators are implements, such as steel pins and rods, used to secure bone fragments together.

Word	Pronunciation	Elements		Definition
alignment	a-**LINE**-ment	S/ P/ R/	-ment *resulting state* a- *variant of ad, into* -lign- *line*	Having a structure in its correct position relative to others
comminuted	**KOM**-ih-nyu-ted	S/ R/	-ed *pertaining to* comminut- *break into pieces*	A fracture in which the bone is broken into pieces
malunion	mal-**YOU**-nee-un	S/ P/ R/	-ion *condition, action* mal- *bad, difficult* -un- *one*	When the two bony ends of the fracture fail to heal together correctly
nonunion	non-**YOU**-nee-un	P/	non- *not*	Total failure of healing of a fracture
osteoblast	**OSS**-tee-oh-blast	S/ R/CF	-blast *immature cell* oste/o- *bone*	A bone-forming cell
osteocyte	**OSS**-tee-oh-site	S/	-cyte *cell*	A bone-maintaining cell
pathologic fracture	path-oh-**LOJ**-ik **FRAK**-chur	S/ R/CF R/ S/ R/	-ic *pertaining to* path/o- *disease* -log- *to study* -ure *result of* fract- *to break*	Fracture occurring at a site already weakened by a disease process, such as cancer
reduction	ree-**DUCK**-shun	S/ P/ R/	-ion *action, condition* re- *backward* -duct- *lead*	Restore a structure to its normal position
traction	**TRAK**-shun		Latin *to pull*	Pulling or dragging force

EXERCISES

A. Deconstruct *the following medical terms into their basic elements. Then provide a brief definition for each term. Fill in the chart.*

Medical Term	Prefix	Root/CF	Suffix	Definition of Medical Term
reduction	1.	2.	3.	4.
alignment	5.	6.	7.	8.
malunion	9.	10.	11.	12.
pathologic	13.	14.	15.	16.
nonunion	17.	18.	19.	20.

B. Demonstrate *your understanding of the terms by finishing this exercise.*

1. What is the difference between an *osteoblast* and an *osteocyte?*

_____

_____

2. Use both *reduction* and *alignment* in one sentence.

_____

_____

3. What is the difference between an open and a closed fracture?

_____

_____

4. What type of preexisting condition might likely cause a pathologic fracture to occur?

_____

_____

5. Briefly explain the difference between a *malunion* and a *nonunion* of a fracture.

_____

_____

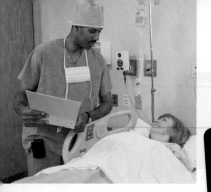

LESSON 4.2

Axial Skeleton

CASE REPORT 4.2

YOU ARE

. . . an orthopedic technologist working in the orthopedic department of Fulwood Medical Center with Dr. Kenneth Stannard.

YOU ARE COMMUNICATING WITH

. . . Ms. Nancy Cardenas, a 27-year-old jeweler, whose car was rear-ended by another car at a traffic light 3 days ago. Ms. Cardenas suffers from severe neck pain radiating down her left arm, as well as dizziness and headaches. She is unable to go to work. Dr. Stannard has examined her and diagnosed her condition as a **whiplash** injury. An MRI shows her-niation (rupture) of intervertebral discs between C5-C6 and C6-C7. Your role is to assist Dr. Stannard and document the care Ms. Cardenas receives to relieve her symptoms. Ms. Cardenas' whiplash injury caused protrusion of two cervical intervertebral discs. The centers of the discs bulge into the vertebral canal and pinch the nerves in such a way that the pain radiates to her left arm.

Structure of the Axial Skeleton (LO 4.1, 4.2, and 4.3)

Your axial skeleton, the upright axis of your body, includes the:

1. **vertebral column,**
2. **skull,**
3. and **rib cage.**

The axial skeleton protects the brain, **spinal cord,** heart, and lungs—most of the major centers of human physiology.

Within the vertebral column, there are 26 bones divided into the following five regions *(Figure 4.7):*

- **Cervical** region, with 7 **vertebrae,** labeled C1 to C7 and curved anteriorly;
- **Thoracic** region, with 12 vertebrae, labeled T1 to T12 and curved posteriorly;
- **Lumbar** region, with 5 vertebrae, labeled L1 to L5 and curved anteriorly;
- **Sacral** region, with 5 bones that in early childhood fuse into 1 bone curved posteriorly; and
- **Coccyx** (tailbone), with 4 small bones fused together into 1 bone curved posteriorly.

The spinal cord lies protected in the vertebral canal of the vertebral column. Spinal nerves travel from the spinal cord to other parts of the body through the intervertebral foramina.

Intervertebral discs consisting of fibrocartilage (a form of cartilage) are also found in the axial skeleton. These discs inhabit the intervertebral space between the bodies of adjacent vertebrae and provide extra support and cushioning (acting as shock absorbers) for the vertebral column.

The vertebral column, like any other body part, is susceptible to injury and disease. One common disorder of the vertebral column is **scoliosis,** an abnormal lateral curvature of the **spine** that occurs in both children and adults. Abnormal curvature of the spine is more common in older people, particularly those with osteoporosis; in this case, the normal anteriorly concave curvature in the thoracic region (**kyphosis**) is exaggerated.

FIGURE 4.7
Vertebral Column, Lateral View.

Cervical region (curved anteriorly)

Thoracic region (curved posteriorly)

Intervertebral disc

Intervertebral foramina
First lumbar vertebra

Lumbar region (curved anteriorly)

Fifth lumbar vertebra
Sacral promontory

Sacral and coccygeal regions (curved posteriorly)

Sacrum

Coccyx

Word	Pronunciation		Elements	Definition
cervical	SER-vih-kal	S/ R/	-al *pertaining to* cervic- *neck*	Pertaining to the neck region
coccyx	KOK-sicks		Greek coccyx	Small tailbone at the lowest end of the vertebral column
kyphosis	ki-FOH-sis	S/ R/	-osis *condition* kyph- *bent, humpback*	A normal posterior curve of the spine that can be exaggerated in disease
kyphotic (adj)	ki-FOT-ik	S/ R/CF	-tic *pertaining to* kyph/o- *bent, humpback*	Pertaining to or suffering from kyphosis
lumbar	LUM-bar		Latin *loin*	The region of the back and sides between the ribs and pelvis
sacrum	SAY-crum		Latin *sacred*	Segment of the vertebral column that forms part of the pelvis
sacral (adj)	SAY-kral	S/ R/	-al *pertaining to* sacr- *sacrum*	Pertaining to or in the neighborhood of the sacrum
scoliosis	skoh-lee-OH-sis	S/ R/	-osis *condition* scoli- *crooked*	An abnormal lateral curvature of the vertebral column
scoliotic (adj)	SKOH-lee-OT-ik	S/ R/CF	-tic *pertaining to* scoli/o- *crooked*	Pertaining to or suffering from scoliosis
spine	SPINE		Latin *spine*	Vertebral column or a short projection from a bone
spinal (adj)	SPY-nal	S/ R/	-al *pertaining to* spin- *spine*	Pertaining to the spine
vertebra vertebrae (pl) vertebral (adj)	VER-teh-brah VER-teh-bree VER-teh-bral	S/ R/	-al *pertaining to* vertebr- *vertebra*	One of the bones of the spinal column Pertaining to a vertebra
whiplash	HWIP-lash	R/ R/	whip- *to swing* -lash *end of whip*	Symptoms caused by sudden, uncontrolled extension and flexion of the neck, often in an automobile accident

EXERCISES

A. Review *the Case Report on this spread before answering the questions.*

1. What are Ms. Cardenas' symptoms? _____

2. What type of accident was she involved in? _____

3. Define the abbreviation MRI in words. _____

4. Describe herniation of a disc. _____

5. What does *intervertebral* mean? _____.

6. Where does the radiating pain in her left arm originate? _____.

7. The "C" in "C5-C6" means _____.

B. Apply *the correct form of the bolded similar terms appropriately in the following documentation, and you will meet a chapter objective! Fill in the blanks.*

vertebra   **vertebral**   **vertebrae**

1. The patient's C5 _____ was fractured in the accident.

2. A part of the axial skeleton is the _____ column.

3. The patient's C5 and C6 _____ were fractured in the accident.

   Now supply the missing terms to complete the following sentence.

4. The designations C5-C6 and C6-C7 are for locations of _____.

LESSON **4.2** Skull and Face

(LO 4.1, 4.2, and 4.3)

The Skull (LO 4.1, 4.2,and 4.3)

When you glance at your face in the mirror, chances are you're not thinking about what's behind your brown eyes or your slightly crooked smile. You see one image—not its layers, pieces, or parts. However, the human skull *(Figure 4.8)* is made up of 22 separate bones. Your **cranium,** the upper part of the skull that encloses the **cranial** cavity and protects the brain, contains 8 of these 22 bones; your facial skeleton contains the rest.

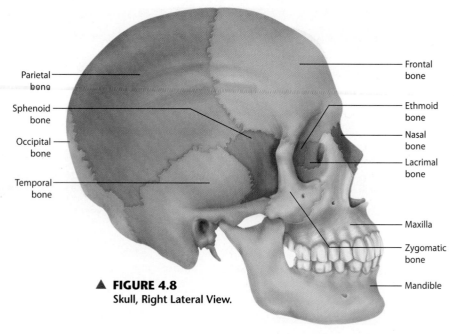

▲ **FIGURE 4.8**
Skull, Right Lateral View.

The bones of the cranium are joined together by sutures (joints that appear as seams), which are covered on the inside and outside by a thin layer of connective tissue. These bones have the following functions:

1. The **frontal** bone forms the forehead, roofs of the (eye) orbits, and part of the floor of the cranium, and contains a pair of right and left frontal sinuses above the orbits.
2. **Parietal** bones form the bulging sides and roof of the cranium.
3. The **occipital** bone forms the back of and part of the base of the cranium.
4. **Temporal** bones form the sides of and part of the base of the cranium.
5. The **sphenoid** bone forms part of the base of the cranium and the orbits.
6. The **ethmoid** bone is hollow and forms part of the nose, the orbits, and the ethmoid sinuses.

The lower part of the skull houses the bones of the facial skeleton *(Figure 4.9).* These bones do the following:

1. **Maxillary** bones form the upper jaw **(maxilla),** hold the upper teeth, and are hollow, forming the maxillary sinuses.
2. **Palatine** bones are located behind the maxilla and cannot be seen on a lateral view of the skull.
3. **Zygomatic** bones are the prominences of the cheeks (cheekbones) below the eyes.
4. **Lacrimal** bones form the medial wall of each orbit.
5. **Nasal** bones form the sides and bridge of the nose.
6. The **mandible** is the lower jawbone, which holds the lower teeth. The mandible articulates (joins) with the temporal bone to form the **temporomandibular joint (TMJ).**

The third component of the axial skeleton, the rib cage, is discussed in Chapter 7, "Respiratory System."

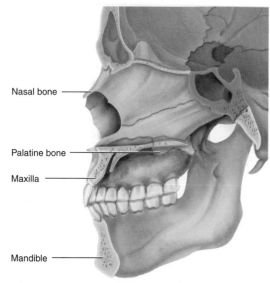

▲ **FIGURE 4.9**
Facial Bones.

Word	Pronunciation		Elements	Definition
cranium	KRAY-nee-um		Greek *skull*	The upper part of the skull that encloses and protects the brain
cranial (adj)	KRAY-nee-al	S/ R/	-al *pertaining to* crani- *skull*	Pertaining to the skull
ethmoid	ETH-moyd	S/ R/	-oid *resembling* ethm- *sieve*	Bone that forms the back of the nose and encloses numerous air cells
lacrimal	LAK-rim-al	S/ R/	-al *pertaining to* lacrim- *tears*	Lacrimal bone forms part of the medial wall of the orbit, *or* pertaining to tears
mandible mandibular (adj)	MAN-di-bel man-DIB-you-lar	S/ R/	Latin *jaw* -ar *pertaining to* mandibul- *mandible*	Lower jaw bone Pertaining to the mandible
maxilla	mak-SILL-ah		Latin *jawbone*	Upper jawbone, containing right and left maxillary sinuses
maxillary (adj)	mak-SILL-ah-ree	S/ R/	-ary *pertaining to* maxilla- *maxilla*	Pertaining to the maxilla
occipital	ock-SIP-it-al	S/ R/	-al *pertaining to* occipit- *back of the head*	The back of the skull
palatine	PAL-ah-tine	S/ R/	-ine *pertaining to* palat- *palate*	Bone that forms the hard palate and parts of the nose and orbits
parietal	pah-RYE-eh-tal	S/ R/	-al *pertaining to* pariet- *wall*	The two bones forming the sidewalls and roof of the cranium
sphenoid	SFEE-noyd	S/ R/	-oid *resemble* sphen- *wedge*	Wedge-shaped bone at the base of the skull
temporal	TEM-pore-al	S/ R/	-al *pertaining to* tempor- *time*	Bone that forms part of the base and sides of the skull
temporomandibular joint (TMJ)	TEM-pore-oh-man-DIB-you-lar JOYNT	S/ R/CF R/	-ar *pertaining to* tempor/o- *temple* -mandibul- *mandible*	The joint between the temporal bone and the mandible
zygoma zygomatic (adj)	zye-GO-mah zye-go-MAT-ik	S/ R/	French *yoke* -ic *pertaining to* zygomat- *cheekbone*	Bone that forms the prominence of the cheek Pertaining to the cheekbone

EXERCISES

A. Roots: *The following medical terms from the WAD box are alike in that they have similar suffixes, but their roots make them different terms. Define each term after you have defined the suffix. Fill in the blanks.*

1. oid means _____.

ethmoid: _____

sphenoid: _____

2. al means _____.

lacrimal: _____

cranial: _____

B. Apply *the language of orthopedics and circle the correct answer.*

1. The mandible is the:

lower jawbone   base of the cranium   upper jawbone

2. Which of these bones is NOT in the facial skeleton?

lacrimal   frontal   patella

3. How many bones are in the cranium?

22   8   14

4. What does *articulate* mean?

stretches   fractures   joins

5. What is a *suture*?

seam   bend   sharp point

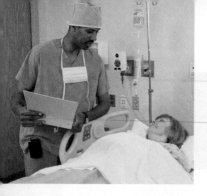

LESSON 4.3

Bones and Joints of the Shoulder Girdle and Upper Limb

OBJECTIVES

Your shoulders, arms, hands, and fingers are used nearly every time you move your body, no matter where you are—at work, at home, at the gym, in the car, or relaxing on the beach. Because these bones and joints get so much use, it's necessary to understand how they work and how to care for them. The information in this lesson will enable you to use correct medical terminology to:

4.3.1 Recognize the structures and functions of the bones and joints of the shoulder girdle.

4.3.2 Explain common disorders of the bones and joints of the shoulder girdle.

4.3.3 Identify the structures and functions of the bones and joints of the arm, elbow, and wrist.

4.3.4 Describe common disorders of the bones and joints of the arm, elbow, and wrist.

4.3.5 Specify the structures and functions of the bones and joints of the hand.

4.3.6 Define common disorders of the bones and joints of the hand.

ABBREVIATION

AC   acromioclavicular

Shoulder Girdle (LO 4.1, 4.2, and 4.3)

The bones and joints of your shoulder girdle connect your axial skeleton to your upper limbs.

The bones of the shoulder girdle are the **scapulae** (shoulder blades) and **clavicles** (collarbones). The scapula extends over the top of the shoulder joint to form a roof called the **acromion,** which is attached to the clavicle at the **acromioclavicular (AC)** joint. Several ligaments hold together the **articulating** surfaces of the humerus and scapula.

The shoulder joint between the scapular and the **humerus** bone of the upper arm *(Figure 4.10)* is a ball-and-socket joint, allowing the head of the humerus greater range of motion than any other joint in the body. This broad range of motion does have one drawback; because the shoulder joint is very unstable, it's prone to **dislocation.**

Disorders of the Shoulder Girdle
(LO 4.1, 4.2, 4.3, and 4.4)

Shoulder separation is a dislocation of the acromio-clavicular joint, often caused by a fall onto the point of the shoulder.

Shoulder dislocation occurs when the ball of the humerus slips out of the scapula's socket, usually anteriorly.

Shoulder subluxation occurs when the ball of the humerus slips partially out of position in the socket, and then moves back in.

CASE REPORT 4.3

YOU ARE

. . . an orthopedic technologist working with Kenneth Stannard, MD, at Fulwood Medical Center.

YOU ARE COMMUNICATING WITH

. . . James Fox, a 17-year-old male who complains of severe pain in his right wrist. While playing soccer a few hours earlier, he fell. James pushed his hand out to break his fall and heard his wrist snap. The wrist is now swollen and deformed.
T 98.2, P 92, R 15, BP 110/76. On examination, his right wrist is swollen, tender, and has a dinner-fork deformity. An IV has been started, and he has been given 3 mg of morphine IV. An X-ray of the wrist has been ordered.

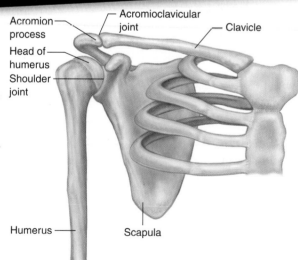

▲ **FIGURE 4.10**
Pectoral Girdle and Humerus.

S = Suffix   P = Prefix   R = Root   R/CF= Combining Form

Word	Pronunciation	Elements		Definition
acromion	ah-**CROW**-mee-on		Greek *tip of the shoulder*	Lateral end of the scapula, extending over the shoulder joint
acromioclavicular	ah-**CROW**-mee-oh-klah-**VICK**-you-lar	S/ R/CF R/	-ar *pertaining to* acromi/o- *acromion* -clavicul- *clavicle*	The joint between the acromion and the clavicle
articulate	ar-**TIK**-you-late	S/ R/	-ate *composed of* articul-*joint*	Two separate bones have formed a joint
articulation	ar-tik-you-**LAY**-shun	S/	-ation *process*	A joint
clavicle	**KLAV**-ih- kul		Latin *collarbone*	Curved bone that forms the anterior part of the pectoral girdle
clavicular (adj)	klah-**VICK**-you-lah	S/ R/	-ar *pertaining to* clavicul- *clavicle*	Pertaining to the clavicle
dislocation	dis-low-**KAY**-shun	S/ P/ R/	-ion *action, condition* dis- *apart, away from* -locat- *place*	Completely out of joint
humerus	**HYU**-mer-us		Latin *shoulder*	Single bone of the upper arm
pectoral	**PEK**-tor-al	S/ R/	-al *pertaining to* pector- *chest*	Pertaining to the chest
pectoral girdle	**PEK**-tor-al **GIR**-del		girdle, Old English *encircle*	Incomplete bony ring that attaches the upper limb to the axial skeleton
scapula scapulae (pl) scapular (adj)	**SKAP**-you-lah **SKAP**-you-lee **SKAP**-you-lar	S/ R/	-ar *pertaining to* scapul- *scapula*	Shoulder blade Pertaining to the shoulder blade
subluxation	sub luck-**SAY**-shun	S/ P/ R/	-ion *action, condition* sub- *under, below, slightly* -luxat- *dislocate*	An incomplete dislocation when some contact between the joint surfaces remains

EXERCISES

A. Review *the Case Report on this spread before answering the questions.*

1. What are Mr. Fox's complaints when he presents at Dr. Stannard's office? _____

2. What is discovered on Mr. Fox's physical examination? _____

3. IV is the abbreviation for the medical term: _____

4. Why are they giving Mr. Fox morphine? _____

5. What diagnostic test has been ordered for Mr. Fox? _____

B Build medical terms *using the language of orthopedics to complete this exercise. Each term is defined and partially complete. Add the rest of the elements to complete the term, and write under the line the element(s) you have used. The first one is done for you. Fill in the blanks*

1. incomplete dislocation _____sub_____ / _____luxat_____ / _____ion_____
                                                  P   R   S

2. joint between acromion and clavicle _____ / _____ / _____ar_____

3. a joint _____ / _____ / _____ation_____

4. pertaining to the shoulder blade _____ / _____ / _____ar_____

LESSON 4.3 Upper Arm and Elbow Joint
(LO 4.1, 4.2, and 4.3)

Your upper arm extends from your shoulder to your elbow and contains only one bone, the humerus *(Figure 4.11)*. The smooth surface of the hemispherical head that articulates with the socket of the scapula is covered with articular cartilage. At the lower end of the humerus, the **trochlea** articulates with the **ulna** bone of the forearm and the **capitulum** articulates with the **radius** *(Figure 4.12)*.

Elbow Joint
(LO 4.1, 4.2, and 4.3)

The elbow joint has two articulations:

1. A hinge joint between the humerus and the ulna bone of the forearm, which allows flexion and extension of the elbow; and

2. A gliding joint between the **humerus** and the radius bone of the forearm, which allows **pronation** and **supination** of the forearm and hand.

Disorders of the Elbow Joint
(LO 4.1, 4.2, 4.3, and 4.4)

When you bend your elbow, you can easily feel the bony prominence (the **olecranon**) that extends from the ulna. The olecranon can be easily fractured by a direct blow to the elbow or by a fall on a bent elbow.

When a child falls on an outstretched arm, the force of hitting the ground can be transmitted up the arm to cause a fracture of the elbow joint. This accounts for about 10% of all fractures in children.

Anterior surface

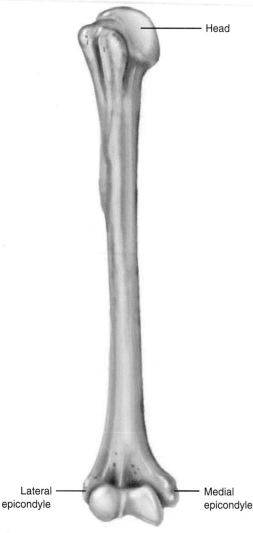

Head

Lateral epicondyle

Medial epicondyle

▲ **FIGURE 4.11**
Humerus.

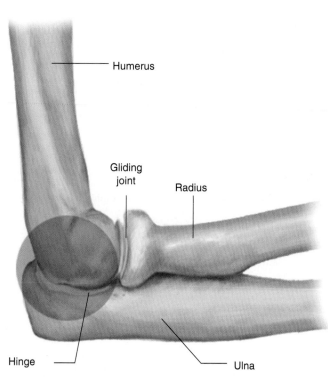

Humerus

Gliding joint

Radius

Hinge

Ulna

▲ **FIGURE 4.12**
Elbow Joint.

Word	Pronunciation	Elements		Definition
capitulum	kah-**PIT**-you-lum	S/ R/CF	-lum *small structure* capit/u *small head*	A small head or rounded extremity of a bone
pronation pronate (verb)	pro-**NAY**-shun **PRO**-nate	S/ R/	-ion *action, condition* pronat- *bend down*	Process of lying face down or of turning a hand or foot with the volar (palm or sole) sur- face down
prone	**PRONE**		Latin, *lying down*	Lying face down, flat on your belly
radius radial (adj)	**RAY**-dee-us **RAY**-dee-al	S/ R/	Latin *spoke of a wheel* -al *pertaining to* radi- *radius*	The forearm bone on the thumb side Pertaining to the radius or to any of the struc- tures (artery, vein, nerve) named after it
supination	soo-pih-**NAY**-shun	S/ R/	-ion *action, condition* supinat- *bend backward*	Process of lying face upward or of turning a hand or foot so that the palm or sole is fac- ing up
supine	soo-**PINE**		Latin *bend backward*	Lying face up, flat on your spine
trochlea	**TROHK**-lee-ah		Latin *pulley*	Smooth articular surface of bone on which another glides
trochlear	**TROHK**-lee-ar	S/ R/	-ar *pertaining to* trochle- *pulley*	Pertaining to a trochlea
ulna ulnar (adj)	**UL**-nah **UL**-nar	S/ R/	Latin *elbow, arm* -ar *pertaining to* uln- *ulna*	The medial and larger bone of the forearm Pertaining to the ulna or to any of the struc- tures (artery, vein, nerve) named after it

EXERCISES

A. Meet lesson *and chapter objectives by answering these questions using the language of orthopedics.*

1. What two types of articulations exist in the elbow?

_____

2. The upper arm has only one bone—the _____

3. What type of joint allows flexion and extension? _____

4. List the common disorders of the elbow joint: _____

5. What does the trochlea articulate with? _____

6. What is the bone of your upper arm that extends from the shoulder to the elbow? _____

7. Based on its shape, what kind of bone is #6? _____

8. What are the two opposite terms in this WAD? _____ and _____

9. Is the radius a forearm bone or an upper arm bone? _____

10. Which is the bigger bone: the radius or the ulna? _____

B. The statement *is either true or false. Circle the correct answer.*

1. The opposite of pronation is supination.   T   F
2. The capitulum articulates with the scapula.   T   F
3. A sports-related injury is very common in the elbow.   T   F
4. The radius is on the thumb side of the hand.   T   F
5. A hinge joint allows pronation of the hand and forearm.   T   F

The Wrist
(LO 4.1, 4.2, and 4.3)

In your forearm, the radius bone on the thumb side and the larger ulna bone on the little-finger side articulate at your wrist joint with the small **carpal** bones *(Figure 4.13)*.

Disorders of the Wrist
(LO 4.1, 4.2, 4.3, and 4.4)

A **Colles fracture** is a common fracture of the radius just above the wrist joint *(Figure 4.14)* that occurs when a person tries to break a fall with an outstretched hand.

Fracture of the scaphoid bone *(Figure 4.13)*—the most common fracture of a carpal bone—also results from breaking a fall with an outstretched hand, but poor blood supply here makes healing slow and difficult.

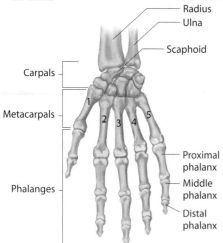

Radius
Ulna
Scaphoid
Carpals
Metacarpals
1 2 3 4 5
Phalanges
Proximal phalanx
Middle phalanx
Distal phalanx

▲ **FIGURE 4.13**
Bones of the Wrist and Hand.

CASE REPORT 4.3 (CONTINUED)

The X-ray of James Fox's wrist showed a **Colles fracture** of the radius, 1 inch above the end of the bone. Dr. Stannard applied a cast with the **distal** fragment of the fracture in palmar flexion and ulnar deviation. Mr. Fox was sent home with Vicodin 500 mg **po, prn,** for pain, and an appointment to return to the clinic in a week.

The Hand (LO 4.1, 4.2, and 4.3)

The five fingers of your single hand have 14 bones called **phalanges.** The thumb has two phalanges, and each of the remaining four fingers has three *(Figure 4.13)*. In your palm, the five bones closest to the fingers are **metacarpals;** these connect to the phalanges at the **metacarpophalangeal** joints. The metacarpals connect at the wrist to eight small carpal bones, which then connect the hand to the bones of the forearm. All of these bones require numerous joints with ligaments to connect and stabilize them.

Disorders of the Hand (LO 4.1, 4.2, 4.3, and 4.4)

Osteoarthritis (OA) in the hand joints occurs from wear and tear leading to deterioration of joint cartilage. Small bony spurs called **Heberden nodes** form over the joint *(Figure 4.15)*.

Rheumatoid arthritis (RA), with destruction of joint surfaces, joint capsules, and ligaments, leads to noticeable deformity and joint instability *(Figure 4.16)*. RA occurs mostly in women, between ages 40 and 60, and affects the synovial membrane lining the joints and tendons. Lumps known as **rheumatic** nodules form over the small joints of the hand and wrist.

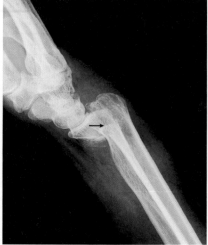

▲ **FIGURE 4.14**
X-Ray of Colles Fracture.

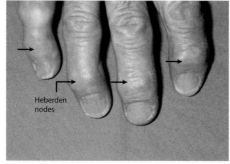

Heberden nodes

▲ **FIGURE 4.15**
Hand with Osteoarthritis.

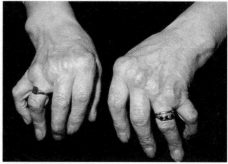

▲ **FIGURE 4.16**
Hands with Rheumatoid Arthritis.

S = Suffix   P = Prefix   R = Root   R/CF= Combining Form

Word	Pronunciation	Elements		Definition
arthritis	ar-**THRI**-tis	S/ R/	-itis *inflammation* arthr- *joint*	Inflammation of a joint or joints
carpus carpal (adj) metacarpal	**KAR**-pus **KAR**-pal **MET**-ah-**KAR**-pal	S/ R/ P/	Greek *wrist* -al *pertaining to* carp- *wrist bones* meta- *after, subsequent to*	The eight carpal bones of the wrist Pertaining to the wrist The five bones between the carpus and the fingers
Colles fracture	**KOL**-ez **FRAK**-chur		Abraham Colles, Irish surgeon, 1773–1843	Fracture of the distal radius at the wrist
eponym	**EH**-po-nim		Greek *epōnymos, meaning eponymous*	A procedure or a diagnosis with a name derived from the name of the person who discovered it (if it is a disease or condition) or originated it (if it is a procedure)
Heberden node	**HEH**-ber-den **NOHD**		William Heberden, English physician, 1710–1801	Bony lump on the terminal phalanx of the fingers in osteoarthritis
metacarpophalangeal	**MET**-ah-**KAR**-poh-fay-**LAN**-jee-al	S/ P/ R/CF R/CF	-al *pertaining to* meta- *after, subsequent to* -carp/o- *bones of the wrist* -phalang/e- *phalanx, finger or toe*	The joints between the metacarpal bones and the phalanges
osteoarthritis	**OSS**-tee-oh-ar-**THRI**-tis	S/ R/CF R/	-itis *inflammation* oste/o- *bone* arthr- *joint*	Chronic inflammatory disease of joints
phalanx phalanges (pl)	**FAY**-lanks fay-**LAN**-jeez		Latin *bone of finger or toe*	One of the bones of the digits (fingers or toes)
rheumatism rheumatic (adj) rheumatoid arthritis	**RU**-mat-izm ru-**MAT**-ik **RU**-mah-toyd ar-**THRI**-tis	S/ R/ S/ S/	-ism *condition* rheumat- *a flow* -ic *pertaining to* -oid *resembling*	Pain in various parts of the musculoskeletal system Pertaining to or characterized by rheumatism Systemic disease affecting many joints

EXERCISES

A. Review *the Case Report on this spread before answering the questions.*

1. What specific type of fx does Mr. Fox have? _____

2. Describe the fracture's location. _____

3. What is the difference between a cast and a splint? _____

4. What is the opposite of *distal?* _____

5. What pain medication was prescribed for Mr. Fox? _____

B. Review Figure 4.13 *on this spread to formulate your answers to the following questions.*

1. What is the difference between the distal and the proximal phalanx? _____

2. What is the only finger with two phalanges instead of three? _____

3. What term can be applied to both fingers and toes? _____

4. What is the most common cause of a Colles fracture? _____

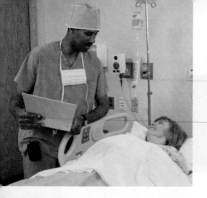

LESSON 4.4

Pelvic Girdle and Lower Limb

You use your legs and feet constantly, every day of your life, whether you are standing, walking, or changing positions. The information in this lesson will enable you to use correct medical terminology to:

4.4.1   Identify the structures and functions of the bones and joints of the pelvic girdle.

4.4.2   Describe common disorders of the bones and joints of the pelvic girdle.

4.4.3   Identify the structures and functions of the bones and joints of the leg, knee, and ankle.

4.4.4   Recognize common disorders of the hip joint, knee, and ankle.

4.4.5   Identify the structures and functions of the bones and joints of the foot.

4.4.6   Name common disorders of the bones and joints of the foot.

The Pelvic Girdle (LO 4.1, 4.2, and 4.3)

Your pelvic girdle consists of your two hip bones that articulate anteriorly with each other at the **symphysis pubis**, and posteriorly with the **sacrum** (a triangular-shaped bone in your lower back). This forms the bowl-shaped **pelvis.** The two joints between your hip bones and the sacrum are called **sacroiliac joints.**

The pelvic girdle has these functions:

1. Supports the axial skeleton;

2. Transmits the upper body's weight to the lower limbs;

3. Provides attachments for the lower limbs; and

4. Protects the internal reproductive organs, urinary bladder, and distal segment of the large intestine.

Each of your hip bones is actually a fusion of three bones; the **ilium, ischium,** and **pubis** *(Figure 4.17a).* This fusion occurs in the region of the **acetabulum,** a cup-shaped cavity on the lateral surface of the hip bone, which receives the head of the **femur,** or thigh bone *(Figure 4.17b).*

The lower part of the pelvis is formed by the lower ilium, ischium, and pubic bones that surround a short canal-like pelvic cavity, through which the rectum, vagina, and urethra pass. In females, the infant passes down this canal during childbirth.

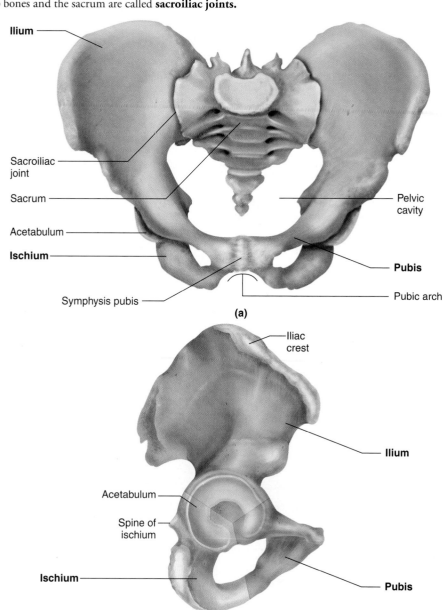

▲ **FIGURE 4.17**
Pelvic Girdle.
(a) Front view. (b) Side view.

Word	Pronunciation		Elements	Definition
acetabulum	ass-eh-**TAB**-you-lum		Latin *vinegar cup*	The cup-shaped cavity of the hip bone that receives the head of the femur to form the hip joint
femur femoral (adj)	**FEE**-mur **FEM**-oh-ral	S/ R/	Latin *thigh* -al *pertaining to* femor- *femur*	The thigh bone Pertaining to the femur
ilium	**ILL**-ee-um		Latin *groin*	Large wing-shaped bone at the upper and posterior part of the pelvis
ischium ischia (pl) ischial (adj)	**IS**-kee-um **IS**-kee-ah **IS**-kee-al	S/ R/	Greek *hip* -al *pertaining to* ischi- *ischium, hip bone*	Lower and posterior part of the hip bone Pertaining to the ischium
pelvis pelvic (adj)	**PEL**-viss **PEL**-vik	S/ R/	Latin *basin* -ic *pertaining to* pelv- *pelvis*	Basin-shaped ring of bones, ligaments, and muscles at the base of the spine. Also, any basin-shaped cavity, like the pelvis of the kidney Pertaining to the pelvis
pubis pubic (adj)	**PYU**-bis **PYU**-bik	S/ R/	Latin *pubis* -ic *pertaining to* pub- *pubis*	Alternative name for the pubic bone Pertaining to the pubic bone
sacroiliac joint	say-kroh-**ILL**-ih-ak **JOINT**	S/ R/CF R	-ac *pertaining to* sacr/o- *sacrum* -ili- *ilium*	The joint between the sacrum and the ilium
symphysis symphyses (pl)	**SIM**-feh-sis **SIM**-feh-sees		Greek *grow together*	Two bones joined by fibrocartilage; in this case, the two pubic bones

EXERCISES

A. Demonstrate your knowledge *of the precise medical term to answer the following questions. Every answer can be found in the above WAD. Write the term that is:*

1. another name for the thigh bone _____

2. a basin-shaped ring of bones _____

3. the joint between the sacrum and the ilium _____

4. the lower posterior part of the hip bone _____

5. the wing-shaped bone in the pelvis _____

B. Meet lesson objectives *and circle the correct medical term based on the statement.*

1. The hip bone is a fusion of three bones: the ilium, the ischium, and the

    femur   pubis   acetabulum

2. The pelvis is shaped like a

    bowl   box   basket

3. One function of the pelvic girdle is to:

    support the cranium   attach lower limbs   transport waste products

4. What organs does the pelvic girdle protect?

    lungs   pancreas and gallbladder   bladder, intestines, reproductive

5. A triangular-shaped bone in the lower back is the

    scapula   sacrum   symphysis

• The sciatic nerve lies directly behind the lower third of the SI joint. Many patients with SI joint strain will have pain radiating down the back of the leg.

CASE REPORT 4.4

YOU ARE

. . . a physical therapist assistant working in the physical therapy department of Fulwood Medical Center.

YOU ARE COMMUNICATING WITH

. . . Sandra Halpin, a 38-year-old female who is complaining of persistent low back pain on her left side. The pain began about two years previously, when she and her husband were moving and she was lifting heavy boxes. Her family physician has prescribed rest, back exercises, muscle relaxants, and painkillers, but she has had no relief.

On examination, she exhibits tenderness over the left sacroiliac joint, and when she presses her left knee to her chest, she experiences considerable pain over the SI joint. X-rays of the pelvis and hips, and an angle study of the SI joints, showed narrowing of the left SI joint space. A diagnosis of left sacroiliac joint strain has been made.

Sacroiliac (SI) joint strain is a common cause of lower back pain. Unlike most joints, the SI joint *(Figure 4.18)* is designed to move only 1/4 of an inch during weight bearing and forward bending movements. Its main function is to provide shock absorption for the spine.

Because stretching in the SI joint ligaments makes this joint overly mobile, it's susceptible to wear and tear, including painful arthritis. Another cause of pain in the SI joint is trauma, when tearing of the joint ligaments allows too much motion.

A clinical examination, joint X-ray **(radiology),** and CT scan may be used to diagnose the presence of sacroiliac strain. For temporary pain relief, a local anesthetic can be injected into the joint. Standard treatment involves stabilizing the joint with a **brace** and strengthening the lower back muscles with physical therapy. Occasionally, **arthrodesis** of the joint is necessary.

Diastasis symphysis pubis sometimes occurs during pregnancy. It is caused by excessive stretching of pelvic ligaments, which widens the joint between the two pubic bones. This leads to pain and difficulty in walking, climbing stairs, and turning over in bed. During pregnancy, however, hormones generally enable connective tissue in the SI joint area to relax so the pelvis can expand enough to allow birth without causing SI joint strain.

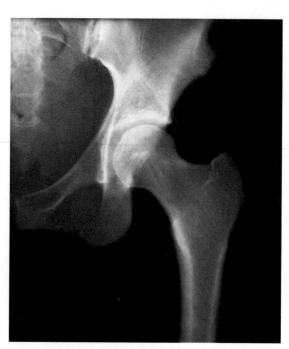

▲ **FIGURE 4.18**
X-ray of Sacroiliac Joint Showing Narrowing of SI Joint Space.

SI   sacroiliac

Word	Pronunciation		Elements	Definition
arthrodesis	ar-**THROW**-dee-sis	S/ R/CF	-desis *to fuse together* arthr/o- *joint*	Fixation or stiffening of a joint by surgery
brace	BRACE		Old English *to fasten*	Appliance to support a part of the body in its correct position
diastasis	die-**ASS**-tah-sis		Greek *separation*	Separation of normally joined parts
radiology	ray-dee-**OL**-oh-jee	S/ R/CF	-logy *study of* radi/o- *radiation, X-rays*	The study of medical imaging
radiologist	ray-dee-**OL**-oh-jist	S/	-logist *one who studies, specialist*	Medical specialist in the use of X-rays and other imaging techniques

EXERCISES

A. Review *the Case Report on this spread before answering the questions.*

1. What is Sandra Halpin's chief complaint? _____

2. How did she injure herself? _____

3. What has *not* helped Ms. Halpin's pain? _____

4. What other specialist besides an orthopedist has seen Ms. Halpin? _____

5. What is Ms. Halpin's final diagnosis? _____

B. Every answer *you need can be found on the two-page spread open in front of you. Fill in the blanks.*

1. What is a common cause of low back pain? _____

2. What two bones form the SI joint? _____ and _____

3. What is the main function of the SI joint? _____

4. Name one cause of pain in the SI joint. _____

5. What diagnostic tests are used to diagnose SI strain? _____

C. Read *the answer choices for each question and immediately discard the ones you know are not correct. Circle the correct answer in the remaining possibilities.*

1. What can provide temporary pain relief from SI joint strain?

  a. stretching   **d.** heat application

  b. a brace   **e.** local anesthetic injected

  c. PT   into the joint

2. The expertise of a radiologist is in:

  a. skin diseases   **d.** interpreting X-rays

  b. tissue study   **e.** lung conditions

  c. disorders of the brain

3. Fixation or stiffening of a joint by surgery is called

  a. arthroscopy   **d.** arthrotomy

  b. arthroplasty   **e.** none of these

  c. arthrodesis

4. What substance allows the SI joint to relax enough for delivery of a baby?

  a. lymph   **d.** synovial fluid

  b. blood   **e.** hormones

  c. enzymes

LESSON 4.4 Bones and Joints of the Hip and Thigh (LO 4.1, 4.2, and 4.3)

Your **hip joint** is a ball-and-socket mechanism formed by the head of your femur (thigh bone) and the acetabulum (cup-shaped hip socket) of your hip bone *(Figure 4.19)*. The **labrum** is the articular cartilage that forms a rim around the hip joint socket, cushioning the joint and helping to keep your femoral head in place in the socket. Finally, the hip joint is secured by a thick joint capsule reinforced by strong ligaments that connect the neck of the femur to the rim of the hip socket.

Disorders and Injuries of the Hip Joint (LO 4.1, 4.2, 4.3, and 4.4)

Hip pointer, often a football-related injury, is a blow to the rim of the pelvis that leads to bruising of the bone and surrounding tissues.

Osteoarthritis is common in the hip as a result of aging, weight bearing, and repetitive use of the joint. The cartilage on both the acetabulum and the head of the femur deteriorates, causing friction between the bones of the femoral head and the acetabulum that leads to pain and loss of mobility.

Rheumatoid arthritis can also affect the hip, beginning in the synovial membrane and progressing to destroy cartilage and bone.

Avascular necrosis of the femoral head is the death (necrosis) of bone tissue when the blood supply is cut off (avascular), usually as a result of trauma.

Fractures of the neck of the femur occur as a result of a fall, most commonly in elderly women with osteoporosis.

Surgical Procedures of the Hip Joint (LO 4.1, 4.2, 4.3, and 4.4)

There are two standard surgical procedures for replacing or repairing the hip joint. **Arthroplasty,** a total replacement of the hip joint with a metal **prosthesis,** is the most common hip surgery today. Here, the diseased parts of the joint are removed and replaced with artificial parts made of titanium and other metals, ceramics, and plastics *(Figure 4.20)*.

Arthrodesis is a surgical procedure that fixates or stiffens a joint.

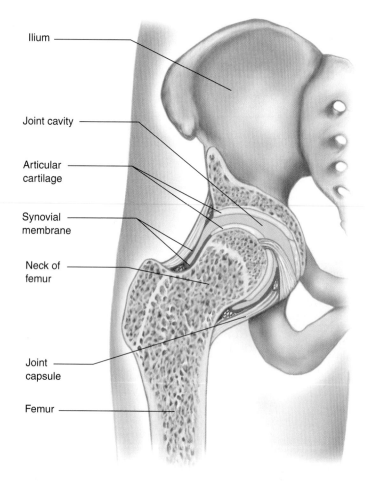

Ilium

Joint cavity

Articular cartilage

Synovial membrane

Neck of femur

Joint capsule

Femur

▲ **FIGURE 4.19**
Hip Joint.
Right frontal view of a section of the hip joint.

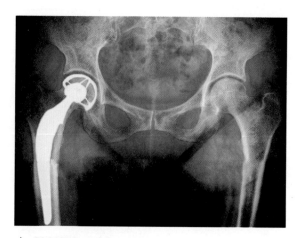

▲ **FIGURE 4.20**
Total Hip Replacement.
Colored x-ray of prosthetic hip.

Word	Pronunciation	Elements		Definition
arthrodesis	ar-**THROW**-dee-sis	S/ R/CF	-desis *to fuse together* arthr/o- *joint*	Fixation or stiffening of a joint by surgery
arthroplasty	**AR**-throw-plas-tee	S/ R/CF	-plasty *reshaping by surgery* arthr/o- *joint*	Surgery to repair, as far as possible, the function of a joint
avascular	a-**VAS**-cue-lar	S/ P/ R/	-ar *pertaining to* a- *without* -vascul- *blood vessel*	Without a blood supply
labrum	**LAY**-brum		Latin *lip-shaped*	Cartilage that forms a rim around the socket of the hip joint
necrosis necrotic (adj)	neh-**KROH**-sis neh-**KROT**-ik	S/ R/CF	Greek *death* -tic *pertaining to* necr/o- *death*	Pathologic death of cells or tissue Pertaining to or affected by necrosis
prosthesis prosthetic (adj)	**PROS**-thee-sis pros-**THET**-ik		Greek *addition*	An artificial part to remedy a defect in the body Pertaining to a prosthesis

EXERCISES

A. Proofread *the following sentences for errors in fact or spelling. Circle the error, then rewrite the sentence correctly.*

1. Rheumatoid arthritis can destroy muscle and bone.

_____

2. Avascular necrosis is the death of cartilage when the blood supply is cut off.

_____

3. Arthrodesis is a total replacement of the hip joint.

_____

4. A joint is replaced with a metal prothesis.

_____

5. The labrum is a mucous membrane that forms a rim around the hip joint socket.

_____

B. Match *the correct medical term in column one with its meaning in column two.*

1. _____ synovial   **A.** artificial body part

2. _____ arthroplasty   **B.** bloodless

3. _____ prosthesis   **C.** death of cells

4. _____ avascular   **D.** lubricating

5. _____ necrosis   **E.** joint repair

C. Circle *the best choice after you have discounted the answers you know are not correct.*

1. What is the purpose of synovial fluid?

  a. balance   **d.** weight bearing

  b. alignment   **e.** mobility

  c. lubrication

2. What is the purpose of a prosthesis?

  a. restore well being   **d.** support the skeleton

  b. remedy a defect in the body   **e.** repair a joint

  c. maintain balance

LESSON 4.4 The Knee Joint

(LO 4.1, 4.2, and 4.3)

Your knees do plenty of bending, whether you're climbing the stairs, exercising, sitting cross-legged, or squatting down to collect something from the floor. Each of your knees is a hinged joint formed with these four bones:

1. **The lower end of the femur,** shaped like a horseshoe;

2. **The flat upper end of the tibia;**

3. **The flat triangular patella** (kneecap), embedded in the **patellar** tendon and articulating with the femur *(Figure 4.21a);* and

4. **The fibula,** which forms a separate joint—the **tibiofibular joint** *(Figure 4.21b)*—by articulating with the tibia.

Mechanically, the patella's role is to provide a 30% strength increase in the extension of the knee joint.

Within the knee joint, two crescent-shaped pads of cartilage—the **medial** and **lateral menisci**—lie on top of the tibia and articulate with the femur. This cartilage helps to distribute weight more evenly across the joint surface to minimize wear and tear.

The knee joint has a fibrous capsule, lined with synovial membrane that secretes synovial fluid to lubricate the joint. Four ligaments hold the knee joint together; the **medial** and **lateral collateral ligaments** located outside the joint, and the **anterior cruciate ligament** (**ACL**) and **posterior cruciate ligament** (**PCL**) located inside the joint cavity, crossing over each other to form an "X" *(Figure 4.21b).*

CASE REPORT 4.5

YOU ARE

. . . an Emergency Technician working in the Emergency Department of Fulwood Medical Center.

YOU ARE COMMUNICATING WITH

. . . Gail Griffith, a 17-year-old high school student and her mother, Mrs. Cindy Griffith. Gail landed awkwardly after jumping for a ball during a basketball game.

Gail: "My knee kinda popped as I landed."

Gail had to be assisted off the court. In the Emergency Department, the knee was swollen and unstable. An MRI showed a partial tear of the medial **collateral** ligament, a complete rupture of the anterior **cruciate** ligament, and a partial tear of the medial **meniscus**. Gail decided to have surgery, even though full recovery would take 6 months to 1 year of rehabilitation.

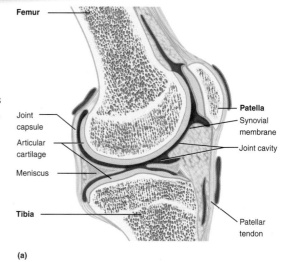

(a)

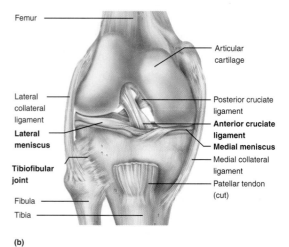

(b)

▶ **FIGURE 4.21**
Knee Joint.
(a) Section of knee joint.
(b) Right knee joint, anterior view.

Word	Pronunciation	Elements		Definition
collateral (Note: *An extra "l" has been inserted.*)	koh-**LAT**-er-al	S/ P/ R/	-al *pertaining to* co- *together* -later- *side*	Situated at the side, often to bypass an obstruction
cruciate	**KRU**-she-ate		Latin *cross*	Shaped like a cross. In this case, the two internal ligaments of the knee joint cross over each other to form an "X"
fibula	**FIB**-you-lah		Latin *clasp* or *buckle*	The smaller of the two bones of the lower leg
fibular (adj)	**FIB**-you-lar	S/ R/	-ar *pertaining to* fibul- *fibula*	Pertaining to the fibula
meniscus menisci (pl)	meh-**NISS**-kuss meh-**NISS**-key		Greek *crescent*	Disc of cartilage between the bones of a joint, in this case, the knee joint
patella (kneecap) patellae (pl) patellar (adj)	pah-**TELL**-ah pah-**TELL**-ee pah-**TELL**-ar	S/ R/	-ar *pertaining to* patell- *patella*	Thin, circular bone in front of the knee joint, embedded in the patellar tendon Pertaining to the patella bone or the tendon
tibia tibial (adj)	**TIB**-ee-ah **TIB**-ee-al	S/ R/	-al *pertaining to* tibi- *tibia*	The larger bone of the lower leg Pertaining to the tibia

EXERCISES

A. Review *the Case Report on this spread before answering the questions.*

1. What are Gail's symptoms when she presents to the ER?

   _____

2. What does MRI mean? _____

3. As a diagnostic test, what did the MRI show? _____

4. What is the meaning of the term "collateral"? _____

5. In her treatment plan, what will Gail be doing after her surgery?

   _____

6. What is the most severe of the injuries to Gail's knee?

   _____

7. Why do you think Gail opted for the surgery?

   _____

B. Spelling: *A medical term must be spelled correctly. Work with a fellow student on this exercise. Cover the WAD box with a sheet of paper while your partner dictates any 5 terms in the above WAD box to you. Write them in the "Test" column, and do your best to spell them correctly. When you are finished, remove the cover and check your spelling. If you have made any errors, rewrite the correct spelling in the "corrections" column.*

Test   Corrections

1. _____   _____

2. _____   _____

3. _____   _____

4. _____   _____

5. _____   _____

OPERATIVE REPORT: FULWOOD MEDICAL CENTER

Patient: Gail Griffith, aged 17.
Preoperative Diagnosis: Traumatic **ACL** tear, medial collateral ligament tear, and tear of medial meniscus, right knee.

CASE REPORT 4.3 (CONTINUED)

Postoperative Diagnosis: Same.
Procedure Performed: **Arthroscopy**, repair of medial collateral ligament, **ACL** reconstruction, repair of torn medial meniscus, right knee.
Operative Findings: An avulsed anterior cruciate ligament **(ACL)** of the femur with a tear of the posterior horn of the medial meniscus and tear of medial collateral ligament.

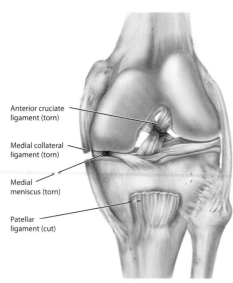

Anterior cruciate ligament (torn)

Medial collateral ligament (torn)

Medial meniscus (torn)

Patellar ligament (cut)

▲ **FIGURE 4.22**
Gail Griffith's Knee Injuries.

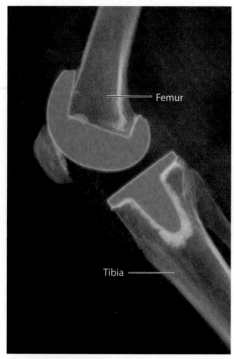

Femur

Tibia

▲ **FIGURE 4.23**
Total Knee Replacement.
Colored X-ray of total knee replacement, left knee.

The Knee Joint (LO 4.1, 4.2, 4.3, and 4.4)

Injuries to the Knee Joint (LO 4.1, 4.2, 4.3, and 4.4)

The **anterior cruciate ligament (ACL)** is the most commonly injured ligament in the knee *(Figure 4.22)*, particularly in football players and female athletes. The injury is often caused by a sudden **hyperflexion** of the knee joint when landing awkwardly on flat ground, as in Gail Griffith's case. Because of its poor vascular (blood) supply, the torn ligament does not heal and has to be surgically mended.

Other commonly injured major ligaments are the medial and lateral collateral ligaments and the posterior cruciate ligament.

Meniscus injuries result from a twist to the knee that tears the meniscus. The torn meniscus flips in and out of the joint as it moves, locking the knee and creating pain. Losing a meniscus leads to arthritic changes, so repair of the meniscus, as in Ms. Griffith's case, instead of removal (a **meniscectomy**) is preferred.

Patellar subluxation or dislocation produces an unstable, painful kneecap.

Prepatellar bursitis ("housemaid's knee") produces painful swelling over the **bursa** at the front of the knee and is seen in people who kneel for extended periods of time, like carpet layers.

Tendinitis of the patellar tendon results from overuse during activities like cycling, running, or dancing. Pain is felt where the tendon is inserted into the tibia, and this is treated with R.I.C.E (rest, ice, compression, elevation).

Surgical Procedures of the Knee Joint (LO 4.1, 4.2, 4.3, and 4.4)

There are several procedures and surgery options for those who sustain knee injuries. **Arthrocentesis** is the aspiration of knee joint fluid, which is examined to establish a diagnosis. Infected fluid may be drained off, or medication, such as local corticosteroids may be inserted.

Arthrography is an X-ray of a joint after injection of a contrast medium (harmless dye) into the joint to make the inside details of the joint visible.

Diagnostic arthroscopy is an exploratory procedure performed using an arthroscope to examine the internal compartments of the knee joint.

Surgical arthroscopy is performed through an arthroscope. This can be a **debridement** or removal of torn tissue like a meniscus or a ligament. It can also be a repair of a torn ligament by suturing, or tendon autograft, or repair of a torn meniscus.

Arthroplasty involves a total replacement of the knee joint *(Figure 4.23)*, usually because of osteoarthritis. The damaged cartilage and bone from the knee joint's surface are removed and replaced with metal and plastic.

Word	Pronunciation	Elements		Definition
arthrocentesis	**AR**-throw-sen-**TEE**-sis	S/ R/CF	-centesis *puncture* arthr/o- *joint*	Aspiration of fluid from a joint
arthrography	ar-**THROG**-rah-fee	S/ R/CF	-graphy *process of recording* arthr/o- *joint*	X-ray of a joint taken after the injection of a contrast medium into the joint
arthroscopy	ar-**THROS**-koh-pee	S/ R/CF	-scopy *the process of using an instrument to examine visually* arthr/o- *joint*	Visual examination of the interior of a joint
arthroscope	**AR**-thro-skope	S/	-scope *instrument to examine visually*	Endoscope used to examine the interior of a joint
bursa bursitis	**BURR**-sah burr-**SIGH**-tis	 S/ R/	Latin *purse* -itis *inflammation* burs- *bursa*	A closed sac containing synovial fluid Inflammation of a bursa
debridement	day-**BREED**-mon ("Mon" is the French pronunciation of *ment*.)	S/ P/ R/	-ment *action* de- *removal, out of* -bride- *rubble, rubbish*	The removal of injured or necrotic tissue
hyperflexion	high-per-**FLEK**-shun	S/ P/ R/	-ion *action, condition* hyper- *excessive* -flex- *bend*	Flexion of a limb or part beyond the normal limits
meniscectomy	men-ih-**SEK**-toh-me	S/ R/	-ectomy *surgical excision* menisc- *crescent, meniscus*	Excision (cutting out) of all or part of a meniscus
prepatellar	pree-pah-**TELL**-ar	S/ P/ R/	-ar *pertaining to* pre- *before, in front of* -patell- *patella*	In front of the patella
rupture	**RUP**-tyur		Latin *break, fracture*	Break or tear of any organ or body part
tendinitis (also spelled tendonitis)	ten-dih-**NYE**-tis	S/ R/	-itis *inflammation* tendin- *tendon*	Inflammation of a tendon

EXERCISES

A. Review *the Case Report on this spread before answering the questions.*

1. What was torn in Gail's knee? _____

2. What does "traumatic" mean? _____

3. Define the procedure performed: _____

4. Which part of Gail's knee has poor blood supply? _____

5. Which terms in the operative report are directional terms? _____

B. Elements: *Recognition of word elements will help you understand a medical term. For each of the following terms, identify the type of the element shown in bold italics, and then define that element. Fill in the chart, and answer the questions below it.*

Remember: An element that begins a term is not necessarily a prefix!

Medical Term	Type of Element (P, R/CF, or S)	Meaning of Element	Meaning of Term
tendin*itis*	1.	2.	3.
*pre*patellar	4.	5.	6.
de*bride*ment	7.	8.	9.
*burs*itis	10.	11.	12.
arthro*centesis*	13.	14.	15.

Lesson 4.4 Bones and Joints of the Lower Leg, Ankle, and Foot
(LO 4.1, 4.2, and 4.3)

Your lower leg has two differently sized bones; the large medial tibia and the thin lateral fibula. The lower end of your tibia on its medial border forms a prominent process called the medial malleolus. The lower end of your fibula forms the lateral malleolus *(Figure 4.24)*. You can palpate (feel) both these prominences at your own ankle, which has two joints:

- One between the lateral malleolus of the fibula and the talus; and

- One between the medial malleolus of the tibia and the talus.

The **talus** is the most superior of the seven **tarsal** bones of the ankle *(Figure 4.24)*, and its upper surface articulates with the tibia. The heel bone is called the **calcaneus.** The tarsal bones help the ankle bear the body's weight. Strong ligaments on both sides of the ankle joint hold the joint together.

Attached to the tarsal bones are the five parallel **metatarsal** bones. These bones form the instep and the ball of the foot, where they bear weight. Each toe has three phalanges, except for the big toe, which has only two. This configuration is identical to the thumb and its relation to the hand.

Disorders and Injuries of the Ankle and Foot
(LO 4.1, 4.2, 4.3, and 4.4)

Podiatry is a health care specialty concerned with the diagnosis and treatment of disorders and injuries of the foot and toenails. A **podiatrist** is not an MD.

Bunions are deformities that appear as swollen bones, which often occur at the base of the big toe. A bunion is also called a **hallux valgus,** and it causes the metatarso-phalangeal joint to misalign and stick out.

Pott fracture is a fracture of the fibula near the ankle, often accompanied by a fracture of the medial malleolus of the tibia.

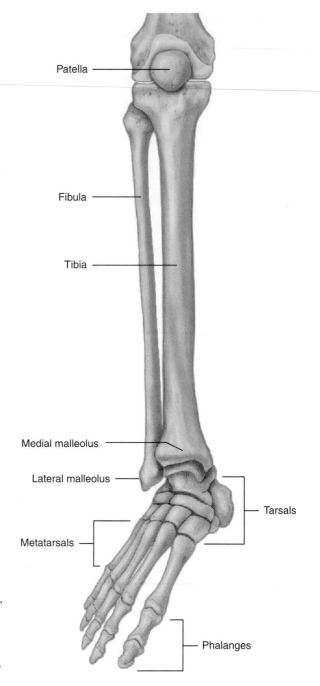

▲ **FIGURE 4.24**
Bones of the Lower Leg and Foot.

Patella

Fibula

Tibia

Medial malleolus

Lateral malleolus

Metatarsals

Tarsals

Phalanges

Word	Pronunciation		Elements	Definition
bunion	BUN-yun		French *bump*	A swelling at the base of the big toe
calcaneus	kal-KAY-knee-us		Latin *the heel*	Bone of the tarsus that forms the heel
calcaneal (adj)	kal-KAY-knee-al	S/ R/	-eal *pertaining to* calcan- *calcaneus*	Pertaining to the calcaneus
hallux valgus	HAL-uks VAL-gus	R/ R/	hallux *big toe* valgus *turn out*	Deviation of the big toe toward the medial side of the foot
metatarsus	MET-ah-TAR-sus	S/ P/ R/	-us *pertaining to* meta- *after, subsequent to* -tars- *ankle*	The five parallel bones of the foot between the tarsus and the phalanges
metatarsal (adj)	MET-ah-TAR-sal	S/	-al *pertaining to*	Pertaining to the metatarsus
podiatry	poh-DIE-ah-tree	S/ R/	-iatry *treatment* pod- *foot*	The diagnosis and treatment of disorders and injuries of the foot
podiatrist	poh-DIE-ah-trist	S/	-iatrist *practitioner*	Practitioner of podiatry
Pott fracture	POT FRAK-shur		Percival Pott, London surgeon, 1714–1788	Fracture of the lower end of the fibula, often with fracture of the tibial malleolus
talus	TAY-luss		Latin *heel bone*	The tarsal bone that articulates with the tibia to form the ankle joint
tarsus	TAR-sus		Latin *ankle*	The collection of seven bones in the foot that form the ankle and instep
tarsal (adj)	TAR-sal	S/ R/	-al *pertaining to* tars- *ankle*	Pertaining to the tarsus

EXERCISES

A. Challenge your knowledge *of the language of orthopedics. Fill in the blanks with the correct medical terms.*

1. Name 3 eponyms that have appeared in this chapter. _____, _____, and _____.

2. Metatarsal bones appear in the foot; what are the similar bones called in the hand? _____

3. Another name for a bunion is _____.

4. What is another name for the heel bone? _____

5. The big toe is similar in construction to the _____ of the hand.

6. What is the prominent process called at the lower end of the tibia on its medial border? _____.

7. Describe the location for the *lateral malleolus*. _____

_____

8. What bones form the instep? _____

9. Write all the suffixes you know from this and previous chapters that all mean *pertaining to*. _____

_____

10. What is the only term in the WAD that has a prefix? _____

11. What element means *foot?* _____

12. Where do bunions frequently occur? _____

13. Why can't a podiatrist write a prescription for pain pills? _____

B. Identify the medical term *based on the brief meaning given to you below. Be sure to check your spelling when you are finished! Fill in the blanks.*

1. swelling at the base of the big toe _____

2. bone of the tarsus that forms the heel _____

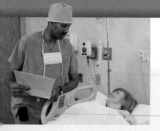

CHAPTER 4 REVIEW

CHALLENGE YOUR KNOWLEDGE

A. Identify the type of element *by placing a ✓ in the appropriate column. Define the element, and then give an example of a medical term using that element. Fill in the chart. The first one is done for you.*

Type of Element

Element	Prefix	Root/CF	Suffix	Meaning of Element	Medical Term Using This Element
toxi		✓		poison	detoxification
ortho	1.			2.	3.
osteo	4.			5.	6.
peri	7.			8.	9.
malacia	10.			11.	12.
chiro	13.			14.	15.
chondro	16.			17.	18.
sarc	19.			20.	21.
pathy	22.			23.	24.
genesis	25.			26.	27.
penia	28.			29.	30.

B. Prefixes: *The following prefixes all appear in this chapter's terms. Use the correct prefix to build the terms; then define the terms.*

There are more prefixes than questions.

a   re   de   inter   trans   non   peri   epi   mal   intra

1. _____ /condyle (upon, above)

   Definition: _____

2. _____ /duct/ion (backward)

   Definition: _____

3. _____ /chondro/plasia (without)

   Definition: _____

4. _____ /union (bad)

   Definition: _____

5. _____ /oste/al (around)

   Definition: _____

6. _____ /toxi/fication (from, out of)

   Definition: _____

7. _____ /union (not)

   Definition: _____

8. _____ /vertebr/al (between)

   Definition: _____

C. Roots and combining forms *are the foundation of every medical term. Deconstruct the following medical terms to discover their basic foundations. Slash the term into its appropriate elements. Notice that not every term needs a prefix.*

1. orthopedic _____ / _____ / _____
                      P   R/CF   S

2. osteopathy _____ / _____ / _____
                      P   R/CF   S

3. epiphysis _____ / _____ / _____
                      P   R/CF   S

4. cortical _____ / _____ / _____
                      P   R/CF   S

5. periosteum _____ / _____ / _____
                      P   R/CF   S

6. chiropractor _____ / _____ / _____
                      P   R/CF   S

7. osteomyelitis _____ / _____ / _____
                      P   R/CF   S

8. osteoporosis _____ / _____ / _____
                      P   R/CF   S

9. sarcoma _____ / _____ / _____
                      P   R/CF   S

10. detoxification _____ / _____ / _____
                       P   R/CF   S

11. epiphysial _____ / _____ / _____
                       P   R/CF   S

12. achondroplasia _____ / _____ / _____
                       P   R/CF   S

13. mandibular _____ / _____ / _____
                       P   R/CF   S

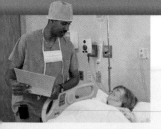

D. Suffixes: *The following suffixes have all appeared in this chapter. The meaning of the suffix is given to you—identify the suffix, and give an example of a medical term that contains that suffix. Fill in the chart.*

Suffix	Meaning of Suffix	Medical Term
1.	condition	2.
3.	resemble	4.
5.	a doer (one who does)	6.
7.	remove	8.
9.	process	10.
11.	specialist	12.
13.	disease	14.
15.	structure	16.
17.	formation	18.
19.	abnormal softening	20.
21.	deficient	22.
23.	inflammation	24.
25.	tumor, mass	26.

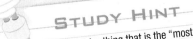

STUDY HINT

"Most." Anything that is the "most powerful," "largest," "smallest," "most common," and so on, is probably going to be a test question! Make sure you know them, and review them before a test.

E. Create a test question *for a fellow student. Write below a multiple-choice or fill-in-the-blank question about anything in this chapter. Make the question a challenge, and try to stump a fellow student! (If the question is multiple choice, it must have five possible answers.)*

Question:

_____

_____

_____

_____

F. Abbreviations *are frequently used in patient documentation. For patient safety, you must know exactly what they mean. Rewrite each sentence, translating the abbreviations into the correct medical terms. Watch your spelling—the answer is not correct unless all the spelling is correct!*

1. Women at risk for osteoporosis should have BMD screening using a DEXA scan.

   _____

   _____

2. An MRI shows herniated discs at C5-C6 and C6-C7, with a fx at C2.

   _____

   _____

G. Build your orthopedic terminology *by completing the medical terms defined. After you fill in the element on the line, write the type of element (prefix, root, combining form, suffix) you have used below the line. Fill in the blanks.*

1. removing poison from tissue   de/ _____ / _____

2. soft bones lacking in calcium   osteo/ _____

3. projection above the condyle   _____ /condyle

4. membrane surrounding a bone   peri/ _____ / _____

5. bone broken in several pieces   _____ /ed

6. having a structure in its correct position   _____ / _____ /ment

7. bone-forming cell   osteo/ _____

8. pertaining to the neck   _____ /al _____

9. space between two vertebrae   _____ /vertebr/ _____

H. Latin and Greek terms *cannot be further deconstructed into prefix, root, or suffix. You must know them for what they are. Test your knowledge of these terms with the following exercise. Match the meaning in column l with the correct medical term in column 2.*

_____ 1. upper jawbone   **A.** cartilage

_____ 2. holds bones together or organs in place   **B.** medulla

_____ 3. outer portion of an organ   **C.** mandible

_____ 4. bone that forms prominence of the cheek   **D.** diaphysis

_____ 5. shaft of a long bone   **E.** coccyx

_____ 6. connective tissue found in joints   **F.** ligament

_____ 7. lower jawbone   **G.** maxilla

_____ 8. small tailbone at the end of the vertebral column   **H.** cortex

_____ 9. attaches muscle to bone   **I.** zygoma

_____ 10. central portion of a structure surrounded by cortex   **J.** tendon

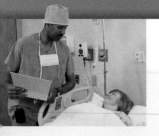

I. Word attack: *First, read the question completely through, including all the possible answer choices. Be careful of words like none, every, and all because they restrict the answer. Remember to cross off what you have determined to be an incorrect answer before you make your final choice.*

What do the terms *epiphysial, osteogenic, mandibular,* and *palatine* have in common?

a. None of them has a prefix.

b. Their suffixes all mean the same thing.

c. They are all diagnostic terms.

d. All three elements (P, R/CF, S) are present in every term.

Questions to ask yourself about the answer choices:

If any one of these terms has a prefix, this answer is not the correct choice because it states that none of them have a prefix.

1. Do any of these terms have a prefix? (yes/no) _____

2. If yes, which one(s)?

_____

3. Determine whether there is a suffix in each term. Do all the suffixes mean the same thing? (yes/no) _____

4. If yes, what do they all mean?

_____

5. Are all these terms diagnoses? (yes/no) _____

6. If no, which ones are not? _____

7. Does every term contain a prefix, root/CF, and suffix? (yes/no) _____

8. Therefore, the answer is (1, 2, 3, or 4) _____ because _____

_____

J. Spelling demons: *The following terms from this chapter are particularly difficult to spell and pronounce. Correct pronunciation and spelling of medical terms is the mark of an educated professional. Circle the correct spelling, and then check (✓) that you have practiced the pronunciation.* **Remember:** *Pronunciations are on the Student Online Learning Center (www.mhhe.com/AllanEss2e).*

Pronunciation ✓

1. cockyx cocyx coccyx coccyz _____

2. cartiledge cartilage carrtilage cartilege _____

3 scoliosis skoliosis scolliosis skolioses _____

4. osteomyilitis osteomielitis osteomyelitis osteomyelites _____

5. kiphosis khyphosis kyphosis kyiphosis _____

6. acondroplasea achondroplasia acondroplasia achodroplasi _____

7. ocipital occipitel ocippital occipital _____

8. sfenoid spenoid sphenoid phenoid _____

9. epiphysial epiphysia epiphyseal epifiseal _____

10. chiropractic chirropractic chiropracctic chiropractice _____

K. Patient education: *Explain the difference among these abnormal spinal curvatures to patients. Be sure to use language a patient can understand.*

1. scoliosis:

_____

_____

_____

_____

2. kyphosis:

_____

_____

_____

_____

3. Which one is the more common defect?

_____

4. Which defect is seen in patients with osteoporosis? _____

5. What is the most common type of bone in the body? _____

6. Where is cartilage found most often in the body? _____

7. What is the most common malignant bone tumor? _____

L. Recall and review: *This exercise on word elements contains elements from the previous chapter. Try to recall the previous elements without turning back in your book. Identify the type of element by placing a ✓ in the appropriate column; then write its meaning. Fill in the blanks.*

Type of Element

Element	Prefix	Root/CF	Suffix	Meaning of Element
vaso	1.			2.
cutane	3.			4.
syn	5.			6.
derm	7.			8.
bi	9.			10.
trans	11.			12.
rrhea	13.			14.
de	15.			16.
necro	17.			18.
plasty	19.			20.

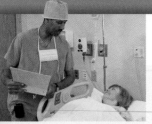

M. Terminology challenge: Suture. *Medical terms can have more than one meaning/usage. Use the Glossary, your library, or an online medical dictionary if you need help answering these questions.*

1   Define *suture* as it is used in this chapter.

   _____

   _____

2. Now use this meaning of *suture* in a sentence that is not a definition or taken directly out of the text.

   _____

   _____

Suture can also be a noun and a verb with another meaning. Can you identify them?

3. *Suture* as a noun (person, place, or thing) can also mean (definition) _____ .

4. Write a sentence using *suture* in this alternate meaning.

   _____

   _____

5. *Suture* as a verb (action) can also mean (definition) _____

   _____

6. Write a sentence with *suture* having this meaning.

   _____

SEE YOUR MEDICAL VOCABULARY INCREASE AS YOU NOW KNOW ONE TERM WITH THREE DIFFERENT MEANINGS!

N. Chapter challenge: *Circle the correct answer.*

1. The medical term for low bone density is:

   a. osteocyte   **d.** osteomalacia

   b. osteomyelitis   **e.** osteopenia

   c. periosteum

2. The four classes of bones are determined by their:

   a. length   **d.** weight

   b. shape   **e.** number

   c. size

3. Which term has a suffix meaning disease?

   a. orthopedist   **d.** osteopath

   b. periosteum   **e.** osteogenic

   c. chiropractor

4. When a bone is fractured, blood vessels bleed into the fracture site and form a(n):

    a. sarcoma

    b. osteosarcoma

    c. hematoma

    d. osteoblast

    e. condyle

5. Find the pair of terms that are both diagnoses:

    a. achondroplasia/medullary

    b. cortex/osteopathy

    c. orthopedic/osteomyelitis

    d. periosteum/osteoporosis

    e. osteomalacia/rickets

6. Which term has neither a suffix nor a prefix?

    a. fracture

    b. sacral

    c. periosteum

    d. osteopath

    e. lacrimal

7. What is the medulla?

    a. the shaft of a long bone

    b. the outer surface covering of bone

    c. the hollow cylinder inside the diaphysis

    d. the end of a bone

    e. the membrane surrounding a bone

8. What does the "O" in the abbreviation DO stand for?

    a. osteopath

    b. orthopedic

    c. orthopedist

    d. osteopathy

    e. orthotic

9. Having a structure in its correct position relative to others is called:

    a. nonunion

    b. alignment

    c. malunion

    d. detoxification

    e. resorption

> **STUDY HINT**
>
> Immediately cross off any answer you know is not correct. Among your remaining choices, there is only one best answer.

10. Which of these is not a bone in the cranium?

    a. frontal

    b. sphenoid

    c. parietal

    d. vomer

    e. occipital

11. Proofread the following statements for spelling and factual errors. Circle the only correct statement.

    a. Ciropractors focus on manual adjustment of joints.

    b. Scoliosis is an abnormal lateral curvature of the vertebral column.

    c. Alignment is removing poison from tissues.

    d. An epicondyle is a medial projection at the ends of flat bones.

    e. A DEXA scan screens for bone marrow.

12. Which disease is a genetic disorder?

    a. osteogenic sarcoma

    b. osteoporosis

    c. osteogenesis imperfecta

    d. osteopenia

    e. osteomalacia

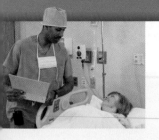

O. Explanation please: *If you really understand a term, you can explain it to someone else. Briefly explain the difference among the following terms.*

1. External manipulation:

_____

_____

_____

2. External fixation:

_____

_____

_____

3. Reduction:

_____

_____

_____

P. Translate *the following sentences into layperson's language a patient can understand.*

1. A patient with osteopenia is at risk for osteoporosis.

_____

_____

_____

_____

STUDY HINT

First, read the sentences and underline or highlight any medical terms (or abbreviations) you will need to explain. Then, rewrite the sentence in nonmedical language.

2. Intervertebral discs consist of fibrocartilage and inhabit the intervertebral space between the bodies of adjacent vertebrae.

_____

_____

_____

_____

3. Osteogenesis imperfecta is a rare genetic disorder producing very brittle bones that are easily fractured, often in utero.

_____

_____

_____

Q. Chapter challenge: *Circle the correct answer.*

1. Rickets is a disease caused by:

    a. poor bone marrow

    b. vitamin A deficiency

    c. excessive potassium

    d. infection

    e. vitamin D deficiency

2. Which term is not a diagnosis?

    a. osteomalacia

    b. osteoporosis

    c. osteopenia

    d. osteoblast

    e. osteomyelitis

3. The terms comminuted, transverse, and impacted all apply to:

    a. dental diagnoses

    b. radiologic procedures

    c. bone fractures

    d. surgical procedures

    e. intervertebral discs

4. Choose the incorrect pair of terms:

    a. curvature/scoliosis

    b. fixation/screws

    c. vertebra/disc

    d. coccyx/tailbone

    e. closed/compound

5. Using the elements as your guide, which term relates to bone marrow?

    a. osteomalacia

    b. osteoblast

    c. osteomyelitis

    d. osteopenia

    e. osteoporosis

6. Which term has a prefix meaning without?

    a. imperfecta

    b. achondroplasia

    c. alignment

    d. reduction

    e. intervertebral

7. Brain teaser: Reduction can be accomplished by:

    a. osteoblasts

    b. external fixation

    c. external manipulation

    d. pathologic fracture

    e. herniation

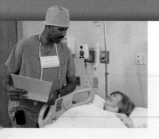

R. Twenty questions: *Challenge your mastery of this chapter's medical vocabulary. Demonstrate your knowledge of the language of orthopedics with correct answers to the following questions.*

1. Which two bones support your teeth? _____ and _____.

2. *In utero* means _____.

3. Name the external fixators that can be used to secure bone fragments together: _____

   _____

4. The _____ is the articular cartilage that forms a rim around the hip joint socket.

5. What is the most commonly injured ligament in the knee? _____

6. The surgical removal of injured or necrotic tissue is _____.

7. According to bone classification, name two short bones: _____ and _____.

8. *TMJ* is the abbreviation for _____.

9. Which type of foot specialist is not a medical doctor? _____

10. What is a *whiplash injury?* _____

11. What covers the outer surface of all bones? _____

12. The collection of bones in the foot that form the ankle and instep is termed the _____.

13. Write the medical term that means *no blood supply:* _____

14. Bringing bones back into alignment is called _____.

15. What is an incomplete dislocation called when some contact between joint surfaces remains? _____

16. A medical procedure that fixates or stiffens a joint is an _____.

17. What is the medical term for the cheekbones? _____

18. *Osteomalacia* in children is known as _____ .

19. Bone marrow produces _____.

20. _____ is aspiration of knee joint fluid.

S. Case Report challenge: *Now that you are more comfortable with the terms in this chapter, you can apply that knowledge and briefly answer the questions about the Case Report. If you read the report through and underline all the medical terminology, this will make it easier to answer the questions.*

CASE REPORT

YOU ARE

> . . . a physical therapist assistant working in the physical therapy department of Fulwood Medical Center.

YOU ARE COMMUNICATING WITH

> . . . Ms. Nancy Cardenas, a 27-year-old jeweler, who was waiting in her car at a traffic light 3 days ago when her car was rear-ended. Ms. Cardenas now has severe neck pain radiating down her left arm, with dizziness and headaches. She is unable to go to work. Dr. Stannard has examined her and diagnosed her condition as a whiplash injury. An MRI shows herniation of intervertebral discs between C5-C6 and C6-C7. Your role is to assist with a regimen of physiotherapy to relieve her symptoms.

1. Define *radiating pain:*

_____

_____

2. The term *whiplash injury* forms a mental picture. Describe that picture:

_____

_____

3. The abbreviation C6-C7 stands for

_____

4. The prefix *inter* in the term intervertebral means that the discs are _____ certain vertebrae in the vertebral column.

5. List the symptoms Ms. Cardenas presented with:

_____

_____

6. What happens when a disc herniates?

_____

_____

7. What diagnosis has the doctor assigned to this patient?

_____

_____

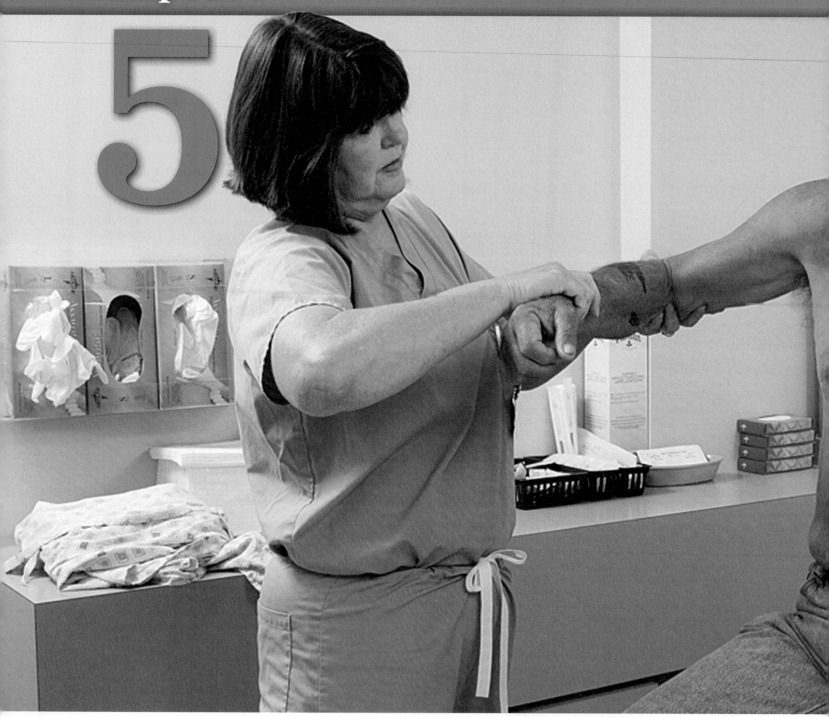

MUSCLES AND TENDONS

**The Essentials of the Languages
of Orthopedics and Rehabilitation**

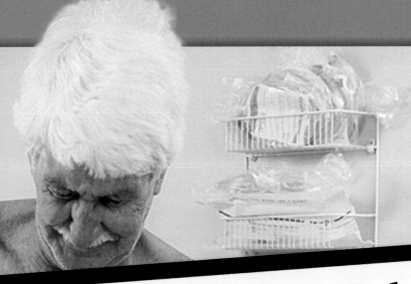

CASE REPORT 5.1

YOU ARE

. . . an orthopedic technologist working with orthopedist Kenneth Stannard, MD, in Fulwood Medical Center.

YOU ARE COMMUNICATING WITH

Mr. Bruce Adams, a 55-year-old construction worker who presents with severe pain in his right shoulder.

Mr. Adams' pain began 3 or 4 months ago; it is worse at the end of the workday and when he lifts his arm above his head. During the past week, the pain has woken him from sleep. Mr. Adams' primary care physician has given him pain medication, advised him to stop working, and referred him to Dr. Stannard for diagnosis and treatment. A physical examination shows that Mr. Adams' pain is noticeably limiting all the passive and active movements of his right shoulder, including his ability to lift weight.

LEARNING OUTCOMES

Your **appendicular skeleton,** which includes the bones of your upper and lower limbs, is attached to the bones of your **axial skeleton** through joints and muscles. Understanding the terminology of the muscles of your limbs and trunk and their disorders is vital to your knowledge of the human body. Information in this chapter will enable you to use correct medical terminology to:

LO 5.1 Describe the functions and structure of skeletal muscle.

LO 5.2 Identify the structures and functions of the muscles and tendons of the shoulder girdle and upper limbs.

LO 5.3 Describe the structures and functions of the muscles and tendons of the pelvic girdle and lower limbs.

LO 5.4 Describe the major diseases of skeletal muscle.

ABBREVIATIONS

ADL activities of daily living
OT occupational therapy
PT physical therapy
ROM range of motion

Rehabilitation programs involve a **multidisciplinary** team approach where each team member manages different rehabilitation activities. The members of a rehabilitation team include the following health professionals and their respective roles (see the WADs in this chapter for these terms):

- A **physiatrist,** often the team leader, is a physician specializing in physical medicine and rehabilitation.

- **Medical specialists** manage acute or chronic illnesses and pain.

- **Occupational therapists** practice occupational therapy **(OT)** to help improve a patient's activities of daily living **(ADLs)** and adapt to visual and other perceptual deficits.

- **Physical therapists** practice **physical therapy (PT)** to help patients improve their strength, range of motion (ROM), balance, and endurance. Physical therapists are assisted by **restorative aids** and teach patients how to use these devices.

- **Rehabilitation psychologists** are specialists who help patients undergoing rehabilitation and those with resulting disabilities to reclaim their sense of belonging, contributing to, and participating in the world around them.

- **Social workers** provide support and assistance with social issues, such as health insurance, care facilities, and employment.

- **Speech therapists** evaluate and treat communication, speech, and swallowing disorders.

- **Orthotists** make and fit orthopedic appliances **(orthotics).**

- **Nutritionists** evaluate and improve a patient's nutritional status.

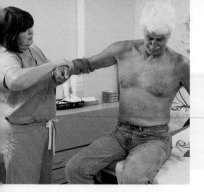

LESSON 5.1

Muscles and Tendons

*In Chapter 4, you learned how the bones of your skeleton support your body and how your joints provide mobility throughout your body. However, neither of these functions can occur without your **muscles,** which provide posture and movement. Information in this lesson will enable you to use correct medical terminology to:*

5.1.1 Identify the functions of skeletal muscle and tendons.

5.1.2 Describe the structure of skeletal muscle and tendons.

5.1.3 Demonstrate an understanding of the major problems and diseases that occur in muscles and tendons.

ABBREVIATIONS

DO	Doctor of Osteopathy
MD	Doctor of Medicine
DC	Doctor of Chiropractic

Functions and Structure of Skeletal Muscle
(LO 5.1, 5.2, and 5.3)

Functions of Skeletal Muscle
(LO 5.1, 5.2, and 5.3)

Skeletal muscles, which are attached to one or more bones, are also called **voluntary** muscles. This means that you have conscious control of your muscles, which perform your movements. Each muscle consists of bundles of muscle cells (often called **fibers** because of their length), blood vessels, and nerves. Connective tissue sheets hold your muscle fibers together and connect the muscles to your bones.

Your skeletal muscle has the following functions:

1. **Movement.** All skeletal muscles are attached to bones so when a muscle **contracts,** your bones move, too *(Figure 5.1).* This allows you to walk, run, and work with your hands.

2. **Posture.** The **tone** of your skeletal muscles holds you straight when sitting, standing, or moving.

3. **Body heat.** When skeletal muscles contract, they produce the heat needed to maintain your body temperature.

4. **Respiration.** Skeletal muscles move the chest wall as you breathe.

5. **Communication.** Skeletal muscles enable you to speak, write, type, gesture, and smile.

Structure of Skeletal Muscle
(LO 5.1, 5.2, and 5.3)

Your skeletal muscle fibers are narrow and measure up to 1½ inches long. Bundles of these fibers create separate muscles, which are held in place by **fascia** *(Figure 5.2),* a thick layer of connective tissue. Fascia extends beyond the muscle to form a tendon, which attaches to a bone's periosteum at the origin and insertion of the muscle.

Because skeletal muscle fibers contain **striations** (alternating dark and light bands of protein filaments responsible for muscle contraction), skeletal muscle can also be called **striated muscle.**

You have the same number of muscle fibers as an adult that you had in late childhood. Exercise and/or weightlifting will enlarge (**hypertrophy**) your muscles, increasing the thickness of your muscle fibers. If you neglect these muscles, they will shrink (**atrophy**).

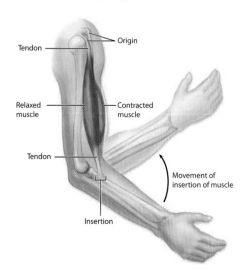

▶ **FIGURE 5.1**
Muscle Contraction.

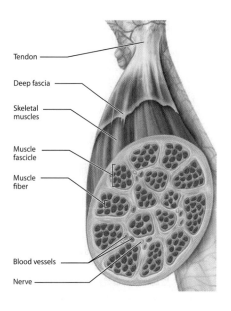

▲ **FIGURE 5.2**
Structure of Skeletal Muscle.

Word	Pronunciation	Elements		Definition
atrophy	**AT**-roh-fee	P/ R/	a- *without* -trophy *nourishment*	The wasting away or diminished volume of tissue, an organ, or a body part
hypertrophy	high-**PER**-troh-fee	P/ R/	hyper- *above, excessive* -trophy *nourishment*	Increase in size, but not in number, of an individual tissue element
contract	kon-**TRAKT**	P/ R/	con- *with, together* -tract *draw*	Draw together or shorten
fascia	**FASH**-ee-ah		Latin *a band*	Sheet of fibrous connective tissue
fiber	**FIE**-ber		Latin *fiber*	A strand or filament
multidisciplinary	mul-tee-**DIS**-ih-plih-**NAR**-ee	S/ P/ R/	-ary *pertaining to* multi- *many* -disciplin- *instruction*	Involving health care providers from more than one profession
muscle	**MUSS**-el		Latin *muscle*	A tissue consisting of cells that can contract
skeletal (adj)	**SKEL**-eh-tal	S/ R/	-al *pertaining to* skelet- *skeleton*	Pertaining to the skeleton
tone	**TONE**		Greek *tone*	Tension present in resting muscles
voluntary muscle	**VOL**-un-tare-ee **MUSS**-el	S/ R/	-ary *pertaining to* volunt- *free will*	Muscle that is under the control of the will

EXERCISES

A. Review *the Case Report on the previous spread before answering the questions. As with any Case Report exercise in this text, first read the report aloud if possible. Read it a second time and underline any medical terms you see in the report. Then answer the questions.*

1. In your own words, explain what an orthopedist specializes in. _____

2. What motivated the patient to see the doctor? _____

3. What makes his pain worse? _____

4. Is there anything about his occupation that may have contributed to his condition? _____

5. Write all the medical terms you have identified in the case report. _____

B. Deconstruct *the following medical terms from the WAD into their basic elements; then define each element. Fill in the chart.*

Medical Term	Prefix	Meaning of Prefix	Root(s)/CF	Meaning of Root(s)/CF	Suffix	Meaning of Suffix
hypertrophy	1.	2.	3.	4.	5.	6.
contract	7.	8.	9.	10.	11.	12.
atrophy	13.	14.	15.	16.	17.	18.
voluntary	19.	20.	21.	22.	23.	24.
skeletal	25.	26.	27.	28.	29.	30.

C. Meet lesson and chapter objectives *and use the correct medical terminology to answer the questions.*

1. Describe the structure of a muscle. _____

2. List the functions of skeletal muscle. _____

3. What connects the appendicular skeleton to the axial skeleton? _____

4. What are the three components of a muscle? _____, _____, and _____ .

5. What is another name for *skeletal muscle*? _____

LESSON 5.1 Disorders of Skeletal Muscles (LO 5.1, 5.2, 5.3, and 5.4)

Because you use so many different muscles for various activities, the likelihood of experiencing some form of skeletal muscle disorder in your lifetime is almost certain. **Muscle soreness** can result from vigorous exercise, particularly if your muscles are not used to it. Exercise increases the lactic acid in your muscle fibers, causing inflammation, and produces soreness in the muscles and nearby connective tissue.

Muscle cramps are sudden, short, painful contractions of a muscle or group of muscles. The cause of these cramps is unknown. A poor diet that leads to low blood potassium, calcium and magnesium levels, caffeine and tobacco use, and reduced blood supply may contribute to muscle cramps. There are no effective medications available.

Muscle strains range from a simple stretch to a partial or complete tear in the muscle, tendon, or muscle-tendon combination. Most strains heal with RICE *(Figure 5.3)*, followed by basic exercises to relieve pain and restore mobility. A complete tear may require surgery.

A **sprain** is a stretch or tear of a ligament, often in the ankle, knee, or wrist, and is also treated by RICE.

Anabolic steroids are related to testosterone but altered to make skeletal muscle hypertrophy. Used illegally in many sports to boost muscle strength, steroids have noticeable, often irreversible side effects. These include stunted growth in adolescents, shrinking testes and reduced sperm counts, masculinization of women's bodies and voices, delusions, and paranoid jealousy. Long-term effects may be increased risk of heart attack and stroke, kidney failure, and liver tumors.

Fibromyalgia affects muscles and tendons all over the body, causing chronic pain, fatigue, and depression. Its cause is unknown and there are currently no laboratory tests for it. The only treatment options are pain management, physiotherapy, and stress reduction.

Myasthenia gravis is a chronic autoimmune disease *(see Chapter 7)* characterized by varying degrees of weakness of the skeletal muscles. The weakness increases with activity and decreases with rest. Facial muscles are often involved, causing problems with eye and eyelid movements, chewing, and talking. Antibodies produced by the immune system block the passage of stimuli from motor nerves to muscles, making movements limited.

Muscular dystrophy is a general term for a group of hereditary, progressive disorders affecting skeletal muscles. **Duchenne muscular dystrophy (DMD)** is the most common in boys, beginning with difficulty walking around the age of 3. Generalized muscle weakness and atrophy progress, and few live beyond 20 years of age. There is no effective treatment.

Rhabdomyolysis is the breakdown of muscle fibers, which releases a protein pigment (**myoglobin**) into the bloodstream. Myoglobin breaks down into toxic compounds that cause kidney failure. Muscle trauma, severe exertion (marathon running), alcoholism, and use of cocaine, heroin, amphetamines, or phencyclidine (**PCP**) can cause this disorder.

Tenosynovitis is an inflammation of the sheath that surrounds a **tendon,** often in the wrist and hands. Repetitive use of these tendons can produce pain, tenderness in the tendon, and difficulty in related joint movement.

▼ **FIGURE 5.3**
RICE Treatment.

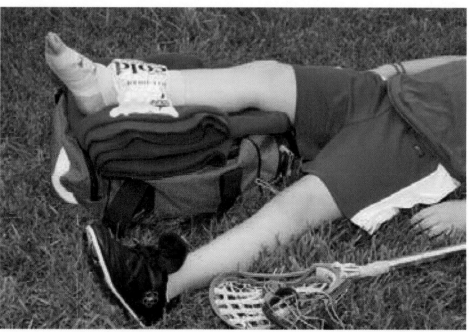

Word	Pronunciation		Elements	Definition
Duchenne muscular dystrophy	DOO-shen MUSS-kyu-lar DISS-troh-fee	P/ R/	Guillaume Benjamin Duchenne, French neurologist, 1806–1875 dys- *bad, difficult* -trophy *nourishment*	A condition with symmetrical weakness and wasting of pelvic, shoulder, and proximal limb muscles
fibromyalgia	fie-broh-my-AL-jee-ah	S/ R/CF R/	-algia *pain* fibr/o- *fiber* -my- *muscle*	Pain in the muscle fibers
myoglobin	MY-oh-GLOW-bin	S/ R/CF R/	-in *substance* my/o- *muscle* -glob- *globe*	Protein of muscle that stores and transports oxygen
rhabdomyolysis	RAB-doh-my-oh-LIE-sis	S/ R/CF R/CF	-lysis *destruction* rhabd/o- *rod shaped* -my/o- *muscle*	Destruction of muscle to produce myoglobin
sprain	SPRAIN		root unknown	A wrench or tear in a ligament
strain	STRAIN		Latin *to bind*	Overstretch or tear in a muscle or tendon
tendon tendinitis *(also spelled tendonitis)*	TEN-dun ten-dih-NYE-tis	S/ R/	Latin *sinew* -itis *inflammation* tendin- *tendon*	Fibrous band that connects muscle to bone Inflammation of a tendon
tenosynovitis	TEN-oh-sine-oh-VIE-tis	S/ R/CF R/	-itis *inflammation* ten/o- *tendon* -synov- *synovial membrane*	Inflammation of a tendon and its surrounding synovial sheath
thymectomy	thigh-MEK-toe-me	S/ R/	-ectomy *surgical excision* thym- *thymus gland*	Surgical removal of the thymus gland

EXERCISES

A. The following elements *are all contained in the WAD above. Circle the best answer.*

1. The suffix *-itis* means: condition   disease   inflammation

2. *Dys* is a: suffix   prefix   root

3. The root *trophy-* means: condition   procedure   nourishment

4. *Fibro* is a: combining form   root   suffix

5. *The root my-* means: tendon   ligament   muscle

6. The suffix *-algia* means: inflammation   pain   swelling

7. *Ectomy* means: fixation   repair   excision

8. Which term has a suffix that means *destruction?*   myoglobin   tenosynovitis   rhabdomyolosis

9. *Teno* is a: prefix   root   combining form

B. Terminology challenge.

1. What term in the WAD has a root and a prefix but no suffix? _____

   Which element in this term functions as a suffix? _____

   Why is that element not called a suffix in this term? _____

2. What is the difference between a *sprain* and a *strain?*

   Sprain: _____

   Strain: _____

3. What term in the WAD has two acceptable spellings? _____   _____

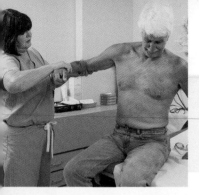

LESSON 5.2

Muscles and Tendons of the Shoulder Girdle, Trunk, and Upper Limb

OBJECTIVES

The muscles and tendons of your shoulders, arms, and hands are nearly always in motion. You shake hands, point your finger, turn doorknobs, and lift various objects throughout the course of any given day. The information in this lesson will enable you to use correct medical terminology to:

5.2.1 Describe the structures and functions of the muscles and tendons of the shoulder girdle.

5.2.2 Identify common disorders of the muscles and tendons of the shoulder girdle.

5.2.3 Specify the major muscles that join the arm to the trunk.

5.2.4 Explain the structures and functions of the muscles of the arm, elbow, forearm, and wrist.

5.2.5 Name a common disorder of the joints, muscles, and tendons of the elbow.

5.2.6 Define common disorders of the joints, and muscles of the hand.

Shoulder Girdle

(LO 5.1, 5.2, and 5.3)

Your **pectoral** (shoulder) **girdle** connects your axial skeleton to your upper limbs and helps you to move these limbs. Without your shoulder girdle, you wouldn't be able to throw a ball, drive a car, or reach that top shelf of your closet or kitchen cabinet. In fact, you wouldn't be able to move your upper limbs.

The muscles and tendons in your shoulder girdle get plenty of use. Four muscles that **originate** on your scapula wrap around the shoulder joint and fuse together. This fusion forms one large tendon (the **rotator cuff**), which is **inserted** into the humerus *(Figure 5.4)*. Your rotator cuff keeps the ball of the humerus tightly in the scapula's socket and provides the kind of strength needed by baseball pitchers.

> ## CASE REPORT 5.1 (CONTINUED)
>
> When Dr. Stannard evaluated Mr. Adams, an MRI revealed a full-thickness tear of his rotator cuff. Mr. Adams has been scheduled for **ambulatory** surgery to repair the tear.

Common Disorder of the Shoulder Girdle (LO 5.1, 5.2, 5.3, and 5.4)

Rotator cuff tears (a frequent injury to the shoulder girdle), are caused by wear and tear from overuse in work situations or in certain sports, such as baseball, football, and golf. These tears can be partial or complete.

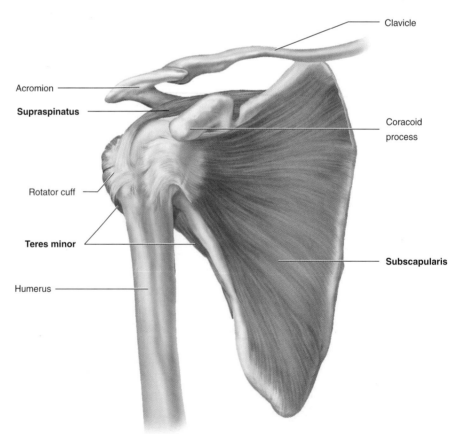

▶ **FIGURE 5.4**
Rotator Cuff Muscles
(labeled in bold).

S = Suffix   P = Prefix   R = Root   R/CF= Combining Form

Word	Pronunciation	Elements		Definition
ambulatory	am-byu-**LAY**-tor-ee	S/ R/	-ory *having the function of* ambulat- *walking*	Surgery or any other care provided without an overnight stay in a medical facility
insertion insert (verb)	in-**SIR**-shun in-**SIRT**	S/ R/	-ion *action, condition* insert- *put together*	The insertion of a muscle is the attachment of a muscle to a more movable part of the skeleton, as distinct from the origin
origin	**OR**-ih-gin		Latin *source of*	Fixed source of a muscle at its attachment to bone
pectoral	**PEK**-tor-al	S/ R/	-al *pertaining to* pector- *chest*	Pertaining to the chest
pectoral girdle	**PEK**-tor-al **GIR**-del		girdle, Old English *encircle*	Incomplete bony ring that attaches the upper limb to the axial skeleton
rotator cuff	roh-**TAY**-tor **CUFF**	S/ R/	-or *one who does* rotat- *rotate* cuff, Old English *band*	Part of the capsule of the shoulder joint

EXERCISES

A. Review *the Case Report on this spread before answering the questions. Apply your knowledge of medical language to fill in the correct answers.*

1. What type of diagnostic test did Mr. Adams have? _____

2. What did the test in question #1 reveal? _____

3. Define *full thickness tear*. Use the glossary or a dictionary. _____

   _____

4. Why does the tear have to be repaired surgically? _____

5. How do you think Mr. Adams may have injured himself? _____

B. Meet *a lesson objective by answering the following questions. Fill in the blanks.*

1. A frequent sports injury to the shoulder girdle is _____

2. The four muscles that originate on the scapula fuse together into the: _____ .

3. The pectoral girdle connects the axial skeleton to _____

4. Is the rotator cuff a tendon, ligament or muscle? _____

5. Where is the insertion point of the rotator cuff? _____

C. Review the WAD *for answers to the questions below.*

1. Explain the terms *origin* and *insertion* in relation to muscles:

   Origin: _____

   Insertion: _____

2. Which suffix means *one who does?* _____

3. If a patient is checked into the hospital as *ambulatory,* what does that mean?

   _____

4. The axial skeleton connects to the limbs, which facilitates what body function? _____

LESSON **5.2** Upper Arm and Elbow Joint (LO 5.1, 5.2, and 5.3)

Your muscles connect your humerus (upper arm bone) to your shoulder girdle, vertebral column, and ribs. These muscles enable your arm to move freely at the shoulder joint. Your major anterior muscles (those at the front of your body) are the **deltoid** (shoulder muscle) and **pectoralis major** (chest muscle) *(Figure 5.5a)*. Among the major posterior muscles is the **latissimus dorsi,** found in your back *(Figure 5.5b)*.

Muscles that move your elbow joint and forearm originate on the upper arm bone or shoulder girdle and are inserted into the bones of your forearm. On the front of the arm, you have a group of three muscles *(Figure 5.5a)*—**biceps brachii, brachialis,** and **brachioradialis.** These muscles flex your forearm at the elbow joint and rotate your forearm and hand sideways or laterally (supination). A single muscle on the back of your arm (the **triceps brachii**) extends your elbow joint and forearm *(Figure 5.5b)*.

ABBREVIATIONS

CTS   carpal tunnel syndrome

Common Disorder of the Elbow (LO 5.1, 5.2, 5.3, and 5.4)

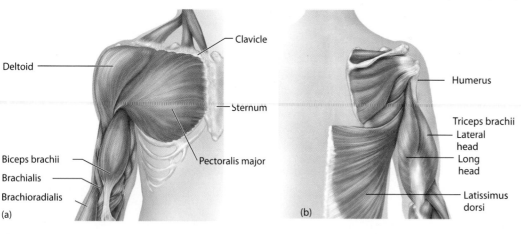

Deltoid

Biceps brachii

Brachialis

Brachioradialis

(a)

Clavicle

Sternum

Pectoralis major

Humerus

Triceps brachii
— Lateral head
— Long head

Latissimus dorsi

(b)

Tennis elbow is a common injury. Upper arm and forearm muscle tendons are inserted into the upper arm bone just above the elbow joint. Small tears in these tendons at their attachments can be caused by trauma or overuse of the elbow joint. Weight lifting, poor tennis skills, and golf frequently overwork the elbow, and straightening it or opening and closing the fingers produces pain. Treatment is rest, ice, pain medication, massage, and stretching exercises.

▲ **FIGURE 5.5**
Muscles Joining Arm to Body.
(a) Anterior view.
(b) Posterior view.

Forearm, Wrist, and Hand (LO 5.1, 5.2, and 5.3)

The muscles of your forearm are responsible for various movements. These muscles supinate and pronate your forearm (turning it upward and downward), flex and extend your wrist joint and hand, and move your hand medially and laterally (back and forth crossways). These terms of movement are detailed in Chapter 2.

Your forearm is bigger near the elbow because the forearm muscles are fleshy and bulky. Your wrist is much thinner because these muscles have become tendons that pass over your wrist on the way to being inserted into your finger bones.

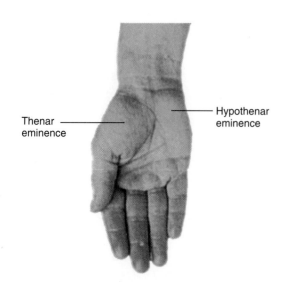

Thenar eminence

Hypothenar eminence

▲ **FIGURE 5.6**
Palmar Surface of the Hand.

Common Disorders of the Wrist (LO 5.1, 5.2, 5.3, and 5.4)

Because you use your hands and wrists almost constantly, your wrists can be prone to disorders and injuries.

Ganglion cysts are fluid-filled cysts on the back of the wrist, which result from irritation or inflammation of the synovial tendon sheaths in this area. These cysts usually disappear on their own.

Stenosing tenosynovitis is a painful inflammation of the synovial sheaths on the back of the wrist.

Carpal tunnel syndrome (CTS) develops on the front of the wrist and results from inflammation and swelling of overused tendon sheaths. Repetitive movements, like typing on a computer keyboard, can lead to CTS. A feeling of "pins and needles" or pain and loss of muscle power in the thumb side of the hand is common.

The Hand (LO 5.1, 5.2, and 5.3)

When you look at the palm of your hand, you'll see a prominent pad of muscles (the **thenar eminence**) at the base of your thumb. A smaller pad of muscles (the **hypothenar eminence**) *(Figure 5.6)* is located at the base of your little finger. The back of your hand is called the **dorsum.**

Word	Pronunciation	Elements		Definition
biceps brachii	BYE-sepz BRAY-key-eye	P/ R/ R/CF	bi- *two* -ceps *head* brachi/i *of the arm*	A muscle of the arm that has two heads or points of origin on the scapula
brachialis	BRAY-kee-al-is	S/ R/	-alis *pertaining to* brachi- *arm*	Muscle that lies underneath the biceps and is the strongest flexor of the forearm
brachioradialis	BRAY-kee-oh-RAY-dee-al-is	S/ R/CF R/	-alis *pertaining to* brachi/o- *arm* -radi- *radius*	Muscle that helps flex the forearm
cyst	SIST		Greek *fluid-filled sac*	An abnormal, fluid-containing sac
deltoid	DEL-toyd	S/ R/	-oid *resembling* delt- *triangle*	Large, fan-shaped muscle connecting the scapula and clavicle to the humerus
dorsum	DOOR-sum		Latin *back*	The back of any part of the body, including the hand
dorsal (adj)	DOOR-sal	S/ R/ R/	-al *pertaining to* dors- *back*	Pertaining to the back of any part of the body
ventral (*opposite of* **dorsal**)	VEN-tral		ventr- *belly*	Pertaining to the belly or situated nearer to the surface of the belly
ganglion	GANG-lee-on		Greek *swelling*	Fluid-containing swelling attached to the synovial sheath of a tendon
latissimus dorsi	lah-TISS-ih-muss DOOR-sigh	S/ R/ R/	-imus *most* latiss- *wide* dorsi *of the back*	The widest (broadest) muscle in the back
stenosis	steh-NOH-sis		Greek *narrowing*	Narrowing of a passage
thenar eminence	THAY-nar EM-in-ens	R/	eminence Latin *stand out* thenar *palm*	The fleshy mass at the base of the thumb
hypothenar eminence	high-poh-THAY-nar EM-in-ens	P/	hypo- *below, smaller*	The fleshy mass at the base of the little finger
triceps brachii	TRY-sepz BRAY-key-eye	P/ R/ R/CF	tri- *three* -ceps *head* brachi/i *of the arm*	Muscle of the arm that has three heads or points of origin

EXERCISES

A. Analyze *the underlined word or part of a word as your clue for the element in the correct term.*

1. arm muscle with <u>three</u> heads _____

2. <u>triangular</u>-shaped muscle _____

3. <u>widest</u> muscle in the back _____

4. arm muscle with <u>two</u> heads _____

5. strongest flexor of the for<u>earm</u> _____

B. Elements *can have more than one meaning and must be applied differently to specific medical terms. Fill in the blanks.*

1. Give an example of a medical term (other than *hypothenar*), from any chapter, that begins with *hypo* and in which *hypo* means *below*.

   Term: _____ means _____.

2. Give an example of a medical term, from any chapter, that begins with *hypo* and in which *hypo* means *deficient* or *less than* (in the sense of location).

   Term: _____ means _____.

STUDY HINT

To help remember the difference between the *thenar* eminence and the *hypothenar* eminence, focus on the prefix *hypo*, which can mean below or smaller. If you hold the hand open, palm facing you, with the thumb straight up, the *hypothenar* eminence is the fleshy mass at the base of the little finger, which is the smallest one on the hand.

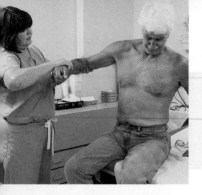

LESSON 5.3

Pelvic Girdle, Thigh, Leg, and Foot

You use the muscles and tendons of your legs and feet so routinely that sometimes you might forget that these "separate pieces" exist until one of them begins to ache or is injured. The information in this lesson will enable you to use correct medical terminology to:

5.3.1 Describe the structures and functions of the muscles of the pelvic girdle.

5.3.2 Define the structures and functions of the muscles and tendons of the thigh, leg, and foot.

5.3.3 Recognize a common disorder of the muscles and tendons of the ankle.

Muscles of the Hip and Thigh (LO 5.1, 5.2, and 5.3)

Some of your body's most powerful muscles support your hip joint and move your thigh. These muscles originate on the pelvic girdle and are inserted into the femur. Among these prominent muscles are your three **gluteus** muscles—**maximus, medius,** and **minimus** *(Figure 5.7)*—and the **adductor** muscles that run down your inner thigh.

Thigh Muscles (LO 5.1, 5.2, and 5.3)

Your thigh muscles move your knee joint and lower leg. Your anterior thigh (the front of your thigh) contains your large **quadriceps femoris** muscle. This muscle has four heads: the rectus femoris, vastus lateralis, vastus medialis, and the vastus intermedius (which lies beneath the rectus femoris). These four muscle heads join into the **quadriceps tendon** (which contains the patella), and continue as the patellar tendon to be inserted into the tibia *(Figure 5.8)*. The quadriceps muscle **extends** (straightens) the knee joint and, because of the lower leg's weight, it has to be a very strong muscle.

Your posterior (rear) thigh is composed mostly of your three **hamstring muscles**—the **biceps femoris, semimembranosus,** and **semitendinosus** *(Figure 5.9)*. These muscles flex (bend) your knee joint and rotate your leg. The hollow area at the back of your knee between your hamstring tendons is the **popliteal fossa.**

Muscles and Tendons of the Lower Leg, Ankle, and Foot (LO 5.1, 5.2, and 5.3)

The muscles of your lower leg move your ankle, foot, and toes. Your front leg muscles bend your foot backward at the ankle and extend your toes. The side or lateral leg muscles turn your foot outward or evert it. Your back leg muscles plantar-flex your foot at the ankle, flex your toes, and turn in or invert your foot. The **gastrocnemius** muscle *(Figure 5.10(a))*, located at the back of your leg, forms a large part of your calf. The distal end of this muscle joins the tendon of the smaller calf (soleus) muscle to create the **Achilles (calcaneal) tendon,** which is attached to the heel bone **(calcaneus)** *(Figure 5.10(b))*. Together, your gastrocnemius muscle and Achilles tendon make it possible for you to "push off" when jumping or running. For more detailed foot movement descriptions, you may review the terms in Chapter 2.

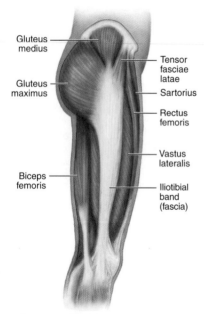

▲ **FIGURE 5.7**
Hip Joint.
Muscles of the hip and thigh, lateral view.

Labels: Gluteus medius, Gluteus maximus, Biceps femoris, Tensor fasciae latae, Sartorius, Rectus femoris, Vastus lateralis, Iliotibial band (fascia)

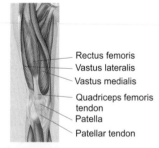

▲ **FIGURE 5.8**
Anterior Muscles of the Thigh.

Labels: Rectus femoris, Vastus lateralis, Vastus medialis, Quadriceps femoris tendon, Patella, Patellar tendon

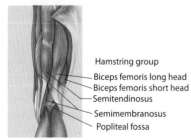

▲ **FIGURE 5.9**
Posterior Thigh Muscles.

Labels: Hamstring group, Biceps femoris long head, Biceps femoris short head, Semitendinosus, Semimembranosus, Popliteal fossa

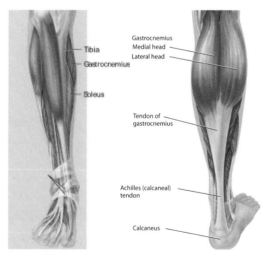

▲ **FIGURE 5.10**
Muscles of Lower Leg and Foot.
(a) Muscles of the front of the right leg.
(b) Muscles of the back of the right leg.

Labels: Tibia, Gastrocnemius, Soleus, Gastrocnemius Medial head, Lateral head, Tendon of gastrocnemius, Achilles (calcaneal) tendon, Calcaneus

Word	Pronunciation	Elements		Definition
abduction abduct (verb)	ab-**DUCK**-shun ab-**DUKT**	S/ P/ R/	-ion *process, action* ab- *away from* -duct- *lead*	Action of moving away from the midline
adductor adduction	ah-**DUCK**-tor ah-**DUCK**-shun	S/ R/ S/ P/	-or *that which does something* -duct- *to lead* -ion *action, condition* ad- *toward*	Muscle that moves the thigh toward the midline Action of moving toward the midline
calcaneal tendon *(same as* Achilles tendon*)*	kal-**KAY**-knee-al ah-**KILL**-eeze	S/ R/	Latin *the heel* -eal *pertaining to* calcan- *calcaneus* mythical Greek warrior	A tendon formed from gastrocnemius and soleus muscles and inserted into the calcaneus
gastrocnemius	gas-trok-**KNEE**-me-us	S/ R/	-ius *pertaining to* gastrocnem- *calf of leg*	Major muscle in back of the lower leg (the calf)
gluteus gluteal (adj)	**GLUE**-tee-us **GLUE**-tee-al	S/ R/	Greek *buttocks* -eal *pertaining to* glut- *buttocks*	Refers to one of three muscles in the buttocks Pertaining to the buttocks
maximus	**MAKS**-ih-mus		Latin *the biggest* or *the greatest*	The gluteus maximus muscle is the largest muscle in the body, covering a large part of each buttock
medius	**ME**-dee-us		Latin *middle*	The gluteus medius muscle is partly covered by the gluteus maximus
minimus	**MIN**-ih-mus		Latin *smallest*	The gluteus minimus is the smallest of the gluteal muscles and lies under the gluteus medius
popliteal fossa	pop-**LIT**-ee-al **FOSS**-ah	S/ R/CF	-al *pertaining to* poplit/e- *ham, back of knee* fossa, Latin *trench, ditch*	The hollow at the back of the knee
quadriceps femoris	**KWAD**-rih-seps **FEM**-or-is	R/ P/ S/ R/	-ceps *head* quadri- *four* -is *belonging to, pertaining to* femor- *femur*	An anterior thigh muscle with four heads (origins)

EXERCISES

A. Spelling: *A medical term must be spelled correctly. Work with a fellow student on this exercise. Cover the WAD with a sheet of paper while your partner dictates any 5 terms in the above WAD to you. Write them in the "Test" column, and do your best to spell them correctly. When you are finished, remove the cover and check your spelling. If you have made any errors, rewrite the correct spelling in the "Corrections" column. After you have corrected your exercise, dictate the remaining 5 terms to your partner.*

Test   **Corrections**

1. _____   _____

2. _____   _____

3. _____   _____

4. _____   _____

5. _____   _____

B. Identify *the medical term, based on the brief meaning given to you. Be sure to check your spelling when you are finished! Fill in the blanks.*

1. Which terms relate to size? _____

2. Another name for the calcaneal tendon is: _____

3. Where is the popliteal fossa? _____

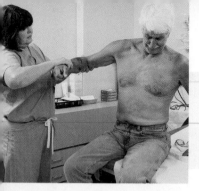

LESSON 5.4

Rehabilitation Medicine

CASE REPORT 5.2

YOU ARE

. . . a **certified occupational therapist** assistant working in the Rehabilitation Unit at Fulwood Medical Center.

YOU ARE COMMUNICATING WITH

. . . Mr. Hank Johnson, a 65-year-old print shop owner.

One year ago, Mr. Johnson had an elective left total-hip replacement for osteoarthritis. Four months later, he had a myocardial infarction. Two weeks ago, while on his exercise bike, he had a stroke. His right arm and leg were paralyzed, he lost his speech, and he had difficulty swallowing. He arrived in the Emergency Department within 3 hours of the stroke and received thrombolytic **therapy** (see Chapter 6). Mr. Johnson is now receiving **physical therapy, occupational therapy,** and speech therapy in the inpatient Rehabilitation Unit. He is able to say some simple words and has begun to have voluntary movements in the arm and leg. Your roles are to help him regain function in his arm and leg and to monitor and record his progress.

Stroke Rehabilitation (LO 5.1, 5.2, 5.3, and 5.4)

The goals of Mr. Johnson's **rehabilitation** program are to enable him to:

- Walk safely using an **assistive device.**
- Use his hands with accuracy.
- Restore his speech abilities.
- Prevent a second stroke.

Because he received thrombolytic therapy (see Chapter 6) within 3 hours of his stroke's onset, he has a 50% chance of being left with little or no residual difficulty, compared to a 35% chance had he not received the therapy.

Social workers are helping Mr. Johnson's wife to make their home safe for his return, including obtaining **adaptive equipment.** Raised toilet seats, handrails in the bath and shower, eating devices, and other adaptive equipment will help Mr. Johnson perform activities of daily living during his recovery. Social workers will also help Mrs. Johnson to work with Medicare to obtain the maximum allowable benefits. Anyone who has had one stroke is at high risk for having a second stroke. Therefore, during this rehabilitative period, Mr. Johnson will be evaluated for such risk factors as narrowing of the carotid arteries with plaque, thrombosis (see Chapter 6), and the presence of atrial fibrillation (see Chapter 6).

Word	Pronunciation		Elements	Definition
assistive device	ah-**SIS**-tiv de-**VICE**	S/ R/	-ive *nature of* assist- *aid, help* device *an appliance*	Tool, software, or hardware to assist in performing daily activities
occupational therapy	**OCK**-you-**PAY**-shun-al **THAIR**-ah-pee	S/ R/ R/	-al *pertaining to* occupation- *work* therapy *treatment*	Use of work and recreational activities to increase independent function
orthotic	or-**THOT**-ik	S/ R/	-ic *pertaining to* orthot- *correct*	Orthopedic appliance to correct an abnormality
orthotist	or-**THOT**-ist	S/	-ist *specialist*	Maker and fitter of orthopedic appliances
physiatry physiatrist	fih-**ZIE**-ah-tree fih-**ZIE**-ah-trist	S/ R/ R/	Greek *science of nature* -ist *specialist* phys- *nature* -iatr- *treatment*	Physical medicine Specialist in physical medicine
physical medicine	**FIZ**-ih-cal **MED**-ih-sin	S/ R/	-al *pertaining to* physic- *body*	Diagnosis and treatment by means of remedial agents, such as exercises, manipulation, heat, etc.
physical therapy *(also known as physiotherapy)*	**FIZ**-ih-cal **THAIR**-ah-pee	S/ R/ R/	-al *pertaining to* physic- *body* therapy *treatment*	Use of remedial processes to overcome a physical defect
physiotherapy (syn)	**FIZ**-ee-oh-**THAIR**-ah-pee	R/CF	physi/o- *body*	Another term for physical therapy
rehabilitation	**REE**-hah-bill-ih-**TAY**-shun	S/ P/ R/	-ion *action, condition* re- *again* -habilitat- *restore*	Therapeutic restoration of an ability to function as before
therapy	**THAIR**-ah-pee		Greek *medical treatment*	Systematic treatment of a disease, dysfunction, or disorder
therapeutic (adj)	**THAIR**-ah-**PYU**-tik	S/ R/	-ic *pertaining to* therapeut- *treatment*	Relating to the treatment of a disease or disorder
therapist	**THAIR**-ah-pist	S/ R/	-ist *specialist* therap- *treatment*	Professional trained in the practice of a particular therapy

EXERCISES

A. Review *the Case Report on this spread before answering the questions. Apply your knowledge of medical language to fill in the correct answers.*

1. Why did Mr. Johnson need a hip replacement? _____

2. What is a *myocardial infarction?* _____

3. What does it mean if you are an *inpatient?* _____

4. What two major medical events has Mr. Johnson suffered recently? _____

5. What are the goals of Mr. Johnson's rehabilitation program? _____

_____

B. Deconstruct *the following medical terms into their word elements. Some terms will not have every element present. Then use any one term in a sentence of patient documentation. Fill in the blanks.*

Medical Term	Prefix	Root/CF	Suffix	Meaning of Term
physiatrist	1.	2.	3.	4.
rehabilitation	5.	6.	7.	8.
orthotic	9.	10.	11.	12.
multidisciplinary	13.	14.	15.	16.
orthotist	17.	18.	19.	20.
physiotherapy	21.	22.	23.	24.

Sentence: _____

_____

LESSON 5.4 Rehabilitation Definitions

(LO 5.1, 5.2, 5.3, and 5.4)

• Coordinated multidisciplinary evaluation, management, and therapy add significantly to the chances of a good recovery.

Definitions (LO 5.1, 5.2, and 5.3)

The following definitions of terms or phrases specific to rehabilitation will help you to understand more precisely the different kinds of rehabilitation in which you may be involved as a health professional.

Rehabilitation medicine focuses on function. Being able to function is essential to an individual's independence and ability to have a good quality of life.

Restorative rehabilitation restores a function that has been lost, such as after a hip fracture, hip replacement, or stroke. This process can be intense but it's also usually short-term.

Maintenance rehabilitation strengthens and maintains a function that is gradually being lost. It is less intense than restorative rehabilitation, but often long-term. Problems of senescence (old age), like difficulty with balance or flexibility, require this long-term approach.

Rehabilitation medicine is also involved with the **prevention** of function loss and the prevention of injury. In sports medicine, an example is the prevention of shoulder and elbow injuries often experienced by baseball pitchers.

Activities of daily living (ADLs) are the routine activities of personal care. The six basic ADLs are eating, bathing, dressing, grooming, toileting, and transferring. Assistive devices are designed to make ADLs easier to perform and help maintain the patient's independence. Examples of these devices include: reachers and grabbers, easy-pull sock aids, long shoehorns, jar openers, and eating aids *(Figure 5.11)*. ADLs are also a measurement to assess therapy needs and monitor its effectiveness.

Instrumental activities of daily living (IADLs) relate to independent living. These activities include; managing money, using a telephone, cooking, driving, shopping for groceries and personal items, and doing housework.

▲ **FIGURE 5.11**
Assistive Device for Dressing.

ADLs	activities of daily living
IADLs	instrumental activities of daily living
BKA	below-the-knee amputation
COTA	certified occupational therapist assistant
PVD	peripheral vascular disease

Amputations

(LO 5.1, 5.2, 5.3, and 5.4)

Seventy-five percent of all amputations are performed on people over 65 years of age with **peripheral vascular disease (PVD).** This includes complications from arteriosclerosis and diabetes. Most of these cases involve **below-the-knee amputations (BKAs).** On the other hand, the war in Iraq has led to soldiers losing their arms and legs from the detonation of explosive devices. In some of these cases, amputations are also required, depending on the level of damage an explosion has caused to the soldier's body.

Rehabilitation after amputation is an increasingly important component in rehabilitation programs. Immediately after surgery, the objectives of the rehabilitation team are to:

• Promote healing of the stump;

• Strengthen the muscles above the site of the amputation;

• Strengthen arm muscles to assist in ambulation or help with walking using a cane, crutches or other assistive devices;

• Prevent **contractures** or **tightening** of the joints above the amputation (knee and hip for BKAs);

• Shrink the post-amputation stump with elastic cuffs or bandages to fit the socket of a temporary **prosthesis** *(Figure 5.12)*; and

• Provide emotional, psychological, and family support.

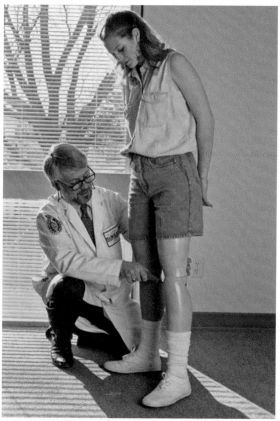

▲ **FIGURE 5.12**
Sixteen-Year-Old Being Fitted with Prosthesis.

Word	Pronunciation	Elements		Definition
contracture	kon-**TRAK**-chur	S/ R/	-ure *result of* **contract-** *pull together*	Muscle shortening due to spasm or fibrosis
prevention	pree-**VEN**-shun	S/ R/	-ion *action, condition* **prevent-** *prevent*	Process to prevent occurrence of a disease or health problem
prosthesis	**PROS**-thee-sis		Greek *an addition*	An artificial part to remedy a defect in the body
restorative rehabilitation	ree-**STOR**-ah-tiv **REE**-hah-bill-ih-**TAY**-shun	S/ R/	-ative *quality of* **restor-** *renew*	Therapy that promotes renewal of health and strength

EXERCISES

A. Rehabilitation *medicine has its own specific goals and terminology. Apply the language of rehabilitation medicine to answer the following questions.*

1. Each of these three types of rehabilitation medicine has a specific focus. Explain what they are.

   a. rehabilitation: _____

   b. restorative rehabilitation: _____

   c. maintenance rehabilitation: _____

2. What does the abbreviation *ADL* stand for? _____

3. List the basic ADLs: _____

   _____

4. What do the IADLs relate to? _____

5. Give an example of an IADL: _____

B. Utilize *the correct language of rehabilitation in the following paragraph. The word bank contains more terms than you need to use—some terms you may use more than once. When you have finished the exercise, proofread it again to see if it makes sense. Fill in the blanks.*

adapt	contracture	amputation(s)	prosthesis
amputee	adaptive equipment	elective	amputate
residual	PVD	assistive	protocol

Seventy-five percent of all (1)_____ are performed on patients over 65 years of age with (2)_____ complicating arteriosclerosis and diabetes. Loss of blood flow to a limb area produces necrotic tissue, which in time can become infected or gangrenous and makes the need for this procedure urgent, rather than (3)_____. A traumatic (4)_____ can occur in an industrial accident, motor vehicle accident, or household accident. The decision to (5)_____ is a serious one and must be undertaken by a qualified surgeon. The (6)_____ will require postoperative training in how to (7)_____ to the use of a (8)_____ and/or (9)_____ Hopefully, there will be no muscle (10)_____ or (11)_____ pain after the surgery.

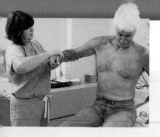

CHAPTER 5 REVIEW

A. Roots/combining forms: *The meaning of the R/CF element is given in the following chart. Identify the R/CF, and list a medical term containing that element. Define the term as well. Fill in the chart.*

Meaning of R/CF	R/CF	Term Containing this R/CF	Definition of the Medical Term
muscle	1.	2.	3.
tendon	4.	5.	6.
chest	7.	8.	9.
arm	10.	11.	12.
palm	13.	14.	15.
thym	16.	17.	18.
calf muscle	19.	20.	21.
buttocks	22.	23.	24.
hollow at back of knee	25.	26.	27.
body	28.	29.	30.

B. Prefixes: *Match the correct medical term in column 1 with the meaning of its prefix in column 2.*

_____ 1. subluxate	**A.** two
_____ 2. hypothenar	**B.** draw together
_____ 3. triceps	**C.** toward
_____ 4. adductor	**D.** after
_____ 5. quadriceps	**E.** without
_____ 6. contract	**F.** under
_____ 7. avascular	**G.** three
_____ 8. abductor	**H.** away from
_____ 9. biceps	**I.** four
_____ 10. postoperative	**J.** below, smaller

> **STUDY HINT**
>
> To help you focus, first underline or highlight only the prefixes in the terms in column 1. Then read all the answer choices in column 2. Finally, go back and do the matching to the highlighted or underlined prefixes. Fill in the blanks.

C. Word attack: *Don't jump to conclusions. Follow the instructions below the question. Any word element you are unsure about can be checked in Appendix A at the back of the book.*

Question:

Circle the term that means *no blood supply:*

a. hematemesis   **b.** hemoptysis

c. avascular   **d.** hemophilia

e. hematoma

Read the question and all the answers twice.

At first glance, you might discount avascular because it is the only answer choice without hem/hemat (which means blood) as a root. Do not do this before you systematically analyze each term.

1. Consider a, b, d, and e as a group since they all have the same R/CF, which you know means blood. The only way to tell them apart is to analyze each suffix. Analyze the suffixes here:

emesis _____

ptysis _____

oma _____

uria _____

2. What is your conclusion after answering question 3?

_____

3. Analyze the remaining choice: *avascular*. Write the meaning of the elements on the second line:

_____ / _____ / _____

_____

4. The correct answer is _____.

D. Recall and review: *This exercise on word elements contains elements from throughout the book. Try to recall the elements without turning back in your book. Indicate the type of element by placing a check mark (✔) in the appropriate column; then write its meaning.*

Element	Type of Element			Meaning of Element
	Prefix	Root/CF	Suffix	
1. ary				2.
3. chondro				4.
5. chiro				6.
7. epi				8.
9. genesis				10.
11. ortho				12.
13. pathy				14.
15. peri				16.
17. plasia				18.
19. sarc				20.

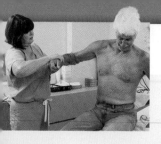

E. Spelling demons: *The following terms from this chapter are particularly difficult to spell and pronounce. Correct pronunciation and spelling of medical terms is the mark of an educated professional. Circle the correct spelling; then check (✔)that you have practiced the pronunciation. (Remember that pronunciations are on the Student Online Learning Center* [www.mhhe.com/AllanEss2e]).

	Terms		Pronunciation ✔
1. tenosynoitis	tenosynovitis	tenosinovitis	_____
2. rhabdomyolysis	rabdomylysis	rhabbomyolysis	_____
3. myogoblin	myoglobolin	myoglobin	_____
4. febromialgia	fibromialgia	fibromyalgia	_____
5. tendonitis	tendinitis	both are correct	_____
6. distrophy	dystrophy	dystrofy	_____

F. Greek and Latin: *Many medical terms come directly from Greek or Latin. Test your knowledge of these terms with this exercise. Fill in the chart with a brief definition of each term.*

Medical Term	Definition
muscle	**1.**
sprain	**2.**
strain	**3.**
origin	**4.**
cyst	**5.**
dorsum	**6.**
ganglion	**7.**
stenosis	**8.**
gluteus	**9.**
maximus	**10.**
medius	**11.**
minimus	**12.**
prosthesis	**13.**
therapy	**14.**
tone	**15.**
tendon	**16.**

G. Terminology challenge: *Think back to elements you have learned throughout the book so far. Fill in the blanks.*

1. The element *pector* means _____ .

   A term using this element is _____ .

   Use this term in a sentence of your choice: _____

   _____

   _____

2. Another element that means the same thing is _____ .

   A term using this element is _____ .

   Use this term in a sentence of your choice: _____

   _____

   _____

H. Create your own test question for this chapter. *It must be a "translate into layperson's terms" or "translate into medical terms" type of question. You may need to draft (practice writing) the question several times before you are satisfied with it. Write the draft of your question below. Then write the finished question, and the answer, on a separate piece of paper, and hand it in to your instructor* 🖐.

_____

_____

_____

_____

_____

_____

_____

Do not forget to write this question and your answer on a separate piece of paper and hand it in to your instructor.

I. Partner exercise: *Ask your study partner to close his or her text. Dictate the following sentences to your partner so that he or she can write them down and then hand them back to you. Check your partner's sentences against the text below. The sentences are not correct unless every word is present and spelled correctly. When you have finished checking your partner's answers, switch places—your partner will dictate, and you will write.*

1. On the front of the arm, a group of three muscles—(1) biceps brachii, (2) brachialis, and (3) brachioradialis—flexes the forearm at the elbow joint and rotates the forearm and hand laterally in supination.

2. The muscles of the forearm supinate and pronate the forearm, flex and extend the wrist joint and hand, and move the hand medially and laterally.

3. The acromion is attached to the clavicle at the acromioclavicular joint, which provides a connection between the axial skeleton, the pectoral girdle, and the arm.

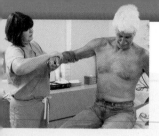

J. Chapter challenge: *Apply the new vocabulary you have learned in this chapter and circle the correct answer.*

1. The correct pair of singular and plural terms is which of the following choices? *(Be precise!)*

   a. scapula/scapulum

   b. clavical/clavicals

   c. phalanx/phalanges

   d. synphysis/synpheses

   e. patela/patellae

2. Which of the following is not a bone?

   a. humerus

   b. brachioradialis

   c. ulna

   d. radius

   e. metacarpal

3. Which of the following is a true statement about the terms *bursitis, tenosynovitis, fasciitis,* and *tendonitis?*

   a. They all involve inflammation.

   b. None of them involves bone.

   c. Every one can be a diagnosis.

   d. Only a and c are true.

   e. Answers a, b, and c are all true.

4. Which group of terms are the *hamstring muscles?*

   a. biceps, triceps, quadriceps

   b. biceps femoris, semimembranosus, semitendinosus

   c. deltoid, pectoralis major, latissimus dorsi

   d. gastrocnemius, soleus, tarsus

   e. biceps brachii, brachialis, brachioradialis

5. Which abbreviation stands for a disease condition?

   a. SI

   b. MRI

   c. CMA

   d. RA

   e. AC

6. Four muscles that originate on the *scapula* wrap around the shoulder joint and fuse to form one large tendon called the:

   a. gastrocnemius

   b. rotator cuff

   c. clavicle

   d. gluteus maximus

   e. humerus

7. What do these terms all have in common: *brachialis, deltoid, latissimus,* and *dorsi?*

   a. They are all tendons.

   b. They are all bones.

   c. They are all muscles.

   d. They are all ligaments.

   e. They have nothing in common.

8. Choose the pair that has both terms spelled correctly:

   a. fasciitis   arthritis

   b. ruhmatoid   rheumatic

   c. phalanx   acetabum

   d. arthrodisis   diastasis

   e. sacroilliac   ischiel

9. Based on the surgical suffix in the term *arthroplasty,* what is being done?

   a. incision into

   b. removal of

   c. repair of

   d. puncture of

   e. fixation of

10. Which two terms relate to *muscles?*

    a. prone   supine

    b. origin   insertion

    c. carpal   metacarpal

    d. thenar   hypothenar

    e. ilium   ischium

11. Where is the *popliteal fossa* located?

    a. in the crook of the elbow

    b. at the back of the neck

    c. at the base of the spine

    d. at the back of the knee

    e. in the pelvic girdle

12. Which two terms contain elements that mean a number?

    a. anterior   posterior

    b. thenar   hypothenar

    c. biceps   triceps

    d. metacarpal   carpal

    e. maximum   medius

K. Case Report challenge: *Now that you are more comfortable with the terms in this chapter, you can apply that knowledge and briefly answer the questions about the Case Report. If you read the report through and underline all the medical terminology, this will make it easier to answer the questions.*

CASE REPORT 5.1

YOU ARE . . . an orthopedic technologist working with orthopedist Kenneth Stannard, MD, in Fulwood Medical Center.

YOU ARE COMMUNICATING WITH

Mr. Bruce Adams, a 55-year-old construction worker who presents with severe pain in his right shoulder.
Mr. Adams' pain began 3 or 4 months ago; it is worse at the end of the workday and when he lifts his arm above his head. During the past week, the pain has woken him from sleep. Mr. Adams' primary care physician has given him pain medication, advised him to stop working, and referred him to Dr. Stannard for diagnosis and treatment. A physical examination shows that Mr. Adams' pain is noticeably limiting all the passive and active movements of his right shoulder, including his ability to lift weight.

1. What is Mr. Adams' main symptom when he presents to Dr. Stannard's office? _____
_____

2. How long has he had this symptom? _____
_____

3. How does this symptom cause difficulty for Mr. Adams? _____
_____

4. Why has the primary care physician referred Mr. Adams to a specialist? _____
_____

5. What recommendations for his condition did Mr. Adams' primary care physician have? _____
_____

6. What does Dr. Stannard observe when he examines Mr. Adams? _____
_____

7. How is this condition affecting Mr. Adams' job performance? _____

8. What likely diagnostic tests or procedures will Mr. Adams probably need? _____
_____

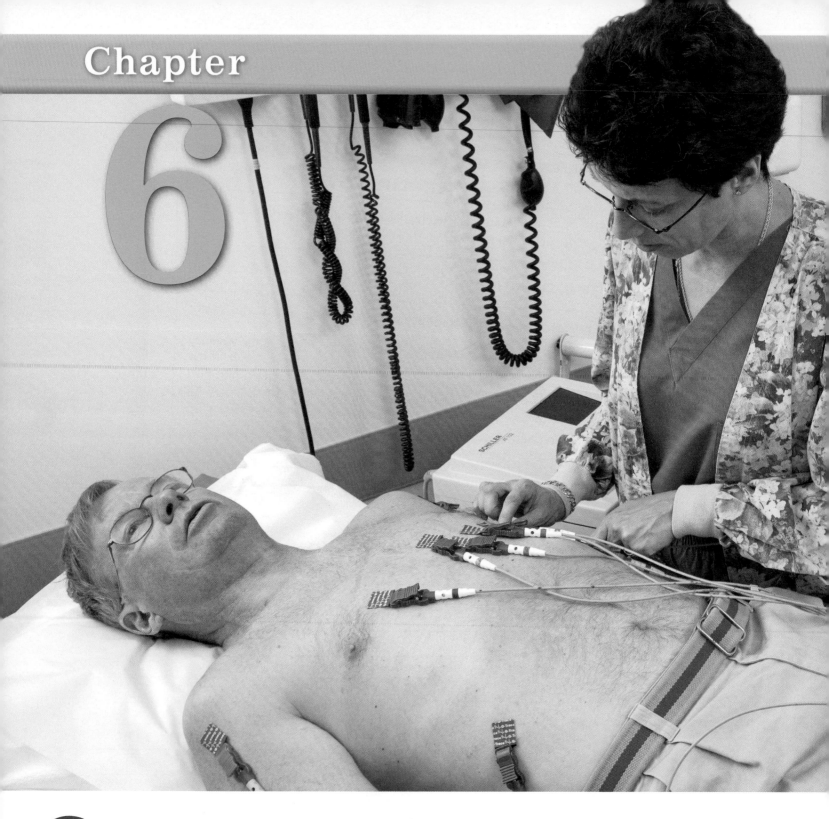

CARDIOVASCULAR AND CIRCULATORY SYSTEMS

The Essentials of the Language of Cardiology

CASE REPORT 6.1

YOU ARE

. . . a cardiovascular technologist (CVT) employed by the **Cardiology** Department at Fulwood Medical Center. You have been called to the Emergency Department (ED) to perform an **electrocardiogram (ECG or EKG)**, STAT.

YOU ARE

COMMUNICATING WITH

. . . Mr. Hank Johnson, a 64-year-old owner of a printing company. Eight months ago, he had a left total hip replacement. In the past 3 months, Mr. Johnson has returned to his daily workouts. This morning, while riding his exercise bike, he felt a tightness in his chest, but continued cycling. He developed pain in the center of his chest, radiating down his left arm and up into his jaw, and became **diaphoretic.** His personal trainer called 911. You perform the ECG and the automatic report describes abnormalities in the chest leads. As you remove the **electrodes,** Mr. Johnson complains that he is feeling faint and short of breath **(SOB).** You are the only person in the room.

The health professionals involved in the diagnosis and treatment of problems with the cardiovascular system include the following:

- **Cardiologists** are medical doctors who specialize in disorders of the cardiovascular system.

- **Cardiovascular surgeons** are surgeons who specialize in surgery of the heart and the peripheral blood vessels.

- **Cardiovascular technologists and technicians** assist physicians in the diagnosis and treatment of cardiovascular disorders.

- **Vascular technologists** are practitioners who assist physicians by performing diagnostic and monitoring procedures using ultrasound.

- **Cardiac sonographers** or echocardiographers are technologists who use ultrasound to observe the heart chambers, valves, and blood vessels.

- **Phlebotomists** or phlebotomy technicians assist physicians by drawing patient blood samples for laboratory testing.

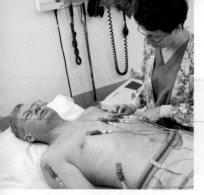

LESSON 6.1
The Heart

OBJECTIVES

Your heart is roughly the size of your fist, weighs approximately 8 to 10 ounces, and pumps around 2,000 gallons of blood each day. Your heart is always working. When your heart fails to work, your blood stops circulating, your tissues stop receiving oxygen and nutrients, your metabolic wastes accumulate, and your cells die. The information in this lesson will enable you to use correct medical terminology to:

6.1.1 Describe the location, structure, and functions of the heart.

6.1.2 Explain the heart cycle.

6.1.3 Identify the blood supply to the heart.

6.1.4 Detail the electrical properties of the heart.

ABBREVIATIONS

CPR	cardiopulmonary resuscitation
CVT	cardiovascular technologist
ECG	electrocardiogram
ED	emergency department
EKG	electrocardiogram
SOB	short(ness) of breath
STAT	immediately

Location of the Heart (LO 6.1, 6.2, and 6.3)

It is important to know precisely where the heart is located so that you can perform effective **cardiopulmonary resuscitation (CPR).** The heart is located in the **thoracic cavity** between the lungs, in an area called the **mediastinum** *(Figure 6.1a)*. The heart is shaped like a blunt cone, pointing down and to the left. It rests at an angle with the majority of its mass to the left of the **sternum** *(Figure 6.1b)*.

▼ **FIGURE 6.1**
Position of Heart in Thoracic Cavity.
(a) Position of heart in mediastinum.
(b) Relationship of heart to sternum.

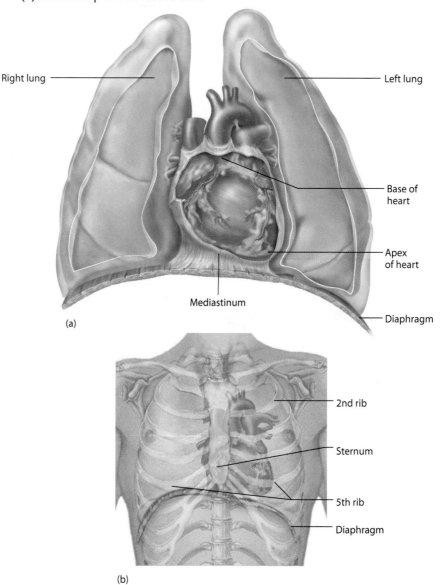

Word	Pronunciation	Elements		Definition
cardiologist	kar-dee-**OL**-oh-jist	S/ R/CF	-logist *one who studies, specialist* cardi/o- *heart*	A medical specialist in the diagnosis and treatment of the heart (cardiology)
cardiology	kar-dee-**OL**-oh-jee	S/	-logy *study of*	Medical specialty of diseases of the heart
cardiopulmonary resuscitation (CPR)	**KAR**-dee-oh-**PUL**-mo-nar-ee ree-sus-ih-**TAY**-shun	S/ R/ R/CF S/ R/-	-ary *pertaining to* -pulmon- *lung* cardi/o- *heart* -ation *a process* resuscit- *revive from apparent death*	The attempt to restore cardiac and pulmonary function
cardiovascular	**KAR**-dee-oh-**VAS**-kyu-lar	S/ R/CF R/	-ar *pertaining to* cardi/o- *heart* -vascul- *blood vessel*	Pertaining to the heart and blood vessels
diaphoresis (noun)	**DIE**-ah-foh-**REE**-sis	R/ S/	diaphor- *sweat* -esis *condition*	Sweat, perspiration, or sweaty
diaphoretic (adj)	**DIE**-ah-foh-**RET**-ic	S/	-etic *pertaining to*	Pertaining to sweat or perspiration
electrocardiogram (ECG, EKG)	ee-lek-troh-**KAR**-dee-oh-gram	S/ R/CF R/CF	-gram *a record* electr/o- *electricity* -cardi/o- *heart*	Record of the electrical signals of the heart
electrocardiograph electrocardiography	ee-lek-troh-**KAR**-dee-oh-graf ee-**LEK**-troh-kar-dee-**OG**-rah-fee	S/ S/	-graph *to record* -graphy *process of recording*	Machine that makes the electrocardiogram The method of recording and the interpretation of electrocardiograms
electrode	ee-**LEK**-trode	S/ R/	-ode *way, road* electr- *electricity*	A device for conducting electricity
mediastinum	**ME**-dee-ass-**TIE**-num	S/ P/ R/	-um *structure* media- *middle* -stin- *partition*	Area between the lungs containing the heart, aorta, venae cavae, esophagus, and trachea
phlebotomist	fleh-**BOT**-oh-mist	S/ R/CF R/	-ist *specialist in* phleb/o- *vein* -tom- *incise, cut*	Person skilled in taking blood from veins
phlebotomy	fleh-**BOT**-oh-me	S/	-tomy *surgical incision*	Taking blood from a vein
sternum	**STIR**-num		Latin *the chest*	Long, flat bone forming the center of the anterior wall of the chest
thoracic cavity	**THOR**-ass-ik **KAV**-ih-tee	S/ R/	-ic *pertaining to* thorac- *chest* cavity, Latin *hollow*	Space within the chest containing the lungs, heart, esophagus, trachea, aorta, venae cavae, and pulmonary vessels

EXERCISES

A. Review *the Case Report on the opening two-page spread before answering the questions.*

1. The following abbreviations all appear in the Case Report. Demonstrate your understanding of the abbreviations by writing out the terms they represent.

   a. EKG _____

   b. ED _____

   c. CVT _____

   d. SOB _____

   e. ECG _____

B. Apply the language *of cardiology in the following documentation. Be sure to use the correct form (noun, adjective) of the term. There is only one best answer for each blank.*

cardiologist   cardiovascular   cardiology   cardiopulmonary

1. The _____ Department sent a specialist to examine the patient in the Emergency Room because of his symptoms. The _____ ordered an angioplasty, which found that the patient had three obstructed arteries in his heart, so the _____ surgeon prepared to operate immediately. Before surgery could begin, the patient suffered a heart attack and _____ resuscitation was needed.

LESSON 6.1 Functions and Structure of the Heart (LO 6.1, 6.2, and 6.3)

Functions of the Heart (LO 6.1, 6.2, and 6.3)

In order to keep your body alive, your heart must work all the time, without stopping. Its three most important functions are to:

1. **Pump blood.** As your heart contracts, it generates pressure that moves your blood through your blood vessels.

2. **Route blood.** Your heart essentially has two pumps: one on the right side that sends blood through the **pulmonary** circulation of your lungs and back to the second pump on your left side, which sends blood through the **systemic** circulation of your body. Your heart valves make this one-way flow of blood possible.

3. **Regulate blood supply.** The changing metabolic needs of your tissues and organs—for example, when you exercise—are met by changes in the rate and force of your heart's contractions.

> ### CASE REPORT 6.1 (CONTINUED)
>
> A **myocardial infarction** (heart attack) is what was happening to Mr. Johnson at the beginning of this chapter. The changes on the ECG showed this event.

Structure of the Heart (LO 6.1, 6.2, and 6.3)

The heart wall consists of three layers *(Figure 6.2):*

1. **Endocardium:** Connective tissue lining the inside of your heart.
2. **Myocardium:** Cardiac muscle cells that contract to enable your heart to pump blood.
3. **Epicardium:** An outer single layer of cells overlying a thin layer of connective tissue.

The **pericardium** is a double-layered connective tissue sac that surrounds and protects your heart.

Blood Supply to Heart Muscle (LO 6.1, 6.2, 6.3, and 6.4)

Because your heart beats continually and forcefully, it requires an abundant supply of oxygen and nutrients. To meet this need, your cardiac muscle has its own blood circulation called the **coronary circulation** *(Figure 6.3).* This system of arteries arises directly from the **aorta.**

If any of your coronary arteries become blocked, the blood supply to a part of your cardiac muscle is cut off **(ischemia)** and the cells supplied by that artery die **(necrosis)** within minutes. This is a **myocardial infarction (MI)** or a "heart attack."

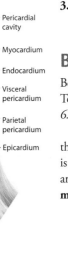

Pericardial cavity
Myocardium
Endocardium
Visceral pericardium
Parietal pericardium
Epicardium

▲ **FIGURE 6.2**
Heart Wall.

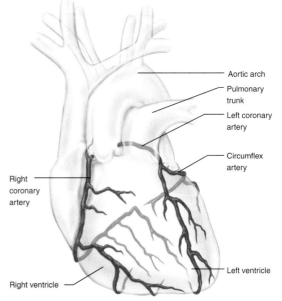

Aortic arch
Pulmonary trunk
Left coronary artery
Circumflex artery
Right coronary artery
Left ventricle
Right ventricle

▲ **FIGURE 6.3**
Coronary Arterial Circulation.

Word	Pronunciation		Elements	Definition
aorta aortic (adj)	a-**OR**-tuh a-**OR**-tik	S/ R/	Greek *lift up* -ic *pertaining to* aort- *aorta*	Main trunk of the systemic arterial system Pertaining to the aorta
coronary circulation	**KOR**-oh-nair-ee **SER**-kyu-**LAY**-shun	S/ R/ S/ R/	-ary *pertaining to* coron- *crown, coronary* -ion *action, condition* circulat- *circular route*	Blood vessels supplying the heart muscle
endocardium endocardial (adj)	**EN**-doh-kar **DEE**-um **EN**-doh-kar-**DEE**-al	S/ P/ R/CF S/	-um *structure* endo- *inside* -card/i- *heart* -al *pertaining to*	The inside lining of the heart Pertaining to the endocardium
epicardium epicardial (adj)	**EP**-ih-kar-**DEE**-um **EP**-ih-kar-**DEE**-al	S/ P/ R/CF S/	-um *structure* epi- *upon, above* -card/i- *heart* -al *pertaining to*	The outer layer of the heart wall Pertaining to the epicardium
infarct infarction	in-**FARKT** in-**FARK**-shun	P/ R/ S/	in- *in* -farct- *area of dead tissue* -ion *action, condition*	Area of cell death resulting from an infarction Sudden blockage of an artery
ischemia ischemic (adj)	is-**KEY**-me-ah is-**KEY**-mik	R/ S/ S/	isch- *to keep back* -emia *a blood condition* -emic *a condition of the blood*	Lack of blood supply to a tissue Pertaining to or affected by the lack of blood supply to a tissue
myocardium myocardial (adj)	**MY**-oh-**KAR**-dee-um my-oh-**KAR**-dee-al	S/ R/CF R/CF S/	-um *structure* my/o- *muscle* -card/i- *heart* -al *pertaining to*	All the heart muscle Pertaining to heart muscle
necrosis necrotic (adj)	neh-**KROH**-sis neh-**KROT**-ik	S/ R/ R/CF S/	-osis *condition* necr- *death* necr/o- *death* -tic *pertaining to*	Pathologic death of cells or tissue Pertaining to or affected by necrosis (death)
pericardium (noun) pericardial (adj)	per-ih-**KAR**-dee-um per-ih-**KAR**-dee-al	S/ P/ R/CF S/	-um *structure* peri- *around* -card/i- *heart* -al *pertaining to*	A double layer of membranes surrounding the heart Pertaining to the pericardium
pulmonary	**PULL**-moh-**NAR**-ee	S/ R/	-ary *pertaining to* pulmon- *lung*	Pertaining to the lungs and their blood supply

EXERCISES

A. Review *the Case Report on this two-page spread before answering the questions.*

1. Based on the patient's ECG, what was his final diagnosis? _____

2. What is the abbreviation for this condition? _____

3. Deconstruct the medical terms in #1 above. _____ / _____ / _____
P   R/CF   S

_____ / _____ / _____
P   R/CF   S

B. Elements: *Solid knowledge of elements will help increase your medical vocabulary. Many of the elements in the WAD above will appear throughout later chapters. Learn these elements now, and you will recognize them later. Put a ✔ in the appropriate column to identify the type of element, and then fill in the last two columns.*

Element	Prefix	Root	CF	Suffix	Meaning of Element	Medical Term with This Element
um	1.				2.	3.
emia	4.				5.	6.
isch	7.				8.	9.
myo	10.				11.	12.

LESSON 6.1 Blood Flow through the Heart (LO 6.1, 6.2, and 6.3)

Your heart has four chambers through which your blood flows *(Figure 6.4)*. These chambers are the:

1. Right **atrium**
2. Right **ventricle**
3. Left atrium
4. Left ventricle

Your right and left atria are separated by a thin muscle wall called the **interatrial septum.** Your right and left ventricles are divided by a thicker muscle wall called the **interventricular septum.**

Your left ventricle pumps blood to all the parts of your body (except the lungs) through the **systemic circulation.** Oxygen (**O₂**) and nutrients are delivered to your body's cells, and carbon dioxide (**CO₂**) and metabolic waste products are removed from the cells. This **deoxygenated** blood, via the veins, returns to the heart where the right ventricle pumps blood into the **pulmonary circulation** to the lungs. In the lungs, the carbon dioxide waste material is exchanged for oxygen from inhaled air *(Figure 6.5)*. This oxygenated blood then travels through the pulmonary veins back to the left side of the heart.

You have four valves that work together to ensure the correct flow of blood through your heart; on the right side are the **tricuspid** and **pulmonary** valves, and on the left side are the **mitral (bicuspid)** and **aortic** valves *(Figure 6.4).*

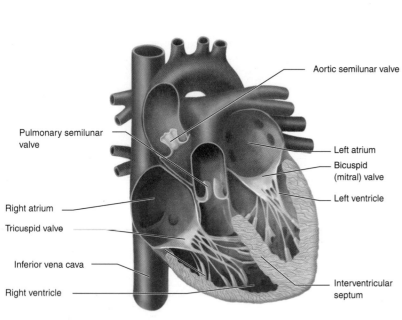

▲ **FIGURE 6.4**
Anatomy of the Heart.

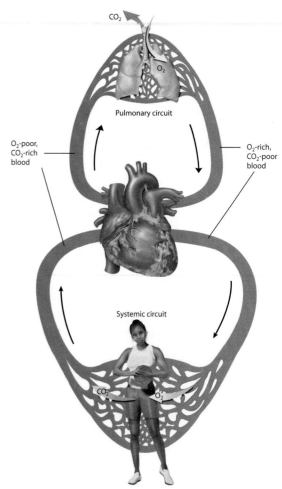

▲ **FIGURE 6.5**
Schematic of Cardiovascular System.

Word	Pronunciation	Elements		Definition
atrium atria (pl) atrial (adj)	A-tree-um A-tree-ah A-tree-al	S/ R/ S/	-um *structure* atri- *entrance, atrium* -al *pertaining to*	Chamber where blood enters the heart on both the right and left sides Pertaining to the atrium
bicuspid	by-**KUSS**-pid	S/ P/ R/	-id *having a particular quality* bi- *two* -cusp- *point*	Having two points; a bicuspid heart valve has two flaps
interatrial	IN-ter-**AY**-tree-al	S/ P/ R/	-al *pertaining to* inter- *between* -atri- *atrium*	Between the atria of the heart
interventricular (IV)	IN-ter-ven-**TRIK**-you-lar	S/ P/ R/	-ar *pertaining to* inter- *between* -ventricul- *ventricle*	Between the ventricles of the heart
mitral	**MY**-tral		Latin *turban*	Shaped like the headdress of a Catholic bishop
septum septa (pl)	**SEP**-tum **SEP**-tah		Latin *partition*	A thin wall dividing two cavities
tricuspid	try-**KUSS**-pid	S/ P/ R/	-id *having a particular quality* tri- *three* -cusp- *point*	Having three points; a tricuspid heart valve has three flaps
ventricle	**VEN**-trih-kel		Latin *small belly*	Chamber of the heart (pumps blood) or a cavity in the brain (produces cerebrospinal fluid)

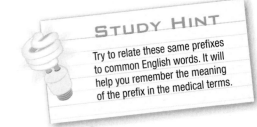

STUDY HINT

Try to relate these same prefixes
to common English words. It will
help you remember the meaning
of the prefix in the medical terms.

EXERCISES

A. Prefixes *can generally answer a question: Where is it? What color is it? How big is it? How many are there? This exercise groups some prefixes from the WAD and asks*

you to identify what makes them similar. Studying elements in similar groups will make them easier to remember. Fill in the chart.

Prefix	Meaning of Prefix	Medical Term with This Prefix	Meaning of Medical Term
bi	1.	2.	3.
tri	4.	5.	6.

These prefixes are similar because: _____

B. This chart has the same prefixes *but is asking for an English word where the prefix means the same as it does in the medical word.*

_____

Prefix	Meaning of Prefix	English Term with This Prefix	Meaning of English Term
bi	1.	2.	3.
tri	4.	5.	6.

C. Meet lesson objectives *and use the language of cardiology to answer the following questions.*

1. Name the four chambers in the heart. _____

2. List the four valves in the heart. _____

3. What is the function of a valve? _____

4. What is the purpose of the systemic circulation? _____

LESSON 6.1 The Heartbeat (LO 6.1, 6.2, and 6.3)

KEYNOTES

- **Vital signs (VS)** measure temperature (T), pulse (P), respiration (R), and blood pressure (BP) to assess cardiorespiratory function.

- A heart rate slower than 60 is called **bradycardia.** A heart rate faster than 100 is called **tachycardia.**

ABBREVIATIONS

AV	atrioventricular
P	pulse
R	respiration
SA	sinoatrial
T	temperature
VS	vital signs

The actions of the four heart chambers are coordinated. When the atria contract (atrial **systole**), the ventricles relax (ventricular **diastole**). When the atria relax (atrial diastole), the ventricles contract (ventricular systole). Then the atria and ventricles all relax briefly. This series of events is a complete cardiac cycle, or heartbeat.

The "lub-dub, lub-dub" sounds heard through the stethoscope are made by the heart valves snapping as they close. If there is an abnormality in valve closure, it will produce an extra, abnormal sound called a **murmur.**

Electrical Properties of the Heart (LO 6.1, 6.2, and 6.3)

As your heart muscles contract, they generate a small electrical current that sustains your heartbeat rhythm through a conduction system *(Figure 6.6)*. Here is how this conduction system works:

1. A small region of specialized muscle cells in the right atrium's **sinoatrial (SA) node** initiates your heartbeat. The SA node is the **pacemaker** of your heart's rhythm.

2. Electrical signals from the SA node spread out through the atria and rejoin at the **atrioventricular (AV) node.** The AV is the electrical gateway to the ventricles.

3. Electrical signals leave the AV node and travel to the ventricular myocardium where they stimulate the ventricular myocardium to contract, creating your heartbeat.

Sinus rhythm is the term used to describe a normal heartbeat, where normal electrical conduction leads to a ventricular rate of about 60 to 80 beats per minute. An abnormal cardiac rhythm is called an **arrhythmia** or a **dysrhythmia.**

An **electrocardiograph** is a device that picks up the heart muscle's electrical changes and amplifies them to record an electrocardiogram in the form of waves *(Figure 6.7)*.

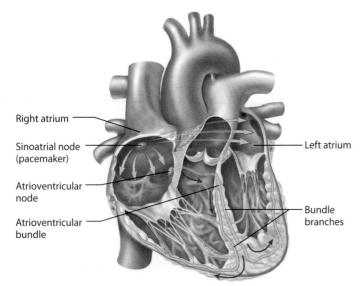

▲ **FIGURE 6.6**
Cardiac Conduction System.

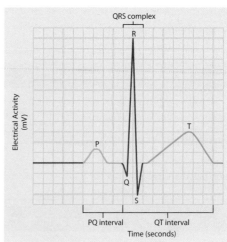

▲ **FIGURE 6.7**
Normal Electrocardiogram.

Word	Pronunciation	Elements		Definition
arrhythmia (Note: double "rr")	a-**RITH**-me-ah	S/ P/ R/	-ia *condition* a- *without* -rrhythm- *rhythm*	Condition when the heart rhythm is abnormal
atrioventricular (AV)	**A**-tree-oh-ven-**TRICK**-you-lar	S/ R/CF R/	-ar *pertaining to* atri/o- *entrance, atrium* -ventricul- *ventricle*	Pertaining to both the atrium and the ventricle
diastole (noun) diastolic (adj)	die-**AS**-toe-lee die-as-**TOL**-ik	 S/ R/	Greek *dilation* -ic *pertaining to* diastol- *diastole*	Dilation of heart cavities, during which they fill with blood Pertaining to diastole
dysrhythmia (Note: single "r")	dis-**RITH**-me-ah	S/ P/ R/	-ia *condition* dys- *bad, difficult* -rhythm- *rhythm*	An abnormal heart rhythm
murmur	**MUR**-mur		Latin *low voice*	Abnormal heart sound heard with a stethoscope when a valve closes or opens abnormally
sinoatrial (SA) node	sigh-noh-**AY**-tree-al NODE	S/ R/CF R/	-al *pertaining to* sin/o- *sinus* -atri- *atrium*	The center of modified cardiac muscle fibers in the wall of the right atrium that acts as the pacemaker for the heart rhythm
sinus rhythm	**SIGH**-nus **RITH**-um		sinus *channel, cavity* rhythm Greek *to flow*	The normal (optimal) heart rhythm arising from the sinoatrial node
systole (noun) systolic (adj)	**SIS**-toe-lee sis-**TOL**-ik	 S/ R/	Greek *contraction* -ic *pertaining to* systol- *systole, contraction*	Contraction of the heart muscle Pertaining to systole
vital signs	**VI**-tal SIGNS		vital Latin *life* signs Latin *mark*	A procedure during a physical examination in which temperature (T), pulse (P), respirations (R), and blood pressure (BP) are measured to assess general health and cardiorespiratory function

EXERCISES

A. Match *the correct element to its meaning.*

_____	**1.** atrio	**a.**	without
_____	**2.** ar	**b.**	contraction
_____	**3.** ia	**c.**	bad, difficult
_____	**4.** systol	**d.**	entrance
_____	**5.** dys	**e.**	condition
_____	**6.** a	**f.**	pertaining to

B. Spelling: *The terms in the WAD can be particularly difficult to spell, yet they occur all the time in a cardiologist's dictation. Circle the correct choice for the documentation.*

1. An (arhythmia/arrhythmia) has been confirmed with the EKG.

2. Her (sysstolic/systolic) blood pressure is dangerously high.

3. The (murrmur/murmur) was detected during ventricular (dyastole/diastole).

4. Cardiac (dysrrhythmia/dysrhythmia) can be a symptom of a serious underlying condition.

5. The (sinoatrial/synoatrial) node is the pacemaker for the heart rhythm.

6. Cardioversion is also called (defibrillation/difribillation).

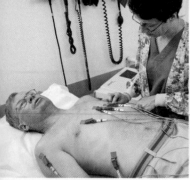

LESSON 6.2

Disorders of the Heart

OBJECTIVES

*Any loss of consciousness precipitated by exertion can be due to a cardiac arrhythmia or a **cardiomyopathy**. In this lesson, the information will enable you to:*

6.2.1 Name common cardiac arrhythmias.

6.2.2 Discuss common disorders of the heart and heart valves.

6.2.3 Describe coronary heart disease.

6.2.4 Explain hypertensive heart disease.

6.2.5 Define the term cardiomyopathy.

CASE REPORT 6.2

YOU ARE

. . . an EMT-P called to the gymnasium of Fulwood University.

YOU ARE COMMUNICATING WITH

. . . Danny Gitlin, a 21-year-old guard on the university basketball team. Danny lost consciousness during a strenuous practice. He had no pulse but was revived by the coach, who used an automatic external **defibrillator (AED)**. Danny has never lost consciousness before, but he has noticed episodes of rapid **palpitations** after games. On examination, he is fully conscious and appears to be fit. His pulse is 70 but irregular in rate and force. His blood pressure is 110/65 mmHg. He has no known family history of heart disease.

Disorders of the Heart
(LO 6.1, 6.2, 6.3, and 6.4)

Abnormal Heart Rhythms
(LO 6.1, 6.2, 6.3, and 6.4)

Arrhythmias are abnormal or irregular heartbeats, and six types are commonly seen:

1. **Premature beats** occur most often in elderly people and are usually associated with caffeine and stress.

2. **Atrial fibrillation (A-fib)** occurs when the two atria quiver rather than contract correctly to pump blood. This causes blood to pool in the atria and sometimes clot.

3. **Ventricular tachycardia (V-tach)** is a rapid heartbeat occurring in the ventricles.

4. **Ventricular arrhythmias** include:
   a. **Premature ventricular contractions (PVCs),** which result when extra impulses arise from a ventricle; and
   b. **Ventricular fibrillation (V-fib),** which occurs when the ventricles lose control, quivering instead of pumping.

5. **Heart block** occurs when interference in cardiac electrical conduction prevents the atria's contractions from coordinating with the ventricles' contractions.

6. **Palpitations** are brief but unpleasant sensations of a rapid or irregular heartbeat. They can be brought on by exercise, anxiety, and stimulants like caffeine.

Arrhythmias can be treated with medications, but some patients require mechanical **pacemakers.** Pacemakers consist of a battery, electronic circuits, and computer memory to generate electronic signals. These signals are carried along thin, insulated wires to the heart muscle. Pacemakers are ideal for patients with a very slow heart rate (bradycardia).

In emergency situations, external **cardioversion** is performed through **automatic external defibrillators,** or **AEDs** *(Figure 6.8).* AEDs send an electric shock to the heart in order to stop the heart temporarily so that a normal contraction rhythm can resume. This procedure was used for Danny Gitlin.

People with life-threatening arrhythmias may need an **implantable cardioverter/defibrillator (ICD),** which senses abnormal rhythms. An ICD gives the heart a small electric shock to return its rhythm to normal.

▶ **FIGURE 6.8**
Automatic External Defibrillator.

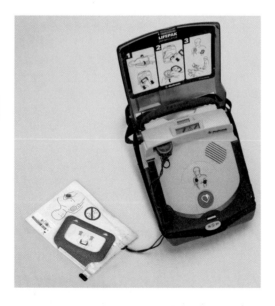

ABBREVIATIONS

AED	automatic external defibrillator
A-fib	atrial fibrillation
EMT-P	Emergency Medical Technician–Paramedic
ICD	implantable cardioverter/defibrillator
PVC	premature ventricular contraction
V-fib	ventricular fibrillation
V-tach	ventricular tachycardia

Word	Pronunciation	Elements		Definition
cardiomyopathy	KAR-dee-oh-my-OP-ah-thee	S/ R/CF R/CF	-pathy *disease* cardi/o *-heart* -my/o- *muscle*	Disease of the heart muscle, the myocardium
cardioversion (also called *defibrillation*)	KAR-dee-oh-VER-shun	R/CF S/	cardi/o- *heart* -version *change*	Restoration of a normal heart rhythm by electric shock
defibrillation	dee-fib-rih-LAY-shun	S/ P/ R/	-ation *process* de- *from, out of* -fibrill- *small fiber*	Restoration of uncontrolled twitching of cardiac muscle fibers to normal rhythm
defibrillator	dee-FIB-rih-lay-tor	S/	-ator *instrument*	Instrument for defibrillation
fibrillation	fi-brih-LAY-shun	S/ R/	-ation *a process* fibrill- *small fiber*	Uncontrolled quivering or twitching of the heart muscle
implantable	im-PLAN-tah-bul	S/ P/ R/	-able *capable* im- *in* -plant- *insert*	A device that can be inserted into tissues
pacemaker	PACE-may-ker	S/ R/	-maker *one who makes* pace- *step*	Device that regulates cardiac electrical activity
palpitation	pal-pih-TAY-shun	S/ R/	-ation *a process* palpit- *throb*	Forcible, rapid beat of the heart felt by the patient

EXERCISES

A. Review *the Case Report on this spread before answering the questions.*

1. What does it mean to *lose consciousness?* _____

2. Danny "had no pulse." What does that mean? _____

3. Where do you see AEDs in public areas? _____

4. What symptom is Danny having? _____

5. What brought on Danny's loss of consciousness? _____

B. Construct *the correct medical terms to match the definitions given. Notice, in particular, that some terms do not have prefixes or suffixes but every term must have a root and/or combining form. Fill in the blanks.*

1. Forceful, rapid beat of the heart

   _____ / _____ / _____
           P   R/CF   S

2. Uncontrolled heart muscle twitching

   _____ / _____ / _____
           P   R/CF   S

3. Device that restores uncontrolled twitching of cardiac muscle to normal rhythm

   _____ / _____ / _____
           P   R/CF   S

4. Implanted device that regulates cardiac electrical activity

   _____ / _____ / _____
           P   R/CF   S

5. Terminology challenge: Find the medical term on this spread that means *slow heart rate*. What element in the term makes you sure it relates to the heart?

   Term: _____ Element: _____

- **Cor pulmonale** is failure of the right ventricle to pump properly. Almost any chronic lung disease causing low blood oxygen (hypoxia) can cause this disorder.

Disorders of Heart Valves
(LO 6.1, 6.2, 6.3, and 6.4)

The heart valves can malfunction in two basic ways. Malfunctions most often occur in the heart's left side.

1. **Stenosis:** The valve cannot open fully, and its opening is narrowed (constricted). Because blood cannot flow freely through the valve, it accumulates in the chamber behind the valve.

2. **Incompetence** or **insufficiency** is a condition where the heart valve cannot close fully, allowing blood to leak or **regurgitate** (flow back) through the valve to the heart chamber from which it came.

Mitral valve stenosis can occur following rheumatic fever. Because the blood cannot flow freely through the valve, the left atrium becomes dilated (enlarged). Eventually, chronic heart failure results.

Mitral valve prolapse occurs when the cusps of the valve bulge back into the left atrium when the left ventricle contracts. This allows blood to flow back into the atrium.

Aortic valve stenosis is common in the elderly when the valves become calcified due to atherosclerosis. Blood flow into the systemic circulation is diminished, leading to dizziness and fainting. The left ventricle dilates, **hypertrophies,** ceases to beat strongly, and ultimately fails.

Aortic valve incompetence initially produces few symptoms other than a murmur. Eventually the left ventricle is unable to cope with the excess volume of blood and fails. (*Figure 6.9* enables you to review the locations of the valves and chambers.)

When a valve replacement is necessary, there are two types of artificial valves available:

1. Mechanical or **prosthetic** valves, which are made from metal alloys and plastics; or

2. **Tissue** valves that can come from a pig or cow, a human cadaver (dead person), or a patient's own pericardium.

Disorders of the Heart Wall
(LO 6.1, 6.2, 6.3, and 6.4)

Endocarditis is an inflammation of the heart's lining, which is usually secondary to an infection elsewhere. Intravenous drug users and people with damaged heart valves are at high risk for endocarditis.

The physical findings on Danny Gitlin suggested a cardiomyopathy, which was confirmed by echocardiography. Exercise testing (a cardiac stress test), with close medical supervision, produced a ventricular arrhythmia that returned to normal on cessation of the test. Danny was treated with beta blockers and restricted to nonstrenuous sports.

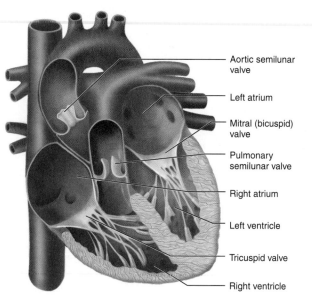

▲ **FIGURE 6.9**
Heart Valves.

- Aortic semilunar valve
- Left atrium
- Mitral (bicuspid) valve
- Pulmonary semilunar valve
- Right atrium
- Left ventricle
- Tricuspid valve
- Right ventricle

Myocarditis is an inflammation of the heart muscle. It can be bacterial, viral, or fungal in origin, or can arise as a complication of other diseases like influenza.

Pericarditis is inflammation of the covering of the heart. The inflammation causes an **exudate** (pericardial effusion) to be released into the pericardial space between the two layers of the pericardium. This interferes with the heart's ability to contract and expand normally, which reduces cardiac output (**CO**) and leads to a life-threatening condition called **cardiac tamponade.**

Cardiomyopathy is a weakening of the heart muscle that makes it pump inadequately. This causes the heart to enlarge (**cardiomegaly**) and leads to heart failure.

Word	Pronunciation		Elements	Definition
cardiomegaly	KAR-dee-oh-MEG-ah-lee	S/ R/CF	-megaly *enlargement* cardi/o- *heart*	Enlargement of the heart
cor pulmonale	KOR pul-moh-NAH-lee	R/ S/ R/	cor *heart* -ale *pertaining to* pulmon- *lung*	Right-sided heart failure arising from chronic lung disease
endocarditis	EN-doh-kar-DIE-tis	S/ P/ R/	-itis *inflammation* endo- *within* -card- *heart*	Inflammation of the lining of the heart
exudate	EKS-you-date	S/ P/ R/	-ate *pertaining to* ex- *out of* -sud- *sweat*	Fluid that has passed out of a tissue or capillaries as a result of inflammation or injury
hypertrophy (can be a noun or a verb)	high-PER-troh-fee	P/ R/	hyper- *above, excessive* -trophy *development*	Increase in size, but not in number, of an individual tissue element
incompetence	in-KOM-peh-tense	S/ P/ R/	-ence *quality of* in- *not* -compet- *strive together*	Failure of a valve to close completely
insufficiency	in-suh-FISH-en-see	S/ P/ R/CF	-ency *quality of* in- *not* –suffic/i- *enough*	Lack of completeness of function; e.g., a heart valve that fails to close properly
myocarditis	MY-oh-kar-DIE-tis	S/ R/CF R/	-itis *inflammation* my/o- *muscle* -card- *heart*	Inflammation of the heart muscle
pericarditis	PER-ih-kar-DIE-tis	S/ P/ R/	-itis *inflammation* peri- *around* -card- *heart*	Inflammation of the pericardium, the covering of the heart
prolapse	pro-LAPS		Latin *a falling*	An organ slips out of its normal position
prosthesis (noun)	PROS-thee-sis		Greek *an addition*	A manufactured substitute for a missing or diseased part of the body
prosthetic (adj)	pros-THET-ik	S/ R/	-ic *pertaining to* prosthet- *artificial part*	Pertaining to a prosthesis
regurgitate	ree-GUR-jih-tate	S/ P/ R/	-ate *pertaining to* re- *back* -gurgit- *flood*	To flow backward; e.g., blood through a heart valve
stenosis	ste-NOH-sis	S/ R/CF	-sis *abnormal condition* sten/o- *narrow*	Narrowing of a canal or passage, e.g., of a heart valve
tamponade	tam-poh-NAID	S/ R/	-ade *a process* tampon- *plug*	Pathologic compression of an organ, such as the heart

EXERCISES

A. Review *the Case Report on this spread before answering the questions.*

1. Translate into layman's language: "The physical findings suggested a cardiomyopathy, which was confirmed by echocardiography." _____

_____

2. The cardiac stress test produced *ventricular arrhythmia* for Danny Gitlin. What made it go away? _____

_____

B. Demonstrate *that you can use the term below correctly. Write a sentence of patient documentation for each of the term's meanings.*

1. *Prosthesis* is a term that appears in chapter 9 relating to orthopedic surgery. Give an example of a heart prosthesis, and another example of an orthopedic prosthesis.

   a. Heart prosthesis: _____

   _____

   b. Orthopedic prosthesis: _____

   _____

- **Risk factors for CAD include:**
  - o Heredity
  - o Age
  - o Obesity
  - o Lack of exercise
  - o Tobacco
  - o Diabetes mellitus
  - o Stress
  - o High blood pressure
  - o Elevated serum cholesterol

- All these risk factors—except heredity and age—can be reduced by lifestyle changes.

Coronary Artery Disease (CAD) (LO 6.1, 6.2, 6.3, and 6.4)

Coronary artery disease occurs when the coronary arteries supplying blood to the myocardium are constricted by **atherosclerotic plaques** called **atheroma** (compare *Figure 6.10(a)* to *6.10(b)*). This reduces the blood supply to the cardiac muscle. Platelet clumping can occur on the plaque and form a blood clot (**coronary thrombosis**). **Atherosclerosis** is the most common form of **arteriosclerosis** (hardening of the arteries), and it can lead to **arteriosclerotic** heart disease (**ASHD**).

Angina pectoris (pain in the chest on exertion) is often the first symptom of a reduced oxygen supply to the myocardium. **Myocardial infarction (MI)** is the death of myocardial cells, caused by the lack of blood supply (**ischemia**) when an artery eventually becomes blocked (**occluded**). If the ischemia is not reversed within 4 to 6 hours, the myocardial cells die (**necrosis**).

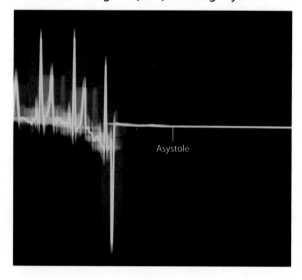

CASE REPORT 6.2 (CONTINUED)

For Mr. Johnson in the Emergency Department, the ECG (EKG) indicated that he was having an MI affecting the anterior wall of his left ventricle. The cardiovascular technician, who did not want to leave the patient alone, used the call system to obtain nursing and medical help.

Circulatory shock occurs when cardiac output is insufficient to meet the body's metabolic needs.

Cardiogenic shock occurs when the heart fails to pump blood effectively through the body's organs and tissues.

Hypovolemic shock occurs from a loss of blood volume, often due to excessive bleeding (hemorrhage) or dehydration.

Cardiac arrest is the sudden cessation of cardiac activity that results from **anoxia** (lack of oxygen in the body tissues). Most patients show **asystole** (no heartbeat) on the cardiac monitor (*Figure 6.11*). A person in cardiac arrest has no pulse, is not breathing, and can be referred to as a **pulseless nonbreather (PNB)**.

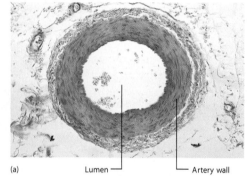

(a)   Lumen ⌐   ⌐ Artery wall

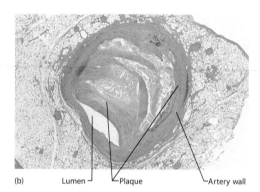

(b)   Lumen ⌐ ⌐Plaque   ⌐Artery wall

▲ **FIGURE 6.10**
Arterial Structure.
(a) Normal coronary artery.
(b) Advanced atherosclerosis.

▼ **FIGURE 6.11**
Electrocardiogram (ECG) Showing Asystole.

Asystole

ASHD	arteriosclerotic heart disease
CAD	coronary artery disease
MI	myocardial infarction
PNB	pulseless nonbreather

Word	Pronunciation	Elements		Definition
anoxia (noun)	an-**OCK**-see-ah	S/ P/ R/	-ia *condition* an- *without* -ox- *oxygen*	Without oxygen
anoxic (adj)	an-**OCK**-sik	S/	-ic *pertaining to*	Pertaining to or suffering from lack of oxygen
arteriosclerosis	ar-**TIER**-ee-oh-skler-**OH**-sis	S/ R/CF R/CF	-sis *abnormal condition* arteri/o- *artery* -scler/o- *hardness*	Hardening of the arteries
arteriosclerotic (adj)	ar-**TIER**-ee-oh-skler-**OT**-ik	S/	-tic *pertaining to*	Pertaining to or affected by arteriosclerosis
asystole	a-**SIS**-toe-lee	P/ R/CF	a- *without* -systol/e *contraction*	Absence of contractions of the heart
atheroma (plaque)	ath-er-**ROE**-mah	S/ R/	-oma *tumor, mass* ather- *porridge, gruel*	Fatty deposit in the lining of an artery
atherectomy	ath-er-**EK**-toe-me	S/	-ectomy *surgical excision*	Surgical removal of the atheroma
atherosclerosis	**ATH**-er-oh-skler-**OH**-sis	S/ R/CF R/CF	-sis *abnormal condition* ather/o- *porridge, gruel* -scler/o- *hardness*	Hardening of the arteries due to atheroma (plaque)
cardiogenic	**KAR**-dee-oh-**JEN**-ik	S/ R/ R/CF	-ic *pertaining to* -gen- *produce* cardi/o- *heart*	Of cardiac origin
hypovolemic	**HIGH**-poh-vo-**LEE**-mick	S/ P/ R/	-emic *a condition in the blood* hypo- *below* -vol- *volume*	Decreased blood volume in the body
hypovolemia	**HIGH**-poh-vo-**LEE**-meah	S/	-ia *a condition*	Pertaining to a decreased blood volume in the body
occlude (verb)	oh-**KLUDE**		Latin *to close*	To close, plug, or completely obstruct
occlusion (noun)	oh-**KLU**-zhun			A complete obstruction
substernal	sub-**STER**-nal	S/ P/ R/	-al *pertaining to* sub- *under* -stern- *chest*	Under (behind) the sternum or breastbone

EXERCISES

A. Review *the Case Report on this spread before answering the questions.*

1. What specific place in Mr. Johnson's heart was affected by his MI?

_____

2. What does an MI do to the living tissue in Mr. Johnson's heart?

_____

3. What is the medical term for this condition in question #2? _____

4. What is the function of the part of the heart which is the answer in question #1 above?

_____

5. What indicated Mr. Johnson was having a heart attack? _____

B. Recall *the use of the prefix in the following terms. You have seen this prefix before, and you will see it again—same prefix, different elements, more terms. Fill in the blanks.*

1. The prefix *sub* means _____.

2. *Substernal* means _____.

3. *Sublingual* means _____.

4. *Subcutaneous* means _____.

5. *Submandibular* means _____.

KEYNOTES

• Hypertension is the major cause of heart failure, stroke, and kidney failure.

• The risk factors for hypertension are:
   o Overweight
   o Alcohol
   o Lack of exercise
   o Tobacco
   o Stress

• All these risk factors can be reduced by lifestyle changes.

Hypertensive Heart Disease (LO 6.1, 6.2, 6.3, and 6.4)

Hypertension (HTN), the most common cardiovascular disorder in this country, affects more than 20% of the adult population. It results from a prolonged elevated blood pressure in the vascular system, which forces the ventricles to work harder to pump blood.

High blood pressure is indicated by a blood pressure reading of 140/90 mmHg (millimeters of mercury) or higher. A normal blood pressure is below 120/80 mmHg. The first number, or **systolic** reading, reflects the blood pressure when the heart is contracting. The second number, or **diastolic** reading, reflects the blood pressure when the heart is relaxed between contractions.

Primary or **essential hypertension** is the most common type of hypertension. Its etiology is **idiopathic** (unknown).

Secondary hypertension results from other diseases like kidney disease, atherosclerosis, and hyperthyroidism.

Malignant hypertension is a rare, severe, life-threatening form of hypertension that involves a blood pressure reading of greater than 200/120 mmHg. Aggressive intervention is mandatory to reduce the blood pressure.

Congestive Heart Failure (CHF) (LO 6.1, 6.2, 6.3, and 6.4)

CHF occurs when the heart is unable to supply enough cardiac output to meet the body's metabolic needs. The most common conditions leading to CHF are:

- Cardiac ischemia
- Severe hypertension
- Valvular regurgitation
- Aortic stenosis
- Cardiomyopathy

Congenital Heart Disease (CHD) (LO 6.1, 6.2, 6.3, and 6.4)

CHD is the result of an abnormal development of the heart in the fetus. Common **congenital** defects or abnormalities can usually be surgically repaired, and can include the following:

1. **Atrial septal defect (ASD)** is a hole in the interatrial septum *(Figure 6.12)*.

2. **Ventricular septal defect (VSD)** is a gap in the interventricular septum *(Figure 6.12)*.

3. **Patent ductus arteriosus (PDA)** arises from a failure of the ductus arteriosus (a normal blood vessel in the fetus) to close within 24 hours of birth.

4. **Coarctation of the aorta** is a narrowing of the aorta shortly after the artery to the left arm branches from the aorta. This causes **hypertension** in the arms behind the narrowing, and **hypotension** in the lower limbs and organs (like the kidney) below the narrowing.

5. **Tetralogy of Fallot (TOF)** is a **syndrome** in which four congenital heart defects all force blood away from the lungs.

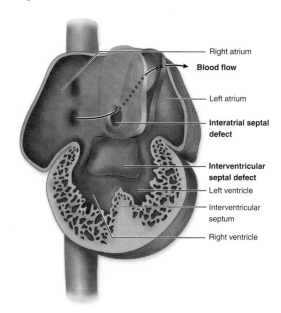

▲ **FIGURE 6.12**
Atrial and Ventricular Septal Defects.

S = Suffix   P = Prefix   R = Root   R/CF= Combining Form

Word	Pronunciation	Elements		Definition
coarctation	koh-ark-**TAY**-shun	S/ R/	-ation *process* coarct- *press together, narrow*	Constriction, stenosis, particularly of the aorta
congenital	kon-**JEN**-ih-tal	S/ P/ R/	-al *pertaining to* con- *together, with* -genit- *bring forth*	Present at birth, either inherited or due to an event during gestation up to the moment of birth
hypertension	HIGH-per-**TEN**-shun	S/ P/ R/	-ion *condition, action* hyper- *excessive* -tens- *pressure*	Persistent high arterial blood pressure
hypotension	HIGH-poh-**TEN**-shun	P/	hypo- *low*	Persistent low arterial blood pressure
idiopathic	ID-ih-oh-**PATH**-ik	S/ R/CF R/	-ic *pertaining to* idi/o- *unknown* -path- *disease*	Pertaining to a disease of unknown etiology
patent ductus arteriosus (PDA) (Note: *This term is composed only of roots.*)	**PAY**-tent **DUK**-tus ar-**TER**-ee-oh-sus	R/ R/ R/	patent *lie open* ductus *leading* arteriosus *artery*	An open, direct channel between the aorta and the pulmonary artery in the newborn
syndrome	**SIN**-drohm	P/ R/	syn- *together* -drome *running*	Combination of signs and symptoms associated with a particular disease process
tetralogy of Fallot (TOF)	te-**TRAL**-oh-jee of fah-**LOW**	P/ R/	tetra- *four* -logy *study of* Etienne-Louis Fallot, French physician, 1850–1911	Set of four congenital heart defects occurring together

EXERCISES

A. Abbreviations *need to be used carefully so that you communicate exactly what is necessary. The following sentences contain abbreviations—translate the abbreviations into their correct medical terms. Rewrite the sentences without the abbreviations and convey the same message. Fill in the blanks.*

1. ASD, TOF, VSD, and PDA are all examples of CHD.

_____

_____

2. The patient's symptoms were HTN and SOB.

_____

_____

3. Aortic stenosis and cardiac ischemia are common conditions leading to CHF.

_____

_____

_____

B. Language: *Answer the questions below.*

1. Translate for your patient from medical to layman's language: "hypertension's etiology is idiopathic."

_____

2. What is the difference between primary and secondary hypertension?

_____

3. Which type of hypertension is life-threatening?

_____

4. Why is it considered life-threatening?

_____

LESSON 6.2 Cardiologic Investigations and Procedures

(LO 6.1, 6.2, 6.3, and 6.4)

Blood Tests (LO 6.1, 6.2, 6.3, and 6.4)

A **lipid profile** helps determine the risk of CAD and comprises:

- Total cholesterol;
- High-density **lipoprotein (HDL)** ("good cholesterol");
- Low-density lipoprotein **(LDL)** ("bad cholesterol"); and
- **Triglycerides.**

Troponin I and **T** are part of a protein complex in muscle that is released into the blood during a muscle injury. Troponin I is found in heart muscle but not in skeletal muscle, which makes it a highly-sensitive indicator of a recent MI.

Diagnostic Tests (LO 6.1, 6.2, 6.3, and 6.4)

Several diagnostic tests are used to measure heart health.

An **electrocardiogram (ECG** or **EKG)** is a paper record of the electrical signals of your heart.

Cardiac stress testing is an exercise tolerance test that raises your heart rate through exercise (like jogging on a treadmill) and monitors its effect on cardiac function. **Nuclear imaging** of the heart, which involves the injection of a radioactive substance, can be used with the stress test.

Echocardiography uses ultrasound waves to study cardiac function.

Magnetic resonance imaging (MRI) can produce detailed images of the heart and identify sections of cardiac muscle that are not receiving an adequate blood supply.

Cardiac catheterization detects pressure and blood flow patterns in the heart. A thin tube is inserted into a vein or artery and is then threaded into the heart under X-ray guidance.

A **coronary angiogram** uses a contrast dye injected during cardiac catheterization to identify coronary artery blockages.

Treatment Procedures (LO 6.1, 6.2, 6.3, and 6.4)

The most immediate need in the treatment of MI is to get blood and oxygen to the affected myocardium. This can be attempted in several ways:

1. **Injection of clot-busting (thrombolytic) drugs:** These drugs are injected within 3½ hours of the MI to dissolve the **thrombus.**
2. **Artery-cleaning angioplasty (percutaneous transluminal coronary angioplasty, or PTCA):** A balloon-tipped **catheter** is guided to the blockage site and inflated. The inflated balloon expands the artery from the inside by compressing the plaque against the artery's walls.
3. **Stent placement:** To reduce the likelihood that the artery will close up again (occlude), a wire-mesh tube, or **stent,** is placed inside the vessel. **Drug-eluting** stents are covered with a special medication to help keep the artery open.
4. **Coronary artery bypass surgery (CABG):** Healthy blood vessels harvested from the leg, chest, or arm are used to bypass (detour) the blood around blocked coronary arteries.
5. **Heart transplant:** The heart of a recently deceased person (donor) is transplanted to the recipient after the recipient's diseased heart has been removed.

KEYNOTES

- A **Holter monitor** is a continuous ECG recorded on a tape-recorder cassette as you work, play, and rest for at least 24 hours.

- An **ambulatory blood pressure** monitor provides a record of your blood pressure over a 24-hour period as you go about your daily activities.

- Other procedures used in cardiology include:

  o **Cardioversion:** An arrhythmia is converted back to normal sinus rhythm with an electric shock from a defibrillator.

  o **Defibrillation:** V-fib is terminated and normal rhythm restored by delivery of an electric shock to the heart.

ABBREVIATIONS

CABG	coronary artery bypass graft
HDL	high-density lipoprotein
LDL	low-density lipoprotein
MRI	magnetic resonance imaging
PTCA	percutaneous transluminal coronary angioplasty

Word	Pronunciation	Elements		Definition
angiogram	AN-jee-oh-gram	S/	-gram *a record*	Radiograph obtained after injection of radi-opaque contrast material into blood vessels
angiography	AN-jee-OG-rah-fee	R/CF S/	angi/o- *blood vessel* -graphy *process of recording*	Radiography of blood vessels after injection of contrast material
angioplasty	AN-jee-oh-PLAS-tee	S/ R/CF	-plasty *surgical repair* angi/o- *blood vessel*	Recanalization of a blood vessel by surgery
catheter	KATH-eh-ter		Greek *to send down*	Hollow tube to allow passage of fluid into or out of a body cavity, organ, or vessel
catheterize (verb)	KATH-eh-teh-RIZE	S/ R/	-ize *action* catheter- *catheter*	To introduce a catheter
catheterization (noun)	KATH-eh-ter-ih-ZAY-shun	S/	-ization *process of inserting*	Introduction of a catheter
echocardiography	EK-oh-kar-dee-OG-rah-fee	S/ R/CF R/CF	-graphy *process of recording* ech/o- *sound wave* -cardi/o- *heart*	Ultrasound recording of heart function
lipoprotein	LIE-poh-pro-teen	R/CF R/	lip/o- *fat* -protein *protein*	Bonding of molecules of fat and protein
percutaneous	PER-kyu-TAY-nee-us	S/ P/ R/CF	-ous *pertaining to* per- *through* -cutan/e- *skin*	Passage through the skin, in this case, by needle puncture
stent	STENT		Charles Stent, English dentist, 19th century	Wire-mesh tube used to keep arteries open
thrombus thrombi (pl) thrombolytic (adj)	THROM-bus THROM-bee throm-boh-LIT-ik	 S/ R/CF R/	Latin *clot* -tic *pertaining to* thromb/o- *blood clot* -ly- *break down*	A clot attached to a diseased blood vessel or heart lining Able to dissolve or break up a blood clot
thrombolysis	throm-BOL-ih-sis	S/	-lysis *dissolve*	Dissolving of a thrombus (clot)
triglyceride	try-GLISS-eh-ride	S/ P/ R/	-ide *having a particular quality* tri- *three* -glycer- *sweet, glycerol*	Lipid containing three fatty acids

EXERCISES

A. Elements *are your best clue to understanding a medical term. Test yourself on the elements in column 1: Write the meaning of the element in its appropriate column. The first one is done for you.*

Element	Meaning of Prefix	Meaning of Root/CF	Meaning of Suffix
per	through		
1. cardio			
2. cutane			
3. tri			
4. lipo			

B. Explain in your own words, *each of the medical terms represented by these abbreviations.*

1. PTCA

P _____

T _____

C _____

A _____

2. CABG

C _____

A _____

B _____

G _____

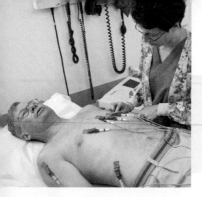

LESSON 6.3

Circulatory Systems

OBJECTIVES

In order to understand the **etiologies** *and effects of Mrs. Jones' problems (see Case Report 6.3), and to clearly communicate with her and Dr. Bannerjee, you first need to have the medical terminology and knowledge to be able to:*

6.3.1 Specify the functions of the systemic and pulmonary circulations.

6.3.2 Identify the major **arteries** and **veins** in the body.

6.3.3 Explain the **hemodynamics** and control of blood flow.

6.3.4 Describe common disorders of the circulatory system.

CASE REPORT 6.3

YOU ARE

. . . a certified medical assistant **(CMA)** working for Dr. Lokesh Bannerjee, a cardiologist in Fulwood Medical Center.

YOU ARE READING THE CONSULTATION REQUEST OF

. . . Mrs. Martha Jones. You are documenting her medical record after Dr. Bannerjee interviewed and examined her.

Fulwood Medical Center
Consultation Request and Report Form

Patient's Name: Jones, MARTHA   Age: 52
To: Dr. LoKESH BANNERJEE   Department: cardiology
From: Dr. Susan Lee   Department: Primary Care
Patient's Location: Fulwood MEDICAL CENTER
Type of Consultation Desired:
    ☐ Consultation Only
    ☐ Consulation and follow Jointly
    ☒ Accept in Transfer
Referring Diagnoses: CLAUDICATION, POSSIBLE DVT
Reason for Consultation: severe pain in both legs on walking

Signature: *[signature]*   Date: 2/21/09   Time 1105 hrs
Consultation Report: by Lokesh Bannerjee
Chief complaint: Pt. c/o severe pain in both legs on walking about 100 yards or climbing a flight of stairs. Pain is so severe she must stop and wait 5 mins. before she can go on. For the past two weeks she has noticed soreness and hardness along a vein in her left calf.
Past medical history: Known type 2 diabetic with hypertension, CAD, diabetic retinopathy, and OA of her hips and knees. Several episodes of ketoacidosis and one of pulmonary edema. Bariatric surgery performed 8 months prior at 275 lbs.
Medications: metformin, verapamil, propanolol, Mevacor
Allergies: NKA
Physical examination: Ht: 5'2" Wt: 190 lbs. BP: 170/100 sitting. P: 80, regular. Both feet show slight pitting edema and skin is pale, cold, and dry. Small ulcer on lateral margin of each big toe. Varicosities, both legs. Tender cord in superficial vein of left calf. Flexion of left foot produces pain in left calf. Chest clear. Heart sounds unremarkable. No loss of sensation in legs or feet.
Impression: 1. varicose veins, both legs.
    2. severe claudication, both legs.
    3. probable deep vein thrombosis, left leg
    4. possible peripheral neuropathy
    5. H/O diabetes type 2, CAD, hypertension, retinopathy, OA
Plan: Admit patient to cardiology unit stat for IV heparin and conversion to oral anticoagulant therapy with Coumadin. Doppler studies, venogram, and angiogram have been ordered.

Signature: *[signature]* MD   Date 2/21/09   Time 1250 hrs

ORDER # 267116 ANDRUS CLINI-REC ® PRIMARY CARE CHARTING SYSTEM • © BIBBERO SYSTEMS, INC. • PETALUMA, CA
TO REORDER CALL TOLL FREE: (800) BIBBERO (800-242-9330)   Mfg IN U.S.A.

ABBREVIATIONS

BP	blood pressure
CMA	certified medical assistant
H/O	history of
NKA	no known allergies
OA	osteoarthritis
P	pulse rate

S = Suffix   P = Prefix   R = Root   R/CF= Combining Form

Word	Pronunciation		Elements	Definition
artery	**AR**-ter-ee		Greek *artery*	Thick-walled blood vessel carrying oxygenated blood away from the heart
claudication	klaw-dih-**KAY**-shun	S/ R/	-ation *a process* claudic- *limping*	Intermittent leg pain and limping
Doppler	**DOP**-ler		Johann Doppler, Austrian mathematician and physician, 1803–1853	Diagnostic instrument that sends an ultrasonic beam into the body
hemodynamics	**HE**-mo-die-**NAM**-iks	S/ R/CF R/	-ics *knowledge* hem/o- *blood* -dynam- *power*	The science of the blood flow through the circulation
vein	VANE		Latin *vein*	Blood vessel carrying blood toward the heart
venous (adj)	**VEE**-nuss	S/ R/	-ous *pertaining to* ven- *vein*	Pertaining to a vein
venogram	**VEE**-noh-gram	S/ R/CF	-gram *recording* ven/o- *vein*	Radiograph of veins after injection of radiopaque contrast material
varix varices (pl) varicose (adj)	**VAIR**-iks **VAIR**-ih-seez **VAIR**-ih-kose	S/ R/	Latin *dilated vein* -ose *full of* varic- *varicosity; dilated, tortuous vein*	Dilated, tortuous vein Characterized by or affected with varices

EXERCISES

A. Review *the Case Report on this spread before answering the questions.*

1. What are Mrs. Jones' symptoms? _____
2. List here Mrs. Jones' other diseases/conditions _____
3. Why did Mrs. Jones have bariatric surgery? _____
4. What's the purpose of anticoagulant therapy? _____
5. Of all the studies ordered for Mrs. Jones, which one uses ultrasound? _____
6. What is *pitting edema?* _____
7. What diagnosis in Mrs. Jones' past medical history relates to her episodes of ketoacidosis? _____
8. What does *peripheral* mean? _____
9. If Mrs. Jones had pulmonary edema, what organs would be involved? _____
10. Describe what a varicose vein might look like. _____

B. Singular and plurals, *nouns and adjectives: Terms from the WAD can all be correctly inserted into the following paragraph of radiology documentation. Fill in the blanks.*

veins   varicosities   varix   vein   varicose   varices   venogram   venous

1. The _____ performed on this patient's left saphenous and popliteal _____ shows the following: One slightly engorged and dilated _____ at the midpoint of the saphenous _____ and several _____ at the terminal end of the popliteal vein where _____ blood is pooling.

   Diagnosis: _____ veins. These _____ need immediate attention by a vascular surgeon.

- All arteries of the systemic circulation arise either directly or indirectly from the aorta.

- Blood flows from arteries to veins through capillary beds.

Circulatory System
(LO 6.1, 6.2, 6.3, and 6.4)

The term **circulatory system** refers to your heart and blood vessels. It has two major divisions:

1. The **pulmonary circulation,** which carries deoxygenated blood from the heart to the lungs, and returns oxygenated blood to the heart; and

2. The **systemic circulation**, which supplies oxygenated blood to every organ except the lungs, and then returns deoxygenated blood to the heart, which pumps it into the pulmonary circulation.

Functions of the Circulatory System (LO 6.1, 6.2, 6.3, and 6.4)

The circulatory system has the following three functions:

- **Transportation.** It carries oxygen, nutrients, hormones, and enzymes that **diffuse** from the blood into the cells. Waste products and carbon dioxide diffuse back from the cells into the system and are carried to the lungs, liver, and kidney for excretion.

- **Homeostasis maintenance.** The systemic circulation directs blood flow to the tissues to enable them to meet their metabolic needs.

- **Blood pressure regulation.** In the systemic circulation, the arteries' ability to expand and contract in coordination with the systole and diastole of the heartbeat maintains a steady flow of blood and blood pressure to the tissues.

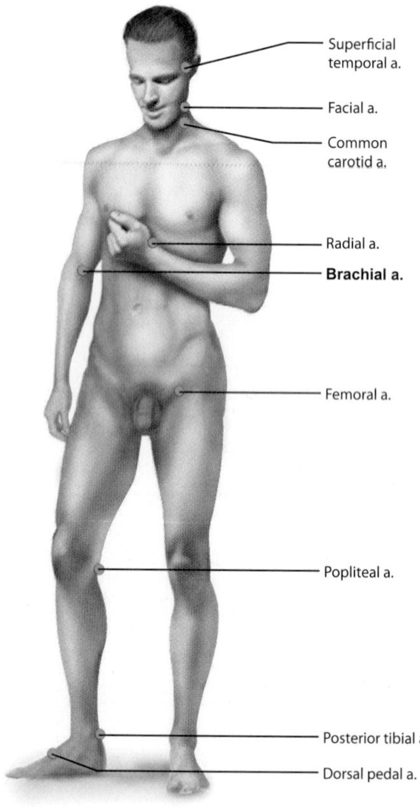

Arterial Pulses
(LO 6.1, 6.2, 6.3, and 6.4)

The pulse is always part of a clinical examination because it can provide information about heart rate, heart rhythm, and the state of the arterial wall by **palpation** *(Figure 6.13)*. The most easily accessible artery is the radial artery at the wrist, where the pulse is usually taken.

Superficial temporal a.

Facial a.

Common carotid a.

Radial a.

Brachial a.

Femoral a.

Popliteal a.

Posterior tibial a.

Dorsal pedal a.

◀ **FIGURE 6.13**
Arterial Pulses—9 locations.
(a. = artery).

Blood Pressure (BP)
(LO 6.1, 6.2, 6.3, and 6.4)

Blood pressure is the force the blood exerts on arterial walls as it is pumped around the circulatory system by the left ventricle. The pressure is measured using a **sphygmomanometer** and a **stethoscope,** usually at the **brachial** artery *(Figure 6.13)*.

Arterioles, Capillaries, and Venules (LO 6.1, 6.2, 6.3, and 6.4)

As the arteries branch farther away from the heart and distribute blood to specific organs, they become smaller, muscular vessels called **arterioles.** By contracting and relaxing, these arterioles are the primary controllers that help the body direct the amount of blood that the organs and structures receive.

From the arterioles, the blood flows into **capillaries** and **capillary beds** *(Figure 6.14)*. Red blood cells flow in single file through the small capillaries

From the capillaries, tiny **venules** accept the blood and merge to form veins. The veins form reservoirs for blood. At any moment, 60% to 70% of the total blood volume is contained in the venules and veins.

Systemic Venous Circulation
(LO 6.1, 6.2, 6.3, and 6.4)

There are three major types of veins:

1. **Superficial,** such as those you can see under the skin of your arms and hands;

2. **Deep,** which run parallel to arteries and drain the same tissues that the arteries supply; and

3. **Venous sinuses,** which are in the head and heart and have specific functions.

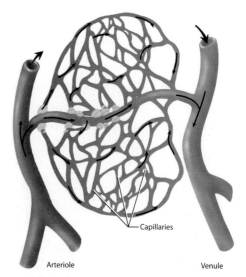

Capillaries

Arteriole

Venule

▲ **FIGURE 6.14**
Capillary Bed.

S = Suffix   P = Prefix   R = Root   R/CF= Combining Form

Word	Pronunciation	Elements		Definition
arteriole	ar-**TER**-ee-ole	S/ R/	-ole *small* arteri- *artery*	Small terminal artery leading into the capillary network
brachial	**BRAY**-kee-al	S/ R/	-al *pertaining to* brachi- *arm*	Pertaining to the arm
capillary capillaries	**KAP**-ih-lair-ee **KAP**-ih-lair-ees	S/ R/	-ary *pertaining to* capill- *hairlike structure*	Minute blood vessel between the arterial and venous systems
diffuse	di-**FUSE**		Latin *to pull in different directions*	To disseminate or spread out
homeostasis	hoh-mee-oh-**STAY**-sis	S/ R/CF	-stasis *stand still* home/o- *the same*	Maintaining the stability, or equilibrium, of a system or the body's internal environment
palpate (verb) palpation (noun)	**PAL**-pate pal-**PAY**-shun	S/ R/	Latin *touch, stroke* -ion *action, condition* palpat- *touch, stroke*	To examine with the fingers and hands Examination with the fingers and hands
sphygmomanometer	**SFIG**-moh-mah-**NOM**-ih-ter	S/ R/CF R/CF	-meter *instrument to measure* sphygm/o- *pulse* -man/o- *pressure*	Instrument for measuring arterial blood pressure
stethoscope	**STETH**-oh-skope	S/ R/CF	-scope *instrument to examine* steth/o- *chest*	Instrument for listening to respiratory and cardiac sounds
vena cava venae cavae (pl)	**VEE**-nah **KAY**-vah **VEE**-nee **KAY**-vee	R/CF R/	ven/a *vein* cava *cave*	One of the two largest veins in the body The two largest veins in the body (superior and inferior venae cavae)
venule	**VEN**-yule or **VEEN**-yule	S/ R/	-ule *small* ven- *vein*	Small vein leading from the capillary network

EXERCISES

A. Build *your knowledge of the elements and terms that make up the language of the cardiovascular system. All your answers can be found in the WAD. Fill in the blanks.*

1. The two suffixes in the WAD that both mean *small* are _____ and _____ .

2. List the three general terms in the WAD that are small *blood vessels*: _____, _____, and _____

3. Name two instruments found in an internal medicine practice: _____ and _____

4. State of equilibrium in the body is called _____ .

5. The two largest veins in the body are the _____ .

B. Construct *the correct medical term to match the definition.*

1. minute blood vessel between the arterial and venous systems:

_____ / _____ / _____
   P   R/CF   S

2. instrument for listening to respiratory and cardiac sounds:

_____ / _____ / _____
   P   R/CF   S

3. pertaining to the arm:

_____ / _____ / _____
   P   R/CF   S

4. instrument for measuring arterial blood pressure:

_____ / _____ / _____
   P   R/CF   S

5. small terminal artery leading into the capillary network:

_____ / _____ / _____
   P   R/CF   S

- All the disorders of the systemic arterial and venous systems are grouped under the term peripheral vascular disease (PVD).

ABBREVIATIONS

DVT	deep vein thrombosis
PVD	peripherial vascular disease

CASE REPORT 6.3 (CONTINUED)

Mrs. Martha Jones, who had been referred to Dr. Bannerjee's cardiovascular clinic, has several circulatory problems related to her diabetes and obesity. She was diagnosed previously with hypertension, CAD, and diabetic retinopathy. She now has severe pain in her legs when walking. Doppler studies and angiograms showed significant blockage of blood flow due to arteriosclerosis of the large arteries in her legs. This blockage produces the pain when walking (intermittent claudication), and is part of her peripheral vascular disease (PVD).

The ulcers on the edges of her big toes are a result of thickening capillary walls and arterioles; this has led to poor circulation in her feet. Mrs. Jones' diabetes has caused these problems.

In addition, in her left leg's venous (vein) system, the tender cord-like lesion is due to **thrombophlebitis** of a superficial vein. A venogram showed a deep vein thrombosis (DVT).

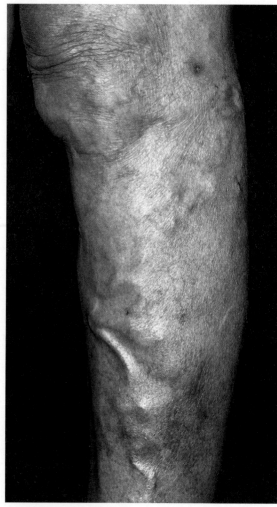

▲ **FIGURE 6.15**
Varicose Veins of the Leg.

Disorders of Veins (LO 6.1, 6.2, 6.3, and 6.4)

Our veins and arteries can be prone to certain disorders, like the DVT experienced by Mrs. Jones in the preceding case report.

Thrombophlebitis is an inflammation of the lining of a vein, allowing clots (thrombi) to form.

Deep vein thrombosis (DVT) is a thrombus formation in a deep vein. The increased pressure in the capillaries due to back pressure from the blocked blood flow in the veins creates a collection of fluid in the tissues called **edema.**

A major complication of thrombus (clot) formation is that a piece of the clot can break off **(embolus)** and be carried in the bloodstream to another organ where it can block blood flow. It often lodges in the lungs, causing a pulmonary embolus or mass *(see Chapter 8).*

Varicose veins are superficial veins that have lost their elasticity and appear swollen and tortuous *(Figure 6.15).* Their valves become incompetent, and blood flows backward and pools. Smaller, more superficial varicose veins are called spider veins. Treatments offered include laser technology and **sclerotherapy,** in which solutions that scar the veins are injected into them. **Collateral** circulations develop to take the blood through alternative routes.

A phlebotomist is a technician who draws blood (phlebotomy).

Disorders of Arteries (LO 6.1, 6.2, 6.3, and 6.4)

An **aneurysm** is a localized **dilation** of an artery, and this commonly occurs in the abdominal aorta. Aneurysms can **rupture,** leading to severe bleeding and hypovolemic shock. Surgical repair consists of excision of the aneurysm and replacement with a **synthetic** graft.

Intracranial aneurysms are an important cause of bleeds into the cranial cavity and brain tissue.

Thromboangiitis obliterans (Buerger disease) is an inflammatory disease of the arteries with clot formation, usually in the legs. The occlusion of arteries and impaired circulation leads to intermittent pain when walking, and a person will often limp to compensate.

Raynaud disease is episodes of spasm (following exposure to cold) of the small arteries supplying the fingers, hands, and feet. It can be associated with connective tissue disorders like scleroderma and lupus.

Carotid artery disease affects the carotid arteries—the two major arteries supplying the brain. They can be involved in arteriosclerosis and the deposition of plaque. This puts the patient at risk for a stroke. A carotid **endarterectomy** can be performed to surgically remove the plaque.

Word	Pronunciation		Elements	Definition
aneurysm	**AN**-yur-izm		Greek *dilation*	Circumscribed dilation of an artery or cardiac chamber
collateral	koh-**LAT**-er-al	P/ R/	col- *with, together* -lateral *at the side*	Situated at the side, often to bypass an obstruction
dilation	die-**LAY**-shun	S/ R/	-ion *action, condition* dilat- *widen, dilate, open up*	Stretching or enlarging an opening
edema (noun)	ee-**DEE**-mah		Greek *swelling*	Excessive accumulation of fluid in cells and tissues
edematous (adj)	ee-**DEM**-ah-tus	S/ R/	-tous *pertaining to* edema- *swelling*	Pertaining to or affected by edema
endarterectomy	**END**-ar-ter-**EK**-toe-me	S/ P/ R/	-ectomy *surgical excision* end- *within* -arter- *artery*	Surgical removal of plaque from an artery
phlebitis	fleh-**BIE**-tis	S/ R/	-itis *inflammation* phleb- *vein*	Inflammation of a vein
rupture	**RUP**-tyur		Latin *break*	Break or tear of any organ or body part
sclerotherapy	**SKLEH-r**oh-**THAIR**-ah-pee	S/ R/CF	-therapy *treatment* scler/o- *hardness*	Injection of a solution into a vein to thrombose it
sclerose (verb)	skleh-**ROSE**	S/ R/	-ose *full of* scler- *hardness*	To harden or thicken
sclerosis (noun)	skleh-**ROH**-sis	S/	-osis *condition*	Thickening or hardening of a tissue
synthetic	sin-**THET**-ik	S/ P/ R/	-ic *pertaining to* syn- *together* -thet-*arrange*	Built up or put together from simpler compounds
thromboembolism	**THROM**-boh-**EM**-boh-lizm	S/ R/CF R/	-ism *condition* thromb/o- *clot* -embol- *plug*	A piece of detached blood clot (embolus) blocking a distant blood vessel
thrombophlebitis	**THROM**-boh-fleh-**BY**-tis	S/ R/CF R/	-itis *inflammation* thromb/o- *clot* -phleb- *vein*	Inflammation of a vein with clot formation

EXERCISES

A. Review *the Case Report on this spread before answering the questions.*

1. What diagnostic tests has Mrs. Jones had? _____

2. What other problems has the patient's diabetes caused? _____

3. Besides her diabetes what other complicating factor did Mrs. Jones have that contributed to her current problems? _____

4. Does Mrs. Jones have atherosclerosis or arteriosclerosis? _____

5. Define a *superficial* vein. _____

6. Define the difference between the two terms mentioned in question #4 above:

_____

7. What skin problem(s) does Mrs. Jones have as a result of the poor blood circulation in her feet? _____

8. What is *thrombophlebitis?* _____

B. Analyze *the italicized terms and their elements to answer the following questions. Review the WAD and circle the correct term.*

1. Its suffix tells you *thrombophlebitis* is:

   a clot   an inflammation   an excision

2. *Endarterectomy* means the plaque has been:

   incised   removed   repaired

3. The combining form *phleb/o* means:

   artery   vein   capillary

4. *Aneurysm* describes a blood vessel that is:

   dilated   constricted   collapsed

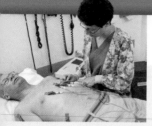

CHALLENGE YOUR KNOWLEDGE

A. Deconstruct *the following medical terms into their basic elements by slashing the terms in the first column. Then fill in the rest of the chart. Knowledge of elements will help you understand the meaning of the term.*

Medical Term	Meaning of Prefix	Meaning of Root/CF	Meaning of Suffix	Meaning of Medical Term
bradycardia	1.	2.	3.	4.
endocardium	5.	6.	7.	8.
cardiomyopathy	9.	10.	11.	12.
bicuspid	13.	14.	15.	16.
pericarditis	17.	18.	19.	20.
diaphoresis	21.	22.	23.	24.
pulmonary	25.	26.	27.	28.
semilunar	29.	30.	31.	32.
arteriosclerosis	33.	34.	35.	36.
ischemia	37.	38.	39.	40

41. Use any one term from the chart in a sentence that is not a definition: _____

_____

B. Elements *remain the single best tool for increasing your medical vocabulary. Identify what the element in column 1 is, and define its meaning in the appropriate column. Then give an example of a medical term with that element. The first one is done for you. Fill in the chart.*

Element	Meaning of Prefix	Meaning of Root/CF	Meaning of Suffix	Medical Term
cardio		heart		cardiovascular
1. a				2.
3. media				4.
5. ism				6.
7. lysis				8.
9. emia				10.
11. thorac				12.
13. myo				14.
15. phleb				16.
17. sclero				18.

C. Translate: *Rewrite the following sentence using medical terms instead of the abbreviations. Make sure you are communicating the same information either way. Check your spelling after you have filled in the blanks.*

1. The CVT started CPR after checking the patient's EKG. He paged the doctor STAT. Apparently, the patient had suffered an MI.

_____

_____

_____

_____

D. Word attack: *Process of elimination can help with multiple-choice questions. Work through the following exercise step-by-step, and practice analyzing multiple-choice questions and answers.*

If a patient is *hypovolemic,* he or she has:

a. decreased blood pressure

b. increased blood pressure

c. decreased blood volume

d. increased blood volume

e. low red blood cells

1. Read the question and all the answer choices. Then read the question again.

2. Look for subtle differences in the answers. Note that some answers relate to "increased" or "decreased." These answers *also* relate to "blood *pressure*" or "blood *volume*" (two different things).

3. Analyze the elements to know whether you are looking for "increased" *or* "decreased" and for "blood pressure" *or* "blood volume."

4. The prefix in the question is _____ and means _____ , so you can immediately discard answer choices _____ because they do not relate to the prefix.

5. Next, analyze the root. The root is _____ and means _____ _____ .

6. Therefore, based on the meanings of the prefix and the root, the answer has to be _____ and the meaning of *hypovolemic* is _____ .

E. Suffixes: *The following procedures could all be performed by a cardiovascular surgeon. First, slash the term into its elements by filling in the blanks. Then use the suffix to help you analyze the meaning of the term. Write a brief description of the procedure on the lines below.*

1. *angioplasty* _____ / _____ / _____
                 P   R/CF   S

  Description:

  _____

2. *endarterectomy* _____ / _____ / _____
                 P   R/CF   S

  Description:

  _____

3. *(cardiac) catheterization* _____ / _____ / _____
                 P   R/CF   S

  Description:

  _____

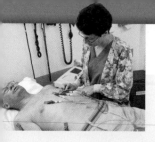

F. Abbreviations *are present throughout medical documentation, and you must be absolutely certain you are interpreting them correctly. Fill in the correct abbreviations in the following patient documentation. All of the abbreviations contain some combination of the following letters. You will have to use some letters more than once:*

A   B   C   D   F   G   H   I   M   O   P   S   T   V

1. Studies show the patient has a hole in the interatrial septum. Diagnosis: _____

2. The pediatric cardiologist was called to the Neonatal Unit because the baby's fetal blood vessel had not closed normally. The baby was diagnosed with _____ .

3. Due to her sedentary lifestyle, obesity, hypertension, and smoking history, the patient is at great risk for _____ .

4. Infant male was born with tetralogy of Fallot (_____) syndrome. This is a form of _____ .

5. This patient's ischemic attack resulted in occlusion of her coronary artery, and a(n) _____ followed.

6. This patient needs a _____ because of blocked coronary arteries.

G. Dictionary or online research: *Look up the term* perfusionist *in a dictionary or online. Write a brief job description for a perfusionist.*

_____

_____

_____

_____

_____

_____

_____

_____

H. Layperson's language: *Mrs. Jones has been given the following diagnoses. Translate them into plain English for her.*

Impression:

1. Varicose veins, both legs.

2. Severe claudication, both legs.

3. Probable deep vein thrombosis, left leg.

4. Possible peripheral neuropathy.

5. H/O CAD, hypertension, retinopathy.

Rewrite the medical terms into layperson's language for your patient.

1. _____

2. _____

3. _____

4. _____

5. _____

_____

I. Interpret *the following paragraph from a patient's chest x-ray report, and answer the questions. Read it once, and then go back and read it again, underlining or highlighting the medical terms.*

The left ventricle is slightly enlarged. Right atrium and right ventricle appear to be dilated. There is tortuosity of the thoracic aorta, with arteriosclerosis. The hilar and interstitial structures are somewhat accentuated. There are large pericardial fat pads.

Tricuspid and pulmonic valves appear normal but are not well seen. Mitral valve appears grossly normal for age. Aortic valve appears grossly normal for age.

Using your knowledge of the terminology in the above report, circle the correct answers for the following questions.

1. Where are the pericardial fat pads?
   - **a.** in the heart
   - **b.** around the heart
   - **c.** beneath the heart
   - **d.** beside the heart
   - **e.** above the heart

2. What is a likely diagnosis for this patient?
   - **a.** CABG
   - **b.** ASHD
   - **c.** PTCA
   - **d.** DVT
   - **e.** MI

3. Which two terms refer to chambers of the heart?
   - **a.** tricuspid/pulmonic
   - **b.** atrium/ventricle
   - **c.** hilar/interstitial
   - **d.** mitral/pulmonic
   - **e.** aortic/pericardial

4. Which heart valve has three flaps?
   - **a.** pulmonic
   - **b.** mitral
   - **c.** tricuspid
   - **d.** hilar
   - **e.** bicuspid

5. A synonym for dilated is:
   - **a.** expanded
   - **b.** twisted
   - **c.** thrombosed
   - **d.** occluded
   - **e.** constricted

J. Prefixes: *Each of the following terms has similar roots and suffixes, but the prefix makes the difference. Deconstruct the term with slashes. Analyze the terms, and explain how they are different.*

1. arrhythmia

_____ / _____ / _____
                  P   R/CF   S

2. dysrhythmia

_____ / _____ / _____
                  P   R/CF   S

3. Describe the difference between *arrhythmia* and *dysrhythmia:*

_____

_____

_____

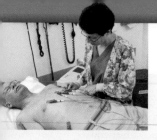

K. Spelling demons: *This chapter contains some particularly difficult terms to pronounce and spell. You can master these terms with practice. Write below the five most difficult terms for you to pronounce and spell correctly. Listen to the Glossary on the Student Online Learning Center* (www.mhhe.com/Allan Ess2e) *for correct pronunciations, and check your spelling.*

Compare your list with your study partner's list to see if you have similar difficult terms.

	Term	Pronunciation Checked	Spelling Checked
1.	_____	_____	_____
2.	_____	_____	_____
3.	_____	_____	_____
4.	_____	_____	_____
5.	_____	_____	_____

L. Seek and find: *The following terms were defined in context in the text but did not necessarily appear in a WAD. Match the appropriate meaning in column 1 with the correct medical term in column 2.*

_____ 1. blocked   **A.** patent

_____ 2. unknown   **B.** hemorrhage

_____ 3. lack of blood supply   **C.** coronary thrombosis

_____ 4. under the tongue   **D.** occluded

_____ 5. detour   **E.** thrombus

_____ 6. excessive bleeding   **F.** necrosis

_____ 7. pain in the chest on exertion   **G.** idiopathic

_____ 8. dead body   **H.** sublingual

_____ 9. open   **I.** ischemia

_____ 10. blood clot in the heart   **J.** angina pectoris

_____ 11. clot   **K.** bypass

_____ 12. death of cells   **L.** cadaver

M. You are mentoring *a new CVT who has just been hired in the Cardiology Department at Fulwood Medical Center. Because you have been on the job for a while, you should be able to explain to him the difference between:*

1. heart valve insufficiency and stenosis

_____

_____

_____

_____

2. a thrombus and an embolus

_____

_____

_____

_____

_____

N. Determine *the correct medical vocabulary to complete the following sentences in patient documentation. An explanation of the term is given in parentheses as a clue. Fill in the blanks.*

1. The (under the tongue) _____ medication did not dissolve completely, so liquid medication was given to the patient instead.

2. The patient's (hardening of the arteries) _____ puts him at risk for a stroke. I have ordered a blood thinner.

3. Schedule the patient for a(n) (surgical removal of plaque deposit in artery lining) _____ as soon as possible.

4. (Absence of heart contractions) _____ occurred at 10:51 p.m., and the patient was pronounced dead.

5. Angioplasty showed a large clot (completely obstructing) _____ his left coronary artery.

6. The bullet entered his left (under the breastbone) _____ area and exited his back.

7. (Being without oxygen) _____ has caused permanent brain damage to this infant.

8. The patient's diagnostic studies show clear evidence of (death of tissue) _____ of the heart muscle.

9. Cardiogenic shock occurred, and the patient's tissues were not (forcing blood through a vascular bed or lumen) _____ adequately.

10. Treatment options offered to the patient for her varicose veins include laser therapy and (injection of a solution into a vein to sclerose it)

_____ .

O. Recall and review: *How well do you remember these word elements from a previous chapter? Try to answer without looking back to check. Fill in the chart.*

Element	Type of Element (P, R, CF, or S)	Meaning of Element
quad	1.	2.
pector	3.	4.
necro	5.	6.
ambulat	7.	8.
trophy	9.	10.

P. Chapter challenge: *Use your knowledge of the language of cardiology and circle the best answer.*

1. Find the abbreviations that are *cardiac diagnoses:*

   a. SOB, ECG, CVT   d. SA, SC, CT

   b. STAT, IV, ASHD   e. CAD, CHF, VSD

   c. CPR, MI, AV

2. The medical term meaning an instrument for measuring arterial blood pressure is:

   a. stethoscope   d. ventilator

   b. sphygmomanometer   e. tonometer

   c. defibrillator

3. Choose the correct abbreviation for "heart attack":

   a. CO   d. MI

   b. AV   e. CAD

   c. ASHD

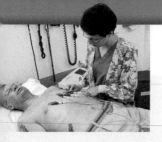

4. Mr. Hank Johnson became *diaphoretic* in the ED. This means he:

    a. began to vomit

    b. started sweating

    c. hemorrhaged

    d. had a fever

    e. became itchy all over

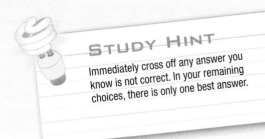

STUDY HINT

Immediately cross off any answer you know is not correct. In your remaining choices, there is only one best answer.

5. Identify the pair of terms that are *incorrectly* spelled:

    a. thrombolytic/arteriosclerosis

    b. substernal/sublingual

    c. oclude/oclusion

    d. plaque/patent

    e. varix/varices

6. The medical term *STAT* means something is to be performed:

    a. after the patient consents

    b. tomorrow

    c. immediately

    d. at the doctor's convenience

    e. when the schedule permits

7. Which phrase best describes the terms *infusion, transfusion,* and *perfusion?*

    a. The suffix is the same.

    b. The root is the same.

    c. There is no combining form.

    d. Only the prefix makes them different.

    e. All these are true.

8. Pick the set of terms that are all blood vessels:

    a. vena cava, arteriole, varix

    b. artery, edema, rupture

    c. venule, arteriole, capillary

    d. aneurysm, phlebitis, sclerose

    e. platelet, thrombocyte, colloid

9. The *thoracic cavity* is in the:

    a. pelvis

    b. abdomen

    c. head

    d. chest

    e. spine

10. A thin wall deviding two cavities:

    a. mediastinum

    b. septum

    c. sternum

    d. endocardium

    e. atrium

Q. Case Report challenge: *Now that you are more comfortable with the terms in this chapter, you can apply that knowledge and briefly answer the questions about the Case Report. If you read the report through and underline or highlight all the medical terminology, this will make it easier to answer the questions.*

CASE REPORT 6.3 (CONTINUED)

Mrs. Martha Jones, who had been referred to Dr. Bannerjee's cardiovascular clinic, has several circulatory problems related to her diabetes and obesity. She was diagnosed previously with hypertension, CAD, and diabetic retinopathy. She now has severe pain in her legs on walking.

Doppler studies and angiograms showed significant blockage of blood flow due to arteriosclerosis of the large arteries in her legs. This blockage produces the pain on walking (intermittent claudication).

The ulcers on the edges of her big toes result from thickening of the walls of her capillaries and arterioles and the resulting poor circulation to her feet. Again, this is due to her diabetes.

In the venous system of her legs, the tender cord-like lesion is due to thrombophlebitis of a superficial vein in her left leg. A venogram showed a deep vein thrombosis (DVT).

---

1. What does the term *hypertension* mean?

_____

2. What part of the patient's body is affected by *retinopathy?*

_____

3. List here all the terms used in the Case Report that relate to different types of blood vessels:

_____

_____

4. What is the opposite of a vein that is *superficial?* _____

_____

5. In layperson's language, what is a *thrombosis?* _____

_____

6. If the patient's pain is *intermittent,* what does that mean? _____

_____

7. Why does Mrs. Jones have pain when she walks? _____

_____

8. With what symptoms did Mrs. Jones present when she saw Dr. Bannerjee?

_____

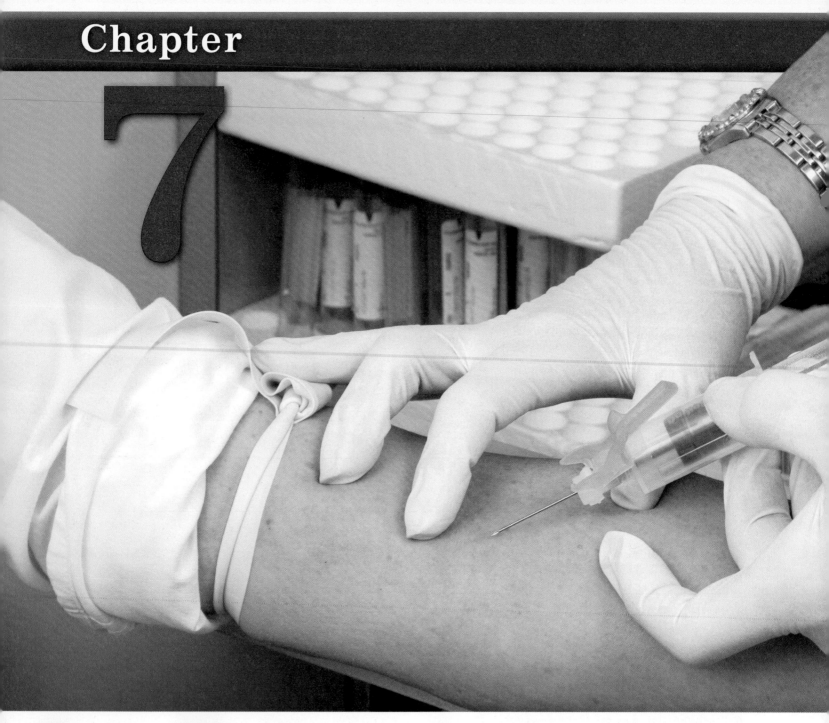

The Blood, Lymphatic, and Immune Systems

The Essentials of the Languages of Hematology and Immunology

YOU ARE

. . . a medical assistant employed by Susan Lee, MD, a primary care physician at Fulwood Medical Center.

YOU ARE COMMUNICATING WITH

. . . Ms. Luisa Sosin, a 47-year-old woman who presented a week ago with fatigue, lethargy, and muscle weakness. A physical examination revealed paleness (pallor) of her skin, a pulse rate of 90, and a respiratory rate of 20. Dr. Lee referred her for extensive blood work. She also determined that Ms. Sosin had been taking aspirin and NSAIDs (nonsteroidal anti-inflammatory drugs) for the past 6 months for lower back pain. Ms. Sosin's laboratory reports show an **iron-deficiency anemia.** You are responsible for documenting her examination and care.

The health professionals involved in the diagnosis and treatment of problems with the blood, lymphatic, and immune systems include the following:

- **Hematologists** are physicians who specialize in the diagnosis, treatment, and prevention of blood and bone marrow diseases.

- **Immunologists** and **allergists** are physicians who specialize in immune system disorders, such as allergies, asthma, and immunodeficiency and autoimmune diseases.

- **Epidemiologists** are medical scientists involved in the study of epidemic diseases and how they are transmitted and controlled.

- **Medical** or **clinical laboratory technicians** perform routine testing procedures on body fluids, blood, and other tissues using microscopes, computers, and other laboratory equipment.

- **Immunology technicians** are certified laboratory technicians with a special interest in immunology who generally work alongside medical researchers.

- **Transfusion technicians** are certified technicians who deal with all phases of blood transfusions.

- **Phlebotomists** assist physicians by drawing patient blood samples for laboratory testing.

LEARNING OUTCOMES

In order to be able to communicate intelligently with Dr. Lee and to appropriately document Ms. Luisa Sosin's medical care, you first need to be familiar with the anatomy, physiology, and medical terminology of hematology. This chapter will provide you with information that enables you to:

LO 7.1 Apply the language of hematology to the anatomy and physiology of the blood.

LO 7.2 Comprehend, analyze, spell, and write the medical terms of hematology so that you can communicate and document accurately and precisely.

LO 7.3 Recognize and pronounce the medical terms of hematology so that you can communicate verbally with accuracy and precision.

LO 7.4 Use correct medical terminology to explain how common blood disorders affect health.

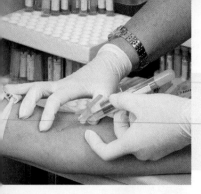

LESSON 7.1

Components and Functions of Blood

OBJECTIVES

The average-sized adult carries about 5 liters (10 pints) of blood in the body at all times. The information in this lesson relates to the composition, functions, and uses of blood, and enables you to use correct medical terminology to:

7.1.1   Identify the components of blood.

7.1.2   Describe plasma and its functions.

7.1.3   Explain the functions of blood.

KEYNOTE

- Serum is identical to plasma except for the absence of clotting proteins.

ABBREVIATIONS

Hct   hematocrit
RBC   red blood cell
WBC   white blood cell

Components of Blood

(LO 7.1, 7.2, and 7.3)

The study of the blood and its disorders—the red and white blood cells within the blood, their proportions, and overall cell health—is called **hematology.** A **hematologist** is a medical specialist who is trained in this area.

Blood is a type of connective tissue that consists of cells contained in a liquid **matrix.** If a blood specimen is collected in a tube and centrifuged, the cells of the blood separate out and fill the bottom 45% of the tube. Ninety-nine percent of these cells are red blood cells **(RBCs)**; white blood cells **(WBCs)** and **platelets** make up the remainder of this sample. The **hematocrit (Hct)** is the percentage of total blood volume composed of red blood cells.

Plasma—a clear, yellowish liquid that is 91% water—makes up the remaining 55% of the blood sample in the tube. Plasma is a **colloid,** a liquid that contains floating particles, most of which are plasma proteins. **Nutrients,** waste products, hormones, and enzymes are dissolved in plasma for transportation. When blood clots, and the solid clot is removed, **serum** remains.

Functions of Blood

(LO 7.1, 7.2, and 7.3)

Your blood travels throughout your body while performing a number of important functions. Your blood:

1. **Maintains your body's homeostasis** *(see Chapter 2).*

2. **Transports nutrients, vitamins, and minerals** from your digestive system and storage areas to your organs and cells. Examples of nutrients are glucose and amino acids *(see Chapter 9).*

3. **Transports waste products** from your cells and tissues to your liver and kidney for excretion. These waste products include creatinine, urea, bilirubin, and lactic acid.

4. **Transports hormones,** like insulin and thyroxine *(see Chapter 12),* from your endocrine glands to target cells.

5. **Transports gases,** like oxygen and carbon dioxide *(see Chapter 8),* to and from your lungs and cells.

6. **Protects against foreign substances, including microorganisms and toxins.** Cells and chemicals in your blood are an important part of your immune system's protective properties.

7. **Forms clots.** Clots provide protection against blood loss. Clotting is the first step in tissue repair and restoration of normal function.

Word	Pronunciation	Elements		Definition
allergist	**AL**-er-jist	S/ R/ R/	-ist *specialist* all- *other, strange* -erg- *work*	Specialist in hypersensitivity reaction
anemia	ah-**NEE**-me-ah	P/ R/	an- *without* -emia *a blood condition*	Decreased number of red blood cells
anemic (adj)	ah-**NEE**-mik	R/	-emic *pertaining to a condition of the blood*	Pertaining to or suffering from anemia
colloid	**COLL**-oyd	S/ R/	-oid *resembling* coll- *glue*	Liquid containing suspended particles
hematocrit (Hct)	**HE**-mat-oh-krit	S/ R/CF	-crit *to separate* hemat/o- *blood*	Percentage of red blood cells in the blood
hematology	he-mah-**TOL**-oh-jee	S/ R/CF	-logy *study of* hemat/o- *blood*	Medical specialty of the blood and its disorders
hematologist	he-mah-**TOL**-oh-jist	S/	-logist *one who studies, specialist*	Specialist in hematology
matrix	**MAY**-triks		Latin mater *mother*	Substance that surrounds and protects cells, is manufactured by the cells, and holds them together
nutrient	**NYU**-tree—ent		Latin *to nourish*	Constituent of food necessary for the body to function normally
nutrition	nyu-**TRISH**-un	S/ R/	-ion *action, condition* nutrit- *nourishment*	The study of food and liquid requirements for normal function of the human body
nutritionist	nyu-**TRISH**-un-ist	S/	-ist *specialist*	A person who specializes in the study of food and liquid requirements for normal function of the human body
plasma	**PLAZ**-mah		Greek *something formed*	Fluid, noncellular component of blood
platelet *(Also called* thrombocyte.)	**PLAYT**-let	S/ R/	-let *little, small* plate- *flat*	Small particle involved in the clotting process
serum	**SEER**-um		Latin *whey*	Fluid remaining after removal of blood cells and the formation of a clot
vitamin (**Note:** *The duplicate letter "a" is omitted. It was originally thought that all vitamins were amines.)*	**VYE**-tah-min	S/ R/	-amin(e) *nitrogen-containing substance* vita- *life*	Essential organic substance necessary in small amounts for normal cell function

EXERCISES

A. Review *Case Report 7.1 before answering the questions.*

1. What are Ms. Sosin's symptoms? _____

2. What additional testing did Dr. Lee order? _____

3. What is the medical term for *paleness?* _____

4. The abbreviation NSAIDs means _____

5. What diagnosis is confirmed with Ms. Sosin's lab results? _____

B. Match *the definition in column 1 with the correct medical term in column 2. Fill in the blanks.*

_____ **1.** decreased number of RBCs   **A.** platelet

_____ **2.** study of blood disorders   **B.** plasma

_____ **3.** fluid remaining after removal of clot   **C.** anemia

_____ **4.** fluid noncellular component of blood   **D.** hematology

_____ **5.** also called a thrombocyte   **E.** serum

Structure, Functions, and Disorders of Red Blood Cells (Erythrocytes)

(LO 7.1, 7.2, 7.3, and 7.4)

- RBCs are unable to move themselves and are dependent on the heart pump and blood flow to move them around the body.

- The average life span of an RBC is 120 days, during which time the cell circulates through the body about 75,000 times.

- Anemia produces **pallor** (pale color) because of the deficiency of the red-colored oxyhemoglobin, the combination of oxygen and hemoglobin.

- Hemolysis liberates hemoglobin from RBCs.

ABBREVIATIONS

CO_2	carbon dioxide
Hb or Hgb	hemoglobin
NO	nitric oxide
O_2	oxygen
PA	pernicious anemia
SOB	short(ness) of breath

Structure of RBCs (Erythrocytes) (LO 7.1, 7.2, and 7.3)

Each RBC is a disk with edges that are thicker than and raised above the flattened center *(Figure 7.1)*. This biconcave surface area enables a more rapid flow of gases into and out of the disk.

The main component of RBCs is **hemoglobin (Hb),** which gives the cells and blood their red color. Hb is composed of the iron-containing pigment **heme** bound to a protein called **globin.** The rest of the red blood cell consists of the cell membrane, water, electrolytes, and enzymes. Mature RBCs do not have a nucleus.

Functions of RBCs (Erythrocytes) (LO 7.1, 7.2, and 7.3)

The functions of the RBCs are to:

1. **Transport oxygen (O_2),** in combination with hemoglobin, throughout the body, from the lungs to the cells;

2. **Transport carbon dioxide (CO_2)** from the tissue cells to the lungs for excretion; and

3. **Transport nitric oxide (NO),** a gas produced by the lining cells of blood vessels that signals smooth muscle to relax, throughout the body.

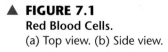

(a) (b)

▲ FIGURE 7.1
Red Blood Cells.
(a) Top view. (b) Side view.

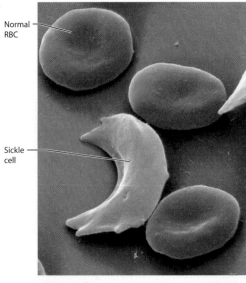

Normal RBC

Sickle cell

▲ FIGURE 7.2
Sickle Cell Disease

Disorders of Red Blood Cells
(LO 7.1, 7.2, 7.3, and 7.4)

Anemia is a red blood cell condition where the number of RBCs or amount of hemoglobin contained in each RBC is reduced. Both of these conditions reduce the blood's oxygen-carrying capacity, producing shortness of breath **(SOB)** and fatigue.

The different types of anemia include:

- **Iron-deficiency anemia** is the diagnosis for Ms. Sosin *(Case Report 7.1 on page 187)*. The cause was chronic bleeding from her gastrointestinal tract due to the aspirin and other painkillers she was taking. Her stools were positive for occult blood. Other causes of iron-deficiency anemia can be heavy menstrual bleeds or a diet deficient in iron.

- **Pernicious anemia (PA)** is due to vitamin B_{12} deficiency. It is caused by a shortage of intrinsic factor, which is normally secreted by cells in the stomach lining *(see Chapter 9)* and binds with B_{12}. This complex is absorbed into the bloodstream. Without B_{12}, hemoglobin cannot form. The number of red cells decreases, hemoglobin concentration decreases, and the size of the red cells increases.

- **Sickle cell anemia** is a genetic disorder found most commonly in African-Americans. Here, the production of abnormal hemoglobin causes the RBCs to form a rigid sickle shape *(Figure 7.2)*. The abnormal cells **agglutinate** (clump together) and block small capillaries. This creates intense pain in the **hypoxic** tissues (a sickle cell crisis) and can lead to stroke, kidney failure, and heart failure. **Sickle cell trait** is a minor form of this disease, and rarely has any symptoms.

- **Hemolytic anemia** is caused by excessive destruction of normal and abnormal RBCs. **Hemolysis** (the destruction of RBCs) can result from toxic substances, such as snake and spider venoms, mushroom toxins, and overdoses of drugs, entering the bloodstream. Trauma to RBCs by hemodialysis or heart-lung machines, or an incompatible blood transfusion can also cause hemolysis.

- **Aplastic anemia** is a condition in which the bone marrow is unable to produce sufficient new cells of all types—red cells, white cells, and platelets. It can be associated with exposure to radiation, benzene, and certain drugs. The diagnosis is made by bone marrow aspiration. Treatment involves suppression of the immune system and, in severe cases, a bone marrow transplant.

S = Suffix   P = Prefix   R = Root   R/CF= Combining Form

Word	Pronunciation	Elements		Definition
agglutinate (verb)	ah-**GLUE**-tin-ate	S/ P/ R/	-ate *composed of, pertaining to* ag- (ad-) *to* -glutin- *stick*	Stick together to form clumps
aplastic anemia	a-**PLAS**-tik ah-**NEE**-me-ah	S/ P/ R/ P/ R/	-tic *pertaining to* a- *without* -plas- *formation* an- *without* -emia *a blood condition*	Condition in which the bone marrow is unable to produce sufficient red cells, white cells, and platelets
erythrocyte	eh-**RITH**-roh-site	S/ R/CF	-cyte *cell* erythr/o- *red*	Red blood cell (RBC)
heme	HEEM		Greek *blood*	The iron-based component of hemoglobin that carries oxygen
hemoglobin oxyhemoglobin hemoglobinopathy	HE-moh-**GLOW**-bin OCK-see-he-moh-**GLOW**-bin HE-moh-**GLOW**-bih-**NOP**-ah-thee	R/ R/CF R/ S/ R/CF R/CF	-globin *protein* hem/o- *blood* oxy- *oxygen* -pathy *disease* -hem/o- *blood* -globin/o- *protein*	Red-pigmented protein that is the main component of red blood cells Combination of hemoglobin and oxygen Disease caused by the presence of an abnormal hemoglobin in red blood cells
hemolysis hemolytic (adj)	he-**MOL**-ih-sis he-moh-**LIT**-ik	S/ R/CF S/ R/	-lysis *destruction* hem/o- *blood* -ic *pertaining to* -lyt- *destroy*	Destruction of red blood cells so that hemoglobin is liberated Pertaining to the destruction of red blood cells
hypoxia (**Note:** *The duplicate letter "o" is omitted.*) hypoxic (adj)	high-**POCK**-see-ah high-**POCK**-sik	S/ P/ R/ S/	-ia *condition* hypo- *below, deficient* -ox- *oxygen* -ic *pertaining to*	Below-normal levels of oxygen in tissues, gases, or blood Deficient in oxygen
pallor	**PAL**-or		Latin *paleness*	Paleness of the skin
pernicious anemia	per-**NISH**-us ah-**NEE**-me-ah	S/ P/ R/ P/ R/	-ous *pertaining to* per- *through* -nici- *lethal* an- *without* -emia *a blood condition*	Chronic anemia due to lack of vitamin B$_{12}$
trait	TRAYT		Latin *an extension*	A discrete characteristic that has a known quality

EXERCISES

A. Review *the Case Report (see bullet under iron deficiency anemia) on page 190 before answering the questions.*

1. The GI tract connects which two organs? _____ and _____

2. Which body system contains the GI tract? _____

3. What caused Ms. Sosin's condition? _____

4. What diagnostic test was positive for the patient? _____

5. Name 2 other causes for the condition Ms. Sosin has. _____ and ____

B. Fill *in the correct disorder that matches the description.*

1. numbers of RBCs reduced _____

2. bone marrow cannot produce sufficient new cells of all types _____

3. genetic disorder found most commonly in African Americans _____

4. caused by excessive destruction of normal and abnormal RBCs _____

5. disorder caused by vitamin B$_{12}$ deficiency _____

LESSON 7.1 Types and Functions of White Blood Cells (Leukocytes) (LO 7.1, 7.2, and 7.3)

KEYNOTE

• Leukocytosis is too many white blood cells and often indicates the presence of an infection.

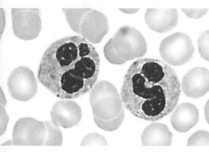

▲ **FIGURE 7.3**
Neutrophils Are Granulocytes.

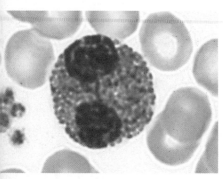

▲ **FIGURE 7.4**
Eosinophils Are Granulocytes.

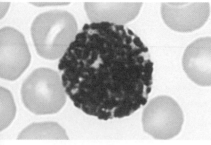

▲ **FIGURE 7.5**
Basophils Are Granulocytes.

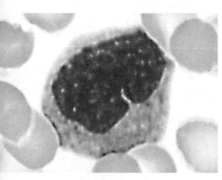

▲ **FIGURE 7.6**
Monocytes Are Agranulocytes.

The types of white blood cells (**WBCs**) can be categorized as **granulocytes** or **agranulocytes**. Granulocytes contain a granular cytoplasm, made up of granules, which are sites for enzyme and chemical production. Agranulocytes do not contain cytoplasmic granules.

Granulocytes
(LO 7.1, 7.2, and 7.3)

1. **Neutrophils** *(Figure 7.3)*, also called **polymorphonuclear leukocytes (PMNLs),** are normally 55% to 65% of the total WBC count. These cells ingest bacteria, fungi, and some viruses. In **neutropenia,** the number of neutrophils is decreased. In **neutrophilia,** the number is increased.
2. **Eosinophils** *(Figure 7.4)* are normally 2% to 4% of the total WBC count. They leave the bloodstream to enter tissue that is undergoing an allergic response. In allergic reactions, the number and percentage of eosinophils increase.
3. **Basophils** *(Figure 7.5)* are normally less than 1% of the total WBC count. Basophils migrate to damaged tissues to release histamine (which increases blood flow) and heparin (which prevents blood clotting).

Agranulocytes
(LO 7.1, 7.2, and 7.3)

4. **Monocytes** *(Figure 7.6)* are the largest blood cells and are normally 3% to 8% of the total WBC count. Monocytes leave the bloodstream and become **macrophages** that ingest bacteria, dead neutrophils, and dead cells in the tissues.
5. **Lymphocytes** *(Figure 7.7)* are the smallest white blood cells and comprise 25% to 35% of the total WBC count. Lymphocytes are produced in red bone marrow and migrate through the bloodstream to lymphatic tissues—lymph nodes, tonsils, spleen, and thymus—where they multiply.
   There are two main types of lymphocytes:

ABBREVIATIONS

DIFF	differential white blood cell count
EBV	Epstein-Barr virus
Ig	immunoglobulin
PMNL	polymorphonuclear leukocyte

a. **B cells** differentiate into plasma cells, which are stimulated by bacteria or toxins to produce antibodies or immunoglobulins (**Ig**) *(Chapter 7).*
b. **T cells** attach directly to foreign antigen-bearing cells like bacteria, which they kill with toxins they secrete.

In a laboratory report, a **differential white blood cell count (DIFF)** lists the percentages of the different leukocytes in a blood sample.

Disorders of White Blood Cells
(LO 7.1, 7.2, 7.3, and 7.4)

A normal cubic millimeter (mm³) of blood contains 5,000 to 10,000 white blood cells. In **leukocytosis,** the total WBC count exceeds 10,000 per cubic millimeter. Other conditions that increase the WBC count beyond the normal range include:

• Allergic reactions, which increase the number of eosinophils;
• Typhoid fever, malaria, and tuberculosis, which increase the number of monocytes; and
• Whooping cough and infectious mononucleosis, which increase the number of lymphocytes.

Infectious mononucleosis occurs in the 15- to 25-year-old population. Its cause—the **Epstein-Barr virus (EBV)**—is a very common virus and a member of the herpes family. The EBV is transmitted by an exchange of saliva, such as a kiss.

Leukemia is cancer of the blood-forming tissues and produces a high number of leukocytes and their precursors. The **leukemic** cells multiply, taking over the bone marrow and causing a deficiency of normal red blood cells, white blood cells, and platelets. This makes the patient anemic and vulnerable to infection and bleeding.

In **leukopenia,** the WBC count drops below 5,000 cells per cubic millimeter of blood. Leukopenia is seen in viral infections like measles, mumps, chickenpox, poliomyelitis, and AIDS.

In **pancytopenia,** the erythrocytes (red blood cells), leukocytes (white blood cells), and thrombocytes (platelets) in the circulating blood are all noticeably reduced. This can occur with cancer chemotherapy.

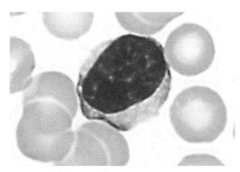

▲ **FIGURE 7.7**
Lymphocytes Are Agranulocytes.

Word	Pronunciation	Elements		Definition
agranulocyte	a-**GRAN**-you-loh-site	R/ P/ R/CF	-cyte *cell* a- *without, not* -granul/o- *granule*	A white blood cell without any granules in its cytoplasm
basophil	**BAY**-so-fill	S/ R/CF	-phil *attraction* bas/o- *base*	A basophil's granules attract a basic blue stain in the laboratory
eosinophil	ee-oh-**SIN**-oh-fill	S/ R/CF	-phil *attraction* eosin/o- *dawn*	An eosinophil's granules attract a rosy-red color on staining
granulocyte	**GRAN**-you-loh-site	R/ R/CF	-cyte *cell* granul/o- *small grain*	A white blood cell that contains multiple small granules in its cytoplasm
leukemia leukemic (adj)	loo-**KEE**-mee-ah loo-**KEE**-mik	S/ R/ S/	-emia *a blood condition* leuk- *white* -emic *pertaining to a blood condition*	Disease when the blood is taken over by white blood cells and their precursors Pertaining to or affected by leukemia
leukocyte leucocyte (syn) (Note: *Either spelling is acceptable.*)	**LOO**-koh-site	R/ R/CF	-cyte *cell* leuk/o- *white*	Another term for a white blood cell
leukocytosis leukopenia	**LOO**-koh-sigh-**TOE**-sis loo-koh-**PEE**-nee-ah	S/ S/	-osis *condition* -penia *deficiency*	An excessive number of white blood cells A deficient number of white blood cells
lymphocyte	**LIM**-foh-site	R/ R/CF	-cyte *cell* lymph/o- *lymph*	Small white blood cell with a large nucleus
monocyte	**MON**-oh-site	R/ P/	-cyte *cell* mono- *single*	Large white blood cell with a single nucleus
mononucleosis	**MON**-oh-nyu-klee-**OH**-sis	S/ P/ R/	-osis *condition* mono- *single* -nucle- *nucleus*	Presence of large numbers of specific, diagnostic mononuclear leukocytes
neutrophil neutropenia neutrophilia	**NEW**-troh-fill **NEW**-troh-**PEE**-nee-ah **NEW**-troh-**FILL**-ee-ah	S/ R/CF S/ S/	-phil *attraction* neutr/o- *neutral* -penia *deficiency* -philia *attraction*	Neutrophils' granules take up purple stain equally, whether the stain is acid or alkaline A deficiency of neutrophils An increase in neutrophils
pancytopenia	**PAN**-site-oh-**PEE**-nee-ah	S/ P/ R/CF	-penia *deficiency* pan- *all* -cyt/o- *cell*	Deficiency of all types of blood cells
polymorphonuclear	**POL**-ee-more-foh-**NEW**-klee-ah	S/ P/ R/CF R/	-ar *pertaining to* poly- *many* -morph/o- *shape* -nucle- *nucleus*	White blood cell with a multilobed nucleus

EXERCISES

A. A suffix *completes a medical term. The element* leuk *or* leuk/o *remains the same in each term below. Review the WAD before you start the exercise.*

Fill in the blanks.

penia   cyte   cytosis   emia

1. An excessive number of white blood cells is: _____

2. The disease when the blood is taken over by the WBCs is: _____

3. Another term for a white blood cell is: _____ .

4. A deficient number of white blood cells is: _____ .

5. What is the difference between leuco and leuko? _____ .

B. Fill *in the blanks.*

1. Write a medical term with the element that means "deficiency." _____/_____/_____

2. Which disorder causes a deficiency of all types of blood cells? _____

3. Where in the body are blood cells produced? _____

4. Name one function of blood. _____

5. What disease is a cancer of the blood-forming tissues? _____

Tissue factors, clotting factors, platelets

↓ That convert

Prothrombin

↓ To

Thrombin

↓ That converts

Fibrinogen

↓ To

Fibrin clot

▲ **FIGURE 7.8**
Blood Coagulation.

CASE REPORT 7.2

YOU ARE

. . . an emergency medical technician (EMT) working in the Fulwood Medical Center Emergency Department.

YOU ARE COMMUNICATING WITH

. . . Janis Tierney, a 17-year-old high school student, who presents with fainting at school. She is pale. Her pulse is 90 and her blood pressure is 100/60. She tells you that she is having a menstrual period with excessive bleeding. Her physical examination is otherwise unremarkable. She has a past history of easy bruising and recurrent nosebleeds, and an episode of severe bleeding after a tooth extraction. Janis has a deficiency of **von Willebrand factor (vWF)**. Her platelets are unable to stick together, and a platelet plug cannot form in the lining of her uterus to help end her menstrual flow.

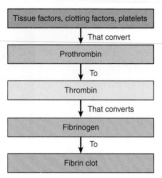

(a)

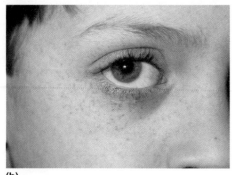

(b)

▲ **FIGURE 7.9**
Subsurface Bleeding.
(a) Purpura. (b) Petechiae.

Hemostasis
(LO 7.1, 7.2, and 7.3)

Hemostasis, the control of bleeding, is a vital issue in maintaining **homeostasis,** the state of the body's equilibrium. Uncontrolled bleeding can offset the body's balance by decreasing blood volume and lowering blood pressure.

Platelets (also called **thrombocytes**) play a key role in hemostasis. They are minute fragments of large bone marrow cells, and consist of a small amount of granular cytoplasm surrounded by a plasma membrane. They have no nucleus.

Hemostasis is achieved through a three-step process:

1. **Vascular spasm,** an immediate but temporary constriction of the injured blood vessels.

2. **Platelet plug formation,** an accumulation of platelets that bind themselves together and adhere to surrounding tissues. The binding and adhesion of platelets is mediated through **von Willebrand factor (vWF),** a protein produced by the cells lining blood vessels.

3. **Blood coagulation** is the process of going through **prothrombin** and **thrombin** to the formation of a blood clot that traps blood cells, platelets, and tissue fluid in a network of **fibrin** *(Figure 7.8).*

After a blood clot forms, platelets adhere to strands of fibrin and contract to pull the fibers and the edges of the broken blood vessel together. **Fibroblasts** invade the clot to produce a fibrous connective tissue that seals the blood vessel.

Disorders of Coagulation (Coagulopathies)
(LO 7.1, 7.2, 7.3, and 7.4)

There are several disorders that can prevent the blood from clotting properly, and these can lead to further health problems.

Hemophilia, in its classical form (hemophilia A), is a disease males inherit from their mothers. It results from a deficiency of the coagulation factor named **factor VIII.**

Von Willebrand disease (vWD)—the most common hereditary bleeding disorder—is a protein deficiency of the factor VIII complex **(vWF)** that is different from the factor deficiency involved in hemophilia.

Disseminated intravascular coagulation (DIC) occurs when a severe bacterial infection activates the clotting mechanism simultaneously throughout the cardiovascular system. Small clots form and obstruct blood flow into tissues and organs, particularly the kidney, leading to renal failure.

Thrombus formation **(thrombosis)** is a clot that forms attached to a diseased or damaged area on the walls of blood vessels or the heart. If part of the thrombus breaks loose and moves through the circulation, it is called an **embolus.**

Thrombocytopenia is a deficiency of platelets.

Purpura is bleeding into the skin from small arterioles that produces a larger individual lesion than the tiny red spots or **petechiae** from capillary bleeds *(Figure 7.9a and b).* **Bruises** (or **hematomas**) are leaks of blood from all types of blood vessels.

Word	Pronunciation	Elements		Definition
coagulant	koh-**AG**-you-lant	S/ R/	-ant *forming, pertaining to* coagul- *clot, clump*	Substance that causes clotting
coagulation	koh-ag-you-**LAY**-shun	S/	-ation *process*	Process of blood clotting
anticoagulant	AN-tee-koh-**AG**-you-lant	P/	anti- *against*	Substance that prevents clotting
embolus	**EM**-boh-lus		Greek *plug, stopper*	Detached piece of thrombus, a mass of bacteria, quantity of air, or foreign body that blocks a blood vessel
fibrin	**FIE**-brin		Latin *fiber*	Stringy protein fiber that is a component of a blood clot
fibroblast	**FIE**-broh-blast	S/ R/CF	-blast *immature cell* fibr/o- *fiber*	Cell that forms collagen fibers
hematoma (also called **bruise**)	he-mah-**TOE**-mah	S/ R/	-oma *mass, tumor* hemat- *blood*	Collection of blood that has escaped from vessels into surrounding tissues
hemophilia	he-moh-**FILL**-ee-ah	S/ R/CF	-philia *attraction* hem/o- *blood*	An inherited disease from a deficiency of clotting factor VIII
hemostasis (**Note:** *Homeostasis has a very different meaning.*)	he-moh-**STAY**-sis	S/ R/CF	-stasis *control, stop* hem/o- *blood*	Control of or stopping bleeding
petechia petechiae (pl)	peh-**TEE**-kee-ah peh-**TEE**-kee-ee		Latin *spot on the skin*	Pinpoint capillary hemorrhagic spot in the skin
prothrombin	pro-**THROM**-bin	S/ P/ R/	-in *substance* pro- *before* -thromb- *blood clot*	Protein formed by the liver and converted to thrombin in the blood-clotting mechanism
purpura	**PUR**-pyu-rah		Greek *purple*	Skin hemorrhages that are red initially and then turn purple
thrombocyte (also called **platelet**)	**THROM**-boh-site	R/ R/CF	-cyte *cell* thromb/o- *blood clot*	Another name for a platelet
thrombocytopenia	**THROM**-boh-site-oh-**PEE**-nee-uh	S/ R/CF	-penia *deficiency* -cyt/o- *cell*	Deficiency of platelets in circulating blood
von Willebrand	VON **WILL**-eh-brand		E.A. Willebrand, Finnish physician, 1870–1949	

EXERCISES

A. **Review** *the Case Report on this spread before answering the questions.*

1. Why is Janis Tierney in the Emergency Department at Fulwood Medical Center?

_____

2. What is causing her blood-related issues? _____

3. What are her symptoms? _____

4. What blood-related issues does she have in her past medical history? _____

5. Translate into medical language: "her blood clotting cells are unable to stick together"

_____

B. Review *the two pages open in front of you to determine the answers to the following questions. Circle the best choice.*

1. In the term *hemostasis*, the suffix means:

   blood   condition   control

2. Which term relates to a color?

   hemophilia   petechia   purpura

3. The process of blood clotting is called:

   homeostasis   coagulation   thrombocytopenia

4. A piece of thrombus that has broken off into the circulation is called:

   an embolus   a fibroblast   a coagulant

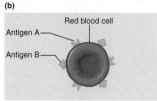

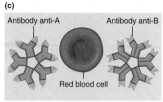

▲ **FIGURE 7.10**
   (a) Type A blood.
   (b) Type B blood.
   (c) Type AB blood.
   (d) Type O blood.

ABBREVIATIONS

Ab   antibody
ABO blood group system

CASE REPORT 7.3

YOU ARE
> . . . an emergency medical technician–paramedic (EMT-P) working in the Level One Trauma Unit at Fulwood Medical Center.

YOU ARE COMMUNICATING WITH
> . . . Ms. Joanne Rodi, an 18-year-old student, who has been admitted to the unit from the operating room. Ms. Rodi has had surgery for multiple fractures sustained in a car accident. She is receiving a blood **transfusion.** You document that her temperature has risen to 102.8°F, her respirations have risen to 24 per minute, and she has chills. You take her blood pressure, and it has fallen to 90/60. What is your next step?

Blood Groups and Transfusions (LO 7.1, 7.2, and 7.3)

Red Cell Antigens (LO 7.1, 7.2, and 7.3)

Antigens are molecules that exist on the surfaces of red blood cells. **Antibodies** are present in the plasma. Each antibody can combine with only a specific antigen. If the plasma antibodies combine with another red cell antigen, bridges form to connect these red cells together. This is called **agglutination,** or clumping, of the cells. Hemolysis (destruction) of the cells also occurs.

The antigens on the surfaces of the cells have been categorized into groups. Two of these groups—the **ABO** and **Rh** blood groups—are the most important.

ABO Blood Group (LO 7.1, 7.2, and 7.3)

The two major antigens on the cell surface are antigen A and antigen B.

A person with only antigen A has *type A* blood.

A person with only antigen B has *type B* blood.

A person with both antigen A and antigen B has *type AB* blood.

A person with neither antigen has *type O* blood and is a universal donor, able to give blood to any other person. Specific antibodies are synthesized in the plasma during the first 8 months after birth:

• Whenever antigen A is absent, anti-A antibody is produced.

• Whenever antigen B is absent, anti-B antibody is produced.

Figure 7.10 shows the different combinations of antigens and antibodies in the different blood types.

A **transfusion** of blood or packed red blood cells replaces lost red blood cells to restore the blood's oxygen-carrying capacity. **Autologous** donation and transfusion occurs when people donate their own blood ahead of time to be given back to them if necessary during a surgical procedure.

CASE REPORT 7.3 (CONTINUED)

> In Joanne Rodi's case, she has type A blood and by mistake received type AB blood, which agglutinated in the presence of her anti-B antibodies. Your immediate response is to stop the transfusion, replace it with a saline **infusion**, call your supervisor, and notify the doctor.

S = Suffix   P = Prefix   R = Root   R/CF= Combining Form

Word	Pronunciation	Elements		Definition
agglutination (noun)	ah-glue-tih-**NAY**-shun	S/ P/ R/	-ation *process* ag- *to (same as ad-)* -glutin- *glue*	Process by which cells or other particles adhere to each other to form clumps
antibody antibodies (pl)	**AN**-tee-body	P/ R/	anti- *against* -body *substance, body*	Protein produced in response to an antigen
antigen	**AN**-tee-gen	P/ R/	anti- *against* -gen *produce, create*	Substance capable of triggering an immune response
autologous	awe-**TOL**-oh-gus	P/ R/	auto- *self, same* -logous *relation*	Blood transfusion with the same person as donor and recipient—self-transfusion
infusion	in-**FYU**-zhun	P/ R/	in- *in* -fusion *to pour*	Introduction intravenously of a substance other than blood
transfusion	trans-**FYU**-zhun	P/ R/	trans- *across* -fusion *to pour*	Transfer of blood or a blood component from donor to recipient

EXERCISES

A. Review *the Case Report on this spread before answering the questions.*

1.   What is the difference between transfusion and infusion? _____

_____

2.   What is the patient's current status regarding her surgery? _____

3.   Is she experiencing hypotension or hypertension now? _____

4.   Who could be involved in the error that caused this problem for the patient? _____

5.   What in Ms. Rodi's type A blood caused the agglutination to occur? _____

6.   What diagnosis originally put Ms. Rodi in the trauma unit? _____

7.   What symptoms signify Ms. Rodi is having a bad reaction? _____

8.   Why should the transfusion be stopped immediately? _____

9.   What is the purpose of the saline solution? _____

10. Critical thinking: Discuss why it is a good idea to know your blood type and the blood type of members of your immediate family. _____

_____

_____

_____

B. Review *the elements in the WAD before starting this exercise. Fill in the blanks.*

_____ 1. trans

_____ 2. anti

_____ 3. fusion

_____ 4. glutin

_____ 5. gen

A. to pour

B. glue

C. against

D. across

E. produce

LESSON 7.1 Blood Groups and Transfusions (continued)

- Rh factor is an antigen on the surface of a red blood cell. Its presence or absence is inherited.

Rh Blood Group
(LO 7.1, 7.2, 7.3, and 7.4)

If an Rh antigen is present on the red cell surface, the blood is said to be Rh-positive (Rh+). This is common, as about 85% of people are Rh-positive. If there is no Rh antigen on the surface, the blood is Rh-negative (Rh–), which is the case for the other 15% of the population.

If an Rh-negative person receives a transfusion of Rh-positive blood, anti-Rh antibodies will be produced. This can cause RBC clumping (agglutination) and destruction (hemolysis).

If an Rh-negative woman and an Rh-positive man conceive an Rh-positive child *(Figure 7.11a),* the placenta normally prevents **maternal** and **fetal** blood from mixing. However, at birth or during a **miscarriage,** fetal cells can enter the mother's bloodstream. These Rh-positive cells stimulate the mother's tissues to produce Rh antibodies *(Figure 7.11b).*

If the mother becomes pregnant with a second Rh-positive fetus, her Rh antibodies can cross the **placenta** and agglutinate and hemolyze the fetal red cells *(Figure 7.11c).* This causes hemolytic disease of the newborn **(HDN,** or **erythroblastosis fetalis).**

Hemolytic disease of the newborn due to Rh incompatibility can be prevented. The Rh-negative mother giving birth to an Rh-positive child should be given Rh-immune globulin **(RhoGAM).**

Other causes of hemolytic disease in newborn include ABO **incompatibility,** incompatibility in other blood group systems, hereditary **spherocytosis,** and infections acquired before birth.

ABBREVIATIONS

HDN	hemolytic disease of the newborn
Rh	Rhesus
RhoGAM	Rhesus immune globulin

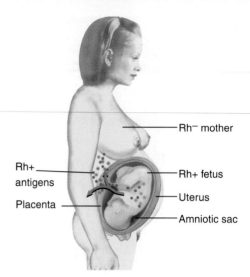

(a) First pregnancy

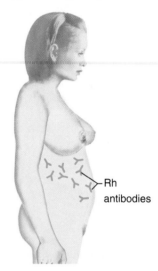

(b) Between pregnancy

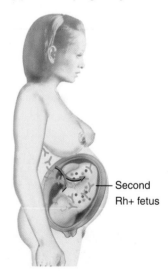

(c) Second pregnancy

▲ **FIGURE 7.11**
Hemolytic Disease of the Newborn.
(a) First pregnancy. (b) Between pregnancies.
(c) Second pregnancy.

S = Suffix   P = Prefix   R = Root   R/CF= Combining Form

Word	Pronunciation	Elements		Definition
erythroblastosis fetalis	eh-**RITH**-roh-blast-oh-sis fee-**TAH**-lis	S/ R/CF R/ S/ R/	-osis *condition* erythr/o- *red* -blast- *immature cell* -is *belonging to* fetal- *fetus*	Erythroblastosis fetalis is a hemolytic disease of the newborn (HDN)
incompatible incompatibility	in-kom-**PAT**-ih-bul in-kom-**PAT**-ih-bul-i-tee	S/ P/ R/	-ible *can do* in- *not* -compat- *tolerate*	Substances that interfere with each other physiologically
fetus fetal (adj)	**FEE**-tus **FEE**-tal	S/ R/	Latin *offspring* -al *pertaining to* fet- *fetus*	Human organism from the end of the eighth week after conception to birth Pertaining to the fetus
maternal	mah-**TER**-nal	S/ R/	-al *pertaining to* matern- *mother*	Pertaining to or derived from the mother
miscarriage	mis-**KAR**-aj	P/	mis- *not, incorrect* -carriage Old English *to carry*	Spontaneous expulsion of the products of pregnancy before fetal viability
placenta	plah-**SEN**-tah		Latin *a cake*	Organ that allows metabolic exchange between the mother and the fetus
spherocyte spherocytosis	**SFEAR**-oh-site **SFEAR**-oh-site-oh-sis	R/ R/CF S/	-cyte *cell* spher/o- *sphere* -osis *condition*	A spherical cell Presence of spherocytes in blood

EXERCISES

A. Apply *the language of hematology and answer the following questions.*

1. For blood to be Rh+ what must it have? _____

2. How are Rh antibodies produced? _____

3. What prevents maternal and fetal blood from mixing? _____

4. What gets destroyed in HDN? _____

5. What is the medical term for HDN? _____

B. Unscramble the letters *for the correct medical term to match the definition.*

1. Presence of spherocytes in blood: rsoyspcosheti _____

2. Substances that interfere with each other: imitlnoeacpb _____

3. Pertaining to the fetus: aetfl _____

4. Spontaneous expulsion of the products of pregnancy: riraamceisg _____

5. Pertaining to the mother: anlrmaet _____

C. Use your knowledge *of medical terminology to answer the following questions.*

1. What is the medical term for *red blood cells clumping together?* _____

2. What is more common: being Rh+ or Rh– ? _____

3. The presence or absence of Rh factor at birth is _____

4. What follows after red blood cells clump together? _____

5. Define *spherocytosis.* _____

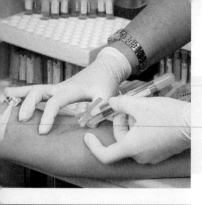

LESSON 7.2

Lymphatic System

As part of your body's defense mechanisms, the lymphatic system and its fluid provide surveillance and protection against foreign materials. In this lesson, the information provided will enable you to use correct medical terminology to:

7.2.1 Detail the anatomy of the **lymphatic** system.

7.2.2 Define the functions of the lymphatic system.

7.2.3 Identify the major cells of the lymphatic system and their functions.

7.2.4 Distinguish the anatomy and functions of the **lymph nodes, tonsils, thymus,** and **spleen.**

7.2.5 Recognize the common disorders of the lymphatic system.

ABBREVIATION

Ab   antibody

CASE REPORT 7.4

YOU ARE

. . . a medical assistant working with Susan Lee, MD, in her primary care clinic.

YOU ARE COMMUNICATING WITH

. . . Ms. Anna Clemons, a 20-year-old waitress, who is a new patient. She has noticed a lump in the left side of her neck. On questioning, you learn that Ms. Clemons has lost about 8 pounds in the past couple of months, has felt tired, and has had some night sweats. Her vital signs are normal. There are two firm, enlarged **lymph nodes** in her left neck in front of the sternocleidomastoid muscle (the long muscle in the side of the neck that extends up to the base of the skull behind the ear). Physical examination is otherwise unremarkable.

Lymphatic System (LO 7.1, 7.2, 7.3, and 7.4)

You live in a world that surrounds you with chemicals and disease-causing organisms waiting for a chance to enter your body and harm you. Your body has three lines of defense mechanisms against foreign organisms (**pathogens**), cells (cancer), or molecules (**pollutants** and **allergens**).

1. **Physical defense mechanisms** include: your skin and mucous membranes; chemicals in your perspiration, saliva, and tears; hairs in your nostrils; and cilia and mucus to protect your lungs. The physical defense mechanisms are further discussed in the individual body system chapters.

2. **Cellular defense mechanisms,** based on defensive cells (**lymphocytes**). These directly attack suspicious cells like cancer cells, transplanted tissue cells, or cells infected with viruses or parasites.

3. **Humoral defense mechanisms** *(see Lesson 7.3),* based on antibodies (**Abs**). These are found in body fluids and bind to bacteria, toxins, and extracellular viruses, tagging them for destruction.

Word	Pronunciation		Elements	Definition
allergen (Note: *The duplicate letter "g" is omitted.*) allergic (adj) allergy	AL-er-jen ah-**LER**-jik AL-er-jee	S/ R/ R/ S/ S/	-gen *create* all- *other, strange* -erg- *work* -ic *pertaining to* -ergy *process of working*	Substance creating a hypersensitivity (allergic) reaction Pertaining to or suffering from an allergy Hypersensitivity to a particular allergen
lymph	LIMF		Latin *clear, spring water*	A clear fluid collected from tissues and transported by lymph vessels to the venous circulation
lymphatic (adj) lymphoid (adj)	lim-**FAT**-ik LIM-foyd	S/ R/ S/	-atic *pertaining to* lymph- *lymph* -oid *resembling*	Pertaining to lymph or the lymphatic system Resembling lymphatic tissue
node	NOHD		Latin *a knot*	A circumscribed mass of tissue
pathogen	PATH-oh-jen	S/ R/CF	-gen *produce, create, form* path/o- *disease*	A disease-causing microorganism
pollutant	poh-**LOO**-tant	S/ R/	-ant *pertaining to* pollut- *unclean*	Substance that makes an environment unclean or impure
spleen	SPLEEN		Greek *spleen*	Vascular, lymphatic organ in left upper quadrant of abdomen
thymus	THIGH-mus		Greek *sweetbread*	Endocrine gland located in the mediastinum
tonsil	TON-sill		Latin *tonsil*	Mass of lymphoid tissue on either side of the throat at the back of the tongue

EXERCISES

A. Review *the Case Report on this spread before answering the questions.*

1. What are Ms. Clemons' symptoms? _____

2. What is present on physical examination of the patient? _____

3. Where is the sternocleidomastoid muscle? _____

4. What was the status of the patient's VS? _____

5. What is a node? _____

B. Build *the correct medical terms that match the definitions given. Fill in the blanks.*

1. substance that makes the environment unclean or impure:

_____ / _____ / _____
        P   R/CF   S

2. substance creating a hypersensitivity reaction:

_____ / _____ / _____
        P   R/CF   S

3. resembling lymphatic tissue:

_____ / _____ / _____
        P   R/CF   S

4. a disease-causing microorganism:

_____ / _____ / _____
        P   R/CF   S

5. hypersensitivity to a particular allergen:

_____ / _____ / _____
        P   R/CF   S

LESSON 7.2 Lymphatic System (continued)
(LO 7.1, 7.2, 7.3, and 7.4)

- Tissues that are the first line of defense against pathogens—for example, the airway passages—have lymphatic tissue in the submucous layers to help protect against invasion.

The lymphatic system (*Figure 7.12*) has three components:

1. A network of thin **lymphatic capillaries and vessels,** similar to blood vessels, that penetrates the **interstitial spaces** (the spaces between tissues) of nearly every tissue in the body except cartilage, bone, red bone marrow, and the CNS;

2. A group of tissues and organs that produce **immune cells;** and

3. **Lymph,** a clear colorless fluid similar to blood plasma but with a composition that varies throughout the body. It flows through the network of lymphatic capillaries and vessels.

The lymphatic system has three functions:

1. **Absorb** excess interstitial fluid and return it to the bloodstream;

2. **Remove** foreign chemicals, cells, and debris from the tissues; and

3. **Absorb** dietary lipids from the small intestine (*see Chapter 9*).

The **lymphatic network** begins with lymphatic capillaries that are closed-ended tubes nestled among **blood capillary networks** (*Figure 7.13*). The lymphatic capillaries are designed to let interstitial fluid enter so it can become lymph. In addition, bacteria, viruses, cellular debris, and traveling cancer cells can enter the lymphatic capillaries with the interstitial fluid. The lymphatic capillaries converge to form the larger **lymphatic collecting vessels,** which resemble small veins and have one-way valves. They travel alongside veins and arteries.

Lymph Nodes
(LO 7.1, 7.2, 7.3, and 7.4)

At irregular intervals, the collecting vessels mentioned above enter into the lymph nodes (*Figure 7.14*). There are hundreds of lymph nodes stationed all over the body (*Figure 7.12*). They are concentrated in the neck, axilla, and groin. Their functions are to filter impurities from the lymph and alert the immune system to the presence of pathogens.

The lymph moves slowly through the nodes, which filter the lymph and remove any foreign matter. Macrophages in the lymph nodes ingest and break down foreign matter and display its fragments to T cells. This alerts the immune system to the presence of an invader. Lymph leaves the nodes when it enters into the **efferent** collecting vessels. All these lymph vessels move lymph toward the thoracic cavity.

Collecting vessels merge into **lymphatic trunks** that drain lymph from a major body region. These lymphatic trunks then merge into two large **lymphatic ducts**—the thoracic duct on the left and the right lymphatic duct, which empty into the veins beneath the collarbone, the subclavian veins (*Figure 7.12*).

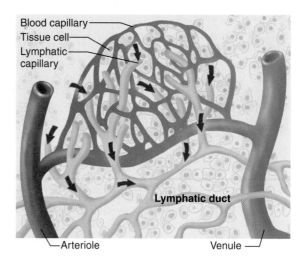

▲ **FIGURE 7.13**
Lymphatic Flow.

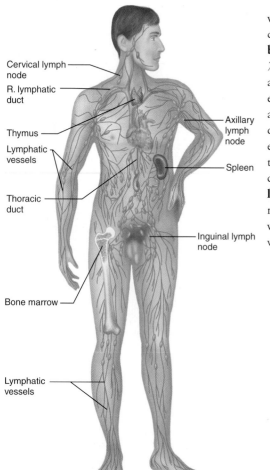

◀ **FIGURE 7.12**
The Lymphatic System.
(R. = right; L. = left)

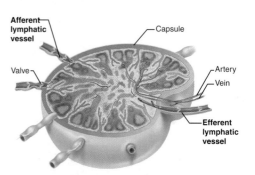

▲ **FIGURE 7.14**
Lymph Node.

Word	Pronunciation		Elements	Definition
efferent	EFF-eh-rent	S/	-ent *end result, pertaining to*	Moving away from a center
		R/	effer- *move away from the center*	
afferent (Note: *These are opposite terms.*)	AFF-eh-rent	R/	affer- *move toward the center*	Moving toward a center
immune	im-YUNE		Latin *protected from*	Protected from an infectious disease
immunity	im-YOU-nih-tee	S/	-ity *condition*	State of being protected
		R/	immun- *immune*	
immunology	im-you-NOL-oh-jee	S/	-logy *study of*	The science and practice of immunity and allergy
		R/CF	immun/o- *immune*	
immunologist	im-you-NOL-oh-jist	S/	-logist *one who studies, specialist*	Medical specialist in immunology
immunize (verb)	IM-you-nize	S/	-ize *affect in a specific way*	Make resistant to an infectious disease
		R/	immun- *immune*	
immunization (noun)	IM-you-nih-ZAY-shun	S/	-ization *process of inserting or creating*	Administration of an agent to provide immunity
interstitial	In-ter-STISH-al	S/	-al *pertaining to*	Pertaining to spaces between cells in a tissue or organ
		R/	interstiti- *space between tissues*	

EXERCISES

A. Precision *in usage is important if you want to communicate correct information. These six terms all contain a common root/combining form.*

Insert the correct term in each sentence.

immune   immunology   immunity   immunologist   immunization   immunize

1. One who specializes in (the study of the science of immunity and allergy) _____ is termed an (type of specialist) _____.

2. The _____ system is a group of specialized cells in different parts of the body that recognize foreign substances and neutralize them.

3. We need to _____ young children before they start school.

4. A prior (injection) _____ obtained before she went overseas boosted her (status of being immune) _____ to the disease.

B. Review *the text on the opposite page and fill in the blanks.*

1. Meet a lesson objective and list the 3 components of the lymphatic system:

   a. _____   **b.** _____   **c.** _____

2. Based on the elements, where are the interstitial spaces? _____

3. Lymph is similar to what other body fluid? _____

4. Name the three functions of the lymphatic system. **a.** _____   **b.** _____   **c.** _____

5. Lymphatic capillaries and vessels penetrate the interstitial spaces nearly everywhere in the body except _____.

6. Where in the body are the major concentrations of lymph nodes? _____

7. What enters lymphatic capillaries to become lymph? _____
   _____

8. Where does the lymphatic network begin? _____
   _____

9. Where do the two large lymphatic ducts empty? _____
   _____

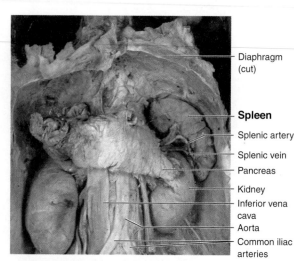

▲ FIGURE 7.15
Position of Spleen.

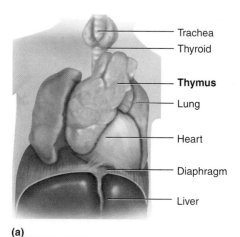

(a)

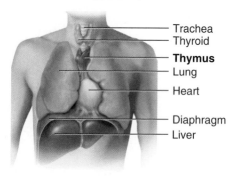

(b)

▲ FIGURE 7.16
Thymus.
(a) Large thymus in infant. (b) Adult thymus.

Lymphatic Tissues and Cells (LO 7.1, 7.2, and 7.3)

In some organs, lymphocytes and other cells form dense clusters called lymphatic **follicles.** These are constant features in the lymph nodes, the tonsils, and the ileum (a part of the small intestine).

Lymphatic tissues are composed of a variety of cells that include:

- **T lymphocytes (T cells):** The "T" stands for thymus, which is where these cells develop and mature. T lymphocytes make up 75% to 85% of body lymphocytes.

- **B lymphocytes (B cells):** These cells mature in the bone marrow. B lymphocytes make up 15% to 25% of lymphocytes. They respond to a specific antigen and become plasma cells to produce antibodies (**immunoglobulins, Ig**) that immobilize, neutralize, and prepare the specific antigen for destruction. Macrophages that have developed from monocytes ingest and destroy antigens, tissue debris, **bacteria,** and other foreign matter (phagocytosis).

Lymphatic Organs (LO 7.1, 7.2, and 7.3)

Spleen (LO 7.1, 7.2, and 7.3)

The **spleen,** a highly vascular and spongy organ, is the largest lymphatic organ. It is located in the left upper quadrant of the abdomen, below the diaphragm and lateral to the kidney *(Figure 7.15).*

The functions of the spleen are to:

- **Phagocytose (consume)** bacteria and other foreign materials.
- **Initiate an immune response** when antigens are found in the blood.
- **Phagocytose old, defective erythrocytes** and platelets.
- **Serve as a reservoir** for erythrocytes and platelets.

Tonsils and Adenoids (LO 7.1, 7.2, and 7.3)

The **tonsils** *(see Chapter 8)* are two masses of lymphatic tissue located at the entrance to the upper part of the throat (the oropharynx) that entrap inhaled and ingested pathogens. **Adenoids** are similar tissues on the posterior wall of the upper pharynx or nasopharynx *(see Chapter 8).* The tonsils and adenoids form lymphocytes and antibodies, trap bacteria and viruses, and drain them into the tonsillar lymph nodes for elimination. Both the tonsils and the adenoids can also become infected.

Thymus (LO 7.1, 7.2, and 7.3)

The thymus, a small organ of the immune system located in the center of the upper chest, has both endocrine *(see Chapter 12)* and lymphatic functions. T lymphocytes develop and mature in the thymus and are released into the bloodstream. The thymus is largest in infancy *(Figure 7.16a)* and reaches its maximum size at puberty. It then shrinks *(Figure 7.16b)* and is eventually replaced by fibrous and fatty (adipose) tissue.

Word	Pronunciation		Elements	Definition
adenoid	ADD-eh-noyd	S/ R/	-oid *resemble* aden- *gland*	Single mass of lymphoid tissue in the midline at the back of the throat
adenoidectomy	ADD-eh-noy-**DEK**-toh-me	S/	-ectomy *surgical excision*	Surgical removal of the adenoid tissue
bacterium bacteria (pl)	bak-**TEER**-ee-um bak-**TEER**-ee-ah		Greek *a staff*	A unicellular, simple, microscopic organism
follicle	**FOLL**-ih-kull		Latin *a small sac*	Spherical mass of cells containing a cavity; or a small cul-de-sac, such as a hair follicle
immunoglobulin	IM-you-noh-**GLOB**-you-lin	S/ R/CF R/	-in *chemical compound, substance* immun/o-*immune* -globul- *globular, protein*	Specific protein evoked by an antigen. All antibodies are immunoglobulins
spleen	SPLEEN		Greek *spleen*	Vascular, lymphatic organ in left upper quadrant of abdomen
splenectomy (Note: *single "e" in* **splen**)	sple-**NECK**-toe-me	S/ R/	-ectomy *surgical excision* splen- *spleen*	Surgical removal of the spleen
splenomegaly	sple-noh-**MEG**-ah-lee	S/ R/CF	-megaly *enlargement* splen/o- *spleen*	Enlarged spleen

EXERCISES

A. Review *all the terms and elements in the WAD above. Pay careful attention to spelling and pronunciation. Answer the following questions by circling the best choice.*

1. In the term *adenoid* one of the elements means:

   tissue   organ   gland

2. The correct plural of bacterium is:

   bacteria   bacteriae   bacteriums

3. In addition to referring to a lymph follicle, the term *follicle* can also apply to:

   digits   bones   hair

4. What do *tonsil* and *adenoid* have in common?

   lymphatic tissue   connective tissue   adipose tissue

5. Immunoglobulin can also be considered:

   tissue collection   pathogens   antibodies

B. Review *all the terms and elements in the WAD above. Pay careful attention to spelling and pronunciation. Answer the following questions by circling the best choice.*

1. The suffix in the term adenoidectomy implies:

   surgical excision   surgical fixation   surgical incision

2. A microscopic organism is:

   bacteria   follicle   bacterium

3. The spleen is located in the:

   ABG   RLQ   LUQ

4. The specific protein evoked by an antigen is:

   bacterium   enzyme   immunoglobulin

5. The element meaning enlargement is:

   megaly   ectomy   oid

Disorders of the Lymphatic System
(LO 7.1, 7.2, 7.3, and 7.4)

- Treatment options for lymphomas include radiation, chemotherapy, and bone marrow transplant.

- The body can function without a spleen but is somewhat more vulnerable to infection.

- Edema due to water retention, when pressed with a finger, leaves a depression (pit). Lymphedema is brawny and pits minimally.

Physicians routinely feel the accessible lymph nodes in the neck (**cervical nodes**), axilla (armpit) (**axillary nodes**), and groin (**inguinal nodes**) for enlargement and tenderness, which indicate disease in the tissues drained by the lymph nodes.

Cancerous lymph nodes are enlarged, firm, and usually painless. Infections in the lymph nodes cause them to be swollen and tender to the touch, a condition called **lymphadenitis.** All lymph node enlargements are collectively called **lymphadenopathy.** When lymph nodes are removed, the process is called **lymphadenectomy.**

Lymphoma is a malignant growth (**neoplasm**) of the lymphatic organs, usually the lymph nodes. Associated symptoms can be fever, night sweats, fatigue, and weight loss. Lymphomas are grouped into two categories by microscopic examination of affected lymphatic tissues:

1. **Hodgkin lymphoma,** or **Hodgkin disease:** The cancer spreads in an orderly manner to adjoining lymph nodes. This enables the disease to be staged depending on how far it has spread; and

2. **Non-Hodgkin lymphomas**: These occur much more frequently than Hodgkin lymphoma. They include some 30 different disease entities in 10 different subtypes.

Diagnostic procedures used to determine lymphoma include; a biopsy of an enlarged node, X-rays, CT and MRI scans, a **lymphangiogram,** and a bone marrow biopsy.

CASE REPORT 7.4 (CONTINUED)

Ms. Anna Clemons has cancerous nodes in her neck. They were caused not by metastatic cancer but by a cancer of the lymph nodes called **Hodgkin lymphoma,** which is detailed later on this page.

Tonsillitis, inflammation of the tonsils and adenoids, occurs mostly in infancy and childhood. The infection can be viral or bacterial, usually streptococcal. It produces enlarged, tender lymph nodes under the jaw. The infection can be recurrent, and a tonsillectomy is sometimes performed (*see Chapter 8*). If the adenoids also show recurrent infection, an adenoidectomy can be performed, often at the same time as the **tonsillectomy.**

Splenomegaly, an enlarged spleen, is not a disease in itself but the result of an underlying disorder. But, when the spleen enlarges, it traps and stores an excessive number of blood cells and platelets (**hypersplenism**), reducing the number of blood cells and platelets in the bloodstream. Occasionally, a splenectomy is necessary.

Ruptured spleen is a common complication from car accidents or other trauma when the abdomen and rib cage are damaged. Intra-abdominal bleeding from the ruptured spleen can be extensive, with a dramatic fall in blood pressure. It is considered a surgical emergency requiring a splenectomy.

Lymphedema is localized, brawny (does not easily pit on finger pressure), minimally-pitting fluid retention caused by a compromised lymphatic system, often after surgery or radiation therapy. It can also be primary, where the cause is unknown.

S = Suffix   P = Prefix   R = Root   R/CF= Combining Form

Word	Pronunciation	Elements		Definition
hypersplenism (Note: *one "e" in this term*)	high-per-**SPLEN**-izm	S/ P/ R/	-ism *condition* hyper- *excessive* -splen- *spleen*	Condition in which the spleen removes blood components at an excessive rate
inguinal	**IN**-gwin-al	S/ R/	-al *pertaining to* inguin- *groin*	Pertaining to the groin
lymphadenectomy	lim-**FAD**-eh-**NECK**-toe-me	S/ R/	-ectomy *surgical excision* lymphaden- *lymph node*	Surgical excision of a lymph node(s)
lymphadenitis lymphadenopathy	lim-**FAD**-eh-neye-tis lim-**FAD**-eh-**NOP**-ah-thee	S/ S/ R/CF	-itis *inflammation* -pathy *disease* lymphaden/o- *lymph node*	Inflammation of a lymph node(s) Any disease process affecting a lymph node(s)
lymphangiogram	lim-**FAN**-jee-oh-gram	S/ R/CF	-gram *recording* lymphangi/o- *lymphatic vessels*	Radiographic images of lymph vessels and nodes following injection of contrast material
lymphedema	**LIMF**-eh-dee-mah	R/ R/	lymph- *lymph* -edema *edema*	Tissue swelling due to lymphatic obstruction
lymphoma	lim-**FOH**-mah	S/ R/	-oma *tumor, mass* lymph- *lymphatic system, lymph*	Any neoplasm of lymphatic tissue
Hodgkin	**HOJ**-kin		Thomas Hodgkin, British physician, 1798–1866	Hodgkin lymphoma is marked by chronic enlargement of lymph nodes spreading to other nodes in an orderly way
neoplasm (noun) neoplastic (adj) neoplasia (Note: *The "m" in -plasm is removed to allow the elements to flow.*)	**NEE**-oh-plazm **NEE**-oh-**PLAS**-tic **NEE**-oh-**PLAY**-zee-ah	P/ R/ S/ S/	neo- *new* -plasm- *to form* -tic *pertaining to* -ia *condition*	A new growth, either a benign or malignant tumor Pertaining to a neoplasm Process that results in formation of a tumor

EXERCISES

A. Review *the Case Report on this spread before answering the questions.*

1. What medical term in the Case Report signifies that the nodes are *malignant?* _____

2. What is the correct medical term for lymph nodes in the neck? _____

3. What is *metastatic* cancer? _____

4. Is this a primary or secondary cancer site? _____

5. What is another term for Hodgkin lymphoma? _____

6. Ms. Clemons does not have cancer anywhere else in her body. What sentence in the Case Report confirms that? _____

_____

B. Elements *remain your best tool for understanding the meaning of a term. Match the meaning of the definition in column 1 with the correct element in column 2.*

_____ **1.** groin   **A.** lymphangio

_____ **2.** lymph node   **B.** gram

_____ **3.** tumor, mass   **C.** inguin

_____ **4.** recording   **D.** oma

_____ **5.** lymph vessels   **E.** lymphadeno

C. Meet lesson objectives *and use the language of immunology to answer the following questions.*

1. Name the diagnostic procedures used to determine lymphoma. _____

2. What is a common injury from a motor vehicle accident? _____

3. What surgery is often performed at the same time as a tonsillectomy? _____

4. What is the difference between *pitting edema* and *lymphedema?* _____

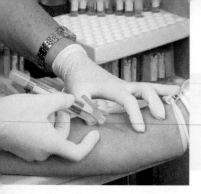

LESSON 7.3

Immune System

OBJECTIVES

Immunology is the study of the immune system. An immunologist is a medical specialist who is involved in the study and research of the immune system, and in treating immune system disorders. The information in this lesson will enable you to use correct medical terminology to:

7.3.1 Define the immune system and its characteristics.

7.3.2 Contrast cellular and humoral immunity.

7.3.3 Explain the structure and actions of antibodies.

7.3.4 Describe some common disorders of the immune system, including **HIV** and **AIDS.**

KEYNOTES

- The immune system is not an organ system but a group of specialized cells in different parts of the body.

- Some antigens are free molecules, such as **toxins.** Others are components of a cell membrane or a bacterial cell wall.

CASE REPORT 7.5

YOU ARE

> . . . a laboratory technician working the night shift at Fulwood Medical Center.

YOU ARE COMMUNICATING WITH

> . . . Mr. Michael Cowan, a 40-year-old homeless man and drug addict, who has presented to the Emergency Department with a high fever, with no obvious cause.
>
> You have been called to the emergency room to take blood from Mr. Cowan. You insert the needle into an **antecubital** vein, but he starts jerking his arm around and trying to get off the gurney. In the struggle, the needle comes out of the vein and pricks your hand through your glove.
>
> You immediately flush and clean your wound, report the incident, seek immediate medical attention, and go through your initial medical evaluation. However, because of your possible exposure to Mr. Cowan's blood, it is essential that you have knowledge about your own immune system and its response to a potential infection. This will help you to make informed decisions about your treatment and future employment.

The Immune System (LO 7.1, 7.2, and 7.3)

The immune system is a group of specialized cells in different parts of the body that recognize and neutralize foreign substances. It is the **third line of defense** listed earlier in this chapter. When the immune system is weak, it allows pathogens, including the viruses that cause common colds and flu, and cancer cells, to successfully invade the body.

Three characteristics distinguish immunity from the first two lines of defense of physical and cellular mechanisms:

1. **Specificity:** The immune response is directed against a specific pathogen. Immunity to one pathogen does not grant immunity to others. Specificity has one disadvantage; if a virus or a bacterium changes a component of its genetic code, it then becomes a new organism to the immune system. This **mutation** occurs, for example, with bacteria in response to antibiotics and in HIV's response to anti-HIV drugs **(development of resistance).**

2. **Memory:** When exposure to the same pathogen occurs again, the immune system recognizes the pathogen and has its responses ready to act quickly.

3. **Discrimination:** The immune system learns to recognize agents (antigens) that represent **"self"** and agents (antigens) that are **"nonself"** (foreign). Most of this recognition is developed prior to birth. A variety of disorders occur when this discrimination breaks down. They are known as **autoimmune disorders.**

An antigen is any molecule that triggers an immune response. Most antigens are unique in their structure. It is this uniqueness that enables your body to distinguish its own (self) molecules from foreign (nonself) molecules.

Word	Pronunciation	Elements		Definition
antecubital	an-teh-**KYU**-bit-al	S/ P/ R/	-al *pertaining to* ante- *in front of, before* -cubit- *elbow*	In front of the elbow
autoimmune	awe-toe-im-**YUNE**	P/ R/	auto- *self, same.* -immune *protected*	Immune reaction directed against a person's own tissue
discrimination	**DIS**-krim-ih-**NA Y**-shun	S/ P/ R/	-ation *process* dis- *away from* -crimin- *distinguish*	Ability to distinguish between different things
mutation	myu-**TAY**-shun		Latin *to change*	Change in the chemistry of a gene
specific	speh-**SIF**-ik	S/ R/	-ic *pertaining to* specif- *species*	Relating to a particular entity
specificity (**Note:** *Has two suffixes.*)	spes-ih-**FIS**-ih-tee	S/	-ity *condition, state*	State of having a specific, fixed relation to a particular entity
toxin	**TOK**-sin		Greek *poison*	Poisonous substance formed by a cell or organism
toxicity	toks-**ISS**-ih-tee	S/ R/	-ity *state, condition* toxic- *poison*	The state of being poisonous

EXERCISES

A. Review *the Case Report on this spread before answering the questions.*

1. If you are taking blood from a patient, what is your occupation? _____

2. Where is the *antecubital* vein? _____

3. What is a gurney? _____

4. Why could this be a future health problem for you? _____

5. What is the main concern about Mr. Cowan's blood? _____

B. Review *the two pages spread open before you. Provide a brief answer to each of the questions below.*

1. What happens when the immune system becomes weak?
_____

2. Does the immune system contain any specific organs?
_____

3. Describe an *autoimmune* disorder:
_____

4. Briefly describe the development of resistance:
_____

5. What occurs when discrimination of the immune system breaks down?
_____

C. Each of these questions *requires a one-word answer. Think carefully before writing the answers.*

1. Use one word to describe the main purpose of the immune system. _____

2. Change in the chemistry of a gene produces a _____.

3. What is a molecule called that triggers a response? _____

LESSON 7.3 Immunity (LO 7.1, 7.2, and 7.3)

KEYNOTES

• Antibodies do not actively destroy an antigen. They render it harmless and mark it for destruction by phagocytes.

• The immune system is thought to be able to produce some 2 million different antibodies.

Immunity is the state of being able to resist a specific infectious disease. It is classified biologically into two types, although these often respond to the same antigen:

1. **Cellular (cell-mediated) immunity:** This is a direct form of defense based on the actions of lymphocytes to attack foreign and diseased cells and destroy them. The many different types of T cells, B cells, and macrophages described in the previous lesson of this chapter are involved in this style of attack *(Figure 7.17)*.

2. **Humoral (antibody-mediated) immunity:** This is an indirect form of attack that employs antibodies produced by plasma cells, which have been developed from B cells. The antibodies bind to an antigen and tag it for destruction. These antibodies are called **immunoglobulins,** present in blood plasma and body secretions.

Complement Fixation (LO 7.1, 7.2, and 7.3)

The complement system is a group of 20 or more proteins continually present in blood plasma. Immunoglobulins bind to foreign cells, initiating the binding of **complement** to the cell and leading to its destruction.

Immunization (LO 7.1, 7.2, and 7.3)

Immunization is the preventive method of stimulating the immune system without exposing the body to an infection. An agent (**vaccine**) composed of the antigenic components of a killed or **attenuated** microorganism or its inactivated toxins is injected into the bloodstream. **Vaccination** is a crucial step in keeping our population healthy. For example, vaccination has eradicated smallpox worldwide. However, if we stop vaccinating against smallpox, our population will again be susceptible to smallpox outbreaks. The same concept applies to the diseases in childhood immunizations *(Table 7.1)*.

▼ **TABLE 7.1**
Recommended Immunizations for Persons Aged 0 to 6 Years

Hepatitis A (HepA)	Hepatitis B (HepB)
Rotavirus (Rota)	Influenza
Inactivated poliovirus (IPV)	Varicella (chickenpox)
Diphtheria, tetanus, pertussis (DTaP)	Pneumococcal (PCV)
Measles, mumps, rubella (MMR)	Meningococcal (MPSV4)
Hemophilus influenza type b (Hib)	

Source: Centers for Disease Control and Prevention, 2009.

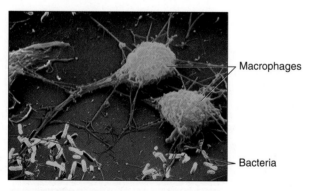
Macrophages
Bacteria

▲ **FIGURE 7.17**
Macrophages Phagocytose Bacteria.
Filamentous extensions of the macrophage snare the rod-shaped bacteria and draw them to the cell surface, where they are engulfed.

Word	Pronunciation	Elements		Definition
attenuate	ah-**TEN**-you-ate	S/	-ate *composed of, pertaining to*	Weaken the ability of an organism to produce disease
		R/	attenu- *weaken*	
attenuated (adj)	ah-**TEN**-you-a-ted	S/	-ated *pertaining to a condition*	Weakened
complement	**KOM**-pleh-ment		Latin *that which completes*	Group of proteins in serum that finish off the work of antibodies to destroy bacteria and other cells
humoral immunity	**HYU**-mor-al im-**YOU**-nih-tee	S/	-al *pertaining to*	Defense mechanism arising from antibodies in the blood
		R/	humor- *fluid*	
		S/	-ity *condition*	
		R/	immun- *immune*	
vaccinate (verb)	**VAK**-sin-ate	S/	-ate *pertaining to, composed of*	To administer a vaccine
		R/	vaccin- *vaccine, giving a vaccine*	
vaccination	vak-sih-**NAY**-shun	S/	-ation *process*	Administration of a vaccine
vaccine	**VAK**-seen		Latin, *related to a cow*	Preparation to generate active immunity

EXERCISES

A. Patient Education. *Explain the following in language your patient can understand.*

1. Explain to your patient how immunization works to protect the body.

_____

_____

2. Give your patient a brief explanation of what the complement system does for the body.

_____

_____

3. Your patient has asked you what *agglutinate* means. Explain the concept to him or her.

_____

_____

4. How is *agglutinate* different from *attenuate?* _____

_____

5. What type of cells produce antibodies? _____

B. Meet lesson and chapter objectives *by using the language of the lymphatic system to fill in the blanks.*

1. If vaccination is the process of injecting the agent, what is the injected agent called? _____

2. What is a toxin? _____

3. What disease has been eradicated worldwide? _____

4. What destroys foreign cells in the body? _____

5. Name three vaccinations a child between 0–6 years should receive. _____

LESSON 7.3 Disorders of the Immune System (LO 7.1, 7.2, 7.3, and 7.4)

- Common food and drug allergens are peanuts, milk, eggs, wheat, shellfish, penicillin and related antibiotics, and sulfa drugs.

- HIV is found in blood, semen, vaginal secretions, saliva, tears, and breast milk of infected mothers.

- The most common means of transmission of HIV are:

  o Sexual intercourse (vaginal, oral, anal).

  o Shared needles for drug use.

  o Contaminated blood products. (All donated blood is now tested for HIV.)

  o Transplacental transmission, from an infected mother to her fetus.

The immune system is prone to very serious disorders, from allergic reactions to life-threatening infections.

Hypersensitivity is an excessive immune response to an antigen that would normally be tolerated. In most allergic (hypersensitivity) reactions, allergens (antigens) stimulate the cells to produce **histamine.** The symptoms produced by these changes include edema, mucus hypersecretion and congestion, watery eyes, and hives (**urticaria).**

Hypersensitivity includes:

- **Allergies**—reactions to environmental antigens like pollens, molds, dusts, foods, and drugs.

- **Autoimmune disorders**—abnormal reactions to your own tissues.

- **Alloimmune disorders**—reactions to tissues transplanted from another person.

Anaphylaxis is an acute, immediate, and severe allergic reaction, which can be relieved by **antihistamines.**

Anaphylactic shock is more severe and is characterized by difficulty in breathing (**dyspnea**) due to bronchiole constriction, circulatory shock, and even death. It is a life-threatening medical emergency.

Asthma is triggered by allergens, listed above, and by air pollutants, drugs, and emotions. Bronchioles constrict spasmodically (**bronchospasm),** leading to the wheezing and coughing of asthma.

Autoimmune disorders are an over-vigorous response of the immune system. Here, the immune system fails to distinguish self-antigens from foreign antigens. These self-antigens produce autoantibodies that attack the body's own tissues. This type of response occurs, for example, in lupus erythematosus, type 1 diabetes, multiple sclerosis, rheumatoid arthritis, and psoriasis.

Immunodeficiency disorders are a deficient response of the immune system where it fails to respond vigorously enough. These disorders are classified into three categories:

1. **Congenital (inborn) disorders** are caused by a genetic abnormality that is often sex-linked, with boys affected more often than girls. An example is **inherited combined immunodeficiency disease,** characterized by an absence of both T cells and B cells *(Figure 7.18).* These children are very susceptible to **opportunistic** infections and must live in protective sterile enclosures.

2. **Immunosuppression** is a common side effect of corticosteroids used in treatment to prevent transplant rejection and in chemotherapy treatment for cancer.

3. **Acquired immunodeficiency** results from diseases like **acquired immunodeficiency syndrome (AIDS),** which involves a severely depressed immune system from infection with the human immunodeficiency virus (**HIV).**

HIV and AIDS
(LO 7.1, 7.2, 7.3, and 7.4)

HIV is one of a group of viruses known as **retroviruses.** Like other viruses, it can replicate only inside a living host cell and it invades helper T cells and cells in the upper respiratory tract and CNS. Inside the cell, the virus can stay **dormant** for months or years. When it is activated (AIDS), the new viruses emerge from the dying host cell and attack more cells. This dormant phase (**incubation**) can range from a few months to 12 years.

As the virus destroys more and more cells, the body cannot produce antibodies. Symptoms appear, including chills, fever, night sweats, fatigue, weight loss, and lymphadenitis. Opportunistic infections by bacteria, viruses, and fungi can occur. These infections include toxoplasmosis, pneumocystitis, tuberculosis, herpes simplex, cytomegalovirus, and candidiasis. Cancers can also invade, and a form of skin cancer called **Kaposi sarcoma** is common.

HIV survives poorly outside the human body. It is destroyed by laundering, dishwashing, chlorination, and the use of disinfectants, alcohol, and germicidal skin cleansers.

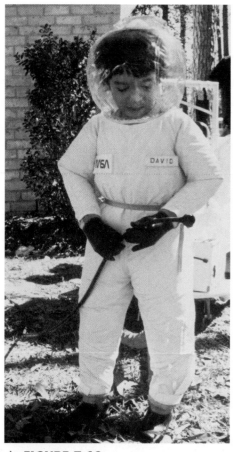

▲ **FIGURE 7.18**
Boy with Combined Immunodeficiency Disease in Protective Sterile Enclosure.

Word	Pronunciation	Elements		Definition
alloimmune	AL-oh-im-**YUNE**	P/ R/	all/o- *other, strange* -immune *immunity*	Immune reaction directed against foreign tissue
anaphylaxis	AN-ah-fih-**LAK**-sis	P/ R/	ana- *excessive* -phylaxis *protection*	Immediate severe allergic response
anaphylactic (adj)	AN-ah-fih-**LAK**-tik	S/ R/	-tic *pertaining to* -phylac- *protect*	Pertaining to anaphylaxis
asthma	**AZ**-mah		Greek *asthma*	Episodes of breathing difficulty due to narrowed or obstructed airways.
asthmatic (adj)	az-**MAT**-ik	S/ R/	-atic *pertaining to* asthm- *asthma*	Suffering from or pertaining to asthma.
dormant	**DOR**-mant	S/ R/	-ant *forming* dorm- *sleep*	Inactive
histamine	**HISS**-tah-mean	R/ R/	hist- *derived from histidine* -amine *nitrogen-containing substance*	Compound liberated in tissues as a result of injury or an immune response
antihistamine	an-tee-**HIS**-tah-mean	P/	anti – *against*	Drug used to treat allergic symptoms because of its action antagonistic to histamine
hypersensitivity	**HIGH**-per-sen-sih-**TIV**-ih-tee	S/ P/ R/	-ity *condition* hyper- *excessive* -sensitiv- *feeling*	Exaggerated abnormal reaction to an allergen
immunodeficiency	IM-you-noh-dee-**FISH**-en-see	S/ R/CF	-ency *quality, state of* immun/o- *immune response*	Failure of the immune system
immunosuppression	IM-you-noh-suh-**PRESH**-un	R/ S/ R/	-defici- *failure, lacking* -ion *action, condition* -suppress- *press under*	Failure of the Immune system caused by an outside agent
incubation	in-kyu-**BAY**-shun	S/ R/	-ation *process* incub- *lie on, hatch*	Process to develop an infection
Kaposi sarcoma	Kah-**POH**-see sar-**KOH**-mah		Moritz Kaposi, Hungarian dermatologist, 1837–1902	A skin cancer often seen in AIDS patients
opportunistic	OP-or-tyu-**NIS**-tik	S/ R/	-istic *pertaining to* opportun- *take advantage of*	An organism or a disease in a host with lowered resistance
retrovirus	**REH**-troh-vie-rus	P/ R/	retro- *backward* -virus *poison*	Virus with an RNA core
urticaria	ur-tee-**KARE**-ee-ah		Latin *nettle*	Rash of itchy wheals (hives)

EXERCISES

A. Build *more medical vocabulary for the language of immunology. Complete the construction of each term by using the following elements to fill in the blanks. There are more answers than you need.*

defici   allo   suppress   sensitiv   ion   hyper   incub   osis   phylaxis   ic   ency   dorm

1. exaggerated, abnormal reaction to an allergen: _____/ _____/ _____ / ity

2. inactive: _____/ _____/ _____ / ant

3. process to develop an infection: _____/ _____/ _____ / ation

4. Terminology challenge: Make a study hint for yourself for dorm = sleep. _____
_____

B. Understanding. *How well do you understand the languages of hematology and immunology?*

1. List every term in the WAD that could be a diagnosis. _____

2. What is the difference between *dormant* and *incubation?* _____

3. What is anaphylaxis? _____

4. What can relieve the condition in #3 above? _____

5. What term is a life-threatening emergency? _____

Infection (LO 7.1, 7.2, 7.3, and 7.4)

- When viruses spread from person to person, they are said to be **contagious.**

- Viral diseases do not respond to antibiotics.

- Nosocomial infections (hospital-acquired infections) are becoming increasingly common and lethal.

- Handwashing is the most important factor in preventing the transmission of infections.

Microbes (microorganisms) are everywhere—in the air, water, and soil and all over our bodies, where they are called **normal flora.** These normal microorganisms are found on your skin, in your nose and respiratory tract, and in your mouth and digestive tract. Your brain and cardiovascular system, however, are microbe-free **(sterile).**

If microorganisms other than the normal flora invade the body, they become pathogens, which cause an **infection.** Pathogens include bacteria, viruses, fungi, and parasites. If the infection harms the body, it creates an **infectious disease.** Bacterial, viral, fungal, and parasitic infections are all caused by pathogens.

Bacterial Infections
(LO 7.1, 7.2, 7.3, and 7.4)

Thousands of different bacteria can cause infections. Bacteria are single-celled microorganisms that reproduce by dividing. Frequently seen bacteria include:

- **Staphylococcus ("staph"),** which can be harmless when present on the skin's surface, but causes infections in wounds or other normally sterile places, like in a joint or the peritoneum;

- **Streptococcus ("strep"),** which is a cause of sore throats;

- **Pneumococcus,** which is a cause of pneumonia; and

- **Coliform** bacteria that normally live in the GI tract but cause infections elsewhere, such as the urinary tract.

In addition, methicillin-resistant *Staphylococcus aureus* **(MRSA)** is a type of bacteria that is resistant to the antibiotics normally used to treat staph infections. MRSA infections occur most frequently in hospitals **(nosocomial** infection), but are now being seen in community health care facilities as community-associated MRSA **(CA-MRSA).**

Viral Infections
(LO 7.1, 7.2, 7.3, and 7.4)

Viruses are the smallest of the microorganisms. They cannot be seen under an ordinary light **microscope** but are visible through electron **microscopy.** Viruses spread from person to person through coughs, sneezes, and unwashed hands.

Viruses cause specific childhood diseases like measles (rubeola), German measles (rubella), chickenpox (varicella), and mumps. They cause upper respiratory infections (see Chapter 8), including modern respiratory infections like **severe acute respiratory syndrome (SARS), avian influenza** (bird flu), and **West Nile virus (WNV).** WNV is a seasonal **epidemic** in North America, which flares up in the summer and fall.

Fungal Infections
(LO 7.1, 7.2, 7.3, and 7.4)

Many fungi are "good fungi," for example, the mushrooms that you eat and the yeasts that ferment beer and bread. Penicillin is derived from a fungus. The most common pathogenic fungi are those that cause skin infections (see Chapter 3).

Opportunistic fungi are normally harmless, but like their name, they pounce on any opportunity to cause disease. People who are on prolonged doses of antibiotics, are receiving chemotherapy or immunosuppressive therapy, or have diabetes mellitus or AIDS are especially susceptible.

Parasitic Infections
(LO 7.1, 7.2, 7.3, and 7.4)

Parasites are organisms that live on or in another organism and steal nourishment from their host. In many rural areas of the world, parasites are **endemic. Malaria** is caused by a parasite that is transmitted from person to person by a single mosquito bite.

Pinworms are the most common parasite in America. Pinworm eggs are introduced into the body through the mouth and hatch in the intestine. The young worms migrate to the anus, where the female deposits her eggs. These eggs can be transferred unknowingly by the fingers from the anus or from infected bedding, to the mouth of the same child or to another child.

CA-MRSA	community-associated methicillin-resistant *Staphylococcus aureus*
MRSA	methicillin-resistant *Staphylococcus aureus*
SARS	severe acute respiratory syndrome
WNV	West Nile Virus

Word	Pronunciation	Elements		Definition
contagious	kon-**TAY**-jus	S/ P/ R/	-ious *pertaining to* con- *with, together* -tag- *touch*	Infection can be transmitted from person to person or from a person to a surface to a person
endemic	en-**DEM**-ik	S/ P/ R/	-ic *pertaining to* en- *in* -dem- *the people*	Pertaining to a disease always present in a community
epidemic	ep-ih-**DEM**-ik	P/	epi- *above, upon*	Pertaining to an outbreak in a community of a disease or a health-related behavior
pandemic	pan-**DEM**-ik	P/	pan- *all*	Pertaining to a disease attacking the population of a very large area
flora	**FLO**-rah		Latin *flower*	Microorganisms covering the exterior and interior surfaces of a healthy animal
infect (verb) infection (noun) infectious (adj)	in-**FEKT** in-**FEK**-shun in-**FEK**-shus	 S/ R/ S/	Latin *invade internally* -ion *condition, action* infect- *internal invasion* -ious *pertaining to*	To invade an organism by a microorganism Invasion of the body by disease-producing microorganisms Capable of being transmitted to a person; or a disease caused by the action of a microorganism
microbe microorganism	**MY**-krohb **MY**-kroh-**OR**-gan-izm	P/ R/ S/ R/	micro- *small* -be *life* -ism *process* -organ- *organ, instrument*	Short for microorganism Any organism too small to be seen by the naked eye
microscope	**MY**-kroh-skope	P/ R/	micro- *small* -scope *instrument for viewing*	Instrument for viewing something small that cannot be seen in detail by the naked eye
microscopic microscopy	**MY**-kroh-**SKOP**-ik my-**CROSS**-koh-pee	S/ R/	-ic *pertaining to* -scopy *to examine, to view*	Visible only with the aid of a microscope Investigation of minute objects through a microscope
nosocomial	noh-soh-**KOH**-mee-al	S/ R/CF R/	-ial *pertaining to* nos/o- *disease* -com- *take care of*	Acquired while in the hospital

EXERCISES

A. Correct usage *of the appropriate grammatical form of a medical term is the mark of an educated professional. Practice your language of immunology in the following sentences. Fill in the blanks.*

1. infect   infection   infectious

This patient has a rarely seen (a) _____. Please refer her to the (b) _____ disease specialist.

2. bacterium   bacteria   bacterial

The (a) _____ streptococcus causes (b) _____ infections in the throat.

3. sterile   sterility   sterilize

An autoclave is used to (a) _____ instruments.

If the (b) _____ of an instrument is in question, it should not be used.

The term (c) _____ can also mean *unable* to *reproduce.*

B. Use the language of immunology *and circle the best answer.*

1. What agent causes infections in wounds and joints?

staph   pneumococcus   heme

2. What term is the same as "microbe free"?

opportunistic   anemic   sterile

3. MRSA occurs most frequently in:

prisons   schools   hospitals

4. Another name for microbes is:

normal flora   bacteria   pollutants

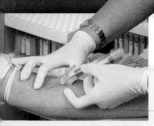

CHAPTER 7 REVIEW THE BLOOD, LYMPHATIC, AND IMMUNE SYSTEMS

CHALLENGE YOUR KNOWLEDGE

A. Prefixes: *Each of the following terms is lacking its prefix. Complete the term with the correct prefix.*

1. protein produced in response to an antigen _____ /body

2. spleen removes blood components at an excessive rate _____ /splen/ism

3. in front of the elbow _____ /cubit/al

4. directed against the person's own tissues_____ /immune

5. immediate, severe, allergic response _____ /phylaxis

6. virus with an RNA core _____ /virus

7. *Anti* means _____ .

   Ante means _____ .

   My study hint to differentiate between *anti* and *ante*: _____

   _____

   _____

B. Suffixes: *Work with the seven terms below from the language of immunology. Their roots/combining forms are similar, and their suffixes help define them. First, deconstruct each of the terms in the chart, and then define the medical term.*

Medical Term	Meaning of Prefix	Meaning of Root/CF	Meaning of Suffix	Meaning of Medical Term
lymphatic	1.	2.	3.	4.
lymphadenectomy	5.	6.	7.	8.
lymphadenitis	9.	10.	11.	12.
lymphadenopathy	13.	14.	15.	16.
lymphangiogram	17.	18.	19.	20.
lymphedema	21.	22.	23.	24.
lymphoma	25.	26.	27.	28.

Using the terms from this chart, answer the following questions.

29. List the terms that can be billed as a diagnosis: _____

    _____

30. Write the term that is a surgical procedure: _____

    _____

31. Write the term that is a radiological procedure: _____

_____

32. List the terms that relate to lymph nodes: _____

_____

33. Name a term that concerns lymphatic vessels (*hint:* check the elements): _____

_____

34. Write an explanation to a fellow student giving the difference between *lymphoma* and *lymphedema*: _____

_____

35. Find the term that is a tumor. _____

36. Name the term that means inflammation. _____

37. Which term is a diagnostic test? _____

38. What have you noticed about all the terms in the chart? _____

C. Immunology terminology: *Increase your knowledge of the language of immunology. The element's meaning is given to you in column 1. Name the element in column 2, and identify the type of element it is in column 3. In the last column, give an example of a medical term containing that element.*

Meaning of Element	Element	Type of Element (P, R, CF, or S)	Medical Term Containing This Element
disease	1.	2.	3.
enlargement	4.	5.	6.
excision	7.	8.	9.
gland	10.	11.	12.
groin	13.	14.	15.
in front of	16.	17.	18.
lymph node	19.	20.	21.
lymphatic vessel	22.	23.	24.
sleep	25.	26.	27.
spaces within tissues	28.	29.	30.
to produce	31.	32.	33.
weaken	34.	35.	36.

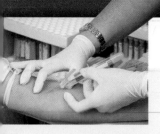

D. Roots and combining *forms are the foundation of every medical term. Slash the term into elements in the first column, identify the R/CF in the second column, and provide the meaning for the R/CF in the third column. Complete the chart with the meaning of the medical term in the last column.*

Medical Term (slash first)	Root/CF	Meaning of Root/CF	Meaning of Medical Term
anaphylactic	1.	2.	3.
immunologist	4.	5.	6.
anemic	7.	8.	9.
hypoxic	10.	11.	12.
pernicious	13.	14.	15.
autoimmune	16.	17.	18.
attenuate	19.	20.	21.
interstitial	22.	23.	24.
hypersplenism	25.	26.	27.
pancytopenia	28.	29.	30.
anaphylaxis	31.	32.	33.
nosocomial	34.	35.	36.

E. What am I? *Each of the following medical terms is a noun, which is the name of a person, place, or thing. Match the meaning in column 1 to the correct medical term in column 2.*

_____ 1. poisonous substance

_____ 2. nonpitting fluid retention

_____ 3. substance producing an allergic reaction

_____ 4. agent intended to prevent disease

_____ 5. lymphatic tissue in the nasopharynx

_____ 6. malignant neoplasm

_____ 7. produced in response to an antigen

_____ 8. has an RNA core

_____ 9. state of being protected

_____ 10. disease-causing microorganism

A. vaccine

B. antibody

C. retrovirus

D. immunity

E. pathogen

F. edema

G. lymphoma

H. allergen

I. adenoid

J. toxin

F. Dictionary exercise: *Look up the word reservoir. Define it, and then give a brief explanation of how the spleen functions as a reservoir.*

1. Definition of reservoir:

_____

2. Spleen as a reservoir:

_____

_____

_____

G. Spelling demons: *Some terms pose difficulty because they may or may not double some letters (or drop some letters) in various forms of the term. Spleen and splenectomy are an example. Test yourself on the correct spelling of the following terms.*

1. lymphatic tissue in oropharynx _____

2. removal of this tissue _____

3. inflammation of this tissue _____

4. vascular, lymphatic organ _____

5. removal of this organ _____

6. enlargement of this organ _____

7. organ removes blood components at an excessive rate _____

H. Recall and review: *How well do you remember these word elements from a previous chapter? Try to answer without looking back to check. Fill in the chart.*

Element	Type of Element (P, R, CF, or S)	Meaning of Element	Term Using Element
diaphor	1.	2.	3.
phlebo	4.	5.	6.
thorac	7.	8.	9.
isch	10.	11.	12.
pulmon	13.	14.	15.
cusp	16.	17.	18.
dys	19.	20.	21.
palpit	22.	23.	24.
steno	25.	26.	27.
sclero	28.	29.	30.

I. Seek and find: *The following terms were defined in context (within the text) and may not always appear in WAD boxes. You are given a brief meaning as the term appeared in the text—write the medical term on the line. Remember to pay attention to these terms—they could be test questions!*

1. clot _____

2. ingest and destroy _____

3. lymph nodes in the neck _____

4. lymph nodes in the armpit _____

5. lymph nodes in the groin _____

6. dormant phase _____

7. hives _____

8. hypersensitivity reactions _____

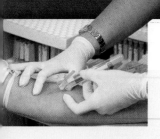

J. Where am I? *Several terms in this chapter denote a place or direction on the body. Challenge yourself to insert the correct term on the line.*

1. pertaining to the groin area _____

2. in front of the elbow _____

3. pertaining to the neck _____

4. in spaces between cells in a tissue or organ _____

5. pertaining to the armpit _____

K. Latin and Greek *terms cannot be further deconstructed into prefix, root, or suffix. You must know them for what they are. Test your knowledge of these terms with this exercise. Match the meaning in column l with the correct medical term in column 2.*

_____ 1. clear fluid	**A.** asthma
_____ 2. mass of tissue	**B.** follicle
_____ 3. change in gene chemistry	**C.** urticaria
_____ 4. that which completes	**D.** lymph
_____ 5. rash of itchy wheals	**E.** mutation
_____ 6. spherical cluster of cells	**F.** complement
_____ 7. hypersensitive lung disorder	**G.** node
_____ 8. paleness	**H.** heme
_____ 9. spot on skin	**I.** embolus
_____ 10. clear spring water	**J.** lymph
_____ 11. blood	**K.** pallor
_____ 12. plug, stopper	**L.** petechia

L. Translation: *Reduce the sentences below to the most basic language that a nonmedical person could understand. First, use your knowledge of medical terminology to understand the statement. Then organize your thoughts and formulate your answer.*

1. "Intra-abdominal hemorrhage from the ruptured spleen can be extensive, with dramatic hypotension, and is a surgical emergency requiring splenectomy."

_____

_____

2. "Hemolysis can be caused by toxic substances or an incompatible blood transfusion."

_____

_____

3. "The abnormal cells agglutinate and block small capillaries, which causes intense pain in the hypoxic tissues."

_____

_____

M. Analyze and discover *the difference. Medical language has many terms that appear similar but have unique meanings all their own. If you can analyze similar terms, you will understand the difference and be able to explain it to your patient.*

1. Alloimmune

Prefix: _____ Means: _____

Root: _____ Means: _____

Autoimmune

Prefix: _____ Means: _____

Root: _____ Means: _____

Write an explanation to your patient of the difference between *alloimmune* and *autoimmune:*

alloimmune: _____

autoimmune: _____

2. Immunodeficiency

Root: _____ Means: _____

CF: _____ Means: _____

Suffix: _____ Means: _____

Immunosuppression

Root: _____ Means: _____

CF: _____ Means: _____

Suffix: _____ Means: _____

Write an explanation to your patient of the difference between *immunodeficiency* and *immunosuppression:*

immunodeficiency: _____

immunosuppresion: _____

N. Review: *Previously, you have studied directional terms that aid you in locating some part of the body. Apply those terms to the following sentence, and briefly explain, in nonmedical terms, the location of the spleen.*

"The spleen, a highly vascular and spongy organ, is the largest lymphatic organ and is located in the LUQ of the abdomen, below the diaphragm and lateral to the kidney."

Read the sentence; then read it again and underline all the medical terms. Be sure you also know the position of the diaphragm and the

kidneys. You may be asked by the instructor to illustrate them on the classroom skeleton.

1. Terms: _____

_____

2. Position of diaphragm: _____

3. Terms: _____

immunodeficiency: _____

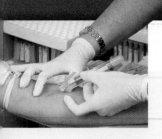

O. Similar but different: *The following terms all contain the word edema, but additional words or elements add new meaning to the term. Give a brief answer that describes each form of edema. Use the Glossary or a dictionary if you are unsure of any term.*

   1. edema:

   _____

   2. peripheral edema:

   _____

   3. pitting edema:

   _____

   4. lymphedema:

   _____

P. Where am I? *Read the brief identifications and supply the correct medical term on the line.*

   1. liquid containing suspended particles _____

   2. percentage of RBCs in the blood _____

   3. fluid, noncellular component of blood _____

   4. also called a thrombocyte _____

   5. paleness of the skin _____

   6. deficient in oxygen _____

   7. substance that causes clotting _____

   8. pinpoint capillary hemorrhage _____

   9. self-transfusion _____

  10. a circumscribed mass of tissue _____

  11. substance that creates an allergic reaction _____

  12. a disease-causing microorganism _____

  13. change in the chemistry of a gene _____

  14. immediate severe allergic response _____

Q. Terminology challenge.

   The challenge element from this chapter is *megaly,* which means

   _____ .

   1. Find a term from this chapter containing this element.

     Term: _____

     Means: _____

2. There are two other terms with this element that have appeared in previous chapters. Can you name them and define them?

Term: _____

Means: _____

Term: _____

Means: _____

R. Chapter challenge: *Circle the correct answer.*

1. Where is a *nosocomial* infection acquired?

    a. in a school

    b. in an airplane

    c. on a cruise ship

    d. in the hospital

    e. where you work

2. "A" in the abbreviation AIDS stands for:

    a. acute

    b. acquired

    c. active

    d. attenuated

    e. asthmatic

3. Choose the pair of correct spellings:

    a. tonsel/tonselectomy

    b. tonsil/tonsillectomy

    c. tonssil/tonsilectomy

    d. tonsill/tonsilectomy

    e. tonnsil/tonsillectomy

4. Identify the term in which a root appears at the end of the term:

    a. anemia

    b. mononucleosis

    c. efferent

    d. agglutinate

    e. interstitial

5. What can be said about the terms *cervical, axillary,* and *inguinal:*

    a. They are all areas accessible to palpation.

    b. Lymph nodes are located in these areas.

    c. Their suffixes all mean pertaining to.

    d. All of these statements are correct.

    e. None of these statements is correct.

6. Which set consists of terms that only contain lymphatic tissue?

    a. spleen, tonsil, adenoid

    b. pancreas, tonsil

    c. spleen, adenoid, adrenal

    d. pancreas, adenoid, tonsil

    e. spleen, pancreas

7. What is the medical term for *hives?*

    a. thrombocytopenia

    b. wheals

    c. hemolysis

    d. hematoma

    e. embolus

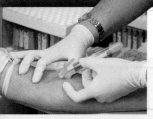

8. The correct plural of *bacterium* is:

   a. bacteriums

   b. bacteriae

   c. bacteria

   d. bacteriaes

   e. bacterias

9. What is the dormant phase of a developing infection called?

   a. incubation

   b. hemoglobinopathy

   c. agglutination

   d. colloid

   e. differential

10. Which disease has been virtually eliminated worldwide by the use of vaccination?

   a. hemophilia

   b. leukopenia

   c. leukemia

   d. smallpox

   e. EBV

11. *Purpura* is bleeding into the skin from small arterioles. What is bleeding from capillary beds called?

   a. thrombosis

   b. embolus

   c. petechiae

   d. hemophilia

   e. thrombocytopenia

12. *Immunosuppressive* drugs are given after:

   a. organ transplant

   b. anaphylactic shock

   c. retrovirus

   d. opportunistic infection

   e. Hodgkin lymphoma

13. *Avian influenza* is another name for what type of flu?

   a. WNV

   b. bird

   c. stomach

   d. respiratory

   e. SARS

14. An *allergic reaction* is one of:

   a. hypoglycemia

   b. hypersensitivity

   c. hypotension

   d. hypersplenism

   e. hypertension

15. *Kaposi sarcoma* is a skin cancer often seen in patients with:

   a. DJD

   b. CF

   c. AIDS

   d. RA

   e. BPH

S. Case Report challenge: *Now that you are more comfortable with the terms in this chapter, you can apply that knowledge and briefly answer the questions about the Case Report. If you read the report through and underline all the medical terminology, this will make it easier to answer the questions.*

CASE REPORT 7.4

YOU ARE

. . . a medical assistant working with Susan Lee, MD, in her primary care clinic.

YOU ARE COMMUNICATING WITH

. . . Ms. Anna Clemons, a 20-year-old waitress, who is a new patient. She has noticed a lump in her left neck. On questioning, you elicit that she has lost about 8 pounds in weight in the past couple of months, has felt tired, and has had some night sweats. Her vital signs are normal. There are two firm, enlarged lymph nodes in her left neck in front of the sternocleidomastoid muscle. Physical examination is otherwise unremarkable. Ms. Clemons has cancerous nodes in her neck. They were not caused by metastatic cancer but by a cancer of the lymph nodes called Hodgkin lymphoma.

1. Where in this Case Report could you substitute an abbreviation for something that has been spelled out?

_____ means _____.

2. The medical term for *enlarged lymph nodes* is

_____.

3. The element oid in *sternocleidomastoid* means

_____.

4. Explain what is meant by *metastatic cancer:*

_____.

5. The suffix in the term *lymphoma* means

_____.

6. What are Ms. Clemons' presenting signs and symptoms?

_____.

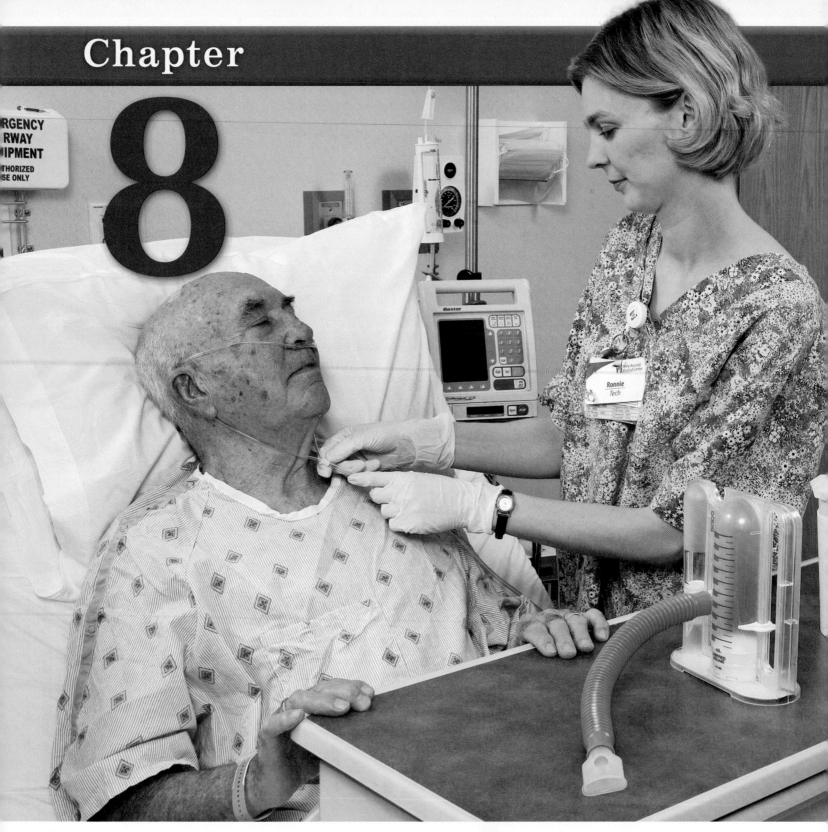

RESPIRATORY SYSTEM
The Essentials of the Language of Pulmonology

CASE REPORT 8.1

YOU ARE

. . . an advanced-level **registered respiratory therapist (RRT)** working with **pulmonologist** Tavis Senko, MD, in the Acute Respiratory Care unit of Fulwood Medical Center.

YOU ARE COMMUNICATING WITH

. . . Mr. Jude Jacobs, a 68-year-old white retired mail carrier, who has chronic obstructive pulmonary disease **(COPD)** and is on continual **oxygen (O₂)** by nasal prongs. He has smoked two packs of cigarettes per day throughout his adult life.

Last night, he was unable to sleep because of increased shortness of breath **(SOB)** and cough. He had to sit upright in bed in order to breathe. His cough produces yellow **sputum.**

Mr. Jacobs' vital signs are temperature **(T)** of 101.6°, pulse **(P)** of 98, respirations **(R)** of 36, and blood pressure **(BP)** 150/90. On examination, he is **cyanotic** and frightened, and he is on oxygen by nasal prongs. Air entry is diminished in both lungs, and there are **rales** (crackles) at the bases of both lungs.

You have been ordered to draw blood for arterial blood gases **(ABGs)** and to measure the amount of air entering and leaving his lungs by using **spirometry.**

LEARNING OUTCOMES

In order to provide optimal care to Mr. Jacobs, determine what is causing his symptoms and signs, and communicate with the other health professionals involved in his care, you need to be able to:

LO 8.1 Apply the language of pulmonology to the functions of the respiratory system.

LO 8.2 Comprehend, analyze, spell, and write the medical terms of pulmonology to communicate and document accurately and precisely.

LO 8.3 Recognize and pronounce the medical terms of pulmonology so that you can communicate verbally with accuracy and precision.

LO 8.4 Explain the effects of common respiratory disorders on health.

LO 8.5 Translate medical terms of pulmonology into everyday language in order to communicate with patients and their families.

In your future career, being able to communicate comfortably, accurately, and effectively with the health professionals involved in the diagnosis and treatment of respiratory problems is key. You may work directly and/or indirectly with one or more of the following:

- **Pulmonologists** are physicians who specialize in the diagnosis and treatment of lung/pulmonary conditions.

- **Registered respiratory therapists (RRT)** or **respiratory care practitioners** assist physicians in evaluating, treating, and caring for patients who have respiratory disorders. They also supervise RT technicians.

- **Respiratory therapy (RT) technicians** assist physicians and RRTs in evaluating, monitoring, and treating patients with respiratory disorders.

- **Sleep technologists** are trained in sleep technology and sleep medicine. These technologists assist sleep specialists in the assessment, monitoring, management, and follow-up care of patients with sleep disorders.

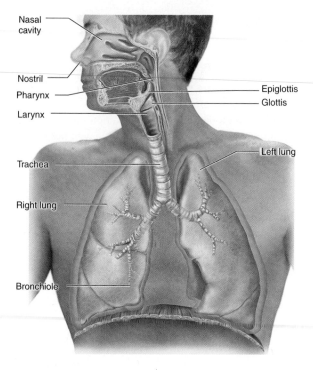

- Nasal cavity
- Nostril
- Pharynx
- Larynx
- Epiglottis
- Glottis
- Trachea
- Left lung
- Right lung
- Bronchiole

▲ **FIGURE 8.1**
The Respiratory System.

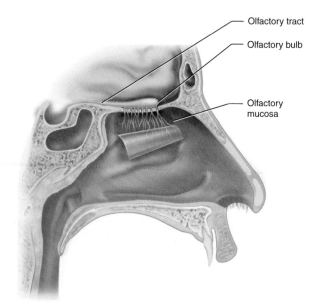

- Olfactory tract
- Olfactory bulb
- Olfactory mucosa

▲ **FIGURE 8.2**
Olfactory Region of the Nose.

ABBREVIATIONS

ABG	arterial blood gas
COPD	chronic obstructive pulmonary disease
O₂	oxygen
RRT	registered respiratory therapist

Introduction to the Respiratory System
(LO 8.1, 8.2, 8.3, and 8.5)

It sounds like a good scheme. Humans and animals breathe in **oxygen** and breathe out **carbon dioxide,** while plants and trees breathe in carbon dioxide and breathe out oxygen. Unfortunately, we continue to generate increasing amounts of carbon dioxide in the air by burning coal, oil, and natural gas, and cutting down forests, thus disturbing this natural balance. In addition, humans have created organic and inorganic chemicals and small particles of solid matter, which float through the air and enter our bodies as we breathe. These **pollutants** can damage our respiratory tracts and cause cancer, brain damage, and birth defects.

The Respiratory Tract (LO 8.1, 8.2, 8.3, and 8.5)

The **respiratory tract** *(Figure 8.1)* has six connected elements:

1. **Nose**
2. **Pharynx**
3. **Larynx**
4. **Trachea**
5. **Bronchi** and **bronchioles**
6. **Alveoli**

   Respiration has two components:

- **Ventilation,** which is the movement of air and its gases into (**inspiration**) and out of (**expiration**) the lungs; and
- The **exchange of gases** between air and blood, and between blood and interstitial fluids.

Functions of the Respiratory System
(LO 8.1, 8.2, 8.3, and 8.5)

Your respiratory system is responsible for the following key functions:

1. **Exchange of gases:** All of your body cells need oxygen and produce carbon dioxide. Your respiratory system allows oxygen from the air to enter the blood and carbon dioxide to leave the blood and enter the air.
2. **Regulation of blood pH:** Regulation occurs by changing carbon dioxide levels in the blood.
3. **Protection:** The respiratory system protects against foreign bodies and against some microorganisms.
4. **Voice production:** Movement of air across the vocal cords makes voice and sound possible.
5. **Olfaction:** The 12 million receptor cells for smell are in a quarter-sized patch of epithelium. These are located in the **olfactory region** *(Figure 8.2)*, the extreme superior region of the nasal cavity. Each cell has 10 to 20 hair-like structures called **cilia** that project into the nasal cavity in a thin mucous film.

Because the olfactory region is right at the top of your nose, you often have to sniff deeply to stimulate the sense of smell. Because dogs have 4 billion receptor cells in their noses, they can be trained to sniff for drugs, explosives, or human scent.

Word	Pronunciation	Elements		Definition
alveolus alveoli (pl) alveolar (adj)	al-**VEE**-oh-lus al-**VEE**-oh-lee al-**VEE**-oh-lar	 S/ R/	Latin *hollow sac* -ar *pertaining to* alveol- *air sac*	Terminal element of respiratory tract where gas exchange occurs Pertaining to the alveoli
bronchus bronchi (pl) bronchiole	**BRONG**-kuss **BRONG**-key **BRONG**-key-ole	 S/ R/CF	Greek *windpipe* -ole *small* bronch/i- *bronchus*	One of two subdivisions of the trachea Increasingly smaller subdivisions of bronchi
cilium cilia (pl)	**SILL**-ee-um **SILL**-ee-ah		Latin *eyelash*	Hairlike motile projection from the surface of a cell
expiration (Note: *The "s" is deleted from the root spirat because the prefix ex already has the "s" sound.*)	**EKS**-pih-**RAY**-shun	S/ P/ R/	-ion *action, condition, process of* ex- *out* -spirat- *breathe*	Breathe out
inspiration (Note: *the opposite of expiration*)	in-spih-**RAY**-shun	S/ P/ R/	-ion *action, condition, process of* in- *into* -spirat- *breathe*	Breathe in
olfaction olfactory (adj)	ol-**FAK**-shun ol-**FAK**-toh-ree	 S/ R/	Latin *to smell* -ory *having the function of* olfact- *smell*	Sense of smell Relating to the sense of smell
oxygen	**OCK**-see-jen	S/ R/	-gen *create* oxy- *oxygen*	The gas essential for life
pharynx pharyngeal (adj)	**FAH**-rinks fah-**RIN**-jee-al	 S/ R/	Greek *throat* -eal *pertaining to* pharyng- *pharynx*	Tube from the back of the nose to the larynx. Pertaining to the pharynx
pulmonary pulmonology pulmonologist	**PULL**-moh-**NAR**-ee **PULL**-moh-**NOL**-oh-jee **PULL**-moh-**NOL**-oh-jist	S/ R/ S/ R/CF S/	-ary *pertaining to* pulmon- *lung* -logy *study of* pulmon/o- *lung* -logist *one who studies, specialist*	Pertaining to the lungs Study of the lungs, or the medical specialty of disorders of the lungs Specialist in treating disorders of the lungs
rale rales (pl)	RAHL RAHLS		French *rattle*	Crackle heard through a stethoscope when air bubbles through liquid in the lungs
respiration respirator respiratory (adj)	RES-pih-**RAY**-shun RES-pih-**RAY**-tor RES-pih-rah-tor-ee	S/ P/ R/ S/ S/	-ation *a process, formed from* re- *again* -spir- *to breathe* -ator *person or thing that does something* -atory *pertaining to, produced by*	Process of breathing; fundamental process of life used to exchange oxygen and carbon dioxide Another name for ventilator Pertaining to respiration
sputum	**SPYU**-tum		Latin *to spit*	Matter coughed up and spat out by individuals with respiratory disorders
trachea trachealis (adj)	**TRAY**-kee-ah tray-kee-**AY**-lis	 S/ R/	Greek *windpipe* -alis *pertaining to* trache- *trachea*	Air tube from the larynx to the bronchi Pertaining to the trachea

EXERCISES

A. Review *Case Report 8.1 before answering the questions.*

1. A pulmonologist is a specialist in diseases of the _____ .

2. Why is Mr. Jacobs receiving continual O₂ by nasal prongs? _____

3. What is *sputum?* _____

4. Which test ordered for Mr. Jacobs involves drawing his blood? _____

5. Describe the sound of rales. _____

6. What in Mr. Jacobs' medical history accounts for the COPD he has today? _____

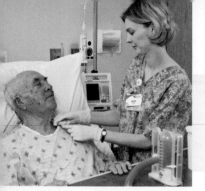

LESSON 8.1

Upper Respiratory Tract

OBJECTIVES

*Your **upper respiratory tract** consists of your nose, pharynx, and trachea. It is the first site that brings air and its pollutants inside your body. The information in this lesson will enable you to use correct medical terminology to:*

8.1.1 Trace the flow of air from the nose through the pharynx and larynx.

8.1.2 Define the protective mechanisms of the upper respiratory tract.

8.1.3 Describe how sound is produced.

8.1.4 Identify common disorders of the upper respiratory tract.

ABBREVIATION

URI   upper respiratory infection

The Nose (LO 8.1, 8.2, 8.3, and 8.5)

When you breathe in air through your nose, the air goes through the nostrils **(nares)** into the **nasal cavity.** Internal hairs guard the nares to prevent large particles from entering your body.

The nasal **septum** divides the nasal cavity into right and left compartments. The **palate** forms the floor of the nose *(Figure 8.3)*. The **paranasal frontal** and **maxillary sinuses** *(Chapter 4)* open into the nose.

Functions of the Nose (LO 8.1, 8.2, 8.3, and 8.5)

Your nose serves as an important part of your respiratory system in several ways:

1. **Passageway for air** to enter or leave the body.

2. **Air cleanser:** The nasal hairs and the mucus (secreted by the nasal mucous membrane) trap particles of dust and solid pollutants.

3. **Air moisturizer:** It adds moisture to the air. Moisture is secreted by the nasal mucosa (mucous membrane) and from tears that drain into the nasal cavity through the nasal lacrimal duct *(see Chapter 11)*.

4. **Air warmer:** The blood flowing through the nasal cavity beneath the mucous membrane lining also warms the air. This prevents damage from cold to the more fragile lower respiratory passages.

5. **Sense of smell (olfaction):** The olfactory region recognizes some 4,000 separate smells *(see previous pages)*.

Disorders of the Nose
(LO 8.1, 8.2, 8.3, 8.4, and 8.5)

A **common cold** is a viral upper respiratory infection **(URI).** It is contagious and easily transmitted in airborne droplets through coughing and sneezing. There is no proven effective treatment.

Rhinitis, also called **coryza,** is an inflammation of the nasal mucosa, which is usually viral.

Allergic rhinitis affects 15% to 20% of the population. The mucous membranes of the nose, pharynx, and sinuses, swell and produce a clear, watery discharge. Treatment entails defining and removing the allergy-causing agent.

Sinusitis is an infection of the paranasal sinuses, often following a viral upper respiratory tract infection. It can also be part of an allergic response. It can be treated with **antibiotics** and **decongestants.**

A **deviated nasal septum** occurs when the partition between the two nostrils is pushed to one side, leading to a partially obstructed airway in one nostril. Treatment is by surgery.

Nasal polyps are benign growths arising from the mucosa of the nasal cavity or a sinus. These can be surgically removed.

Epistaxis (a nosebleed) is bleeding from the septum of the nose, usually as a result of trauma.

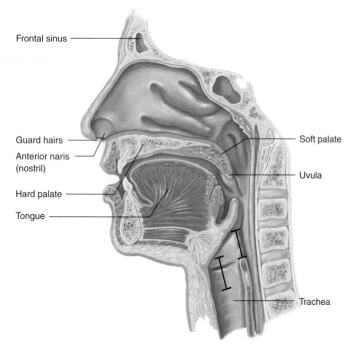

Frontal sinus

Guard hairs

Anterior naris (nostril)

Hard palate

Tongue

Soft palate

Uvula

Trachea

▲ FIGURE 8.3
Upper Respiratory Tract.

Word	Pronunciation		Elements	Definition
coryza *(also called* **rhinitis***)*	koh-**RYE**-zah		Greek *catarrh*	Acute inflammation of the mucous membrane of the nose
decongestant	dee-con-**JESS**-tant	S/ P/ R/	-ant *pertaining to* de- *take away, remove* -congest- *accumulation of fluid*	Agent that reduces the swelling and fluid in the nose and sinuses
epistaxis	ep-ih-**STAK**-sis	S/ P/ R/	-is *pertaining to* epi- *above, upon* -stax- *fall in drops*	Nosebleed
naris nares (pl) nasal	**NAH**-ris **NAH**-rez **NAY**-zal	 S/ R/	Latin *nostril* -al *pertaining to* nas- *nose*	Nostril Pertaining to the nose
palate	**PAL**-ate		Latin *palate*	Roof of the mouth, floor of the nose
paranasal	**PAR**-ah **NAY**-zal	S/ P/ R/	-al *pertaining to* para- *adjacent to* -nas- *nose*	Adjacent to the nose
polyp	**POL**-ip		Latin *many feet*	Any mass of tissue that projects outward
rhinitis *(also called* **coryza***)*	rye-**NIE**-tis	S/ R/	-itis *inflammation* rhin- *nose*	Acute inflammation of the nasal mucosa
septum septa (pl)	**SEP**-tum **SEP**-tah		Latin *partition*	Thin wall separating two cavities or tissue masses
sinus	**SIGH**-nus		Latin *cavity*	Cavity or hollow space in a bone or other tissue
sinusitis	sigh-nyu-**SIGH**-tis	S/ R/	-itis *inflammation* sinus- *sinus*	Inflammation of the lining of a sinus

EXERCISES

A. Elements: *Work with elements to build your knowledge of the language of pulmonology. One element in each of the following medical terms is boldfaced. Identify the type of element (P, R, CF, or S) in column 2; then write the meaning of that element in column 3. Finally, write the meaning of the complete term in column 4.*

Medical Term	Type of Element	Meaning of Element	Meaning of the Term
1. **nas**al	_____	_____	_____
2. decongest**ant**	_____	_____	_____
3. **rhin**itis	_____	_____	_____
4. epi**stax**is	_____	_____	_____
5. **para**nasal	_____	_____	_____
6. sinus**itis**	_____	_____	_____

B. Apply *the language of pulmonology to answer the following questions correctly.*

1. There are two elements in the WAD that have the same meaning. Which are they? _____ and

   _____ both mean _____ .

2. List all the terms in this WAD that are a diagnosis. _____

3. Where else in the body would the term *septa* apply? _____

4. Which elements in the WAD mean *inflammation?* _____

5. What is another term for *nostril?* _____

6. What is the difference between *rhinitis* and *sinusitis?* _____

CASE REPORT 8.2

YOU ARE

. . . a sleep technologist in the Sleep Disorders Clinic at Fulwood Medical Center. You are about to position the electrodes on your patient for an overnight **polysomnography** (sleep study).

YOU ARE COMMUNICATING WITH

. . . Mr. Tye Gawlinski, a 29-year-old professional football player, and his wife. Mrs. Helen Gawlinski states that her husband snores loudly and has 40 or 50 periods in the night when he stops breathing. The snoring is so loud that she cannot sleep, even in the adjoining bedroom. Mr. Gawlinski complains of being tired all day and not having the energy he needs for his job. The sleep study is being performed to confirm a diagnosis of obstructive sleep **apnea.**

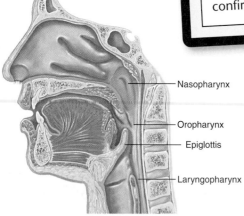

▲ **FIGURE 8.4**
Regions of the Pharynx.

Nasopharynx
Oropharynx
Epiglottis
Laryngopharynx

The Pharynx (LO 8.1, 8.2, 8.3, and 8.5)

Your pharynx is a muscular funnel that receives air from the nasal cavity, and food and drink from the oral cavity. It is divided into three regions *(Figure 8.4):*

1. **Nasopharynx:** Located at the back of the nose and above the soft palate and uvula. The posterior surface contains the pharyngeal **tonsil (adenoid).** Only air moves through this region;

2. **Oropharynx:** Located at the back of the mouth, and below the soft palate and above the epiglottis. It contains two sets of tonsils called the palatine and lingual tonsils. Air, food, and drink all pass through this region; and

3. **Laryngopharynx:** Located below the tip of the epiglottis. It is the pathway to the esophagus. Only food and drink pass through the laryngopharynx.

Disorders of the Pharynx (LO 8.1, 8.2, 8.3, 8.4, and 8.5)

Snoring occurs regularly in 25% of normal adults and is most common in overweight males. It worsens with age. Snoring noises are made at the back of the mouth and nose where the tongue and upper pharynx meet the soft palate and uvula *(Figure 8.5).*

Obstructive sleep apnea is the condition Mr. Gawlinski has. Bulky neck tissue from his football training causes an obstruction by the soft tissues at the back of his nose and mouth. This leads to frequent episodes of gasping for breath, followed by complete cessation of breathing **(apnea).** These episodes reduce the level of oxygen in the blood **(hypoxemia),** making his heart pump harder. If this problem goes untreated for several years, it can cause hypertension and cardiac enlargement.

Pharyngitis is an acute or chronic infection involving the pharynx, tonsils, and uvula. It is usually viral in children. Increasing air humidity and getting extra rest are effective treatments.

Tonsillitis is usually a viral infection of the tonsils in the oropharynx. In less than 20% of cases, this infection is caused by a streptococcus. A rapid strep test and throat culture are used to identify the strep sore throat or pharyngitis.

Nasopharyngeal carcinoma is a rare form of cancer that occurs mostly in males between the ages of 50 and 60. Treatment includes radiation and chemotherapy.

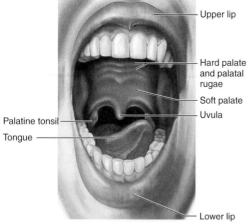

Upper lip
Hard palate and palatal rugae
Soft palate
Uvula
Palatine tonsil
Tongue
Lower lip

▲ **FIGURE 8.5**
Soft Tissues at the Back of the Mouth.

CASE REPORT 8.2 (CONTINUED)

Initially, Mr. Gawlinski was instructed to sleep on his side and to use a device that, through a mask over his nose and mouth, produces a continuous positive airway pressure **(CPAP)** in his airways. He found this very uncomfortable, and it kept him awake. Instead, he chose to have the pillar procedure, in which three tiny pillars were placed in the back of his throat to support the tissues. Subsequently, Mr. Gawlinski has stopped snoring and Mrs. Gawlinski is back in the same bed.

ABBREVIATION

CPAP   continuous positive airway pressure

Word	Pronunciation	Elements		Definition
adenoid	ADD-eh-noyd	S/ R/	-oid *resembling* aden- *gland*	Single mass of lymphoid tissue in the midline at the back of the throat
apnea	AP-nee-ah	P/ R/	a- *without* -pnea *breathe*	Absence of spontaneous respiration
hypoxemia	high-pock-SEE-me-ah	S/ S/	-emia *condition of the blood* -ia *condition*	Low oxygen level in arterial blood
hypoxia (noun)	high-POCK-see-ah	P/ R/	hyp- *below* -ox- *oxygen*	Decreased below normal levels of oxygen in tissues, gases, or blood
hypoxic (adj)	high-POCK-sik	S/	-ic *pertaining to*	Deficient in oxygen
laryngopharynx	lah-RIN-go-FAH-rinks	R/ R/CF	-pharynx *pharynx, throat* laryng/o- *larynx*	Region of the pharynx below the epiglottis that includes the larynx
nasopharynx	NAY-zoh-FAH-rinks	R/ R/CF	-pharynx *pharynx, throat,* nas/o- *nose*	Region of the pharynx at the back of the nose and above the soft palate
nasopharyngeal (adj)	NAY-zoh-fah-RIN-jee-al	S/ R/CF	-eal *pertaining to* -pharyng- *pharynx, throat*	Pertaining to the nasopharynx
oropharynx	OR-oh-fah-rinks	R/ R/CF	-pharynx *pharynx, throat* or/o- *mouth*	Region at the back of the mouth between the soft palate and the tip of the epiglottis.
oropharyngeal (adj)	OR-oh-fah-RIN-jee-al	S/ R	-eal *pertaining to* -pharyng- *pharynx, throat*	Pertaining to the oropharynx
pharyngitis	fair-in-JIE-tis	S/ R/	-itis *inflammation* pharyng- *pharynx, throat*	Inflammation of the pharynx
polysomnography	POLL-ee-som-NOG-rah-fee	S/ P/ R/CF	-graphy *process of recording* poly- *many* -somn/o- *sleep*	Test to monitor brain waves, muscle tension, eye movement, and oxygen levels in the blood as the patient sleeps
tonsil	TON-sill		Latin *tonsil*	Mass of lymphoid tissue on either side of the throat at the back of the tongue
tonsillitis (Note: *double "ll"*)	ton-sih-LIE-tis	S/ R/	-itis *inflammation* tonsill- *tonsil*	Inflammation of the tonsils
tonsillectomy	ton-sih-LEK-toh-me	S/	-ectomy *surgical excision*	Surgical removal of the tonsils

EXERCISES

A. Review *the Case Report on this spread before answering the questions.*

1. What are Mr. Gawlinski's chief complaints? _____

2. What does polysomnography measure? _____

3. If apnea is complete cessation of breathing, what is dyspnea? _____

4. Hypoxia refers to the level of _____ in the blood.

5. Is the answer to question #4 above too high or too low? _____

B. Use the medical terms *from this spread to fill in the blanks.*

1. Two terms that mean "inflammation of" are _____
   and _____.

2. If left untreated, chronic obstructive sleep apnea could cause _____.

3. The medical term for a common sore throat is _____.

4. Surgical excision of the tonsils is _____.

5. Mr. Gawlinski underwent the diagnostic procedure of _____.

6. What is a nonmedical term for question #5 above? _____

LESSON 8.1 The Larynx (LO 8.1, 8.2, 8.3, and 8.5)

The flow of inhaled air moves on from your pharynx to your **larynx.** The upper opening into the larynx from the oropharynx is called the **glottis.** The spoon-shaped **epiglottis** guards the glottis. When you swallow food, your tongue pushes down the epiglottis to close the glottis and direct the food into the esophagus behind it *(Figure 8.6).* The **thyroid** cartilage, or the Adam's apple, forms the anterior and lateral walls of the larynx. Inside the larynx, two pairs of horizontal ligaments—your **vocal** cords *(Figures 8.7 and 8.8)*—stretch across the lateral walls and enable sounds to be made as air passes between them.

Functions of the Larynx (LO 8.1, 8.2, 8.3, and 8.5)

Two major roles of your larynx are:

1. Maintaining an open passage for the movement of air to and from the trachea *(Figure 8.7);* and

2. Producing sounds through the vocal cords.

Sound Production Air moving past the vocal cords makes them vibrate to produce sound. The force of the air moving past the vocal cords determines the loudness of the sound. Muscles in the cords pull them closer together with varying degrees of tautness *(Figure 8.8).* A high-pitched sound is produced by taut cords and a low-pitched sound is made by more relaxed cords. Males' vocal cords are longer and thicker than those of females. They vibrate more slowly and produce lower-pitched sounds.

The crude sounds produced by the larynx are transformed into words by the actions of the pharynx, tongue, teeth, and lips.

Disorders of the Larynx (LO 8.1, 8.2, 8.3, 8.4, and 8.5)

Laryngitis is an inflammation of the mucosal lining of the larynx, which produces hoarseness and sometimes progresses to a loss of voice.

Epiglottitis is an inflammation of the epiglottis. **Acute epiglottitis** is seen most commonly in children between the ages of 2 and 7 years. It can cause acute airway obstruction, which requires a tube to be inserted into the windpipe **(intubation).** It is preventable by vaccine.

Croup (laryngotracheobronchitis) is a group of viral diseases causing an inflammation and obstruction of the upper airway. It's most common in children between the ages of 3 months and 5 years. In severe cases, a child makes a high-pitched, squeaky, inspiratory noise called **stridor.** Humidity is the initial treatment.

Papillomas or polyps are benign tumors of the larynx due to overuse or irritation. These are surgically removed using a **laryngoscope.**

Carcinoma of the larynx produces a persistent hoarseness. Its incidence peaks among people in their 50s and 60s. Treatment can be radiation and/or chemotherapy.

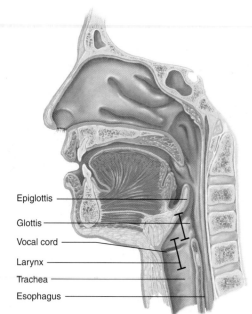

Epiglottis
Glottis
Vocal cord
Larynx
Trachea
Esophagus

▲ **FIGURE 8.6**
Larynx Location..

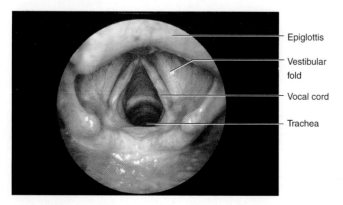

Epiglottis
Vestibular fold
Vocal cord
Trachea

▲ **FIGURE 8.7**
View of Larynx Using Laryngoscope.

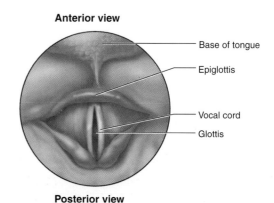

Anterior view

Base of tongue
Epiglottis
Vocal cord
Glottis

Posterior view

▲ **FIGURE 8.8**
Vocal Cords Pulled Close and Taut.

Word	Pronunciation	Elements		Definition
croup (also called laryngotracheobronchitis)	KROOP		Old English *to cry out loud*	Infection of the upper airways in children characterized by a barking cough
epiglottis	ep-ih-**GLOT**-is	P/ R/	epi- *above* -glottis *mouth of windpipe*	Leaf-shaped plate of cartilage that shuts off the larynx during swallowing
epiglottitis	ep-ih-**GLOT**-eye-tis	S/ R/	-itis *inflammation* -glott- *mouth of windpipe*	Inflammation of the epiglottis
glottis	**GLOT**-is		Greek *opening of larynx*	The opening from the oropharnyx into the larynx
intubation	IN-tyu-**BAY**-shun	S/ P/ R/	-ation *a process* in- *in* -tub- *tube*	Insertion of a tube into the trachea
laryngotracheobronchitis (also called **croup**)	lah-**RING**-oh-**TRAY**-kee-oh-brong-**KIE**-tis	S/ R/CF R/CF R/	-itis *inflammation* laryng/o- *larynx* -trache/o-*trachea* -bronch- *bronchus*	Inflammation of the larynx, trachea, and bronchi
larynx laryngeal (adj)	**LAH**-rinks lah-**RIN**-jee-al	S/ R/	Greek *larynx* -eal *pertaining to* laryng- *larynx*	Organ of sound production Pertaining to the larynx
laryngitis laryngoscope	lah-rin-**JEYE**-tis lah-**RING**-oh-skope	S/ R/CF S/	-itis *inflammation* laryng/o- *larynx* -scope *instrument for viewing*	Inflammation of the larynx Hollow tube with a light and camera used to visualize or operate on the larynx
papilla papillae (pl) papilloma	pah-**PILL**-ah pah-**PILL**-ee pap-ih-**LOH**-mah	S/ R/CF	Latin *small pimple* -oma *tumor, mass* papill/o- *pimple*	Any small projection Benign projection of epithelial cells
stridor	**STRY**-door		Latin *a harsh, creaking sound*	High-pitched noise made when there is a respiratory obstruction in the larynx or trachea
vocal	**VOH**-kal	S/ R/	-al *pertaining to* voc- *voice*	Pertaining to the voice

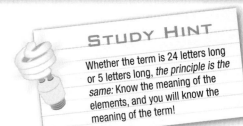

STUDY HINT

Whether the term is 24 letters long or 5 letters long, *the principle is the same*: Know the meaning of the elements, and you will know the meaning of the term!

EXERCISES

A. Deconstruction: *For long or short medical terms, deconstruction into word elements is your key to solving the meaning of the term. Follow the directions and fill in the blanks.*

1. *laryngotracheobronchitis*

   Slash all the elements of this term. _____/_____/_____

2. Combine the meanings of the elements, and define the term.

   _____

3. *vocal*

   Slash all the elements of this term. _____/_____/_____

4. Combine the meanings of the elements, and define the term.

   _____

B. Apply *the language of pulmonology to answer the following questions correctly.*

1. What is another term meaning *croup?* _____

2. What body parts are involved in speech production? _____

3. What is the squeaky noise on *inspiration* termed? _____

4. What is the medical term for a benign tumor of the *larynx?* _____

5. To aid in breathing, what can be inserted into the windpipe? _____

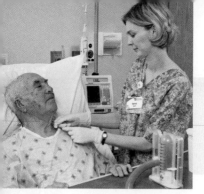

LESSON 8.2

Lower Respiratory Tract

Once the air you inhale has passed through the upper airway and many of the pollutants and impurities have been filtered out, the major needs still remain: to get oxygen (O_2) into the blood and remove carbon dioxide (CO_2) from the blood. To make this possible, the inhaled air has to travel into the alveoli of the lungs, where these exchanges can occur. In this lesson, you will learn to use correct medical terminology to:

8.2.1 Trace the passage of air from the larynx into the alveoli and back.

8.2.2 Describe the mechanics of ventilation.

8.2.3 Integrate the functions of the different elements of the lower airway with their structures.

8.2.4 Discuss the effects of common disorders of the lungs on health.

Trachea (LO 8.1, 8.2, 8.3, and 8.5)

The flow of inhaled air now moves into your trachea (windpipe). This is a rigid tube that descends from the larynx and divides into the two main **bronchi** *(Figure 8.9)*, which serve as airways going to your right and left lungs.

The Lungs (LO 8.1, 8.2, 8.3, and 8.5)

Your two lungs are the main organs of respiration and are located in the thoracic cavity. Each lung is a soft, spongy, cone-shaped organ with its **base** resting on the **diaphragm** and its top **(apex)** above and behind the clavicle. Its outer convex, costal surface presses against the **rib cage.** Its inner concave surface presses against the chest region **(mediastinum).**

The right lung has three **lobes:** superior, middle, and inferior. The left lung has two lobes; superior and inferior *(Figure 8.9a).* Each lobe is separated from the others by **fissures.**

Tracheobronchial Tree
(LO 8.1, 8.2, 8.3, and 8.5)

The tracheobronchial tree is an upside-down, tree-like structure that conducts air in your chest. It is comprised of the trachea, bronchi, and bronchial tubes. As inhaled air continues down the respiratory tract, the main bronchi divide into a **secondary (lobar)** bronchus for each lobe. Each secondary bronchus then divides into tertiary (third) bronchi that supply **segments** of each lobe *(Figure 8.10).* These divisions create branch-like airways.

Bronchioles and Alveoli
(LO 8.1, 8.2, 8.3, and 8.5)

The tertiary bronchi further divide into **bronchioles,** which in turn divide into several thin-walled **alveoli.** Each **alveolus** is a thin-walled sac supported by a thin **respiratory membrane.** This membrane allows the exchange of gases with the surrounding pulmonary capillary network.

The Pleura
(LO 8.1, 8.2, 8.3, and 8.5)

The **pleura** is a double-layered serous membrane that covers the surface of both lungs. The space between these two layers is called the **pleural cavity,** which contains a thin film of lubricant fluid. This lubricant enables the lungs to expand (inspiration) and deflate (expiration) with minimal friction.

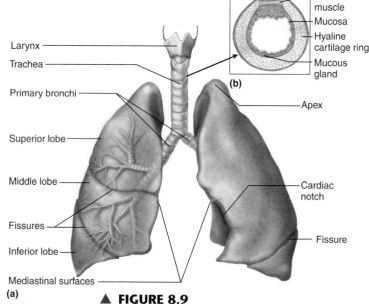

▲ **FIGURE 8.9**
Lower Respiratory Tract.
(a) Gross anatomy. (b) C-shaped tracheal cartilage.

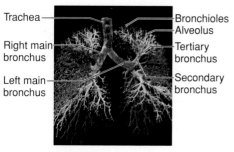

▲ **FIGURE 8.10**
Latex Cast of Tracheobronchial Tree.

S = Suffix   P = Prefix   R = Root   R/CF= Combining Form

Word	Pronunciation		Elements	Definition
diaphragm	DIE-ah-fram		Greek *diaphragm*	The muscular sheet separating the abdominal and thoracic cavities
diaphragmatic (adj)	DIE-ah-frag-**MAT**-ik	S/ R/CF	-tic *pertaining to* diaphragm/a- *diaphragm*	Pertaining to the diaphragm
fissure fissures (pl)	FISH-ur	S/ R/	-ure *process, result of* fiss- *split*	Deep furrow or cleft
lobe lobar (adj)	LOBE **LOW**-bar	S/ R/	Greek *lobe* -ar *pertaining to* lob- *lobe*	Subdivision of an organ or other part Pertaining to a lobe
lobectomy	low-**BECK**-toe-mc	S/	-ectomy *surgical excision*	Surgical removal of a lobe
mediastinum	ME-dee-ass-**TIE**-num	S/ P/ R/	-um *structure* media- *middle* -stin- *partition*	Area between the lungs containing the heart, aorta, venae cavae, esophagus, and trachea
mediastinal (adj)	ME-dee-ass-**TIE**-nal	S/	-al *pertaining to*	Pertaining to the mediastinum
pleura pleurae (pl) pleural (adj)	PLUR-ah PLUR-ee PLUR-al	S/ R/	Greek *rib* -al *pertaining to* pleur- *pleura*	Membrane covering the lungs and lining the ribs in the thoracic cavity Pertaining to the pleura
pleurisy	PLUR-ih-see	S/	-isy *inflammation*	Inflammation of the pleura

EXERCISES

A. Precision *in communication means using the correct form of the medical term, as well as the correct spelling. Test your knowledge of plurals, adjectives, and spelling with this exercise. Circle the correct choice.*

1. The median partition of the thoracic cavity is the:

    mediastenum   mediasternum   mediastinum   midiasternum

2. The patient was diagnosed with _____ pneumonia.

    lobe   lobular   lobar   lumbar

3. The _____ tissue was sent to pathology for a diagnosis.

    plural   pleural   ploral   pliral

4. The muscle separating the abdominal and thoracic cavities is the:

    diaphram   diaphragm   diaphracum   diaphragmm

5. Removal of a portion of a lung is a:

    lobotomy   lobectomy   lobarectomy   lobarotomy

STUDY HINT

Frequent errors are made on test questions regarding the term *pleural*, meaning *pertaining to the pleura*. It is not spelled "plural," which means *more than one*. Be especially careful when dealing with this term, and always check your spelling. Both terms sound alike, are spelled differently, and have very different meanings. The right answer (pleural) is wrong if it is spelled "plural." Don't lose points on a test because of carelessness.

B. Meet lesson objectives *and practice the language of pulmonology with your answers below.*

1. Trace the passage of air from the nose into the alveoli. _____

_____

2. What are the basic components of the lower respiratory tract? _____

_____

3. Which component of the respiratory system allows exchange of gases? _____

4. What are the two gases that need to be exchanged in the respiratory system? _____

LESSON 8.2 Mechanics of Respiration (LO 8.1, 8.2, 8.3, and 8.5)

A resting adult breathes 10 to 15 times per minute and **inhales** about 500 mL of air during inspiration and **exhales** it during expiration. The mission is to get air into and out of the alveoli so that oxygen can enter the bloodstream and carbon dioxide can exit.

Your diaphragm does most of the work. In inspiration, it drops down and flattens to expand the thoracic cavity and reduce the pressure in the airways. The external intercostal muscles also help by lifting the chest wall up and out to further expand the thoracic cavity *(Figure 8.11a)*.

Expiration is a process of letting go. The diaphragm and the intercostal muscles relax, and the thoracic cavity springs back to its original size *(Figure 8.11b)*.

Common Signs and Symptoms of Respiratory Disorders (LO 8.1, 8.2, 8.3, 8.4, and 8.5)

The common signs and symptoms of respiratory disorders are often visible and audible, and they include the following:

1. **Cough** is triggered by irritants in the respiratory tract. Irritants include cigarette smoke (as with Mr. Jacobs), infection, or tumors, as in lung cancer. A productive cough produces **sputum,** which can be swallowed or **expectorated.** Bloody sputum is called **hemoptysis.** Thick, yellow **(purulent)** sputum indicates infection. A **nonproductive** cough is dry and hacking.

   Abnormal amounts of mucus arising from the upper respiratory tract and expectorated or coughed up are called **phlegm.**

2. **Dyspnea,** or shortness of breath **(SOB),** can occur from exertion or, in severe disorders, during rest when all the respiratory muscles are used to exchange only a small volume of air.

3. **Cyanosis** is seen when the blood has increased levels of **unoxygenated hemoglobin** and has a characteristic dark red-blue color.

4. **Changes in the rate of breathing** may occur. **Eupnea** is the normal, easy respiration (around 15 breaths per minute) in a resting adult. Both **tachypnea** (rapid rate of breathing) and **hyperpnea** (breathing deeper and more rapidly than normal) are signs of respiratory difficulty, as is **bradypnea** (slow breathing).

5. **Sneezing** is caused by irritants in the nasal cavity.

6. **Hiccups** are reflex spasms of the diaphragm. The etiology is unknown, and there is no specific medical cure.

7. **Yawning** is a reflex that originates in the brainstem in response to hypoxia, boredom, or sleepiness. The exact mechanisms are not known.

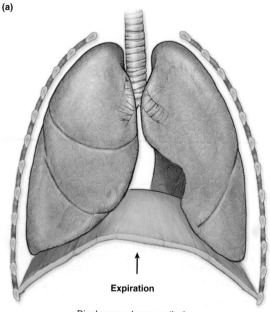

Inspiration

Diaphragm contracts; vertical dimensions of thoracic cavity increase.

(a)

Expiration

Diaphragm relaxes; vertical dimensions of thoracic cavity decrease.

(b)

▲ **FIGURE 8.11**
Inspiration and Expiration.

ABBREVIATION

SOB   short(ness) of breath

Word	Pronunciation	Elements		Definition
bradypnea *(opposite of* **tachypnea***)*	brad-ip-**NEE**-ah	P/ R/	brady- *slow* -pnea *breathe*	Slow breathing
cyanosis	sigh-ah-**NO**-sis	S/ R/	-osis *condition* cyan- *dark blue*	Blue discoloration of the skin, lips, and nail beds due to low levels of oxygen in the blood
cyanotic (adj)	sigh-ah-**NOT**-ik	S/ R/CF	-tic *pertaining to* cyan/o *dark blue*	Pertaining to or marked by cyanosis
dyspnea	disp-**NEE**-ah	P/ R/	dys- *bad, difficult* -pnea *breathe*	Difficult breathing
eupnea	yoop-**NEE**-ah	P/ R/	eu- *normal, good* -pnea *breathe*	Normal breathing
exhale	**EKS**-hail	P/ R/	ex- *out* -hale *breathe*	Breathe out
expectorate	ek-**SPEK**-toh-rate	S/ P/ R/	-ate *pertaining to* ex- *out* -pector- *chest*	Cough up and spit out mucus from the respiratory tract
hemoptysis	he-**MOP**-tih-sis	R/CF R/	hem/o- *blood* -ptysis *spit*	Bloody sputum
hyperpnea	high-perp-**NEE**-ah	P/ R/	hyper- *excessive* -pnea *breathe*	Deeper and more rapid breathing than normal
inhale	**IN**-hail	P/ R/	in- *in* -hale *breathe*	Breathe in
phlegm	**FLEM**		Greek *flame*	Abnormal amounts of mucus expectorated from the respiratory tract
tachypnea *(opposite of* **bradypnea***)*	tak-ip-**NEE**-ah	P/ R/	tachy- *rapid* -pnea *breathe*	Rapid breathing

EXERCISES

> **STUDY HINT**
>
> The English word *breath* is a noun and is the air you inhale and exhale. ("Take a deep breath.") The English word *breathe* has an "e" on the end of it and is the verb meaning to *inhale and exhale*. ("She was unable to breathe.").

A. Construct terms: *Knowing just one element will enable you to build more terms with the addition of other elements. Practice building your pulmonology terms with the following root and various prefixes. Fill in the blanks.*

1. The root *pnea* means _____.

   Add the following prefixes to the root pnea to form the new terms.

   tachy   brady   dys   eu   hyper

2. difficult breathing   _____ /pnea

3. deeper breathing than normal   _____/ pnea

4. slow breathing   _____ /pnea

5. normal breathing   _____ /pnea

6. rapid breathing   _____ /pnea

B. Apply *the language of pulmonology to answer the following questions correctly.*

1. Demonstrate that you can use *breath* and *breathe* correctly. Write a brief sentence for each.

1a._____

1b._____

2. How do *exhale* and *inhale* relate to respiration? _____

3. Respiration takes place in which body cavity? _____

LESSON 8.2 Disorders of the Lower Respiratory Tract

(LO 8.1, 8.2, 8.3, 8.4, and 8.5)

There are a number of disorders that are specific to your lower respiratory tract. These disorders are described below.

Acute bronchitis can be viral or bacterial, leading to the production of excess mucus with some obstruction of airflow. It resolves without significant residual damage to the airway.

Chronic bronchitis is the most common obstructive disease, caused by cigarette smoking or repeated episodes of acute bronchitis. Along with excess mucus production, cilia are destroyed. A pattern develops, involving chronic cough, dyspnea, and recurrent acute infections.

In advanced chronic bronchitis, hypoxia and **hypercapnia** (excess carbon dioxide) are produced and heart failure follows.

Bronchiolitis is a viral inflammation of the small airway bronchioles. It occurs in adults as the early and often unrecognized start of airway changes in cigarette smokers or in those exposed to "secondhand smoke." Bronchiolitis also affects children under the age of 2 because their small airways become blocked very easily. In severe cases, this disease can cause noticeable respiratory distress.

Pulmonary emphysema is a disease of the respiratory bronchioles and alveoli. These airways become enlarged, and the septa between the alveoli are destroyed, forming large sacs **(bullae).** There is a loss of surface area for gas exchange.

Chronic airway obstruction (CAO) is also called chronic **obstructive pulmonary disease (COPD).** It is a progressive disease, as Mr. Jacobs' history shows. It involves both chronic bronchitis and emphysema. A history of heavy cigarette smoking *(Figure 8.12),* with chronic cough and sputum production, is followed by increasing dyspnea and need for oxygen. Right-sided heart failure (cor pulmonale, *see Chapter 6)* is the end result, due to pulmonary hypertension and backup of blood into the right ventricle.

Bronchiectasis is the abnormal dilation of the small bronchioles due to repeated infections. The damaged, dilated bronchi are unable to clear secretions, making them prone to further infections and increased damage.

Bronchial asthma is a disorder with recurrent acute episodes of bronchial obstruction. This results from a constriction of bronchioles **(bronchoconstriction),** a **hypersecretion** of mucus, and an inflammatory swelling of the bronchiolar lining. Between attacks, breathing can be normal. The etiology of asthma is an allergic response to substances like pollen, animal dander, or the feces of dust mites.

Cystic fibrosis (CF) is a genetic disorder caused by an increased **viscosity** (thickness and stickiness) of secretions from the pancreas, salivary glands, liver, intestine, and lungs. In the lungs, a very thick mucus obstructs the airways and causes repeated infections. Many CF patients die before the age of 30 from respiratory failure.

Pulmonary edema is the collection of fluid in the lung tissues and alveoli. It commonly results from left ventricular failure or mitral valve disease with congestive heart failure **(CHF).**

During **auscultation** (examination by stethoscope) of the chest, the air bubbling through abnormal fluid in the alveoli and small bronchioles, as in pulmonary edema, produces a noise called **rales.** When the bronchi are partly obstructed and air is being forced past the obstruction, a high-pitched noise called a **rhonchus** is heard.

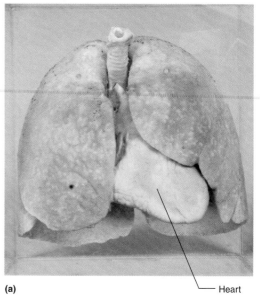

(a) — Heart

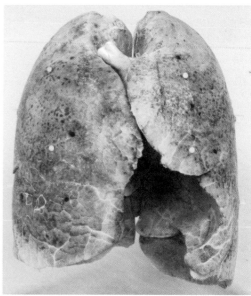

(b)

▲ FIGURE 8.12
Whole Lungs.
(a) Nonsmoker's lungs. (b) Smoker's lungs.

ABBREVIATIONS

CAO	chronic airway obstruction
CF	cystic fibrosis
COPD	chronic obstructive pulmonary disease
CHF	congestive heart failure

Word	Pronunciation		Elements	Definition
asthma asthmatic (adj)	**AZ**-mah az-**MAT**-ic	 S/ R/	Greek *asthma* -atic *pertaining to* asthm- *asthma*	Episodes of breathing difficulty due to narrowed or obstructed airways Pertaining to or suffering from asthma
auscultation	aws-kul-**TAY**-shun	S/ R/	-ation *a process* auscult- *listen to*	Diagnostic method of listening to body sounds with a stethoscope
bronchiectasis	brong-key-**ECK**-tah-sis	S/ R/CF	-ectasis *dilation* bronch/i- *bronchus*	Chronic dilation of the bronchi following inflammatory disease and obstruction
bronchiolitis (Note: *This term has two suffixes—the "e" is dropped before the "i" in* itis.)	brong-key-oh-**LYE**-tis	S/ S/ R/CF	-itis *inflammation* -ole *small* bronch/i- *bronchus*	Inflammation of the small bronchioles
bronchitis	brong-**KI**-tis	S/ R/	-itis *inflammation* bronch- *bronchus*	Inflammation of the bronchi
bronchoconstriction	**BRONG**-koh-kon-**STRIK**-shun	S/ R/CF R/	-ion *action, condition* bronch/o- *bronchus* -constrict- *to narrow*	Reduction in diameter of a bronchus
bulla bullae (pl)	**BULL**-ah **BULL**-ee		Latin *bubble*	Bubble-like dilated structure
cystic fibrosis	**SIS**-tik fie-**BRO**-sis	S/ R/ S/ R/	-ic *pertaining to* cyst- *cyst* -osis *abnormal condition* fibr- *fiber*	Genetic disease in which excessive viscid mucus obstructs passages, including bronchi
emphysema	em-fih-**SEE**-mah	P/ R/	em- *in, into* -physema *blowing*	Dilation of respiratory bronchioles and alveoli
hypercapnia	**HIGH**-per-**KAP**-nee-ah	S/ P/ R/	-ia *condition* hyper- *excessive* -capn- *carbon dioxide*	Abnormal increase of carbon dioxide in the arterial bloodstream
hypersecretion	**HIGH**-per-seh-**KREE**-shun	S/ P/ R/	-ion *action, condition* hyper- *excessive* -secret- *secrete*	Excessive secretion of mucus (or enzymes or waste products)
rhonchus rhonchi (pl)	**RONG**-kuss **RONG**-key		Greek *snoring*	Wheezing sound heard on auscultation of the lungs; made by air passing through a constricted lumen
viscosity viscous (adj) (cf. **viscus,** *any internal organ*)	viss-**KOS**-ih-tee **VISS**-kus	S/ R/	-ity *condition* viscos- *viscous, sticky*	The resistance of a fluid to flow Sticky fluid that is resistant to flow

EXERCISES

A. Elements. *The elements below all appear in the language of pulmonology. Challenge your knowledge of these elements, and make the correct match. Fill in the blanks.*

_____ **1.** ectasis

_____ **2.** capn

_____ **3.** physema

_____ **4.** viscos

_____ **5.** auscult

_____ **6.** ole

A. listen to

B. sticky

C. carbon dioxide

D. blowing

E. small

F. dilation

B. Apply *the language of pulmonology to answer the following questions correctly.*

1. A sticky fluid that is resistant to flow: _____

2. If hypoxia and hypercapnia are both present, what condition will likely follow? _____

3. *Hypercapnia* is excessive _____

4. *Hypoxia* is deficient _____

Disorders of the Lower Respiratory Tract *(continued)*

Pneumonia *(Figure 8.13)* is an acute infection of the alveoli and lung parenchyma (functional cells of the lung). Bacterial infections focus on the alveoli; viral infections, on the parenchyma. **Lobar pneumonia** is an infection limited to one lung lobe. **Bronchopneumonia** is an infection in the bronchioles that spreads to the alveoli.

When an area of the lung (**segment**) or a lobe becomes airless as a result of the infection, the lung is **consolidated.** When an area of the lung collapses as a result of bronchial obstruction, this is called **atelectasis.**

Pleurisy, an inflammation of the pleurae, can be a complication of pneumonia. This condition makes breathing painful because the parietal pleura is very pain-sensitive. The inflammation often leads to fluid accumulating in the pleural cavity. This is a **pleural effusion.** If the pleural effusion contains pus, the condition is called **empyema.** If it contains blood, the condition is called **hemothorax.** When pleural fluid is drawn off for therapeutic reasons or for laboratory analysis, the procedure is **aspiration** or **thoracentesis.**

Lung abscess can be a complication of bacterial pneumonia or cancer. Long-term antibiotics are used, and partial surgical excision of the abscess may be necessary.

Pneumothorax is the entry of air into the pleural cavity *(Figure 8.14).* The cause can be unknown, called a **spontaneous pneumothorax,** but it often results from trauma when a fractured rib, knife blade, or bullet lacerates the pleura.

Adult respiratory distress syndrome (ARDS) is sudden, life-threatening lung failure caused by a variety of underlying conditions from major trauma to sepsis. The alveoli fill with fluid and collapse, shutting down gas exchange. Hypoxia results. **Mechanical ventilation** is mandatory. The mortality rate is 35% to 50%.

Neonatal respiratory distress syndrome (NRDS) is seen in premature babies whose lungs have not matured enough to produce surfactant, a substance secreted in the lungs *(see Bonus Chapter).* The alveoli collapse, and mechanical ventilation is needed to keep them open.

Chronic infections of the lung parenchyma are the result of prolonged exposure to infection or to occupational irritant dusts or droplets. These disorders are called **pneumoconioses.** Levels of dust inhalation overwhelm the airways' particle-clearing abilities. The dust particles accumulate in the alveoli and parenchyma, leading to fibrosis. **Asbestosis** results from inhaling asbestos particles and can lead to a cancer in the pleura called **mesothelioma. Silicosis** from silica particles is called "stonecutters' disease." **Anthracosis** from coal dust particles is called "coal miners' disease." (**Anthrax** is a different disease, caused by toxins produced by the anthrax bacillus.) **Sarcoidosis** produces lesions and is a fibrotic (scarring) disorder of the lung parenchyma.

Pulmonary tuberculosis is a chronic, infectious disease of the lungs.

Lung cancer, related to tobacco use, was once only a male disease. Now, fatalities in women from lung cancer exceed those from breast cancer. Ninety percent of lung cancers arise in the mucous membranes of the larger bronchi and are called **bronchogenic carcinomas.** A subgroup of bronchogenic carcinomas called **adenocarcinoma** accounts for 30% to 50% of all lung cancers and is the most common in women. The lung cancer obstructs the bronchus, spreads into the surrounding lung tissues, and metastasizes to the lymph nodes, liver, brain, and bone. This disease is associated with cigarette smoking.

ABBREVIATIONS

ARDS	adult respiratory distress syndrome
NRDS	neonatal respiratory distress syndrome

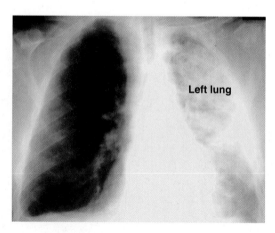

▲ **FIGURE 8.13**
Chest X-ray of Patient with Pneumonia in the Left Lung.
A normal lung appears as a cloudy, black space on an x-ray because its spongy structure is filled with air. In contrast, a pneumonia lung appears white or opaque on an x-ray due to accumulation of fluid and cells in the alveoli.

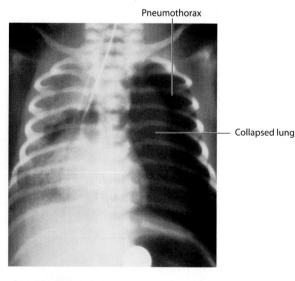

▲ **FIGURE 8.14**
Left Pneumothorax.
There are no lung markings seen in the area of the pneumothorax.

Word	Pronunciation	Elements		Definition
adenocarcinoma	ADD-eh-noh-kar-sih-NOH-mah	S/ R/CF R/	-oma *tumor* aden/o- *gland* -carcin- *cancer*	A cancer arising from glandular epithelial cells
anthracosis	an-thra-KOH-sis	S/ R/	-osis *condition* anthrac- *coal*	Lung disease caused by the inhalation of coal dust
anthrax	AN-thraks		Greek *carbuncle*	A severe, malignant infectious disease
asbestosis	as-bes-TOE-sis	S/ R/	-osis *condition* asbest- *asbestos*	Lung disease caused by the inhalation of asbestos particles
aspiration	as-pih-RAY-shun	S/ R/	-ion *process* aspirat- *to breathe on*	Removal by suction of fluid or gas from a body cavity
atelectasis	at-el-ECK-tah-sis	S/ R/	-ectasis *dilation* atel- *incomplete*	Collapse of part of a lung
bronchogenic	BRONG-koh-JEN-ik	S/ R/CF	-genic *creation* bronch/o- *bronchus*	Arising from a bronchus
bronchopneumonia	BRONG-koh-new-MOH-nee-ah	S/ R/ R/CF	-ia *condition* -pneumon- *air, lung* bronch/o- *bronchus*	Acute inflammation of the walls of smaller bronchioles with spread to lung parenchyma
empyema	EM-pie-EE-mah	S/ P/ R/	-ema *quality of, quantity of* em- *in, into* -py- *pus*	Pus in a body cavity, particularly in the pleural cavity
hemothorax	he-moh-THOR-ax	R/CF R/	hem/o- *blood* -thorax *chest*	Blood in the pleural cavity
pneumoconiosis pneumoconioses (pl)	new-moh-koh-nee-OH-sis	S/ R/ R/CF	-osis *condition* -coni- *dust* pneum/o- *lung, air*	Fibrotic lung disease caused by the inhalation of different dusts
pneumonia	new-MOH-nee-ah	S/ R/	-ia *condition* pneumon- *lung, air*	Inflammation of the lung parenchyma (tissue)
pneumonitis (same as **pneumonia**)	new-moh-NI-tis	S/	-itis *inflammation*	
pneumothorax	new-moh-THOR-ax	R/CF R/	pneum/o- *air, lung* -thorax *chest*	Air in the pleural cavity
sarcoidosis (**Note:** *two suffixes*)	sar-koy-DOH-sis	S/ S/ R/	-osis *condition* -oid- *resembling* sarc- *sarcoma, flesh*	Granulomatous lesions of the lungs and other organs; cause is unknown
silicosis	sil-ih-KOH-sis	S/ R/	-osis *condition* silic- *silicon, glass*	Fibrotic lung disease from inhaling silica particles
thoracentesis (same as **pleural tap**)	THOR-ah-sen-TEE-sis	S/ R/	-centesis *to puncture* thora- *chest*	Insertion of a needle into the pleural cavity to withdraw fluid or air
tuberculosis	too-BER-kyu-LOW-sis	S/ R/	-osis *condition* tubercul- *nodule, swelling, tuberculosis*	Infectious disease that can infect any organ or tissue

EXERCISES

A Suffixes The WAD above contains a lot of suffixes you will see again in other medical terms you will meet in later chapters. Confirm your knowledge of suffixes by filling in the chart with the correct meaning for the element.

Suffix	Meaning of Suffix	Medical Term with This Suffix
centesis	1.	2.
oma	3.	4.
osis	5.	6.
ia	7.	8.

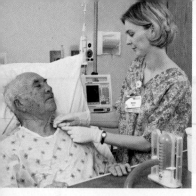

LESSON 8.3

Diagnostic and Therapeutic Procedures

OBJECTIVES

Specific diagnostic and therapeutic procedures, as well as a wide range of pharmacologic agents, are available to help patients with lung diseases. In this lesson, the information will enable you to use correct medical terminology to:

8.3.1 Identify specific pulmonary function tests (PFTs) and other diagnostic procedures.

8.3.2 Describe common therapeutic procedures.

8.3.3 List different classes of pharmacologic agents and their effects on the lungs.

KEYNOTES

- Measure pulmonary function with a spirometer, a peak flow meter, and arterial blood gases.

- **Bronchoscopy** is a procedure for inserting a fiber optic tube into the bronchial tubes to visually examine the tubes, take a tissue biopsy, or do a washing for secretions.

- **Mediastinoscopy** is used to stage lung cancer and diagnose mediastinal masses. The mediastinoscope is inserted through an incision in the suprasternal notch.

- **Thoracentesis** is the insertion of a needle through an intercostal space to remove fluid from a pleural effusion for laboratory study or to relieve pressure. The procedure is also called a **pleural tap.**

CASE REPORT 8.1 (CONTINUED)

Mr. Jacobs' forced expiratory volume was only 40% of normal because the fibrotic (scarring) effects of his repeated lung infections had reduced the volume of his airways. When he was off oxygen, his arterial oxygen levels were below 50% of normal. Even with nasal prongs and oxygen, his arterial oxygen levels were still only 75% of normal.

Diagnostic Procedures (LO 8.1, 8.2, 8.3, 8.4, and 8.5)

Pulmonary Function Tests (PFTs) (LO 8.1, 8.2, 8.3, 8.4, and 8.5)

Pulmonary function can be measured by the following PFTs to estimate the quality of a patient's respiratory function. A **spirometer** is a device for measuring the volume of air that patients move in and out of their respiratory systems. The volume of air expired at the end of the test is the patient's **forced expiratory vital capacity (FVC).** The spirometer also measures **flow rates.** For example, the **forced expiratory volume in 1 second (FEV1)** is the amount of air expired in the first second of the test.

A **peak flow meter** records the greatest flow of air that can be sustained for 10 milliseconds on forced expiration, the **peak expiratory flow rate (PEFR).** This test is valuable in following the course of asthma, and in postoperative care to monitor the return of lung function after anesthesia.

Arterial blood gases, the measurement of oxygen and carbon dioxide levels in the blood, are good indicators of respiratory function.

A **pulse oximeter** is a sensor placed on the finger to measure the oxygen saturation of the blood.

Other Diagnostic Procedures (LO 8.1, 8.2, 8.3, 8.4, and 8.5)

Chest x-ray (CXR) is a radiographic image of the chest taken in **anteroposterior (AP), posteroanterior (PA),** lateral, and sometimes oblique and lateral decubitus positions.

Computed tomography (CT), angiography of the pulmonary circulation using contrast materials, **magnetic resonance angiography (MRA)** to define emboli in the pulmonary arteries, and **ultrasonography** of the pleural space are chest-imaging techniques in modern use. **Position emission tomography (PET)** can sometimes distinguish benign from malignant lesions.

Tracheal aspiration uses a soft catheter that allows brushings and washings to be performed to remove cells and secretions from the trachea and main bronchi. The catheter can be passed through a tracheostomy or **endotracheal** (windpipe) tube, or through the mouth and nose.

Percutaneous transthoracic needle aspiration is the insertion of a needle with a cutting chamber through an intercostal space (between the ribs) to take a specimen of parietal pleura for examination.

Thoracotomy is used to obtain an open biopsy of tissue from the lung, hilum, pleura, or mediastinum. It is performed through an intercostal incision under general anesthesia.

ABBREVIATIONS

AP	anteroposterior	FVC	forced vital capacity	PET	positron emission tomography
CT	computed tomography	MRA	magnetic resonance angiography	PFTs	pulmonary function tests
CXR	chest x-ray	PA	posteroanterior		
FEV1	forced expiratory volume in 1 second	PEFR	peak expiratory flow rate		

Word	Pronunciation	Elements		Definition
bronchoscopy	brong-**KOS**-koh-pee	S/ R/CF	-scopy *to examine, view* bronch/o *bronchus*	Examination of the interior of the tracheobronchial tree with an endoscope
bronchoscope	**BRONG**-koh-skope	S/	-scope *instrument for viewing*	Endoscope used for bronchoscopy
endotracheal	en-doh-**TRAY**-kee-al	S/ P/ R/	-al *pertaining to* endo- *inside* -trache- *trachea*	Pertaining to being inside the trachea
mediastinoscopy	**ME**-dee-ass-tih-**NOS**- koh-pee	S/ R/CF	-scopy *to examine, view* mediastin/o *mediastinum*	Examination of the mediastinum using an endoscope
spirometer	spy-**ROM**-eh-ter	S/ R/CF	-meter *measure* spir/o- *to breathe*	An instrument used to measure respiratory volumes
spirometry	spy-**ROM**-eh-tree	S/	-metry *process of measuring*	Use of a spirometer
thoracotomy	thor-ah-**KOT**-oh-me	S/ R/CF	-tomy *surgical incision* thorac/o *chest*	Incision through the chest wall
tomography	toe-**MOG**-rah-fee	S/ R/CF	-graphy *process of recording* tom/o- *cut, slice, layer*	Radiographic image of a selected slice of tissue
transthoracic	tranz-thor-**ASS**-ik	S/ P/ R/	-ic *pertaining to* trans- *across* -thorac- *chest*	Going through the chest wall
ultrasonography	**UL**-trah-soh-**NOG**-rah-fee	S/ P/ R/CF	-graphy *process of recording* ultra- *beyond* -son/o- *sound*	Delineation of deep structures using sound waves

EXERCISES

A. Review *the Case Report on this spread before answering the questions.*

1. Where can you substitute an abbreviation in the Case Report? _____

2. In what blood vessels is O$_2$ measured? _____

3. What is the noun form for *fibrotic?* _____

4. What has reduced the volume of Mr. Jacobs' airways? _____

5. Will supplemental oxygen improve Mr. Jacobs' condition 100%? _____

6. What is a medical term for *scarred* tissue? _____

7. Reference a keynote and define the location of the suprasternal notch. _____

_____

B. Abbreviations *are helpful only if you know how to interpret them. This exercise asks questions about the abbreviations in the Abbreviations box on this spread. Your knowledge of the language of pulmonology will assist you. Fill in the blanks.*

1. Insert the abbreviations that are directional terms:

_____

2. List the abbreviations that stand for diagnostic radiological procedures:

_____

3. Name the abbreviations that are measurements of PFTs:

_____

4. Write a sentence (that is not directly out of the text) using any of the abbreviations listed on the left-hand page.

_____

_____

LESSON 8.3 Therapeutic Procedures

(LO 8.1, 8.2, 8.3, 8.4, and 8.5)

Many effective therapeutic procedures are available for successfully treating pulmonary function disorders. These procedures are outlined below.

Pulmonary rehabilitation includes education, breathing exercises and retraining, exercises for the upper and lower extremities, and psychosocial support.

Nutritional support is critical for patients who have difficulty breathing, or who need to lose or have lost a lot of weight.

Immunizations are available against influenza, and the pneumococcus bacterium—the most common cause of bacterial pneumonia.

Postural drainage therapy (PDT) uses gravity (by positioning and tilting the patient) to promote the drainage of secretions from lung segments. Chest **percussion** (tapping) on the chest wall can help loosen, mobilize, and drain any retained secretions. These two procedures are part of **chest physiotherapy.**

Constant positive airway pressure (CPAP) is an attempt to keep alveoli open by maintaining a positive pressure in the airways. A mask is fitted over the patient's nose and mouth and attached to a **ventilator.** This can be used at night when sleeping or for acute situations in COPD.

Positive end expiratory pressure (PEEP) is a ventilation technique to keep the alveoli from collapsing in ARDS and neonatal respiratory distress syndrome.

An **oropharyngeal airway** is used in the unconscious patient during bag and mask ventilation to maintain an open airway. A tube is inserted to prevent the tongue from falling back and obstructing the airway, and to facilitate suctioning the airway. An **endotracheal intubation** involves the placement of a tube into the trachea. This allows the patient to be placed on a ventilator so their breathing can be controlled.

Pulmonary resection is the surgical removal of lung tissue.

- **Wedge resection** is the removal of a small, localized area of diseased lung.
- **Segmental resection** is the removal of lung tissue attached to a bronchiole.
- **Lobectomy** is the removal of a lobe.
- **Pneumonectomy** is the removal of an entire lung.

Tracheotomy is an incision made into the trachea (windpipe) so that a temporary or permanent opening into the windpipe, called a **tracheostomy,** is created (*Figure 8.15*). A tube is placed into the opening to provide an airway. A tracheostomy is used to maintain an airway when there is obstruction or paralysis in the respiratory structures above it.

Mechanical ventilation is a process involving the movement of gases into and out of the lungs via a device programmed to meet the patient's respiratory requirements. A tracheostomy or endotracheal tube must be attached to the mechanical device (**ventilator**). This procedure can augment or replace the patient's own **ventilatory** efforts.

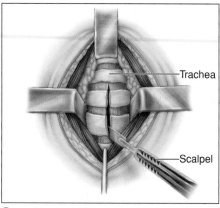

① Tracheotomy incision is made superior to sternal notch.

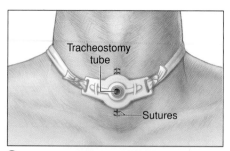

② Retractors separate the tissue, and an incision is made through the third and fourth tracheal rings.

③ A tracheostomy tube is inserted, and the remaining incision is sutured closed.

▲ **FIGURE 8.15**
Tracheostomy Procedure.

Pulmonary Pharmacology

- **Bronchodilators** relax the smooth muscles of the bronchioles. Examples are theophylline, beta2-agonists such as salbutamol and terbutaline, and anticholinergics such as ipratropium bromide.

- **Anti-inflammatory** drugs, such as corticosteroids, are best given by inhalation, but can be used orally or intravenously in acute episodes of asthma or COPD.

- **Mucolytics** are agents that attempt to break up mucus so it can be cleared more effectively from the airways. Examples are guaifenesin (common in over-the-counter cough medications), potassium iodide, and N-acetylcysteine taken through a **nebulizer.**

- **Antibiotics** are used when a bacterial infection is present. Penicillin, erythromycin, cefotaxime, and flucloxacillin are frequently used.

- **Oxygen** is used in hypoxemia and can be given by nasal **cannula** or by mask and intubation. Patients with severe, chronic COPD can be attached to a portable oxygen cylinder.

Word	Pronunciation	Elements		Definition
bronchodilator	BRONG-koh-die-LAY-tor	S/ R/CF R/	-or *one who does, that which does something* bronch/o- *bronchus* -dilat- *expand, open up*	Agent that increases the diameter of a bronchus
cannula	KAN-you-lah		Latin *reed*	Tube inserted into a blood vessel or cavity as a channel for fluid or gas
immunization	im-you-nih-ZAY-shun	S/ R/	-ation *process* immuniz- *make immune*	Administration of an agent to provide immunity
mucolytic	MYU-koh-LIT-ik	S/ R/CF R/	-ic *pertaining to* muc/o- *mucus* -lyt- *dissolve*	Agent capable of dissolving or liquefying mucus
nebulizer	NEB-you-liz-er	S/ R/	-izer *line of action, affects in a particular way* nebul- *cloud*	Device used to deliver liquid medicine in a fine mist
pneumonectomy	NEW-moh-NECK-toe-me	S/ R/	-ectomy *surgical excision* pneumon- *lung, air*	Surgical removal of a lung
resection resect (verb)	ree-SEK-shun ree-SEKT	S/ P/ R/	-ion *action, condition* re- *back* -sect- *cut off*	Removal of a specific part of an organ or structure
tracheostomy tracheotomy	tray-kee-OST-oh-me tray-kee-OT-oh-me	S/ R/CF S/	-stomy *new opening* trache/o- *trachea* -tomy *surgical incision*	Insertion of a tube into the windpipe to assist breathing Incision made into the trachea to create a tracheostomy
ventilation ventilator	ven-tih-LAY-shun VEN-tih-lay-tor	S/ R/ S/	-ation *a process* ventil- *wind* -ator *person or thing that does something*	Movement of gases into and out of the lungs Device that breathes for the patient

EXERCISES

A. Deconstruct: *Define the elements, and then use any two terms in one sentence each (that is not directly out of the text) to demonstrate that you understand the term's meaning. Fill in the blanks.*

Medical Term	Meaning of Prefix	Meaning of Root/CF	Meaning of Suffix
immunization	1.	2.	3.
nebulizer	4.	5.	6.
mucolytic	7.	8.	9.
bronchodilator	10.	11.	12.

13. _____

_____

14. _____

B. Meet lesson and chapter objectives *by applying the language of pulmonology to answer the following questions correctly.*

1. Describe the process of *mechanical ventilation:*

_____

_____

2. What is the difference between *antibiotic* and *antinflammatory* medication?

_____

_____

3. A *tracheotomy* creates an opening. What goes in that opening? _____

4. What is the medical term for the *windpipe?* _____

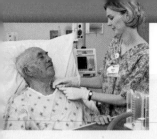

CHAPTER 8 REVIEW RESPIRATORY SYSTEM

CHALLENGE YOUR KNOWLEDGE

A. Word elements *will always remain the best tool for deconstructing medical terminology. Test your knowledge of respiratory word elements by breaking down the following medical terms. Fill in the chart.*

Medical Term	Prefix	Root/Combining Form	Suffix	Meaning of Term
hemothorax	1.	2.	3.	4.
aspiration	5.	6.	7.	8.
pneumonia	9.	10.	11.	12.
bronchitis	13.	14.	15.	16.
empyema	17.	18.	19	20.
pneumoconiosis	21.	22.	23.	24.
tachypnea	25.	26.	27.	28.
bronchogenic	29.	30.	31.	32.

Take five of the above terms and apply them appropriately in the following sentences:

33. Rapid breathing is _____ .

34. Another term for *thoracentesis* is _____ .

35. *Pleural effusion* containing pus is also termed _____ .

36. *Anthracosis* is a form of _____ .

37. *Bloody pleural effusion* is also termed _____ .

B. Suffix: *The suffix itis is one that you will encounter over and over again in this text. Build the correct medical term to match its definition. Fill in the blanks.*

1. inflammation of the bronchus _____ / itis

2. inflammation of the organ of voice production _____ / itis

3. inflammation of the tonsils _____ / itis

4. inflammation of the throat _____ / itis

5. inflammation of the nose _____ / itis

6. inflammation of the epiglottis _____ / itis

7. croup _____ / itis

8. inflammation of the small bronchioles _____ / itis

9. synonym for pneumonia _____ / itis

10. inflammation of the sinuses _____ / itis

C. Roots: *Sometimes in medical terminology there can be two roots or combining forms with the same meaning. Pneum/o and pulmon/o are examples. These elements are not interchangeable—the medical term takes either one combining form or the other. Demonstrate your knowledge of the difference between the two elements by choosing the correct form for the terms listed below.*

1. PFT is the abbreviation for what diagnostic test? _____

2. Acute infection affecting the alveoli and lung parenchyma is _____ .

3. Entry of air into the pleural cavity is called _____ .

4. A specialist in the study of the lung is called a _____ .

5. Surgical removal of a lung is called a _____ .

6. COPD is the abbreviation for what lung disease? _____

7. Sarcoidosis is a form of the disease called _____ .

8. Study of the lungs and lung diseases is _____ .

D. Construct medical terms *with the correct combination of elements. Write each term on the line provided after the definition. Some elements you will use more than once; some elements you will not use at all.*

endo	ectomy	tomy	ation
bronch/o	trans	scopy	trache/o
lob	al	graphy	thorac/o
re	pneum/on	ventil	tom/o
son/o	osis	stomy	ion
ic	ator	ia	mediastin/o

1. surgical removal of a lung _____ / _____ / _____
                        P   R/CF   S

2. examination of a bronchus _____ / _____ / _____
                        P   R/CF   S

3. image of a selected slice of tissue _____ / _____ / _____
                        P   R/CF   S

4. pertaining to being inside the trachea _____ / _____ / _____
                        P   R/CF   S

5. examination of the mediastinum _____ / _____ / _____
                        P   R/CF   S

6. incision through the chest wall _____ / _____ / _____
                        P   R/CF   S

7. mechanical device that breathes
   for the patient _____ / _____ / _____
                        P   R/CF   S

8. pertaining to across the chest _____ / _____ / _____
                        P   R/CF   S

9. removal of part of a lung _____ / _____ / _____
                        P   R/CF   S

10. new opening in the neck to the trachea _____ / _____ / _____
                        P   R/CF   S

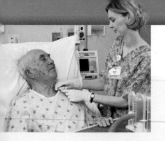

E. Word attack: *This is an exercise in the thought process required to arrive at the correct answer to a multiple-choice question. Look at the roots of the following terms to find the clues. Fill in the blanks.*

Abnormal increase of carbon dioxide in the arterial bloodstream is:

  a. hypertension

  b. hyperglycemia

  c. hypercapnia

  d. hypersecretion

  e. hyperpnea

Read the question and all the possible answers.

1. Read the question and answers again. Look for key words in the question. In this particular case, "abnormal" and "increase" should catch your eye. An increase of anything will require _____ as an element.

   All of these terms begin with the same element, so you need to look at other elements for your clues.

2. Ask yourself: What is there an increase of? _____

   _____

   That is an important part of the question. Since a root is the foundation of every term, check your roots.

3. tens   =   _____

   glyc   =   _____

   capn   =   _____

   secret =   _____

   pnea   =   _____

4. Therefore, an "abnormal increase of carbon dioxide in the arterial bloodstream" is _____.

F. Recall and review: *How well do you remember these word elements from a previous chapter? Try to answer without looking back to check. Fill in the blanks.*

Element	Type of Element (P, R, CF, or S)	Meaning of Element
1. retro	_____	_____
2. media	_____	_____
3. emia	_____	_____
4. myo	_____	_____
5. peri	_____	_____
6. ic	_____	_____
7. hypo	_____	_____
8. intra	_____	_____

G. Terminology challenge: *For this exercise, remember terminology from a body system studied previously. Fill in the blanks.*

What is the difference between the following terms?

hyperpnea

hypertension

1. What do both these terms have in common? _____

2. Which two different body systems do they represent? _____

_____

H. Explain the difference: *Do you understand the following terms well enough to explain the difference to patients if they should ask? Write a brief explanation of each term.*

What is the difference between:

1. *inspiration* _____

expiration _____

aspiration _____

2. *pneumothorax* _____

hemothorax _____

I. Noun, adjective, verb: *Meet a chapter objective by using the correct form of a term in precise communication. Insert the appropriate terms ON the line. UNDER the line, write the form (noun, adjective, verb) that you have used.*

1. resect   resection

The patient is scheduled for a lung _____ tomorrow.

The surgeon is not sure he can _____ the tumor.

2. cyanosis   cyanotic

This patient is showing signs of _____ .

Mr. Jacobs appeared _____ to the respiratory therapist.

3. respirator   respiratory

_____ illnesses can spread quickly.

The comatose patient will be taken off the _____ .

4. Take the terms (a) pharynx and (b) pharyngeal and compose a sentence for each term. At the end of each sentence, write which form of the term you have used (noun, adjective, verb).

Sentence:

a. _____

_____

_____

This form of the term is a(n) _____ .

Sentence:

b. _____

_____

_____

This form of the term is a(n) _____ .

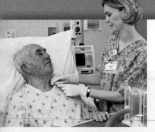

J. Suffixes: *Knowledge of elements aids you in choosing the appropriate medical term for the correct meaning you want to convey either verbally or in documentation. Suffixes will help you choose the correct term. Use the following medical terms to fill in the statements relating to the bronchus.*

bronchogenic	bronchi
bronchopneumonia	bronchioles
bronchiolitis	bronchus
bronchoconstriction	bronchial
bronchitis	bronchiectasis

NOTE: *In the term bronchopneumonia, the combining form is used, and it is one word. In the term bronchial asthma, the suffix al makes it an adjective, and the two words are separated.*

1. One of 2 subdivisions of the trachea _____

2. Plural of the word above _____

3. Pertaining to the bronchus_____

4. Increasingly smaller subdivisions of bronchi _____

5. Inflammation of the bronchus _____

6. Chronic dilation of bronchi following inflammatory disease _____

7. Inflammation of the small bronchioles _____

8. Reduction in diameter of a bronchus _____

9. Arising from a bronchus _____

10. Acute inflammation of bronchioles with spread to lung parenchyma _____

Now, **build new terms,** *also relating to the bronchus, using the word elements below. Your root or combining form will be bronch/o. You have more elements than you need. Fill in the blanks.*

stenosis	plasty	gram
scope	pathy	pulmonary
dilation	dilator	scopy

11. An instrument used to view into the bronchus _____

12. Drug meant to open bronchial passages _____

13. Surgical procedure doing plastic repair on a bronchus _____

14. Examination of the bronchus _____

15. Pertaining to the bronchus and lung _____

K. Explain *in the language of pulmonology the role of the diaphragm in the process of respiration.*

1. The diaphragm's role in respiration is:

_____

_____

I. **Translate** *these physician's orders into medical terms, and test how well you understand what the physician has written. Fill in the blanks.*

1. Physician order: This patient is to have AP and PA CXRs, followed by a CT, MRI, and PET scan STAT.

   _____

   _____

   _____

2. Physician order: Schedule the patient with COPD for ABGs and PFTs as soon as possible.

   _____

   _____

   _____

M. **Translate** *the following statements into layperson's language. Reconstruct each sentence into language a nonmedical person could understand. Fill in the blanks, and then check your spelling!*

1. Sputum from a productive cough should be expectorated.

   _____

   _____

   _____

2. Tachypnea, hyperpnea, and bradypnea are all signs of respiratory difficulty.

   _____

   _____

   _____

3. Acute respiratory failure results in inadequate tissue oxygenation or carbon dioxide elimination.

   _____

   _____

   _____

N. **Train your eye and ear** *to see and hear the difference in medical terms. Remember that patient safety depends on you! Describe the difference in the following terms:*

1. emphysema:_____

   empyema: _____

2. rhonchus: _____

   bronchus:_____

3. mucous:_____

   mucus:_____

4. aspiration: _____

   inspiration: _____

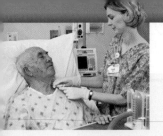

O. Chapter challenge: *Circle the correct answer.*

1. *Epistaxis* is the medical term for:

   a. fainting

   b. vomiting

   c. nosebleed

   d. difficulty breathing

   e. productive cough

2. Another term for *heart failure* is:

   a. cyanosis

   b. conchae

   c. choana

   d. cor pulmonale

   e. chordae tendineae

3. What is the total number of *lobes* in *both* lungs?

   a. 4

   b. 5

   c. 6

   d. 2

   e. 3

4. What term is used for a reflex spasm of the diaphragm?

   a. coughing

   b. sneezing

   c. hiccups

   d. yawning

   e. blinking

5. The medical term for *croup* is:

   a. bronchiectasis

   b. bronchitis

   c. laryngotracheobronchitis

   d. laryngitis

   e. pharyngitis

6. Identify the pair of terms that both have elements meaning *lung:*

   a. pneumonectomy   pulmonologist

   b. bronchitis   laryngitis

   c. pulmonology   pharynx

   d. trachea   pneumonia

   e. pneumonic   mediastinal

7. *Stridor, rales,* and *rhonchi* can all be considered:

   a. fissures

   b. signs

   c. diseases

   d. conditions

   e. infections

8. Which sentence is correct? Proofread carefully.

   a. Lung abcess can be a complication of bacterial pnemonia.

   b. Pneumonconiosis is caused by the inhalation of certain dusts.

   c. The cause of sarcoidossis is unknown.

   d. The synonym for *thoracentesis* is *plural tap.*

   e. Tuberculosis can affect any organ or tissue.

9. When a lung segment becomes airless as a result of infection, the lung is said to be:

a. constricted

d. congested

b. consolidated

e. choked up

c. compromised

10. What is the commonality of the abbreviations *CXR, PFT,* and *PET?*

a. They are all surgical procedures.

d. They are all symptoms.

b. They are all diagnostic tests.

e. They are all drugs.

c. They are all diseases.

11. An element in *hemothorax* can tell you that the pleural cavity contains:

a. pus

d. blood

b. mucus

e. water

c. phlegm

12. Which set of terms is spelled correctly?

a. oropharingeal   bronchoscopy

b. canula   ventilator

c. sinusitis   decongestant

d. spitum   polyp

e. tonsil   tonsilectomy

13. *Polysomnography* is:

a. a diagnostic test

d. both a and b

b. a sleep study

e. none of these

c. a surgical procedure

P. **Meet lesson objectives** *and use the language of pulmonology to answer the following questions.*

1. What are the main functions of the *respiratory system?*

_____

_____

2. Where is the *olfactory region?*_____

3. Describe a *deviated nasal septum.*

_____

_____

4. What is another medical term for *croup?* _____

5. Benign tumors of the larynx are called _____ and _____ .

6. Which two gases are constantly being exchanged in the respiratory system? _____ and _____ .

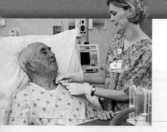

Q. Chapter challenge: *Circle the correct answer.*

1. Identify the pair of terms that can be diagnoses:

   a. epiglottis   pleura

   b. intubation   fissure

   c. alveoli   bronchioles

   d. pleurisy   epiglottitis

   e. diaphragm   eupnea

2. What can be said about the terms *endotracheal, transthoracic,* and *pulmonary?*

   a. All their suffixes mean the same thing.

   b. None of them has a prefix.

   c. All of them are adjectives.

   d. Answers a, b, and c are all correct.

   e. Answers a and c are correct.

3. *Bradypnea, dyspnea, eupnea, tachypnea,* and *hyperpnea* all describe:

   a. auscultation   d. respiration

   b. bronchoconstriction   e. viscosity

   c. cor pulmonale

4. Only one pair of terms has the correct spelling *and* plural form. Which is it?

   a. rhoncus   rhonci

   b. ronkus   ronki

   c. rhonchus   rhonchi

   d. ronchus   ronchi

   e. runchus   runchi

5. Brain teaser: When an area of the lung collapses as a result of bronchial obstruction, this is called:

   a. pneumoconiosis   d. hemothorax

   b. asbestosis   e. mesothelioma

   c. atelectasis

6. Find the medical term with an element that means *puncture:*

   a. thoracotomy   d. thoracentesis

   b. pneumonectomy   e. rhinoplasty

   c. tomography

7. Benign tumors of the larynx can be:

   a. polyps   d. neither a nor b

   b. papillomas   e. both a and b

   c. malignant

R. Case Report challenge: *Now that you are more comfortable with the terms in this chapter, you can apply that knowledge and briefly answer the questions about the Case Report. If you read the report through and underline all the medical terminology, this will make it easier to answer the questions.*

YOU ARE COMMUNICATING WITH

. . . Mr. Jude Jacobs, a 68-year-old white retired mail carrier, who has chronic obstructive pulmonary disease (COPD) and is on continual oxygen by nasal prongs. He has smoked two packs per day during all his adult life.

Last night, he was unable to sleep because of increased shortness of breath and cough. His cough is productive of yellow sputum. He had to sit upright in bed to be able to breathe.

Vital signs are temperature (T) 101.6, pulse (P) 98, respirations (R) 36, blood pressure (BP) 150/90. On examination, he is cyanotic and frightened and is on oxygen by nasal prongs. Air entry is diminished in both lungs, and there are rales at both bases.

You have been ordered to draw blood for arterial blood gases and to measure the amount of air entering and leaving his lungs by using spirometry.

1. What disease appears in Mr. Jacobs' medical history?

_____

2. Which particular symptom indicates Mr. Jacobs has an infection?

_____

3. Cyanotic indicates an outward sign the physician can detect. What is it?

_____

4. *Rales* heard through a stethoscope indicate the presence of what in the lungs?

_____

5. Where can abbreviations be substituted in this documentation? Write them here:

_____

6. Define what makes a condition "chronic."

_____

7. What is the opposite of a chronic condition?

_____

THE DIGESTIVE SYSTEM

The Essentials of the Language of Gastroenterology

In your future career, being able to communicate comfortably, accurately, and effectively with the health professionals involved in the diagnosis and treatment of problems in the **gastroenterological** system is key. You may work directly and/or indirectly with one or more of the following:

- **Gastroenterologists** are medical specialists in the field of gastroenterology.

- **Proctologists** are surgical specialists in diseases of the anus and rectum.

- **Dentists** are qualified practitioners in the anatomy, physiology, and pathology of the oral-facial complex.

- **Periodontists** are specialists in disorders of the tissues surrounding the teeth.

- **Nutritionists** are professionals who prevent and treat illness by promoting healthy eating habits.

- **Dietitians** manage food services systems and promote sound eating habits.

LEARNING OUTCOMES

As a medical transcriptionist (MT), your job is to accurately transcribe the voice-recorded reports of physicians and any other healthcare professionals into readable text. To ensure that Mrs. Jones receives the best possible care, you and the healthcare professionals directly and indirectly involved with her care, need to be able to:

LO 9.1 Apply the language of gastroenterology to the gastrointestinal tract, liver, gallbladder, and pancreas.

LO 9.2 Comprehend, analyze, spell, and write the medical terms of gastroenterology.

LO 9.3 Recognize and pronounce the medical terms of gastroenterology.

LO 9.4 Discuss the cause, diagnosis, and treatment of common disorders of the gastrointestinal tract.

Fulwood Medical Center
3333 Medical Parkway, Fulwood, MI 01234
555-247-6100

Center for Bariatric Surgery

Charles Leavenworth, MD
Medical Director
Lombard Insurance Company
One Lombard Place
Haverson, MI 01233

10/06/11
Request for authorization of surgery
Mrs. Martha Jones   Subscriber ID: 056437

Dear Doctor Leavenworth,
 Mrs. Jones is a 52-year-old former waitress, recently divorced. She is 5 feet 4 inches tall and weighs 275 pounds. She has type 2 diabetes with frequent episodes of hypoglycemia and also ketoacidosis, requiring three different hospitalizations. She now has diabetic retinopathy and peripheral vasculitis. Complicating this are hypertension (185/110), coronary artery disease, and pulmonary edema. In spite of monthly meetings with our nutritionist, she has gained 25 pounds in the past six months.
 To reduce and control her weight, I am proposing to perform a gastric bypass using a laparoscopic approach. We will need to admit her two days prior to surgery to control her blood sugar and cardiovascular problems, and we anticipate that she will remain in the hospital for two days after surgery, barring any complications. She is also very aware of the necessary follow-up to the procedure and the counseling required for a new lifestyle.
 We believe not only that this is an essential procedure medically but that it will reduce in the long term the financial burden of her multiple therapies and improve the quality of the patient's life. Enclosed is supportive documentation of her current history and medical problems.
 Your company has designated our hospital as a Center of Excellence for weight-loss surgery, and I look forward to your prompt agreement with this approach for this patient.

 Sincerely,

 Stewart Walsh, MD, FACS
 Chief of Surgery

CASE REPORT 9.1

YOU ARE

. . . a medical transcriptionist at Fulwood Medical Center.

YOU ARE COMMUNICATING WITH

. . . one of Fulwood's physicians, Dr. Stewart Walsh, who has dictated this letter to request authorization for a surgical procedure:

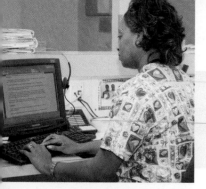

LESSON 9.1

The Digestive System

OBJECTIVES

There are basic terms and elements of medical terminology that apply throughout the different parts of the digestive system. Understanding these basic terms and elements of the digestive system will enable you to use correct medical terminology to:

9.1.1 Name the health professionals involved in gastroenterology.

9.1.2 List the organs and accessory organs of the digestive system.

9.1.3 Identify the components of the alimentary canal.

9.1.4 Describe the structure and functions of the digestive system.

CASE REPORT 9.1 (CONTINUED)

In Mrs. Jones's case, the **gastric** bypass procedure reduced the size of her stomach from 2 quarts to 2 ounces. The bypass was taken to the mid-ileum (middle part of the small intestine). This resulted in her being able to eat less and to absorb less. She had no complications from the **laparoscopic** procedure and lost 15 pounds In the 2 months that followed.

Alimentary Canal and Accessory Organs (LO 9.1, 9.2, and 9.3)

Every cell in your body requires a constant supply of nourishment in a form that can be absorbed across its cell membrane. The **digestive system** breaks down the **nutrients** in food into elements that can be transported to the cells via the blood and lymphatics.

The digestive system consists of the **alimentary canal,** or digestive tract, which extends from the mouth to the **anus,** and **accessory organs** connected to the canal to assist in digestion.

Gastroenterology is the study of the digestive system. A **gastroenterologist** is a physician who specializes in diseases of the digestive tract. The **gastrointestinal (GI)** tract is another name for your stomach and intestines, but is often used to mean the whole digestive system.

The **alimentary canal** *(Figure 9.1)* includes the:

- **Mouth**
- **Pharynx**
- **Esophagus**
- **Stomach**
- **Small intestine**
- **Large intestine**

The **accessory organs** of digestion include the:

- **Teeth**
- **Tongue**
- **Salivary glands**
- **Liver**
- **Gallbladder**
- **Pancreas**

ABBREVIATION

GI   gastrointestinal

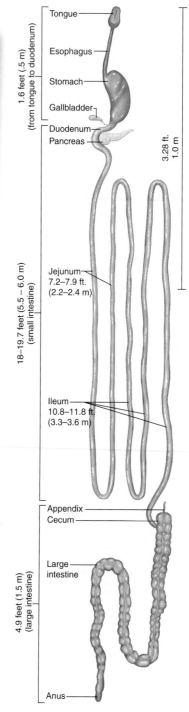

▲ **FIGURE 9.1**
Alimentary Canal.

Word	Pronunciation	Elements		Definition
alimentary	al-ih-**MEN**-tar-ee	S/ R/	-ary *pertaining to* aliment- *nourishment, food*	Pertaining to the digestive tract
alimentary canal	kah-**NAL**		canal, Latin *a duct or channel*	Digestive tract
anus	**A**-nus		Latin *a ring*	Terminal opening of the digestive tract through which feces are discharged
anal (adj)	**A**-nal	S/ R/	-al *pertaining to* an- *anus*	Pertaining to the anus
bariatric	bar-ee-**AT**-rik	S/ R/	-atric *treatment* bari- *weight*	Treatment of obesity
digestion	die-**JEST**-shun	S/ R/	-ion *action* digest- *to break down food*	Breakdown of food into elements suitable for cell metabolism
digestive (adj)	die-**JEST**-iv	S/	-ive *nature of, quality of*	Pertaining to digestion
esophagus	ee-**SOF**-ah-gus		Greek *gullet*	Tube linking the pharynx and the stomach
gastric (adj)	**GAS**-trik	S/ R/	-ic *pertaining to* gastr- *stomach*	Pertaining to the stomach
gastroenterology	**GAS**-troh-en-ter-**OL**-oh-gee	S/ R/CF R/CF	-logy *study of* gastr/o- *stomach* -enter/o- *intestine*	Medical specialty of the stomach and intestines
gastroenterologist gastrointestinal	**GAS**-troh-en-ter-**OL**-oh-jist **GAS**-troh-in-**TESS**-tin-al	S/ S/ R/CF R/	-logist *one who studies, specialist* -al *pertaining to* gastr/o- *stomach* intestin- *gut, intestine*	Medical specialist in gastroenterology Pertaining to the stomach and intestines
intestine intestinal (adj)	in-**TESS**-tin in-**TESS**-tin-al	S/ R/	Latin *intestine, gut* -al *pertaining to* intestin- *gut*	The digestive tube from stomach to anus Pertaining to the intestines
laparoscopy	lap-ah-**ROS**-koh-pee	S/	-scopy *to view, to examine*	Examination of contents of abdomen using an endoscope
laparoscope	**LAP**-ah-roh-skope	R/CF S/	lapar/o- *abdomen in general* -scope *instrument for viewing*	Instrument (endoscope) used for viewing abdominal contents
laparoscopic (adj)	**LAP**-ah-roh-**SKOP**-ik	S/	-ic *pertaining to*	Pertaining to laparoscopy
nutrient	**NYU**-tree-ent	S/ R/	Latin *to nourish* -ive *nature of, pertaining to* nutrit- *nourishment*	A substance in food required for normal physiologic function
nutritive (adj)	**NYU**-trih-tiv		Latin *to nourish*	Providing nourishment
nutrition	nyu-**TRISH**-un	S/	-ion- *action, condition*	The study of food and liquid requirements for normal function of the human body
nutritionist	nyu-**TRISH**-un-ist	S/	-ist *specialist in*	Certified professional in nutrition science

EXERCISES

A. Review *the Case Report on this, and the chapter opening, spread before answering the questions.*

1. What is the term for Mrs. Jones being severely overweight for her height? _____

2. What is the difference between hypoglycemia and hypertension? _____

3. What disease has previously caused Mrs. Jones to be hospitalized? _____

4. What are her complications from the disease in question 3? _____

5. Why does she need to be admitted 2 days prior to her surgery? _____

B. Analyzing *elements can tell you a lot about a medical term. Look closely at the following medical terms, and let the elements be your guide. Review the WAD before you start the exercise. Fill in the blanks.*

gastric   gastroenterology   gastrointestinal   gastroenterologist   gastroscope

1. Based on the root, the term *gastric* pertains to the _____ .

2. Analyzing the two combining forms, the term *gastroenterology* pertains to the _____ and the _____ .

3. In the term *gastrointestinal*, the root intestin has the same meaning as the combining form _____ in *gastroenterology*.

4. A *gastroscope* would be inserted into the _____ for examination or biopsy.

LESSON 9.1 Actions and Functions of the Digestive System

(LO 9.1, 9.2, and 9.3)

The actions and functions of your digestive system have these five components:

1. **Propulsion:** The mechanical movement of food from the mouth to the anus. Normally, this takes 24 to 36 hours.

2. **Digestion:** The breakdown of foods into forms that can be transported to cells and absorbed into these cells. This process has two parts:

   a. **Mechanical digestion** breaks larger pieces of food into smaller ones without altering their chemical composition. **Mastication** (chewing) breaks down the food into smaller particles so that digestive enzymes have a larger surface area with which to interact. **Deglutition** (swallowing) moves the **bolus** (mass or lump) of food from the mouth into the esophagus. **Peristalsis** (waves of contraction and relaxation) moves food material through most of the alimentary canal.

   b. **Chemical** digestion breaks down large molecules of food into smaller and simpler chemicals by way of digestive enzymes (made by the salivary glands, stomach, small intestine, and pancreas).

3. **Secretion:** The addition of secretions like mucus, that lubricate, liquefy, and digest food throughout the digestive tract, while also keeping the tract's lining lubricated.

4. **Absorption:** The movement of nutrient molecules out of the digestive tract, through the epithelial cells lining the tract, and into the blood or lymph for transportation to body cells.

5. **Elimination:** The process by which the body removes undigested food residue.

Word	Pronunciation	Elements		Definition
bolus	BOH-lus		Greek *lump*	A single mass of a substance
deglutition	dee-glue-TISH-un	S/ R/	-ion *action, condition* deglutit- *to swallow*	The act of swallowing
masticate (verb)	MAS-tih-kate	S/ R/	-ate *pertaining to, composed of* mastic- *chew*	To chew
mastication (noun)	mas-tih-KAY-shun	S/	-ation *process*	The process of chewing
peristalsis	per-ih-STAL-sis	P/ R/	peri- *around* -stalsis *constrict*	Waves of alternate contraction and relaxation of the intestinal wall to move food along the digestive tract

EXERCISES

A. Match *the correct medical term in column 2 to the definition in column 1. The body process, or action, is described for you below. Fill in the blanks.*

_____ **1.** swallowing

_____ **2.** releasing products of metabolism

_____ **3.** chewing

_____ **4.** removal of waste material

A. mastication

B. elimination

C. deglutition

D. secretion

B. Review *the text to obtain answers to the following questions.*

1. What is the mechanical movement of food from mouth to anus called? _____

2. Which organs produce digestive enzymes? _____

3. What lubricates the food in the digestive tract? _____

4. What liquefies the food in the digestive tract? _____

5. What breaks down food in the digestive tract? _____

6. Which body process removes undigested food residue? _____

C. Meet chapter and lesson objectives *by explaining to a fellow student the difference between mechanical and chemical digestion. Be sure to include the appropriate medical terms in your explanation.*

1. Medical digestion: _____

_____

_____

2. Chemical digestion: _____

_____

_____

3. List here all the medical terms you have included in your explanations: _____

_____

_____

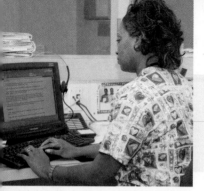

LESSON 9.2

Mouth, Pharynx, and Esophagus

The Mouth and Mastication (LO 9.1, 9.2, and 9.3)

Your **mouth** *(Figure 9.2)* is the gateway to your digestive tract. It's the first site of mechanical digestion, through mastication (chewing), and of chemical digestion, through an **enzyme** in your **saliva.**

The roof of your mouth is called the **palate,** and its anterior two-thirds is the bony **hard palate.** The posterior one-third is the muscular **soft palate.** The skeletal muscle of the soft palate has a projection or flap called the **uvula,** which closes off the **nasopharynx** (upper pharynx) when swallowing.

Your **tongue** moves food around your mouth and helps the cheeks, lips, and gums hold food in place while you chew it. Small, rough, raised areas on the tongue, called **papillae,** contain some 4,000 taste buds that react to the chemical nature of food to give you different taste sensations *(Figure 9.3).* A taste-bud cell lives for 7 to 10 days before it's replaced.

Adult Teeth (LO 9.1, 9.2, and 9.3)

The average adult has 32 teeth—16 rooted in the upper jaw (maxilla) and 16 in the lower jaw (mandible) *(Figure 9.4).* The bulk of a tooth is composed of **dentine** (also spelled *dentin),* a substance like bone but harder, that is covered in **enamel.** The dentine surrounds a central **pulp** cavity, containing blood vessels, nerves, and connective tissue. The blood vessels and nerves reach this cavity from the jaw through tubular root canals.

Salivary Glands (LO 9.1, 9.2, and 9.3)

Salivary glands secrete saliva. The two **parotid** glands (beside the ears), the two **submandibular** glands (beneath the mandible), the two **sublingual** glands (beneath the tongue) *(Figure 9.4),* and numerous minor salivary glands scattered in the mucosa of the tongue and cheeks, secrete more than a quart of saliva daily.

Saliva is 95% water, and its major functions are to begin the digestion of starch and fat and to lubricate food so it's easier to swallow.

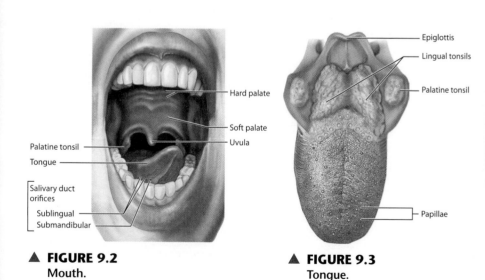

▲ **FIGURE 9.2**
Mouth.

▲ **FIGURE 9.3**
Tongue.

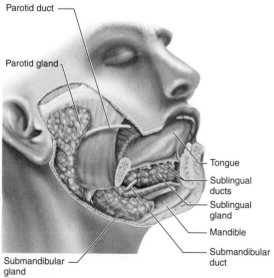

▲ **FIGURE 9.4**
Salivary Glands.

Word	Pronunciation		Elements	Definition
dentine (also spelled dentin)	**DEN**-tin	S/ R/	-ine *pertaining to, substance* dent- *tooth*	Dense, ivory-like substance located under the enamel in a tooth
dentist	**DEN**-tist	S/ R/	-ist *specialist* dent- *tooth*	A qualified practitioner in the anatomy, physiology, and pathology of the oral-facial complex
enamel	ee-**NAM**-el		French *enamel*	Hard substance covering a tooth
enzyme	**EN**-zime	P/ R/	en- *in* -zyme *enzyme, fermenting*	Protein that induces changes in other substances
mouth	**MOWTH**		Old English *mouth*	External opening of a cavity or canal
nasopharynx	**NAY**-zoh-**FAIR**-inks	R/CF R/	nas/o- *nose* -pharynx *throat*	Region of the pharynx at the back of the nose and above the soft palate
oral	**OR**-al	S/ R/	-al *pertaining to* or- (os) *mouth*	Pertaining to the mouth
palate	**PAL**-ate		Latin *palate*	Roof of the mouth
papilla papillae (pl)	pah-**PILL**-ah pah-**PILL**-ee		Latin *small pimple*	Any small projection
parotid	pah-**ROT**-id	S/ P/ R/	-id *having a particular quality* par- *beside* -ot- *ear*	The parotid gland is the salivary gland beside the ear
pulp	**PULP**		Latin *flesh*	Dental pulp is the connective tissue in the cavity in the center of the tooth
saliva (noun) salivary (adj)	sa-**LIE**-vah **SAL**-ih-var-ee	S/ R/	Latin *spit* -ary *pertaining to* saliv- *saliva*	Secretion in mouth from salivary glands Pertaining to saliva
sublingual	sub-**LING**-wal	S/ P/ R/	-al *pertaining to* sub- *underneath* -lingu- *tongue*	Underneath the tongue
submandibular	sub-man-**DIB**-you-lar	S/ P/ R/	-ar *pertaining to* sub- *underneath* -mandibul- *mandible*	Underneath the mandible
tongue	**TUNG**		Latin *tongue*	Mobile muscle mass in the mouth; bears the taste buds
uvula	**YOU**-vyu-lah		Latin *grape*	Fleshy projection of the soft palate

EXERCISES

A. Apply *your knowledge of the same elements to various terms, and increase your medical vocabulary. Focus on what is the same and what is different about the following terms. Fill in the chart.*

Medical Term	Meaning of Prefix	Meaning of Root	Meaning of Suffix	Meaning of Term
submandibular	1.	2.	3.	4.
sublingual	5.	6	7.	8
subcutaneous (from Chapter 3)	9.	10.	11.	12.

B. Answer *the following questions based on the above chart.*

1. What is similar about every term? _____

2. Which element makes every term different? _____

3. Do all these terms describe size, number, location, or color? _____

LESSON 9.2 Disorders of the Mouth
(LO 9.1, 9.2, 9.3, and 9.4)

The human mouth is the entrance to the digestive system, and since so many elements pass through it, the human mouth is prone to tooth disorders and a host of other conditions.

A buildup of **dental plaque** (a collection of oral microorganisms and their products), or **tartar** (calcified deposits at the margin of the teeth along the gums), is a precursor to invasion by dental disease-causing bacteria.

Dental caries, which are tooth decay and cavity formation, are erosions of the tooth surface caused by bacteria *(Figure 9.5)*. If untreated, it can lead to an abscess at the root of the tooth. **Gingivitis** is an infection of the gums. **Periodontal disease** occurs when the gums and the jawbone are involved in a disease process. In **periodontitis,** infection causes the gums to pull away from the teeth, forming pockets that become sources of infection that can spread to underlying bone. Infection of the gums with a purulent or pus-like discharge is called **pyorrhea.**

The term **stomatitis** is used for any infection of the mouth, including:

- **Mouth ulcers,** also called **canker** sores, are erosions of the mucous membrane lining the mouth. **Aphthous** ulcers are the most common and occur in clusters of small ulcers that last for 3 or 4 days. These are usually stress- or illness-related but can also be caused by trauma.

- **Cold sores,** or fever blisters *(Figure 9.6),* are recurrent ulcers of the lips, lining of the mouth, and gums due to infection with the virus **herpes simplex type 1 (HSV-1).** These ulcers usually clear up spontaneously.

- **Thrush** *(Figure 9.7)* is an infection occurring anywhere in the mouth that is caused by the fungus *Candida albicans.* This fungus is normally found in the mouth, but it can multiply out of control as a result of prolonged antibiotic or steroid treatment, cancer chemotherapy, or diabetes. Newborn babies can acquire oral thrush from the mother's vaginal yeast infection during the birth process. Treatment with antifungal agents is usually successful.

- **Oral cancer** *(Figure 9.8)* occurs most often on the lip, but it can also occur on the tongue. Eighty percent of oral cancers are associated with smoking or chewing tobacco. Metastasis occurs to lymph nodes, bones, lungs, and liver.

Halitosis is the medical term for bad breath, which occurs in association with any of the above mouth disorders.

ABBREVIATION

HSV-1   Herpes simplex virus, type 1

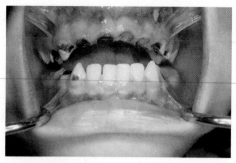

▲ **FIGURE 9.5**
Dental Caries.

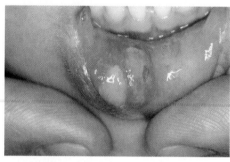

▲ **FIGURE 9.6**
Cold Sores.
Ulcer inside lower lip.

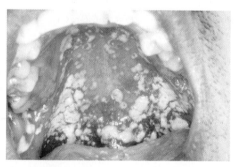

▲ **FIGURE 9.7**
Oral Thrush.

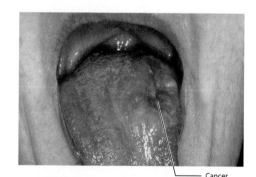

Cancer

▲ **FIGURE 9.8**
Oral Cancer.
Cancer of the tongue.

Word	Pronunciation	Elements		Definition
aphthous	**AF**-thus		Greek *ulcer*	Painful small oral ulcers (canker sores)
canker	**KANG**-ker		Latin *crab*	Nonmedical term for aphthous ulcer
caries	**KARE**-eez		Latin *dry rot*	Bacterial destruction of teeth
gingiva	**JIN**-jih-vah		Latin *gum*	Tissue surrounding the teeth and covering the jaw
gingival (adj)	**JIN**-jih-val	S/ R/	-al *pertaining to* gingiv- *gum*	Pertaining to the gums
gingivitis gingivectomy	jin-jih-**VI**-tis jin-jih-**VEC**-toe-me	S/ S/	-itis *inflammation* -ectomy *surgical excision*	Inflammation of the gums Surgical removal of diseased gum tissue
halitosis	hal-ih-**TOE**-sis	S/ R/	-osis *condition* halit- *breath*	Bad odor of the breath
periodontal	**PER**-ee-oh-**DON**-tal	S/ P/ R/	-al *pertaining to* peri- *around* -odont- *tooth*	Around a tooth
periodontics	**PER**-ee-oh-**DON**-tiks	S/	-ics *knowledge*	Branch of dentistry specializing in disorders of tissues around the teeth
periodontist periodontitis	**PER**-ee-oh-**DON**-tist **PER**-ee-oh-don-**TIE**-tis	S/ S/	-ist *specialist* -itis *inflammation*	Specialist in periodontics Inflammation of tissues around a tooth
plaque	PLAK		French *plate*	Patch of abnormal tissue
pyorrhea	pie-oh-**REE**-ah	R/ R/CF	-rrhea *flow* py/o- *pus*	Purulent discharge
tartar	**TAR**-tar		Latin *crust on wine casks*	Calcified deposit at the gingival margin of the teeth
thrush	**THRUSH**		Root unknown	Infection with *Candida albicans*

EXERCISES

A. Suffixes: *Find the correct suffix to complete the medical terms, which all appear on this two-page spread. Fill in the blanks.*

ist   itis   ectomy   rrhea   osis   al   ics

1. inflammation of the gums   gingiv/ _____

2. specialized branch of dentistry   periodont/ _____

3. around a tooth   periodont/ _____

4. bad breath   halit/ _____

5. surgical removal of diseased gum tissue   gingiv/ _____

6. specialist in periodontics   periodont/ _____

7. purulent discharge   pyo/ _____

B. Identify *the following medical terms that have their origin in Greek, Latin, or French.*

1. patch of abnormal tissue _____

2. canker sores _____

3. pertaining to the gums _____

4. nonmedical term for a mouth ulcer _____

5. bacterial destruction of teeth _____

C. Terminology challenge: *Recall and review terms from other chapters.*

1. In which other body system vocabulary does the medical term *plaque* appear? System: _____

   Define *plaque* in that system: _____

LESSON 9.2

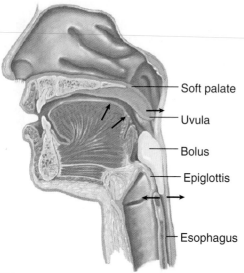

▲ FIGURE 9.9
Swallowing.
The bolus of food is in the oropharynx.

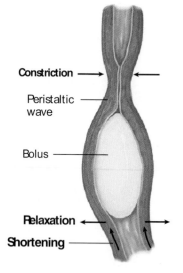

▲ FIGURE 9.10
Swallowing.
The bolus of food is in the esophagus.

Esophagus (LO 9.1, 9.2, and 9.3)

The chicken and vegetables that you ingested earlier have now been sliced and ground into small particles by the teeth. These particles are partly digested and lubricated by saliva, and rolled into a bolus between the tongue and the hard palate, the bony roof of the mouth. The bolus is now ready to be swallowed down the oropharynx (upper part of the throat) *(Figure 9.9)* into the **esophagus.**

The bolus enters the esophagus from the lower end of the pharynx. In the esophagus, peristaltic, or wavelike, contractions of the esophageal wall muscles move it downward *(Figure 9.10)*. At the lower end of the esophagus, the **cardiac sphincter** relaxes to allow the bolus to enter the stomach.

The **esophagus** *(Figure 9.11)* is a tube 9 to 10 inches long. It pierces the diaphragm at the esophageal **hiatus** to go from the thoracic cavity to the abdominal cavity *(Figure 9.11)*.

Disorders of the Esophagus (LO 9.1, 9.2, 9.3, and 9.4)

Just like the mouth, the esophagus, too, can be prone to illness. **Esophagitis** is an inflammation of the lining of the esophagus, producing a burning chest pain **(heartburn)** after eating, pain on swallowing, and occasional vomiting of blood **(hematemesis).** The most common cause is **reflux** of the stomach's acid contents into the esophagus, also known as **gastroesophageal reflux disease (GERD).**

Hiatal hernia occurs when a portion of the stomach protrudes through the diaphragm alongside the esophagus at the esophageal hiatus. Surgical repair—a hiatal **herniorrhaphy**—may be necessary.

Esophageal varices are varicose veins of the esophagus. They are **asymptomatic** until they rupture, causing massive bleeding and hematemesis. They are a complication of cirrhosis of the liver *(see later this chapter)*.

Cancer of the esophagus arises from the tube's lining. Symptoms are **dysphagia** (difficulty swallowing), a burning sensation in the chest, and weight loss. Risk factors include: cigarettes, alcohol, betelnut chewing, and esophageal reflux. The cancer metastasizes to the liver, bones, and lungs.

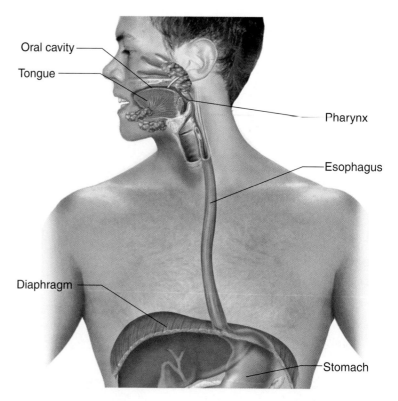

▲ FIGURE 9.11
Esophagus.

Word	Pronunciation	Elements		Definition
asymptomatic	A-simp-toe-**MAT**-ik	S/ P/ R/	-ic *pertaining to* a- *without* symptomat- *symptom*	Without any symptoms or abnormalities experienced by the patient
symptomatic *(with* **symptoms***)*	simp-toe-**MAT**-ik			Pertaining to the symptoms of a disease
dysphagia	dis-**FAY**-jee-ah	P/ R/	dys- *difficulty* -phagia *swallowing*	Difficulty in swallowing
emesis hematemesis	**EM**-eh-sis he-mah-**TEM**-eh-sis	 R/ R/	emesis Greek *to vomit* hemat- *blood* -emesis *to vomit*	Vomit Vomiting of red blood
esophagus esophageal (adj)	ee-**SOF**-ah-gus ee-**SOF**-ah-**JEE**-al	 S/ R/	Greek *gullet* -eal *pertaining to* esophag- *esophagus*	Tube linking pharynx to stomach Pertaining to the esophagus
esophagitis	ee-**SOF**-ah-**JI**-tis	S/	-itis *inflammation*	Inflammation of the lining of the esophagus
hernia	**HER**-nee-ah		Latin *rupture*	Protrusion of a structure through the tissue that normally contains it
herniorrhaphy	**HER**-nee-**OR**-ah-fee	S/ R/CF	-rrhaphy *suture* herni/o- *hernia*	Repair of a hernia
hiatus (noun) hiatal (adj)	high-**AY**-tus high-**AY**-tal	 S/ R/	Latin *an aperture* -al *pertaining to* hiat- *opening*	An opening through a structure Pertaining to a hiatus
postprandial	post-**PRAN**-dee-al	S/ P/ R/	-ial *pertaining to* post- *after* -prand- *breakfast*	Following a meal
reflux	**REE** fluks	P/ R/	re- *back* -flux *flow*	Backward flow
sphincter	**SFINK**-ter		Greek *a band*	A band of muscle that encircles an opening; when it contracts, the opening squeezes closed
varix varices (pl) varicose (adj)	**VAIR**-iks **VAIR**-ih-seez **VAIR**-ih-kose	 S/ R/	Latin *dilated vein* -ose *full of* varic- *varicosity; dilated, tortuous vein*	Dilated, tortuous vein Characterized by or affected with varices

EXERCISES

A. Knowledge *of elements is your best tool for increasing your medical vocabulary. Each of the following terms has an element in bold. Identify that element and give its meaning. Fill in the chart.*

Medical Term	Identity of Element (P, R, CF, or S)	Meaning of Element	Meaning of Term
reflux	1.	2.	3.
dysphagia	4.	5.	6.
herniorrhaphy	7.	8.	9.
hematemesis	10.	11.	12.
asymptomatic	13.	14.	15.

B. Apply *the language of gastroenterology and fill in the blanks.*

1. What is another term for *varicose veins* of the esophagus? _____

2. What is a *bolus*? _____

3. What structure does the esophagus travel through from the *thoracic cavity* to the abdominal cavity? _____

4. What is burning chest pain called? _____

5. What are you vomiting in *hematemesis?* _____

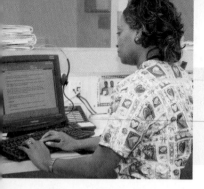

LESSON 9.3

Digestion—Stomach and Small Intestine

OBJECTIVES

The bolus of food that you swallowed has now passed down your esophagus and into your stomach. The process of digestion begins in earnest. The stomach continues the mechanical breakdown of the food particles and initiates the chemical digestion of protein and fats. The small intestine is where the greatest amount of food digestion and absorption occurs. The information in this lesson will enable you to use correct medical terminology to:

9.3.1 Define the functions of the stomach and small intestine in digestion.

9.3.2 Explain how food is propelled through the stomach and small intestine.

9.3.3 Describe the process of digestion.

ABBREVIATIONS

HCl	hydrochloric acid
ml	milliliter

CASE REPORT 9.2

YOU ARE

. . . a medical interpreter working in Fulwood Medical Center.

YOU ARE COMMUNICATING WITH

. . . Mr. Xavier Ramirez, a 45-year-old farm worker, who has come to Dr. Susan Lee's primary care clinic. Mr. Ramirez complains of experiencing persistent, burning epigastric pain for several months. He has been a chain-smoker since the age of 14. His pain is eased by antacids but quickly returns. He has been taking aspirin because of joint pain in his fingers while he works. Dr. Lee has decided to refer him to a gastroenterologist for a gastroscopy. Your role is to explain the procedure to Mr. Ramirez and ensure that he keeps his appointments.

Digestion: The Stomach (LO 9.1, 9.2, and 9.3)

Your stomach's peristaltic contractions mix different boluses of food together and push these contents toward the **pylorus** (the stomach opening that leads to the bowel) *(Figure 9.12)* to produce a mixture of semi-digested food called **chyme.**

The cells of your stomach's lining secrete *(Figure 9.13)*:

1. **Mucus,** which lubricates food and protects the stomach lining;

2. **Hydrochloric acid (HCl),** which breaks up the connective tissue of meat and the cell walls of vegetables (think of the chicken-and-vegetables meal you ate earlier);

3. **Pepsin** (an active enzyme), which digests chicken and vegetable proteins;

4. **Intrinsic factor,** which is essential for vitamin B_{12} absorption in the small intestine; and

5. **Gastrin** (a chemical), which stimulates HCl and **pepsinogen** production, and encourages the stomach's peristaltic contractions.

A typical meal like chicken and vegetables takes 3 to 4 hours to exit the stomach as chyme. Peristaltic waves squirt 2 to 3 milliliters **(ml)** of this chyme at a time through the **pyloric sphincter** into the **duodenum** (the first part of the small intestine) *(Figure 9.12)*.

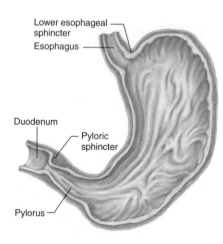

▲ **FIGURE 9.12**
Stomach.

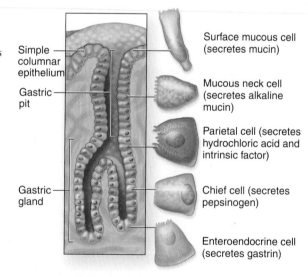

▲ **FIGURE 9.13**
Gastric Cells and Their Secretions.

S = Suffix   P = Prefix   R = Root   R/CF= Combining Form

Word	Pronunciation	Elements		Definition
chyme	KYME		Greek *juice*	Semifluid, partially digested food passed from the stomach into the duodenum
duodenum	du-oh-**DEE**-num	S/ R/	-um *structure* duoden- *twelve*	The first part of the small intestine; approximately twelve finger-breadths (9 to 10 inches) in length
duodenal (adj)	du-oh-**DEE**-nal	S/	-al *pertaining to*	Pertaining to the duodenum
gastrin	**GAS**-trin	S/ R/	-in *substance, chemical compound* gastr- *stomach*	Hormone secreted in the stomach that stimulates secretion of HCl and increases gastric motility
hydrochloric acid (HCl)	high-droh-**KLOR**-ic **ASS**-id	S/ R/CF R/	-ic *pertaining to* hydr/o- *water* -chlor- *green*	The acid of gastric juice
intrinsic factor	in-**TRIN**-sik **FAK**-tor	S/ R/ R/	-ic *pertaining to* intrins- *on the inside* factor *maker*	Makes the absorption of vitamin B₁₂ happen
mucus (noun)	**MYU**-kus		Latin *slime*	Sticky secretion of cells in mucous membranes
mucous (adj) mucin	**MYU**-kus **MYU**-sin			Relating to mucus or the mucosa Protein element of mucus
pepsin	**PEP**-sin		Greek *to digest*	Enzyme produced by the stomach that breaks down protein
pepsinogen	pep-**SIN**-oh-jen	S/ R/CF	-gen *produce* pepsin/o- *pepsin*	Converted by HCl in the stomach to pepsin
pylorus	pie-**LOR**-us	S/ R/	-us *pertaining to* pylor- *gate, pylorus*	Exit area of the stomach
pyloric (adj)	pie-**LOR**-ik	S/	-ic *pertaining to*	Pertaining to the pylorus

EXERCISES

A. Review *the Case Report on this spread before answering the questions.*

1. What are the patient's complaints when he presents to the clinic? _____

2. What is not healthy in the patient's past medical history? _____

3. What do antacids help? _____

4. Why is Mr. Ramirez taking aspirin? _____

5. What is a gastroscopy? _____

B. Grammatical forms *can change with the addition of just one letter. Be aware of the correct spelling of these forms and also how they are used in a sentence. For example, mucus is the noun (person, place, or thing) form of the term, and mucous is the adjective (descriptive) form of the term. Insert the correct grammatical form (noun or adjective) in each of the following sentences. Check your spelling when you are finished.*

1. The sticky secretion of the _____ membranes is _____.

2. A sinus infection will produce a lot of _____ in the nasal passages.

3. Some internal organs have a _____ lining or covering.

Demonstrate that you know the difference in the forms of these terms. Create a sentence of patient documentation using any form of one of these terms.

Sentence:

_____

KEYNOTE

- Difficulty in swallowing is called dysphagia.

Disorders of the Stomach

(LO 9.1, 9.2, 9.3, and 9.4)

CASE REPORT 9.2 (CONTINUED)

A **gastroscopy** on Mr. Ramirez reveals a gastric ulcer.

Gastroesophageal reflux disease (GERD) refers to the regurgitation of stomach contents back into the esophagus. The acidity of regurgitated food can irritate and ulcerate the esophageal lining and cause bleeding. Scar tissue can cause an esophageal **stricture** and **dysphagia.**

Vomiting can result from over-expansion or irritation of any part of the digestive tract. The muscles of the diaphragm and abdominal wall forcefully contract and expel the stomach contents upward into the esophagus and mouth.

Gastritis is an inflammation of the stomach lining, producing symptoms of epigastric pain, feeling of fullness, nausea, and occasional bleeding. It can be acute or chronic, and is caused by common medications like aspirin and **NSAIDs,** by radiotherapy and chemotherapy, and by alcohol and smoking. Treatment involves removing the factors causing the gastritis, acid neutralization, and suppression of gastric acid *(see below).*

Peptic ulcers occur in the stomach and duodenum when the mucosal lining breaks down *(Figure 9.14).* Most peptic ulcers are caused by the bacterium *Helicobacter pylori (H. pylori),* which produces enzymes that weaken the protective mucus. These ulcers respond to antibiotics. **Dyspepsia** (epigastric pain with bloating and nausea) is the most common symptom.

Gastric ulcers are peptic ulcers that occur in the stomach. If a blood vessel erodes,

ABBREVIATIONS

GERD	Gastroesophageal reflux disease
NSAID	Nonsteroidal anti-inflammatory drug

bleeding may also be present. If untreated, the ulcer can eat into the entire wall, causing a **perforation.**

Gastric cancer can be asymptomatic for a long period and then cause **indigestion, anorexia,** abdominal pain, and weight loss. It affects men twice as often as women. It metastasizes to the lymph nodes, liver, peritoneum, chest, and brain. It is usually treated with surgery and chemotherapy.

Small Intestine

(LO 9.1, 9.2, and 9.3)

The small intestine, called *small* because of its diameter, completes the chemical digestion process. It is responsible for the **absorption** of most of the nutrients. The small intestine extends from the pylorus of the stomach to the beginning of the large intestine, and it has three segments *(Figure 9.15),* as listed below:

1. The **duodenum** is the first 9 to 10 inches of the small intestine. It receives chyme from the stomach, together with pancreatic juices and bile;

2. The **jejunum** makes up about 40% of the small intestine's length. It is the primary region for chemical digestion and nutrient absorption; and

3. The **ileum** makes up about 55% of the small intestine's length. It ends at the **ileocecal** valve, a **sphincter** that controls entry into the large intestine.

Digestion in the Small Intestine

(LO 9.1, 9.2, and 9.3)

After leaving the stomach as chyme, the food spends 3 to 5 hours in the small intestine, where most of the nutrients are absorbed.

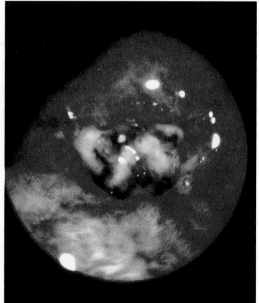

▲ **FIGURE 9.14**
Bleeding Peptic Ulcer.

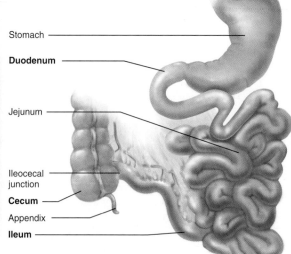

Stomach

Duodenum

Jejunum

Ileocecal
junction

Cecum

Appendix

Ileum

▲ **FIGURE 9.15**
Small Intestine.

Word	Pronunciation	Elements		Definition
absorption	ab-**SORP**-shun	S/ R/	-ion *action, condition* absorpt- *to swallow*	Uptake of nutrients and water by cells in the GI tract
anorexia	an-oh-**RECK**-see-ah	S/ P/ R/	-ia *condition* an- *without* -orex- *appetite*	Without an appetite; or an aversion to food .
cecum (noun)	**SEE**-kum	S/ R/	-um *structure* cec- *cecum*	Blind pouch that is the first part of the large intestine
cecal (adj)	**SEE**-kal	S/	-al *pertaining to*	Pertaining to the cecum
dyspepsia	dis-**PEP**-see-ah	S/ P/ R/	-ia *condition* dys- *difficult, bad* -peps- *digestion*	"Upset stomach," epigastric pain, nausea, and gas
gastritis	gas-**TRY**-tis	S/ R/	-itis *inflammation* gastr- *stomach*	Inflammation of the lining of the stomach
gastroesophageal	**GAS**-troh-ee-sof-ah-**JEE**-al	S/ R/CF R/CF	-al *pertaining to* gastr/o- *stomach* -esophag/e- *esophagus*	Pertaining to the stomach and esophagus
gastroscope	**GAS**-troh-skope	S/ R/CF	-scope *instrument for viewing* gastr/o- *stomach*	Endoscope for examining the inside of the stomach
gastroscopy	gas-**TROS**-koh-pee	S/	-scopy *to examine, to view*	Endoscopic examination of the stomach
ileum	**ILL**-ee-um	S/ R/	-um *structure* ile- *ileum*	Third portion of small intestine
ileocecal	**ILL**-ee-oh-**SEE**-cal	S/ R/CF R/	-al *pertaining to* ile/o- *ileum* cec- *cecum*	Pertaining to the junction of the ileum and cecum
indigestion	in-dih-**JESS**-chun	S/ P/ R/	-ion *action, condition* in- *in, not* -digest- *to break down*	Symptoms resulting from difficulty in digesting food
jejunum (noun)	je-**JEW**-num	S/ R/	-um *structure* jejun- *jejunum*	Segment of small intestine between the duodenum and the ileum.
jejunal (adj)	je-**JEW**-nal	S/	-al *pertaining to*	Pertaining to the jejunum
peptic	**PEP**-tik	S/ R/	-ic *pertaining to* pept- *digest*	Relating to the stomach and duodenum
perforation	per-foh-**RAY**-shun	S/ R/	-ion *action, condition* perforat- *bore through*	A hole through the wall of a structure
stricture	**STRICK**-shur		Latin *draw tight*	Narrowing of a tube

EXERCISES

A. Review *the Case Report on this spread before answering the questions.*

1. Mr. Ramirez was diagnosed with a gastric ulcer. What is the difference between a peptic ulcer and a gastric ulcer? _____

2. What type of "scope" did the surgeon use to find the ulcer? _____

3. Name one complication Mr. Ramirez could develop from his gastric ulcer. _____

4. What bacterium causes most peptic ulcers? _____

B. Practice *the language of gastroenterology. Review this spread and the WAD before you start the exercise. Use the terms found there to answer the following questions.*

1. Write the three segments of the small intestine in their correct order of location in the intestine.

_____ , _____ , _____

2. A term can often designate more than one area of the gastrointestinal tract (example: *gastrointestinal*).

Find a similar term in the WAD above. _____

The two organs referred to in this term are: _____ and _____

3. Patient education: Explain to your patient the function of a *stricture* in the intestine.

_____

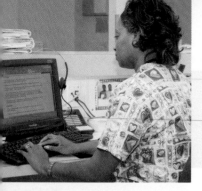

LESSON 9.4

Digestion—Liver, Gallbladder, and Pancreas

CASE REPORT 9.3

YOU ARE

. . . a coder in the Health Information Management department at Fulwood Medical Center.

YOU ARE COMMUNICATING WITH

. . . Dr. Susan Lee, and you are questioning the documentation of Mrs. Sandra Jacobs's care. Mrs. Jacobs, a 46-year-old mother of four, presented in Dr. Lee's primary care clinic with episodes of cramping pain in her upper abdomen associated with nausea and vomiting. A physical examination reveals an obese white woman with tenderness over her gallbladder. Her BP is 170/90 and she has slight pedal edema. A **provisional diagnosis** of gallstones has been made. She has been referred for an ultrasound examination and an appointment has been made to see Dr. Walsh in the surgery department.

The Liver (LO 9.1, 9.2, and 9.3)

Your **liver** is your largest internal organ. It is a complex structure located under your right ribs just below your diaphragm *(Figure 9.16)*.

As a complex organ, your liver's multiple functions include:

• Manufacturing and excreting **bile;**

• Removing **bilirubin** (a pigment) from the bloodstream;

• Storing excess sugar as **glycogen;** and

• Manufacturing blood proteins, including those needed for clotting *(see Chapter 7)*.

Disorders of the Liver
(LO 9.1, 9.2, 9.3, and 9.4)

Hepatitis is an inflammation of the liver causing **jaundice,** where the skin and sometimes the eyes have a yellowish hue. Viral hepatitis is the most common cause of hepatitis and is related to three major types of virus:

1. **Hepatitis A virus (HAV)** is highly contagious and causes a mild to severe infection. It is transmitted by contaminated food.

2. **Hepatitis B virus (HBV),** or serum hepatitis, is transmitted through contact with blood, semen, vaginal secretions, or saliva, as well as by a needle prick and the sharing of contaminated needles.

3. **Hepatitis C virus (HCV)** is the most common blood-borne infection in the United States. Like HBV, the disease is transmitted by blood and body fluids.

In addition, **hepatitis D** can occur in association with hepatitis B, making the infection worse. **Hepatitis E** is similar to hepatitis A and occurs mostly in underdeveloped countries.

Chronic hepatitis occurs when the acute hepatitis is not healed after 6 months. It progresses slowly, can last for years, and is difficult to treat.

Cirrhosis of the liver is a chronic irreversible disease, replacing normal liver cells with hard, fibrous scar tissue. Its most common cause is alcoholism. There is no known cure.

Cancer of the liver as a primary cancer usually arises in patients with chronic liver disease, often from HBV infection.

Sternum   5th rib

Liver

▲ **FIGURE 9.16**
Location of Liver.

Word	Pronunciation		Elements	Definition
bile	BILE		Latin *bile*	Fluid secreted by the liver into the duodenum
bile acids	**BILE AH**-sids			Steroids synthesized from cholesterol
biliary (adj)	**BILL**-ee-air-ee	S/ R/CF	-ary *pertaining to* bil/i- *bile*	Pertaining to bile or the biliary tract
bilirubin	bill-ee-**RU**-bin	S/ R/CF	-rubin *rust colored* bil/i- *bile*	Bile pigment formed in the liver from hemoglobin
cirrhosis	sir-**ROE**-sis	S/ R/	-osis *condition* cirrh- *yellow*	Extensive fibrotic liver disease
glycogen	**GLYE**-koh-gen	S/ R/CF	-gen *produce, create* glyc/o- *sugar, glycogen*	The body's principal carbohydrate reserve, stored in the liver and skeletal muscle
hepatic	hep-**AT**-ik	S/ R/	-ic *pertaining to* hepat- *liver*	Pertaining to the liver
hepatitis	hep-ah-**TIE**-tis	S/	-itis *inflammation*	Inflammation of the liver
jaundice	**JAWN**-dis		French *yellow*	Yellow staining of tissues with bile pigments, including bilirubin
liver	**LIV**-er		Old English *liver*	Body's largest organ, located in the right upper quadrant of the abdomen
provisional diagnosis *(also called* **preliminary diagnosis***)*	pro-**VISH**-un-al die-ag-**NO**-sis	S/ R/ P/ R/	-al *pertaining to* provision- *provide* dia- *complete* -gnosis *knowledge of an abnormal condition*	A temporary diagnosis pending further examination or testing The determination of the cause of a disease

EXERCISES

A. Review *the Case Report on this spread before answering the questions.*

1. What symptoms did Mrs. Jacobs have when she presented to Dr. Lee's clinic?

_____

2. What does the physical examination reveal? _____

3. Does Mrs. Jacobs have hypertension or hypotension? _____

4. What is pedal edema? _____

5. What is another term for a provisional diagnosis? _____

B. Elements: *Use this exercise as a quick review of the elements in the WAD. Circle the correct choices, and then answer the question.*

1. In the term *hepatic,* the root means:

    pancreas   stomach   liver

2. The suffix in *cirrhosis* indicates this is:

    a condition   a surgical excision   a structure

3. *Bilirubin* is the color of:

    blood   milk   rust

4. The root in cirrhosis indicates a:

    color   size   location

5. Which three terms in the WAD refer to color?

    _____, _____, _____

LESSON 9.4 Gallbladder, Biliary Tract, and Pancreas (LO 9.1, 9.2, and 9.3)

Gallbladder and Biliary Tract (LO 9.1, 9.2, and 9.3)

On the underside of your liver is your **gallbladder,** which stores and concentrates the bile produced by the liver. The **cystic duct** from the gallbladder joins with the **hepatic duct** to form the **common bile duct.** This duct system, which moves the bile from the liver to the duodenum, is called the **biliary tract** *(Figure 9.17a and b).*

Disorders of the Gallbladder (LO 9.1, 9.2, 9.3, and 9.4)

Gallstones (cholelithiasis) can form in the gallbladder from excess cholesterol, bile salts, and bile pigment *(Figure 9.18).* The stones can vary in size and number. Risk factors are obesity, high-cholesterol diets, multiple pregnancies, and rapid weight loss.

Choledocholithiasis occurs when small stones become impacted in the common bile duct. This can cause biliary colic and jaundice *(see below).*

Cholecystitis is an acute or chronic inflammation of the gallbladder, usually associated with cholelithiasis and obstruction of the cystic duct with a stone.

Jaundice (icterus) is a symptom of many different diseases in the biliary tract and liver. It is a yellow discoloration of the skin and sclera of the eyes caused by deposits of bilirubin just below the skin's outer layers.

CASE REPORT 9.3 (CONTINUED)

Mrs. Jacobs presented in the emergency department with the classic gallstone symptoms of severe waves of right upper quadrant pain (biliary colic), nausea, and vomiting.

The Pancreas (LO 9.1, 9.2, and 9.3)

Your **pancreas** is a spongy, exocrine gland. **Exocrine** glands secrete fluids. In fact, many of the glands in your body are exocrine glands, including your sweat glands, mammary glands, and other digestive enzyme-releasing glands. The majority of the pancreas secretes digestive juices, but smaller areas of **pancreatic islet cells** secrete the hormones **insulin** and **glucagon** *(see Chapter 12).*

The pancreas produces pancreatic digestive juices that are excreted through the pancreatic duct. This duct joins the common bile duct shortly before it opens into the duodenum *(Figure 9.17b),* which encircles the top or head of the pancreas *(Figure 9.17b).* Pancreatic and bile juices then enter the duodenum. Other pancreatic cells secrete insulin and glucagon, which go directly into the bloodstream. This part of the pancreas is an **endocrine** (hormone-secreting) gland.

Pancreatic juices contain alkaline electrolytes, which help neutralize the acid chyme as it comes from the stomach, and enzymes, which break down starches, fats, and proteins into simpler elements.

Disorders of the Pancreas (LO 9.1, 9.2, 9.3, and 9.4)

Pancreatitis is an inflammation of the pancreas. The acute disease ranges from a mild, self-limiting episode to an acute life-threatening emergency. In the chronic form, there is a progressive destruction of pancreatic tissue leading to malabsorption and diabetes.

Pancreatic cancer is the fourth leading cause of cancer-related death. Treatment is surgical resection of the cancer. The prognosis is poor.

Cystic fibrosis (CF) is an inherited disease that becomes apparent in infancy or childhood. With CF, the pancreas, liver, intestines, sweat glands, and lungs all produce abnormally thick mucous secretions. The malabsorption of fat and protein leads to large, bulky, foul-smelling stools. Problems with thick mucous secretions in the lungs lead to chronic lung disease.

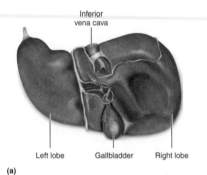

Inferior vena cava

Left lobe   Gallbladder   Right lobe

(a)

Cystic duct

Hepatic duct

Common bile duct

Pancreatic duct

Gallbladder

Duodenum

Tail of pancreas

Body of pancreas

Jejunum

(b)

▲ **FIGURE 9.17**
(a) Underside of liver.
(b) Anatomy of gallbladder, pancreas, and biliary tract.

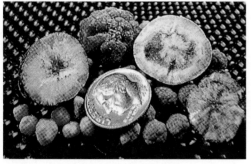

◀ **FIGURE 9.18**
Gallstones. The dime is included to illustrate the relative size of the gallstones.

Word	Pronunciation	Elements		Definition
cholecystitis	KOH-leh-sis-TIE-tis	S/ R/CF R/	-itis *inflammation* chol/e - *bile* -cyst- *bladder*	Inflammation of the gallbladder
cholecystectomy	KOH-leh-sis-TECK-toe-me	S/	-ectomy *surgical excision*	Surgical removal of the gallbladder
choledocholithiasis	koh-leh-**DOH**-koh-lih-**THIGH**-ah-sis	S/ R/CF R/	-iasis *condition* choledoch/o- *common bile duct* -lith- *stone*	Presence of a gallstone in the common bile duct
cholelithiasis	KOH-leh-lih-THIGH-ah-sis	S/ R/CF R/CF	-iasis *condition* chol/e- *bile* -lith/o- *stone*	Condition of having bile stones (gallstones)
cholelithotomy	KOH-leh-lih-THOT-oh-me	S/	-tomy *surgical incision*	Surgical removal of a gallstone(s)
endocrine	EN-doh-krin	P/ R/	endo- *within, inside* -crine *secrete*	A gland that produces an internal or hormonal substance and secretes it into the bloodstream
exocrine	EK-soh-krin	P/	exo- *outward, outside*	A gland that secretes substances outwardly through excretory ducts
gallstone	GAWL-stone	R/ R/	gall- *bitter* -stone *pebble*	Hard mass of cholesterol, calcium, and bilirubin that can be formed in the gallbladder and bile duct
gallbladder	GAWL-blad-er		bladder, Old English *receptacle*	Receptacle on the inferior surface of the liver for storing bile
glucagon	GLU-kah-gon	R/ R/	gluc- *glucose, sugar* -agon *to fight*	Hormone that mobilizes glucose from body storage
insulin	IN-syu-lin	S/ R/	-in *chemical compound* insul- *island*	Pancreatic hormone that suppresses blood glucose levels and transports glucose into cells
pancreas	PAN-kree-as		Greek *sweetbread*	Lobulated gland, the head of which is tucked into the curve of the duodenum
pancreatic (adj)	pan-kree-**AT**-ik	S/ R/	-ic *pertaining to* pancreat- *pancreas*	Pertaining to the pancreas
pancreatitis	PAN-kree-ah-TIE-tis	S/	-itis *inflammation*	Inflammation of the pancreas

EXERCISES

A. Review the *Case Report on this spread before answering the questions.*

1. What abbreviation could be used in the case report? _____

2. Define "biliary colic." _____

3. What is the difference between "cholelithiasis" and "choledocholithiasis"? _____
_____

4. Do both of the terms above involve a stone? _____

5. What type of surgery will Mrs. Jacobs most likely have? _____

B. Roots or combining forms *can remain the same, but the addition of other elements will construct entirely different medical terms. Use this group of elements, in addition to chol/e, to form the medical terms that are defined. Some elements you will use more than once; some elements you will not use at all. Fill in the blanks.*

The element chol/e means _____.

Add these elements to chol/e to form the medical terms defined below:

lith   choledoch/o   iasis   chol   ectomy   osis   cyst   otomy   cyst/o   itis

1. condition of gallstones: _____ / _____ / _____

2. surgical removal of gallbladder: _____ / _____ / _____

3. gallstone in the common bile duct: _____ / _____ / _____

4. surgical incision into gallbladder to remove gallstones: _____ / _____ / _____

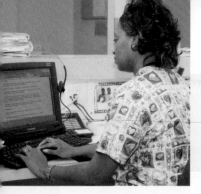

LESSON 9.5

Absorption and Malabsorption

OBJECTIVES

In the previous lessons in this chapter, you learned about the digestive secretions of the different segments of the digestive tract, liver, and pancreas. This information can now be brought together to review the overall process of digestion so that you will be able to use correct medical terminology to:

9.5.1 Explain the chemical digestion and absorption of proteins, carbohydrates, and fats.

9.5.2 Describe disorders of chemical digestion, absorption, and **malabsorption.**

CASE REPORT 9.4

YOU ARE

. . . a dietitian working at Fulwood Medical Center.

YOU ARE COMMUNICATING WITH

. . . Mrs. Jan Stark, a 36-year-old pottery maker, and her husband, Mr. Tom Stark. From her medical record, you see that Mrs. Stark has been referred to you by Dr. Cameron Grabowski, a gastroenterologist.
For the past 10 years, Mrs. Stark has had spasmodic episodes of **diarrhea** and **flatulence** associated with severe headaches and fatigue. During those episodes, her stools were greasy and pale. She has seen several physicians who have recommended low-fat, high-carbohydrate diets but she has had no relief. Dr. Grabowski has performed an intestinal biopsy through an oral **endoscopy** and diagnosed **celiac disease.** This condition is a sensitivity to the protein **gluten** that is found in wheat, rye, barley, and oats. Dr. Grabowski has asked you to ensure that Mrs. Stark accepts a diet free of gluten-containing foods like breads, cereals, cookies, and beer.

Chemical Digestion, Absorption, and Transport
(LO 9.1, 9.2, and 9.3)

Carbohydrates (LO 9.1, 9.2, and 9.3)

In your small intestine, carbohydrates like **starches** are broken down into simple sugars—glucose and fructose—which are absorbed by the lining cells and transferred to the capillaries of the **villi** *(Figure 9.19)*. The most commonly consumed carbohydrates are bread, soft drinks, cookies, cakes, doughnuts, syrups, jams, potatoes, and rice. From the capillaries of the villi, the simple sugars are carried to the liver by the **portal vein,** where the nonglucose sugars are converted to glucose. Glucose is the major source of energy for all cells.

Glycogen, the storage form of carbohydrate, is found in the liver and skeletal muscle. Glycogen in muscles supplies glucose during high-intensity and endurance exercise.

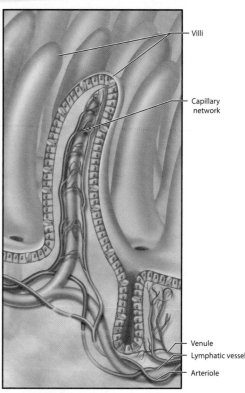

Villi

Capillary network

Venule
Lymphatic vessel
Arteriole

▲ **FIGURE 9.19**
Intestinal Villi.

Word	Pronunciation	Elements		Definition
celiac disease	SEE-lee-ack diz-EEZ	S/ R/ P/ R/	-ac *pertaining to* celi- *abdomen* dis- *apart* -ease *normal function*	Disease caused by sensitivity to gluten
diarrhea	die-ah-REE-ah	P/ R/	dia- *complete* -rrhea *flow, discharge*	Abnormally frequent and loose stools
endoscopy	en-DOS-koh-pee	P/ R/	endo- *inside, within* -scopy *to examine, view*	The use of an endoscope
endoscope	EN-doh-skope	R/	-scope *instrument for viewing*	Instrument used to examine the interior of a tubular or hollow organ
flatulence	FLAT-you-lents	S/ R/	-ence *forming* flatul- *excessive gas, flatus*	Excessive amount of gas in the stomach and intestines
flatus	FLAY-tus		Latin *blowing*	Gas or air expelled through the anus
gluten	GLU-ten		Latin *glue*	Insoluble protein found in wheat, barley, and oats
glycogen	GLYE-koh-jen	S/ R/CF	-gen *to produce* glyc/o- *sugar/glucose*	The body's principal carbohydrate reserve, stored in the liver and skeletal muscle
malabsorption	mal-ab-SORP-shun	S/ P/ R/	-ion *action, condition* mal- *bad, difficult* -absorpt- *swallow, take in*	Inadequate gastrointestinal absorption of nutrients
portal vein	POR-tal VANE		portal, Latin *gate* vein, Latin *vein*	The vein that carries blood from the intestines to the liver
starch	STARCH		Anglo-Saxon *stiffen*	Complex carbohydrate made of multiple units of glucose attached together
villus villi (pl)	VILL-us VILL-eye		Latin *shaggy hair*	Thin, hairlike projection, particularly of a mucous membrane lining a cavity

EXERCISES

A. Review *the Case Report on this spread before answering the questions.*

1. What is the meaning of the term *spasmodic episodes?* _____

2. What kind of specialist referred Mrs. Stark to the nutritionist?

   _____

3. When Mrs. Stark's condition flares up, what symptoms are present?

   _____

4. What procedure did Dr. Grabowski perform to get a definitive diagnosis for Mrs. Stark?

   _____

5. Why did Mrs. Stark not get any relief from her previous doctor's recommendations for a low-

   fat, high-carbohydrate diet? _____

STUDY HINT

Endoscope is a generic (general) term that means any instrument *(scope)* used to examine the inside *(endo)* of a tubular or hollow organ. The instrument obtains its specific name from the organ it is used to examine. Thus, an instrument used to view a stomach is a gastroscope specifically, but it is also an endoscope in general.

B. Construct *the correct medical term to match the definitions. Review the WAD before you fill in the blanks.*

1. inadequate gastrointestinal absorption of nutrients   _____ / _____ / _____

                                                                            P   R/CF   S

2. abnormally frequent and loose stools   _____ / _____ / _____

                                                        P   R/CF   S

3. examination of a hollow structure with a special instrument   _____ / _____ / _____

                                                                                 P   R/CF   S

4. excessive amount of gas in stomach and intestines   _____ / _____ / _____

                                                                      P   R/CF   S

5. the instrument used for endoscopy   _____ / _____ / _____

                                                      P   R/CF   S

Proteins (LO 9.1, 9.2, and 9.3)

Proteins are only 10% to 20% digested when they arrive in the duodenum and small intestine. Enzymes produced by cells in the small intestine, and the pancreatic enzyme trypsin, break down the remaining proteins into **amino acids.**

The amino acids are carried away in the blood and are transported to cells all over the body to be used as building blocks for new tissue formation.

Lipids (LO 9.1, 9.2, and 9.3)

Lipids (fats) enter the duodenum and small intestine as large globules. These have to be **emulsified** by the bile salts into smaller droplets so that pancreatic **lipase** (fat-reducing enzymes) can digest them into very small droplets of free **fatty acids** and **monoglycerides.**

These small droplets are taken up by the **lacteals** (lymphatic vessels) inside the villi and then move into the lymphatic system. The droplets now comprise a milky, fatty lymphatic fluid called **chyle,** which eventually reaches the thoracic duct and moves into the bloodstream *(see Chapter 7)*. Chyle is stored in adipose tissue. The fat-soluble vitamins A, D, E, and K are absorbed with the lipids.

Water (LO 9.1, 9.2, and 9.3)

Water has no caloric value and makes up approximately 60% of your body weight (about 10 gallons). Your small intestine absorbs 92% of your body's water, which is taken into the bloodstream through the capillaries in the villi *(Figure 9.20)*. Water-soluble vitamins, C and the B complex, are absorbed with water except for B_{12}. This is a large molecule that has to bind with intrinsic factor in the stomach so that cells in the distant ileum can receive it and absorb it into the bloodstream.

You can survive six to eight weeks without food, but only a few days without water. Although water is an integral part of all tissues, it is not stored in one particular place from which it can be released.

Minerals (LO 9.1, 9.2, and 9.3)

Minerals are absorbed along the whole length of the small intestine. Iron and calcium are absorbed according to the body's needs. The other minerals are absorbed regardless of need, and the kidneys excrete the surplus.

The major minerals are sodium **(Na)**, potassium **(K)**, calcium **(Ca)**, and magnesium **(Mg).**

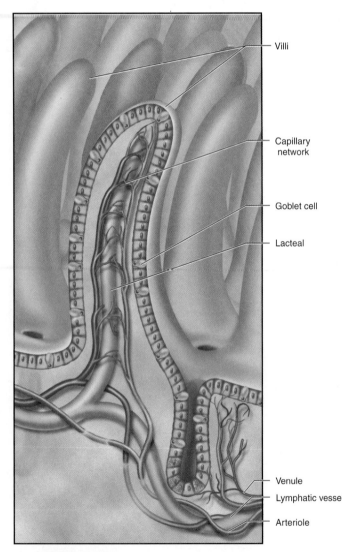

Villi

Capillary network

Goblet cell

Lacteal

Venule
Lymphatic vessel
Arteriole

▲ **FIGURE 9.20**
Intestinal Villi.

Word	Pronunciation		Elements	Definition
amino acid	ah-**ME**-no **ASS**-id	R/CF	amin/o- *nitrogen containing* acid, Latin *sour*	The basic building block for protein
chyle	KYLE		Greek *juice*	A milky fluid that results from the digestion and absorption of fats in the small intestine
emulsify	ee-**MUL**-sih-fye	S/ R/	-ify *to become* emuls- *suspend in a liquid*	Break up into very small droplets to suspend in a solution (emulsion)
emulsion (noun)	ee-**MUL**-shun	S/	-ion *condition, action*	The system that contains small droplets suspended in a liquid
lacteal	**LAK**-tee-al	S/ R/CF	-al *pertaining to* lact/e- *milk*	A lymphatic vessel carrying chyle away from the intestine
lipase	**LIE**-paze	S/ R/	-ase *enzyme* lip- *fat*	Enzyme that breaks down fat
lipid	**LIP**-id		Greek *fat*	General term for all types of fatty compounds; e.g., cholesterol, triglycerides, and fatty acids
mineral	**MIN**-er-al	S/ R/	-al *pertaining to* miner- *mines*	Inorganic compound usually found in the earth's crust

EXERCISES

A. Seek and find *the correct medical terms to fill in the blanks. The answers to the following questions can all be found on the two-page spread open in front of you.*

1. What proteins break down into: _____

2. Another name for minerals: _____

3. Milky fluid that results from the digestion and absorption of fats: _____

4. Term used to describe all types of fatty compounds: _____

5. Break up into small droplets to suspend in a liquid: _____

B. Continue searching *for the correct answer.*

1. Lymphatic vessel that carries chyle away from the intestine: _____

2. Inorganic compounds found in the earth's crust: _____

3. Number of calories in an ounce of water: _____

4. Percentage of the body's weight that is water: _____

5. List the four major minerals: _____

C. Rewrite *the only false statement in the exercise.*

Amino acids build new tissue formation.

Chyle is stored in bone marrow.

Another name for sodium is salt.

Water is absorbed back into your body in the small intestine.

Fat soluble vitamins are A, D, E, and K.

1. Corrected statement: _____

- In malnutrition, the body breaks down its own tissues to meet its nutritional and metabolic needs.

- Milk sugar is lactose. The enzyme lactase breaks down lactose into glucose.

- Diarrhea is caused by irritation of the intestinal lining that causes feces to pass through the intestine too quickly for adequate amounts of water to be reabsorbed.

CASE REPORT 9.4 (CONTINUED)

Mrs. Jan Stark, who presented in the emergency department (ED) with **dehydration**, was found to have celiac disease, a sensitivity to the protein gluten. This disease involves the destruction of epithelial cells of the digestive tract lining, so intestinal enzymes are not being produced and absorption is not taking place.

This diagnosis was made through an intestinal biopsy by oral endoscopy. A diet free of gluten-containing foods, like breads, cereals, cookies, and beer, relieved her symptoms.

Disorders of Absorption (LO 9.1, 9.2, 9.3, and 9.4)

The term **malabsorption syndromes** refers to a group of diseases in which intestinal absorption of nutrients is impaired.

Malnutrition can arise from malabsorption, but can also result from a lack of food, as with famine and poverty. Malnutrition can also result from a loss of appetite in people with cancer or a terminal illness.

Lactose intolerance occurs when the small intestine is not producing enough of the enzyme **lactase** to break down the milk sugar lactose. The result is diarrhea and cramps. Lactase can be taken in pill form before eating dairy products, and milk products can be avoided.

Crohn disease (or **regional enteritis**) is an inflammation of the small intestine, frequently in the ileum and occasionally also in the large intestine. The symptoms are abdominal pain, diarrhea, fatigue, and weight loss. There is no cure.

Constipation occurs when fecal movement through the large intestine is slow and thus too much water is reabsorbed by the large intestine. The feces become hardened. Constipation can be caused by lack of dietary fiber, lack of exercise, and emotional upset.

Gastroenteritis (stomach "flu") is an infection of the stomach and intestine that can be caused by a large number of bacteria and viruses. It causes vomiting, diarrhea, and fever. An outbreak of gastroenteritis can sometimes be traced to contaminated food or water.

Dysentery is a severe form of bacterial gastroenteritis with blood and mucus in frequent, watery stools.

Malnutrition, malabsorption, and severe forms of diarrhea and vomiting can cause dehydration and an electrolyte imbalance, possibly leading to coma and death.

S = Suffix   P = Prefix   R = Root   R/CF= Combining Form

Word	Pronunciation	Elements		Definition
constipation	kon-stih-**PAY**-shun	S/ R/	-ation *process* constip- *press together*	Hard, infrequent bowel movements
Crohn disease	**KRONE** diz-**EEZ**		Burrill Crohn, New York gastroenterologist, 1884–1983	Narrowing and thickening of terminal small bowel
(*also known as* **regional enteritis**)	**REE**-jun-al en-ter-I-tis	S/ R/	-itis *inflammation* enter- *intestine*	
dehydration	dee-high-**DRAY**-shun	S/ P/ R/	-ation *a process* de- *without* -hydr- *water*	Process of losing body water
dysentery	**DIS**-en-tare-ee	P/ R/	dys- *bad, difficult* -entery *condition of the intestine*	Disease with diarrhea, bowel spasms, fever, and dehydration
gastroenteritis	**GAS**-troh-en-ter-I-tis	S/ R/ R/CF	-itis *inflammation* -enter- *intestine* gastr/o- *stomach*	Inflammation of the stomach and intestines
lactose lactase	**LAK**-toes **LAK**-tase	S/ R/	Latin *milk sugar* -ase *enzyme* lact- *milk*	The disaccharide found in cow's milk Enzyme that breaks down lactose (milk sugar) to glucose and galactose
malnutrition	mal-nyu-**TRISH**-un	S/ P/ R/	-ion *process* mal- *bad, difficult, inadequate* -nutrit- *nourishment*	Inadequate nutrition from poor diet or inadequate absorption of nutrients

EXERCISES

A. Review *the Case Report on this spread before answering the questions.*

1. What is dehydration? _____

2. What is Mrs. Stark's final diagnosis? _____

3. Translate the following sentence into layman's language: "This diagnosis was made through an intestinal biopsy by oral endoscopy." _____
_____
_____

4. What types of food should Mrs. Stark avoid? _____

5. What sensitivity does Mrs. Stark have as a result of her disease? _____

B. Construct *the correct medical term based on the definition.*

1. inflammation of the stomach and intestines _____ / _____ / _____

2. process of losing body water _____ / _____ / _____

3. severe form of bacterial gastroenteritis _____ / _____ / _____

4. inadequate nutrition from poor diet _____ / _____ / _____

5. enzyme that breaks down lactose to glucose _____ / _____ / _____

C. Use the language *of gastroenterology for your answers.*

1. Because celiac disease destroys the digestive tract lining, what two things are *not* happening? a. _____
  b. _____

2. One letter can make a difference. Define *lactose* and *lactase*. _____
_____

3. Which element makes them different? _____

4. What is the difference between *gastroenteritis* and *regional enteritis?* _____
_____

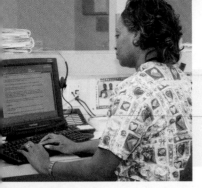

LESSON 9.6

The Large Intestine and Elimination

OBJECTIVES

Once your small intestine has digested and absorbed the nutrients, the residual materials must be prepared in your large intestine so they can be eliminated from your body. The information in this lesson will enable you to use correct medical terminology to:

9.6.1 Describe the structure and functions of the large intestine.

9.6.2 Outline disorders of the large intestine.

KEYNOTES

- A **sphincter** is a ring of smooth muscle that forms a one-way valve.

- Colon: Ascending to transverse to descending to sigmoid to rectum to anus.

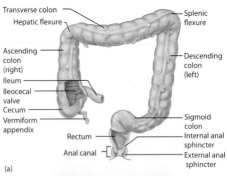

(a)

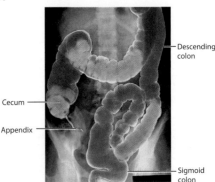

(b)

Structure and Functions of the Large Intestine
(LO 9.1, 9.2, and 9.3)

Structure of the Large Intestine
(LO 9.1, 9.2, and 9.3)

Your **large intestine** is so named because its diameter is much greater than that of your small intestine. In your abdominal cavity, the large intestine forms a perimeter around the central mass of the small intestine.

At the junction between the small and large intestines, a ring of smooth muscle called the **ileocecal sphincter** forms a one-way valve. This allows chyme to pass into the large intestine and prevents the large intestine's contents from backing into the ileum.

The **cecum** is located at the beginning of the large intestine. It is a pouch in the abdomen's right lower quadrant. A narrow tube with a closed end (the **vermiform appendix**) projects downward from the cecum (*Figure 9.21a and 9.21b*). The function of the appendix is not known.

The ascending **colon** begins at the cecum and extends upward to underneath the liver. Here, it makes a sharp turn at the hepatic **flexure** and becomes the transverse colon. At the left side of the abdomen, near the spleen at the splenic flexure, the transverse colon turns downward to form the descending colon. At the pelvic brim, the descending colon forms an S-shaped curve called the **sigmoid** colon. This descends in the pelvis to become the rectum and then the **anal canal.**

The **rectum** has three transverse folds—rectal valves that enable it to retain **feces** while passing gas (flatus).

◀ **FIGURE 9.21**
Large Intestine.
(a) Surface anatomy.
(b) X-ray of large intestine following barium enema.

The anal canal (*Figure 9.22*) is the last 1 to 2 inches of the large intestine, opening to the outside as the **anus.** An internal anal sphincter, composed of smooth muscle from the intestinal wall, and an external anal sphincter, composed of skeletal muscle that can be controlled voluntarily, guard the exit of the anus.

Functions of the Large Intestine
(LO 9.1, 9.2, and 9.3)

Your large intestine has the following key functions:

- **Absorption** of water and electrolytes. The large intestine receives more than 1 liter (1,000 ml) of chyme each day from the small intestine. It reabsorbs water and electrolytes to reduce the volume of chyme to 100 to 150 ml of feces, which are eliminated by **defecation;**

- **Secretion** of mucus that protects the intestinal wall and holds particles of fecal matter together;

- **Digestion** (by the bacteria that inhabit the large intestine) of any food remnants that have escaped the small intestine's digestive enzymes;

- **Peristalsis** happens a few times a day in the large intestine to produce mass movements toward the rectum; and

- **Elimination** of materials that were not digested or absorbed.

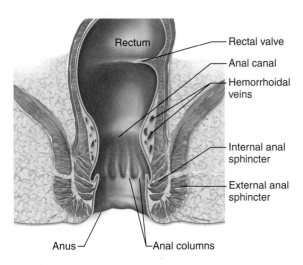

▶ **FIGURE 9.22**
Anal Canal.

S = Suffix   P = Prefix   R = Root   R/CF= Combining Form

Word	Pronunciation		Elements	Definition
anus	A-nus		Latin *ring*	Terminal opening of the digestive tract through which feces are discharged
anal (adj)	A-nal	S/ R/CF	-al *pertaining to* an/o- *anus*	Pertaining to the anus
anorectal junction	A-no-**RECK**-tal **JUNK**-shun	R/ S/ R/	-rect- *rectum* -ion *condition, action* junct- *joining together*	The junction between the anus and rectum
appendix	ah-**PEN**-dicks		Latin *appendage*	Small blind projection from the pouch of the cecum
appendicitis	ah-pen-dih-**SIGH**-tis	S/ R/	-itis *inflammation* appendic- *appendix*	Inflammation of the appendix
appendectomy *(note elimination of "Ic" prior to "ec" of -ectomy)*	ah-pen-**DEK**-toe-me	S/	-ectomy *surgical excision*	Surgical removal of the appendix
colon	**KOH**-lon		Greek *colon*	The large intestine, extending from the cecum to the rectum
colic (adj)	**KOL**-ik	S/ R/	-ic *pertaining to* col- *colon*	Spasmodic, crampy pains in the abdomen
colitis	koh-**LIE**-tis	S/	-itis *inflammation*	Inflammation of the colon
feces	**FEE**-sees		Latin *dregs*	Undigested, waste material discharged from the bowel
fecal (adj)	**FEE**-kal	S/ R/	-al *pertaining to* fec- *feces*	Pertaining to feces
defecation	def-eh-**KAY**-shun	S/ P/	-ation *process* de- *removal*	Evacuation of feces from rectum and anus
flexure	**FLEK**-shur		Latin *bond*	A bend in a structure
Ileum ileocecal sphincter	**ILL**-ee-um **ILL**-ee-oh-**SEE**-cal **SFINK**-ter	S/ R/CF R/	Latin *roll up, twist* -al *pertaining to* ile/o- *ileum* -cec- *cecum* sphincter, Greek *band*	Third portion of the small intestine Band of muscle that encircles the junction of ileum and cecum
rectum	**RECK**-tum	R/	Latin *straight* rect- *rectum*	Terminal part of the colon from the sigmoid to the anal canal
rectal (adj)	**RECK**-tal	S/	-al *pertaining to*	Pertaining to the rectum
sigmoid	**SIG**-moyd		Greek *letter "S"*	Sigmoid colon is shaped like an "S"

EXERCISES

A. Apply *the language of the digestive system and answer the following questions.*

1. What part of the digestive system contains both an internal and external sphincter? _____

2. What body part has no known use or function? _____

3. What is a ring of smooth muscle that forms a one-way valve called? _____

4. How did the "large" intestine get its name? _____

5. Where is the cecum located? _____

6. The *hepatic flexure* is near what major body organ? _____

B. Deconstruct: *Attack a medical term with your analytical skills. Break down these terms into their elements to define the word. Know the meaning of the elements = know the meaning of the term. Fill in the chart.*

Medical Term	Meaning of Prefix	Meaning of Root/CF	Meaning of Suffix	Meaning of Term
colitis	1.	2.	3.	4.
defecation	5.	6.	7.	8.
anorectal	9.	10.	11.	12.
ileocecal	13.	14.	15.	16.

Disorders of the Large Intestine and Anal Canal
(LO 9.1, 9.2, and 9.3)

- A **proctologist** is a surgical specialist in diseases of the anus and rectum.

- **Fissures** are tears; **fistulas** are abnormal passages.

- Consuming black licorice, Pepto-Bismol, or blueberries can produce black stools.

Disorders of the Large Intestine
(LO 9.1, 9.2, 9.3, and 9.4)

Appendicitis is the most common cause of acute abdominal pain in the right lower quadrant. If neglected, the inflamed appendix can rupture, leading to **peritonitis.** Appendicitis is treated with a surgical appendectomy, usually performed through laparoscopy.

Diverticulosis is the presence of small pouches bulging outward through weak spots in the large intestine's lining (*Figure 9.23*). The pouches are asymptomatic until they become infected and inflamed, a condition called **diverticulitis.** The most likely cause of **diverticular disease** (diverticulosis and diverticulitis) is a low-fiber diet.

Ulcerative colitis is an extensive inflammation and ulceration of the large intestine's lining. It produces bouts of bloody diarrhea, crampy pain, weight loss, and an electrolyte imbalance.

Irritable bowel syndrome (IBS) is an increasingly common large-bowel disorder presenting with crampy pain, gas, and changes in bowel habits to either constipation or diarrhea. There are no anatomical changes seen in the bowel. The cause is unknown.

Polyps, which vary in size and shape, are masses of tissue arising from the large intestine's wall and protruding into the bowel lumen. Although most polyps are benign, an endoscopic biopsy can determine if they are precancerous or cancerous.

Colon and rectal cancers are the second cause of cancer deaths after lung cancer. The majority of these cancers occur in the rectum and sigmoid colon. They can spread through the bowel wall, extend down the lumen, and metastasize to regional lymph nodes and to liver, lungs, bones, and brain through the bloodstream.

Obstruction of the large bowel can be caused by cancers, large polyps, or diverticulitis.

Intussusception is a form of obstruction that occurs when one segment of bowel slips inside another segment, causing an obstruction.

Proctitis is an inflammation of the rectum's lining, often associated with ulcerative colitis, Crohn disease, or radiation therapy.

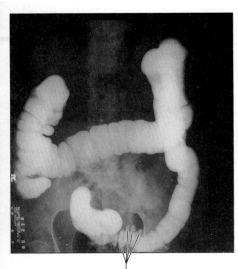

▲ **FIGURE 9.23**
Barium Enema Showing Diverticulosis.

Diverticula

Disorders of the Anal Canal
(LO 9.1, 9.2, 9.3, and 9.4)

Hemorrhoids are dilated veins in the submucosa (connective tissue layer) of the anal canal, often associated with pregnancy, chronic constipation, diarrhea, or aging. They protrude into the anal canal (**internal**) or bulge out along the edge of the anus (**external**) *(Figure 9.24),* producing pain and bright red blood from the anus. A **thrombosed** hemorrhoid, in which blood has clotted, is very painful.

Anal fissures are tears in the anal canal's lining, perhaps from difficult bowel movements (**BMs**). **Anal fistulas** occur following abscesses in the anal glands and are an abnormal passage (fistula) between the anal canal and the skin outside the anus. Surgical procedures—a **fistulectomy** and a **fistulotomy**—are used to treat anal fistulas.

Gastrointestinal (GI) Bleeding
(LO 9.1, 9.2, and 9.3)

GI tract bleeding can have a variety of causes, which are not always easy to recognize. Sometimes, the bleeding can be internal and painless. It can present in different ways, however, to provide a clue as to the site of bleeding:

- **Hematemesis** is the vomiting of bright red blood, which indicates an upper GI source of bleeding (esophagus, stomach, duodenum) that is brisk.

- **Vomiting of "coffee grounds"** occurs when bleeding from an upper GI source has slowed or stopped.

- **Melena,** the passage of black, tarry stools, usually indicates upper GI bleeding.

- **Occult blood** cannot be seen in the stool, but when a chemical fecal occult blood test (**Hemoccult**) is positive, the source of the bleeding can be anywhere in the GI tract.

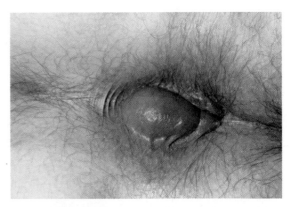

▲ **FIGURE 9.24**
External Hemorrhoid.

BM   bowel movement
IBS   irritable bowel syndrome

Word	Pronunciation	Elements		Definition
bowel	BOUGH-el		Latin *sausage*	Another name for intestine
diverticulum	die-ver-**TICK**-you-lum	S/ R/	-um *tissue, structure* diverticul- *byroad*	A pouchlike opening or sac from a tubular structure (e.g., intestine)
diverticula (pl) diverticulosis	di-ver-**TICK**-you-lah DIE-ver-tick-you-**LOW**-sis	S/	-osis *condition*	Presence of a number of small pouches in the wall of the large intestine
diverticulitis	DIE-ver-tick-you-**LIE**-tis	S/	-itis *inflammation*	Inflammation of the diverticula
fissure	**FISH**-ur		Latin *slit*	Deep furrow or cleft
fistula	**FIS**-tyu-lah		Latin *pipe, tube*	Abnormal passage
hemorrhoid hemorrhoids (pl) hemorrhoidectomy (Note: *This term has two suffixes.*)	**HEM**-oh-royd **HEM**-oh-roy-**DEK**-toh-me	S/ R/CF S/	-rrhoid *flow* hem/o- *blood* -ectomy *surgical excision*	Dilated rectal vein producing painful anal swelling Surgical removal of hemorrhoids
intussusception	**IN**-tuss-sus-**SEP**-shun	S/ P/ R/	-ion *action, condition* intus- *within* -suscept- *to take up*	The slipping of one part of bowel inside another to cause obstruction
melena	mel-**EN**-ah		Greek *black*	The passage of black, tarry stools
occult blood Hemoccult test	oh-**KULT BLUD** **HEEM**-o-kult **TEST**		occult, Latin *to hide*	Blood that cannot be seen in the stool but is positive on a fecal occult blood test Trade name for a fecal occult blood test
peritoneum peritoneal (adj) peritonitis	per-ih-toe-**NEE**-um **PER**-ih-toe-**NEE**-al **PER**-ih-toe-**NIE**-tis	S/ R/CF S/ S/	-um *tissue* periton/e- *stretch over* -al *pertaining to* -itis *inflammation*	Membrane that lines the abdominal cavity Pertaining to the peritoneum Inflammation of the peritoneum
polyp polyposis polypectomy	**POL**-ip pol-ih-**POH**-sis pol-ip-**ECK**-toh-mee	S/ R/ S/	-osis *condition* polyp- *polyp* -ectomy *surgical excision*	Mass of tissue that projects into the lumen of bowel Presence of several polyps Excision or removal of a polyp
proctitis proctologist	prok-**TIE**-tis prok-**TOL**-oh-jist	S/ R/ S/ R/CF	-itis *inflammation* proct- *rectum* -logist *specialist* proct/o- *rectum*	Inflammation of the lining of the rectum A surgical specialist in diseases of the anus and rectum

EXERCISES

A. Suffixes: *This is a two-part exercise. First, insert the correct suffix to complete the term. Then circle the word in the definition that has the same meaning as the suffix. (There are more suffixes than you need.)*

osis   ectomy   um   itis   al   ion

1. excision or removal of a polyp   polyp/ _____

2. inflammation of the diverticula   diverticul/ _____

3. membranous structure lining the abdominal cavity   peritone/ _____

4. condition of having multiple polyps   polyp/ _____

5. pertaining to the peritoneum   peritone/ _____

B. Apply *the language of the digestive system and answer the following questions.*

1. List all the terms on this spread that mean *inflammation of:* _____

2. What is the difference between *diverticulitis* and *diverticulosis?* _____

_____

3. Where else in the body can you have polyps? _____

4. What are dilated veins in the anal canal called? _____

LESSON 9.6

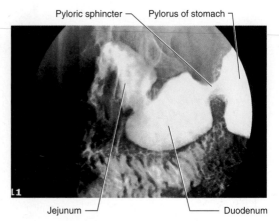

Pyloric sphincter — Pylorus of stomach

Jejunum — Duodenum

▲ **FIGURE 9.25**
Barium Meal.

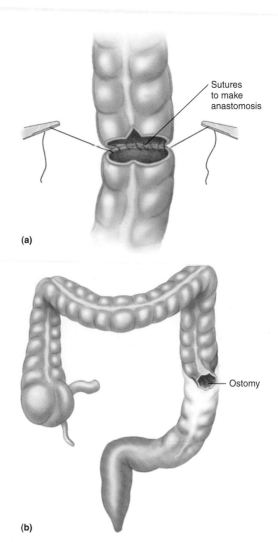

Sutures to make anastomosis

(a)

Ostomy

(b)

▲ **FIGURE 9.26**
Intestinal Resections.
(a) Anastomosis. (b) Ostomy.

Diagnostic and Therapeutic Procedures
(LO 9.1, 9.2, and 9.3)

Procedures for the Biliary System (LO 9.1, 9.2, and 9.3)

Specific diagnostic and therapeutic procedures for the bile duct or biliary system include the following three approaches.

A **cholangiography** requires the intravenous injection of a dye, followed by an X-ray of the biliary system so that the biliary system can be viewed.

A **cholecystectomy** is the surgical removal of the gallbladder through an open incision or by laparoscopic cholecystectomy.

A **cholelithotomy** is the surgical removal of gallstones.

Diagnostic Procedures for the Digestive Tract
(LO 9.1, 9.2, and 9.3)

A number of diagnostic procedures can be used to effectively determine issues related to the digestive tract.

Barium swallow involves ingestion of barium sulfate, a contrast material, to show details of the pharynx and esophagus on an X-ray.

Barium meal *(Figure 9.25)* uses barium sulfate to study the distal esophagus, stomach, and duodenum on an X-ray.

Enteroscopy through an oral endoscope is used to visualize and biopsy tumors and ulcers, and to control bleeding from the esophagus, stomach, and duodenum. This procedure is also called **esophagogastroduodenoscopy.**

Angiography uses dye to highlight blood vessels. It can be used to define the site of a bleed.

Fecal occult blood test (Hemoccult) is used to detect the presence of blood not visible to the naked eye.

Nasogastric aspiration and **lavage** that shows bright red blood indicates active upper GI bleeding. Vomiting of coffee-ground material indicates the bleeding has slowed or stopped.

Upper GI barium X-rays are less accurate than **panendoscopy** at identifying the bleeding lesion.

Barium enema involves the injection of a radiographic contrast material into the large intestine as an enema, and X-ray films are taken.

Endoscopy enables direct visual examination of the intestine with a flexible tube containing light-transmitting glass fibers or a video transmitter. Endoscopy can also be used to perform a biopsy, remove polyps (polypectomy), and coagulate bleeding lesions. **Panendoscopy** examines the esophagus, stomach, and duodenum.

Anoscopy examines the anus and lower rectum with a rigid instrument. **Flexible sigmoidoscopy** examines the rectum and sigmoid colon. **Colonoscopy** examines the whole length of the colon. **Gastroscopy** examines the stomach. **Proctoscopy** examines the anus.

Digital rectal exam is performed by the physician, who palpates the rectum and prostate gland with an index finger.

Surgical Procedures for the Digestive Tract
(LO 9.1, 9.2, and 9.3)

Once a digestive tract problem has been accurately diagnosed using one or more of the above procedures, several surgical options are available.

Intestinal resections are used to surgically remove diseased portions of the intestine. The remaining portions of the intestine can be joined together through an **anastomosis** *(Figure 9.26a)*. If there is insufficient bowel remaining, an **ostomy** *(Figure 9.26b)* can be performed, in which the end of the bowel opens onto the skin at a **stoma** (a surgical, artificial opening). **Ileostomy** and **colostomy** are two common procedures.

Word	Pronunciation	Elements		Definition
anastomosis	ah-**NAS**-toh-**MOH**-sis	S/ R/	-osis *condition* anastom- *provide a mouth*	A surgically made union between two tubular structures
anastomoses (pl)	ah-**NAS**-toh-**MOH**-seez			
endoscope	**EN**-doh-skope	P/ R/	endo- *within, inside* -scope *instrument for viewing*	Instrument to examine the inside of a hollow or tubular organ
endoscopy	en-**DOS**-koh-pee	P/ R/	endo- *within, inside* -scopy *to examine, to view*	The use of an endoscope
colonoscopy	koh-lon-**OSS**-koh-pee	R/CF	colon/o *colon*	Examination of the inside of the colon by endoscopy
panendoscopy (Note: *two* *prefixes*) proctoscopy (*also called* anoscopy) sigmoidoscopy	pan-en-**DOS**-koh-pee prok-**TOSS**-koh-pee sig-moi-**DOS**-koh-pee	P/ P/ R/CF R/ R/ R/CF	pan- *all* endo- *within, inside* proct/o- *anus* -scopy *to examine, to view* sigm- *Greek "S"* sigmoid/o- *sigmoid colon*	Examination of the inside of the esophagus, stomach, and upper duodenum using a flexible fiber-optic endoscope Examination of the inside of the anus by endoscopy Examination of the sigmoid colon by endoscopy
gastroscopy	gas-**TROSS**-koh-pee	R/CF	gastr/o- *stomach*	Examination of the inside of the stomach by endoscopy
enema	**EN**-eh-mah		Greek *injection*	An injection of fluid into the rectum
ostomy	**OSS**-toe-me	S/- R/	-stomy *new opening* os- *mouth*	Artificial opening into a tubular structure
colostomy ileostomy	koh-**LOSS**-toe-me ill-ee-**OS**-toe-me	R/CF R/CF	col/o- *colon* ile/o- *ileum*	Artificial opening from the colon to the outside of the body Artificial opening from the ileum to the outside of the body
stoma	**STOW**-mah		Greek *mouth*	Artificial opening

EXERCISES

A. Test yourself *on the elements contained in the WAD. The prefixes and suffixes you will see again in terms in other chapters. Match the element in column 1 with its definition in column 2.*

_____ **1.** os	**A.** colon	
_____ **2.** gastro	**B.** instrument for viewing	
_____ **3.** endo	**C.** all	
_____ **4.** colo	**D.** mouth	
_____ **5.** scope	**E.** condition	
_____ **6.** procto	**F.** ileum	
_____ **7.** stomy	**G.** stomach	
_____ **8.** ileo	**H.** within	
_____ **9.** pan	**I.** new opening	
_____ **10.** osis	**J.** anus	

B. Cover the WAD *with a piece of paper and spell the following terms correctly. Circle the best answer.*

1. procktologist   proctologist   practologist

2. intuception   intussception   intussusception

3. polyp   polip   polypp

4. anastomossis   anastamossis   anastomosis

5. peritineum   peritoneum   peritonium

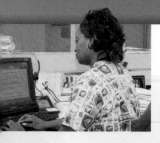

CHAPTER 9 REVIEW THE DIGESTIVE SYSTEM

CHALLENGE YOUR KNOWLEDGE

A. Roots/Combining forms *are the core meaning of every term. These terms all end in itis, which means inflammation. The root will tell you exactly what is inflamed. If you slash the term first, this will help isolate the roots. Fill in the chart.*

Medical Term	Root	Meaning of Root	Meaning of Medical Term
appendicitis	1.	2.	3.
cholecystitis	4.	5.	6.
colitis	7.	8.	9.
diverticulitis	10.	11.	12.
esophagitis	13.	14.	15.
gastritis	16.	17.	18.
gastroenteritis	19.	20.	21.
gingivitis	22.	23.	24.
hepatitis	25.	26.	27.
pancreatitis	28.	29.	30.
periodontitis	31.	32.	33.
peritonitis	34.	35.	36.
proctitis	37.	38.	39.

B. Spelling demons: *Have a fellow student dictate the following terms to you. Cover 1–10 with a piece of paper, and write your terms on the lines Try your best to spell them correctly on the first attempt!*

1. intussusception _____

2. hemorrhoidectomy _____

3. dyspepsia _____

4. gastroenterologist _____

5. peristalsis _____

6. cirrhosis _____

7. aphthous _____

8. pyorrhea _____

9. herniorrhaphy _____

10. hematemesis _____

C. Roots: *Master all forms of the same term, including the plurals. Always analyze a term beginning with the suffix. Fill in the blanks.*

1. **diverticulitis**   **diverticulum**   **diverticulosis**   **diverticula**

   What starts out as a single _____, if left untreated, can lead to many _____.

   The condition of having a number of these small pouches in the wall of the large intestine is known as _____.

   Should these pouches become inflamed, _____ will result.

2. **polypectomy**   **polyposis**   **polyp (singular)**

   The first polyp was found on sigmoidoscopy. A follow-up colonoscopy 6 months later found several more (plural)

   _____ in the large intestine. Diagnosis is _____.

   Proposed treatment is _____.

3. **peritoneum**   **peritonitis**   **peritoneal**

   The _____ laceration sliced completely through the _____.

   Because of an infection in the wound, the patient developed _____.

4. **gingivectomy**   **gingival**   **gingivitis**   **gingiva**

   The patient's _____ tissue is severely infected. Diagnosis is _____.

   A _____ has been scheduled; I will try to preserve as much of the healthy _____

   as possible.

D. Greek and Latin are the origins for many medical terms. *Give a meaning for each term; then use any three terms in sentences of your choice that are not directly out of this book. Fill in the chart.*

Medical Term	Meaning
bolus	1.
canker	2.
caries	3.
esophagus	4.
intestine	5.
pulp	6.
saliva	7.
ulcer	8.
uvula	9.

1. _____

   _____

   _____

2. _____

   _____

   _____

3. _____

   _____

   _____

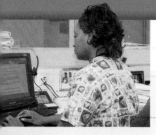

E. Prefixes make the difference *in precision. Analyze the two medical terms in each pair below. Write a brief description of how they differ, based on their prefixes.*

1. *emesis* and *hematemesis* _____

_____

2. *symptomatic* and *asymptomatic* _____

_____

F. Recall and review: *How well do you remember these word elements from a previous chapter? Try to answer without looking back to check. Fill in the chart.*

Element	Medical Term with this Element	Type of Element (P, R, CF, or S)	Meaning of Element	Meaning of Term
brady	1.	2.	3.	4.
pector	5.	6.	7.	8.
ptysis	9.	10.	11.	12.
cyano	13.	14.	15.	16.
ectasis	17.	18.	19.	20.

G. Construct medical terms *to match the definitions given. You are given more elements than you need for possible answers. Fill in the blanks.*

bari	abdomino	heme	deglutit	par	ary
ar	ot	mastic	lingu	dys	halit
laparo	odont	emesis	peri	mandibul	gingiv
phagia	rrhea	sub	rrhaphy	hemat	hiat

1. pertaining to food or nutrition   *aliment/*_____

2. removal of diseased gum tissue   _____/*ectomy*

3. salivary gland beside the ear   _____/*id*

4. underneath the tongue   *sub/*_____/*al*

5. examination of the contents of the abdomen   _____/*scopy*

6. around a tooth   _____/*ondont/al*

7. purulent discharge   *pyo/* _____

8. process of swallowing   _____/*ion*

9. bad breath   _____/*osis*

10. management of obesity   _____/*atrics*

H. Word attack: *Work through this exercise step-by-step for tips on how to apply your knowledge of elements to answer multiple-choice questions.*

Circle the term with the element meaning *difficult* or *bad:*

  a. anorexia

  b. perforation

  c. indigestion

  d. dyspepsia

  e. stricture

1. First, discard any answer choice(s) that do not break down into elements, since you are looking for a term with an element.

Discard: _____

2. Since prefixes are the most usual element for description (size, color, location, etc.), start by analyzing the prefixes. The prefixes are:

_____ means _____

_____ means _____

_____ means _____

_____ means _____

3. The correct answer is _____.

I. Identification: *The following word bank contains identifications for the terms in the chart. Put the correct identification next to each term in the chart. There are more words in the bank than medical terms.*

  Word Bank:

procedure	symptom	disease
adjective	plural term	noun
singular term	structure	instrument
process	inflammation	organ

Medical Term	Identification
diarrhea	**1.**
duodenum	**2.**
dysentery	**3.**
endoscope	**4.**
gingivectomy	**5.**
mucus	**6.**
tongue	**7.**
varicose	**8.**
villi	**9.**

J. Precision in documentation: *Get the stone in the right place: cholelithiasis or choledocholithiasis? Make the correct choice of medical terminology. Fill in the blanks.*

1. Patient's films revealed a stone in the common bile duct. Diagnosis: _____

2. The presence of a stone in the patient's gallbladder was confirmed by the radiologist. Diagnosis: _____

3. Acute or chronic inflammation of the gallbladder. Diagnosis: _____

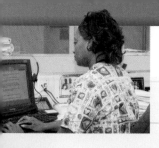

K. *Some of the terms in this chapter are particularly hard to spell and pronounce. Refer to the Student Online Learning Center (www.mhhe.com/AllanEss2e) for pronunciation practice, and remember that spelling is important! Read these sentences aloud after you have circled your choices for the correct spelling.*

1. The (nasopharynx/nasopharyix) is behind the nose and above the soft palate.

2. (Hyatus/Hiatus) is rooted in the Latin word for opening and is the *opening* through the diaphragm for the (esophagis/esophagus).

3. (Sphincter/Sphinchter) is a root meaning *a band* and is a band of muscle that encircles a tube.

4. (Uvula/Vuvula) comes from the Latin meaning *small grape*.

5. (Postprandial/Postperandial) medication, meaning medication *taken after meals,* has been ordered.

6. (Hemotemasis/Hematemesis) is the (vomiting/vomitting) of blood.

7. Throat cancer would produce (dysphagia/dyspagia).

8. (Varricces/Varices) is the plural of (varix/varex) and means *dilated vein*. The adjective is (varicose/varricose).

9. (Hernioraphy/Herniorrhaphy) is the surgical fixation of a hernia.

L. Translate these sentences, *which come directly from this chapter. Express the same thought in language your patient can understand.*

"Choledocholithiasis can cause biliary colic and jaundice."

_____

_____

_____

_____

_____

_____

"Endoscopy can be used to perform a biopsy of a polyp, polypectomy, and to coagulate bleeding lesions."

_____

_____

_____

_____

_____

_____

M. Chapter challenge: *Circle the best answer.*

1. The "R" in the abbreviation *GERD* stands for:

   a. reflex

   b. removal

   c. reflux

   d. resection

   e. resorption

2. What do all these terms have in common: *diarrhea, flatulence, pyorrhea?*

   a. They are all symptoms.

   b. None of them has a prefix.

   c. They are all misspelled.

   d. They all relate to the large intestine.

   e. They have all of the above in common.

3. The one term that is *not* a body process is:

   a. peristalsis

   b. secretion

   c. deglutition

   d. mastication

   e. halitosis

4. *Regional enteritis* is another name for:

   a. diverticulosis

   b. IBS

   c. celiac disease

   d. peritonitis

   e. Crohn disease

5. Hiatal hernia occurs when:

   a. a portion of the intestine telescopes in on itself

   b. a portion of the stomach protrudes through the diaphragm

   c. a portion of the liver protrudes through the stomach

   d. a portion of the stomach protrudes through the intestine

   e. a portion of the bowel protrudes through the stomach

6. The term that contains two prefixes is:

   a. panendoscopy

   b. gastroenterology

   c. nasopharynx

   d. submandibular

   e. periodontal

7. *Cholecystectomy* and *cholelithotomy* are both procedures on the:

   a. small intestine

   b. pancreas

   c. liver

   d. large intestine

   e. gallbladder

8. Proofread the following sentences. Which is the only one that is correct?

   a. A gingivectomy creates a new opening outside the body.

   b. Melena is the passage of black, tarry stools.

   c. Dysphagia is difficulty in chewing.

   d. The roof of the mouth is called the uvula.

   e. The maxilla is the lower jaw.

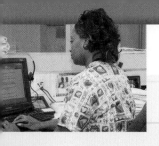

N. The two suffixes *scope* and *scopy* are attached to many medical terms you will meet in later chapters. Scope *is the actual instrument used in the procedure. The procedure itself is the* scopy. *Start by slashing the terms into elements in the first column, and then utilize the language of gastroenterology to fill in the chart for this exercise.*

Name of Instrument	Name of Procedure	Definition of Procedure
anoscope	1.	2.
colonoscope	3.	4.
endoscope	5.	6.
gastroscope	7.	8.
laparoscope	9.	10.
panendoscope	11.	12.
proctoscope	13.	14.
sigmoidscope	15.	16.

O. Terminology challenge: *Train your eye and ear to know the difference. Words can be very similar looking or sounding but mean entirely different things. If you really understand the following medical terms, you can explain them to a fellow student. Explain to your classmate the difference between them.*

1. *chyle* and *chyme*

_____

_____

2. *fissure* and *fistula*

_____

_____

3. *stricture* and *sphincter*

_____

_____

P. Chapter challenge: *Circle the best answer.*

1. What is the adjective used to describe a *dilated vein?*

   a. adipose   **d.** alimentary

   b. varicose   **e.** sublingual

   c. edematous

2. What substance in the body is harder than bone?

   a. dentine   **d.** plaque

   b. papilla   **e.** tartar

   c. pulp

3. The fungus *Candida albicans* causes:

   a. caries

   b. aphthous ulcers

   c. thrush

   d. canker sores

   e. fever blisters

4. Icterus is another term for:

   a. peristalsis

   b. cirrhosis

   c. jaundice

   d. diverticulosis

   e. GERD

5. The set of terms that are all diagnoses is:

   a. cholangiography, jaundice, cholelithiasis

   b. endoscopy, icterus, cholecystectomy

   c. hepatitis, diverticulosis, choledocholithiasis

   d. pancreatitis, polypectomy, anoscopy

   e. diabetes, cystic fibrosis, cholelithotomy

6. If you have *postprandial* burning chest pain, it is coming:

   a. after you go to bed

   b. before a meal

   c. when you wake up

   d. after a meal

   e. at none of these times

7. Which is the only term that signifies the *bile duct*?

   a. cholelithiasis

   b. cholecystitis

   c. cholelithotomy

   d. choledocholithiasis

   e. cholecystectomy

Q. Where am I? *Use the language of the digestive system to answer the following questions.*

   1. Where are the taste buds located? Be specific.

   _____

   _____

   2. Where is the *splenic flexure* found?

   _____

   _____

   3. Where is the *alimentary canal?*

   _____

   _____

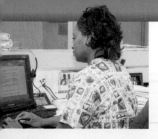

R. Case Report challenge: *Now that you are more comfortable with the terms in this chapter, you can apply that knowledge and briefly answer the questions about the Case Report.*

You may someday find yourself doing medical transcription in a hospital or physician's office. Proofread the beginning of the letter Dr. Walsh has sent to the patient's insurance company, asking for preauthorization for her surgery. Underline or highlight *all the errors;* then rewrite the correct terms on the lines below the letter. Then add a brief definition of the term, using the Glossary or a medical dictionary.

> *Dear Doctor Leavenworth,*
> *Request for Authorization of Surgery*
> *Re: Mrs. Martha Jones.*
> *Subscriber ID # FMC 056437*
> *Mrs. Jones is a 52-year-old former waitress, recently divorced. She is 5 feet 4 Inches tall and weighs 275 pounds. She has Type III diabeetes with frequent episodes of hyperglycemia and also ketoacidoses requiring three different hospitalizations. She now has diabetick retinnopathy and peripheral vascullitis. Complicating this is hypertension (185/110), coronery artery disease, and pulmonary edema.*

1. Write the correct form of the misspelled words and a brief definition here:

_____

_____

_____

_____

_____

_____

_____

_____

2. Critical thinking: Analyze the questions, formulate your answers, and be prepared to discuss in class:

a. Why are precertifications necessary for surgery? _____

_____

_____

b. What types of information will the insurance company need to determine Mrs. Jones' need for this surgery?_____

_____

_____

c. Assuming this is not an electronic medical record, what are your thoughts on why precision in communication is important in a patient's

medical record?_____

_____

_____

S. Case Report challenge: *Reread the following Case Report on Mrs. Jan Stark. Remember to highlight or underline the medical terms before you answer the questions.*

> For the past 10 years she has had spasmodic episodes of **diarrhea** and **flatulence** associated with severe headaches and fatigue. During those episodes her stools were greasy and pale. She has seen several physicians who have recommended low-fat, high-carbohydrate diets without relief.

Dr. Grabowski has performed an intestinal biopsy through oral endoscopy and diagnosed celiac disease.

1. List all of Mrs. Stark's signs:

   _____

2. Define *flatulence*:

   _____

   _____

3. If this was an *intestinal biopsy*, what *specific* type of endoscope was used?

   _____

   _____

4. *Oral endoscopy* means the scope was inserted through the patient's _____.

5. What does the term *spasmodic* mean? Check the Glossary or a medical dictionary, and write the definition on the lines below.

   _____

   _____

   _____

6. What does Mrs. Stark need to eliminate from her diet to improve her condition?

   _____

   _____

   _____

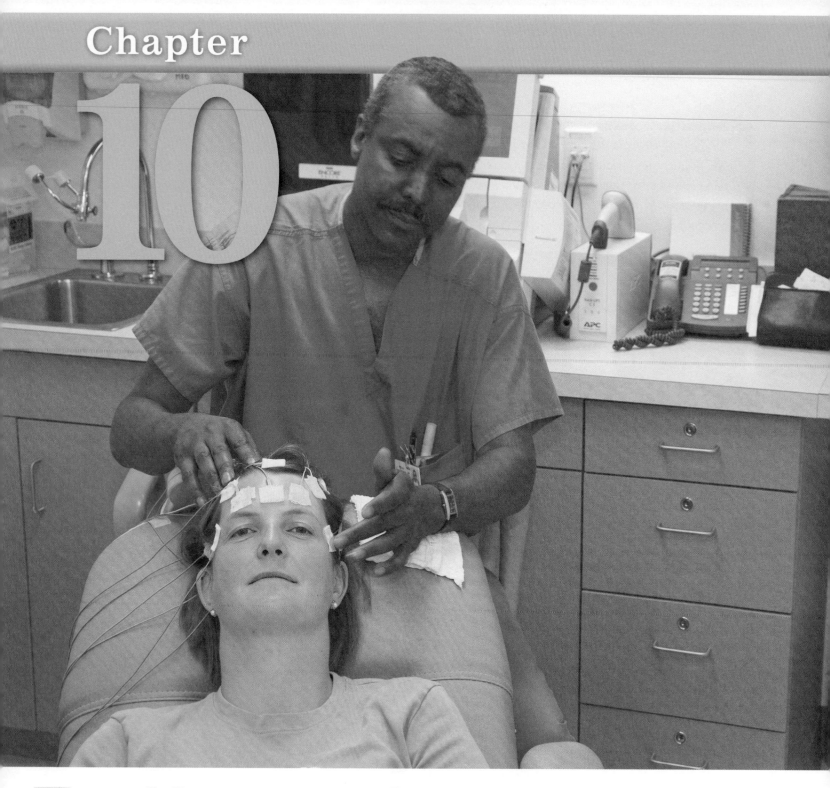

THE NERVOUS SYSTEM AND MENTAL HEALTH

The Essentials of the Languages of Neurology and Psychiatry

CASE REPORT 10.1

YOU ARE

> . . . an **electroneurodiagnostic** technologist working with Gregory Solis, MD, a **neurosurgeon** at Fulwood Medical Center.

YOU ARE COMMUNICATING WITH

> . . . Ms. Roberta Gaston, a 39-year-old woman, who has been referred by Raul Cardenas, MD, a **neurologist**, for evaluation for possible **neurosurgery**. Ms. Gaston has had **epileptic** seizures since the age of 16. She also has daily minor spells in which she stops interacting and blinks rhythmically for about 20 seconds, after which she returns to normal. She is unable to work and is cared for by her parents. Her neurologic examination is normal. Her **electroencephalogram** (**EEG**) shows diffuse epileptic discharges in the left frontal region. Her CT scan is normal. An MRI shows a 20-mm-diameter mass adjacent to her left ventricle.

LEARNING OUTCOMES

Your roles are to perform electroneurodiagnostic evaluations, communicate with Ms. Gaston and her parents, communicate with other health professionals, and maintain and document Ms. Gaston's history and care. To perform these roles, you must be able to:

LO 10.1 Apply the language of neurology to the structures and functions of the nervous system.

LO 10.2 Comprehend, analyze, spell, and write the medical terms of neurology and mental health.

LO 10.3 Recognize and pronounce the medical terms of neurology and mental health.

LO 10.4 Explain the effects of common disorders of the nervous system on health.

The health professionals involved in the diagnosis and treatment of problems with the neurological system and mental health include the following:

- **Neurologists** are medical doctors who specialize in disorders of the nervous system.

- **Neurosurgeons** are medical doctors who perform surgical procedures on the nervous system.

- **Psychiatrists** are medical doctors who are licensed in the diagnosis and treatment of mental disorders.

- **Anesthesiologists** are medical doctors who are certified to administer anesthetics and can also be responsible for pain management.

- **Psychologists** are professionals who are licensed in the science concerned with the behavior of the human mind.

- **Neuropsychologists** are individuals who evaluate the patient's memory, language, and cognitive functions, and develop appropriate treatment plans.

- **Electroneurodiagnostic technicians** (also called EEG technicians) are professionals who operate specialized equipment that measures the electrical activity of the brain, peripheral nervous system, and spinal cord.

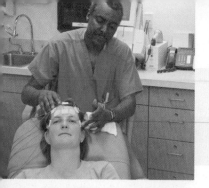

LESSON 10.1

Functions and Structure of the Nervous System

OBJECTIVES

*The trillions of cells in your body must communicate and work together for you to function effectively. This communication is done through your **nervous system**, so it is essential that you understand how this system operates. In this lesson, you will learn to use correct medical terminology to:*

10.1.1 Describe the functions of the nervous system.

10.1.2 Relate the functions of the nervous system to the structures of its components.

10.1.3 List the subdivisions of the nervous system, their different functions, and their basic cells.

ABBREVIATIONS

CT   computed tomography
EEG   electroencephalogram
MRI   magnetic resonance
       imaging

Functions of the Nervous System (LO 10.1, 10.2, and 10.3)

Optimal communication between your nervous system and all the cells in your body requires that the following five functions are always working smoothly:

1. **Sensory input** to the brain comes from receptors all over your body at both the conscious and subconscious levels *(Figure 10.1)*. You are conscious of external stimuli that you receive from your body as it interacts with your environment. Inside your body, internal stimuli concerning the amount of oxygen and carbon dioxide in your blood, and other homeostatic variables like your body temperature, are being processed continually at the subconscious level.

2. **Motor output** from your brain stimulates the skeletal muscles to contract, which enables you to move. Your nervous system controls the production of sweat, saliva, and digestive enzymes without active input from you.

3. **Evaluation and integration** occur in your brain and spinal cord to process the **sensory** input, initiate a response, and store the event in memory.

4. **Homeostasis** is maintained by your nervous system taking in internal sensory input and responding to it. For example, the nervous system responds by stimulating the heart to deliver the correct volume of blood to ensure oxygenation of and removal of waste products from cells.

5. **Mental activity** occurs in your brain so that you can think, feel, understand, respond, and remember.

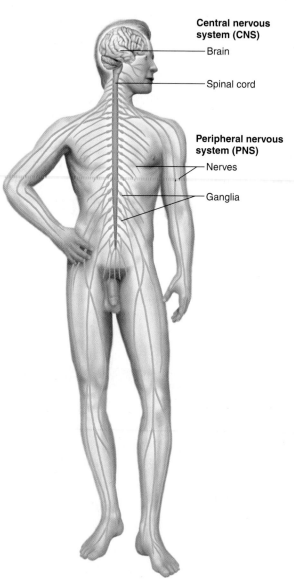

▲ **FIGURE 10.1**
The Nervous System.

Word	Pronunciation	Elements		Definition
electroencephalogram (EEG)	ee-**LEK**-troh-en-**SEF**-ah-low-gram	S/ R/CF R/CF	-gram *recording* electr/o- *electricity* -encephal/o- *brain*	Record of the electrical activity of the brain
electroencephalograph	ee-**LEK**-troh-en-**SEF**-ah-low-graf	S/	-graph *to write, record*	Device used to record the electrical activity of the brain
electroencephalography	ee-**LEK**-troh-en-**SEF**-ah-**LOG**-rah-fee	S/	-graphy *process of recording*	The process of recording the electrical activity of the brain
electroneurodiagnostic (adj)	ee-**LEK**-troh-**NYUR**-oh-die-ag-**NOS**-tik	S/ R/CF R/CF R/	-ic *pertaining to* electr/o- *electricity* -neur/o- *nerve* -diagnost- *decision*	Pertaining to the use of electricity in the diagnosis of a neurologic disorder
epilepsy	**EP**-ih-**LEP**-see		Greek *seizure*	Chronic brain disorder due to paroxysmal excessive neuronal discharges
epileptic (adj) (Note: *An epileptic episode is called a* seizure.)	**EP**-ih-**LEP**-tik **SEE**-zhur	S/ R/	-ic *pertaining to* epilept- *seizure*	Pertaining to or suffering from epilepsy
motor	**MOH**-tor		Latin *to move*	Structures of the nervous system that send impulses out to cause muscles to contract or glands to secrete
nerve	NERV		Latin *nerve*	A cord of nerve fibers bound together by connective tissue
nervous system	**NER**-vus **SIS**-tem	S/ R/	-ous *pertaining to* nerv- *nerve* system, Greek *an organized whole*	The whole, integrated nerve apparatus
neurology	nyu-**ROL**-oh-jee	S/ R/CF	-logy *study of* neur/o- *nerve*	Medical specialty of disorders of the nervous system
neurologist	nyu-**ROL**-oh-jist	S/	-logist *one who studies, specialist*	Medical specialist in disorders of the nervous system
neurologic (adj)	**NYUR**-oh-**LOJ**-ik	S/ R/	-ic *pertaining to* -log- *to study*	Pertaining to the nervous system
neurosurgeon	**NYU**-roh-**SUR**-jun	S/ R/	-eon *one who does* -surg- *operate*	One who operates on the nervous system
neurosurgery	**NYU**-roh-**SUR**-jer-ee	S/	-ery *process of*	Operating on the nervous system
sensory	**SEN**-soh-ree	S/ R/	-ory *having the function of* sens- *feel*	Pertaining to sensation; structures of the nervous system that carry impulses to the brain

EXERCISES

A. Review *the Case Report at the beginning of this chapter before answering the questions.*

1. Why does Ms. Gaston have to be cared for by her parents? _____

2. What is the medical term for an "epileptic episode"? _____

3. Translate into layman's language for Ms. Gaston's parents the sentence, "Her EEG shows diffuse epileptic discharges in the left frontal region."

_____

4. Which diagnostic tests for Ms. Gaston are reported as normal? _____

5. Which diagnostic tests are reported as abnormal? _____

B. Documentation: *Fill in the following paragraph with the appropriate language of neurology. Review the WAD before starting this exercise.*

electroencephalography	**electroneurodiagnostic**	**epilepsy**	**electroencephalograph**
neurologist	**electroencephalogram**	**neurosurgeon**	

Roberta Gaston and her parents were sent to this office by her (1) _____.

Dr. Solis has ordered some (2) _____ tests because of her (3) _____.

The particular type of test is an (4) _____, which will produce an EEG on the (device) (5) _____.

After the results of the (6) _____, if Ms. Gaston needs surgery, it will be performed by a(n) (7) _____.

LESSON 10.1   Components of the Nervous System
(LO 10.1, 10.2, and 10.3)

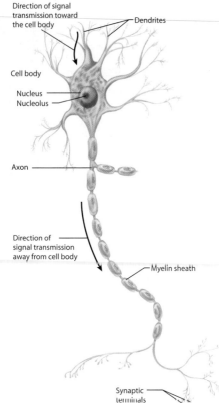

▲ **FIGURE 10.2**
Neuron.

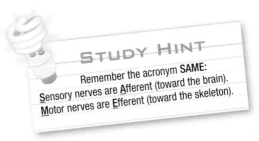

STUDY HINT

Remember the acronym **SAME:**
Sensory nerves are **A**fferent (toward the brain).
Motor nerves are **E**fferent (toward the skeleton).

Your nervous system has two major anatomical subdivisions:

1. The **central nervous system (CNS),** consisting of the brain and spinal cord; and
2. The **peripheral nervous system (PNS),** consisting of all the neurons and nerves outside the central nervous system. It includes 12 pairs of cranial nerves originating from the brain and 31 pairs of spinal nerves originating from the spinal cord.

The peripheral nervous system is further subdivided into:

  i. The **sensory division,** in which sensory nerves (**afferent** nerves) carry messages toward the spinal cord and brain from sense organs; and

  ii. The **motor division,** in which motor nerves (**efferent** nerves) carry messages away from the brain and spinal cord to muscles and organs.

  a. The **visceral motor division** is called the **autonomic nervous system (ANS).** It carries signals to glands and to cardiac and smooth muscle. It operates at a subconscious level outside your voluntary control, and it has two subdivisions:

- The **sympathetic division** arouses the body for action by increasing the heart and respiratory rates to increase oxygen supply to the brain and muscles.
- The **parasympathetic division** calms the body, slowing down the heartbeat but stimulating digestion.

  b. The **somatic motor division** carries signals to the skeletal muscles and is within your voluntary control.

Cells of the Nervous System
(LO 10.1, 10.2, and 10.3)

Neurons (nerve cells) receive stimuli and transmit impulses to other neurons or to organ receptors. Each neuron consists of a cell body and two types of processes or extensions, called **axons** and **dendrites** *(Figure 10.2).*

Dendrites are short, multiple, highly branched extensions of the neuron's cell body. They direct impulses toward the cell body. A single axon, or nerve fiber, arises from the cell body, is covered in a fatty **myelin** sheath, and carries the impulse away from the cell body. Each axon measures a few millimeters to a meter in length.

Bundles of axons appear white in color and create the **white matter** of the brain and spinal cord. Neuron cell bodies, dendrites, and synapses appear gray and create the **gray matter.**

The axon terminates in a network of small branches that ends at a **synapse** (junction) with a dendrite from another neuron, or with a receptor on a muscle cell or gland cell *(Figure 10.3).* **Neurotransmitters** cross the synapse to stimulate or inhibit another neuron or the cell of a muscle or gland. Examples of neurotransmitters are norepinephrine, serotonin, and **dopamine.**

Groups of cell bodies cluster together to form ganglia, and groups of cell bodies and axons collect together to form nerves.

The trillion neurons in the nervous system are outnumbered 50 to 1 by the supportive **glial** cells **(neuroglia).**

The blood-brain barrier is a physical barrier—composed of glial cells and the capillary blood vessel walls—that prevents foreign substances, toxins, and infections from leaving the bloodstream and affecting the brain cells.

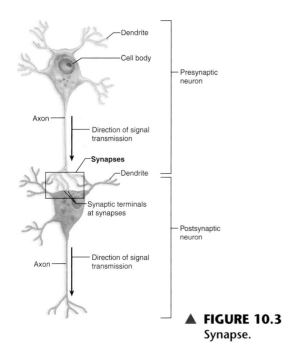

▲ **FIGURE 10.3**
Synapse.

Word	Pronunciation		Elements	Definition
afferent (Note: *also called* sensory; *opposite of* efferent)	AFF-eh-rent		Latin *to bring to*	Moving toward a center; for example, nerve fibers conducting impulses to the spinal cord and brain.
autonomic	awe-toh-**NOM**-ik	S/ P/ R/	-ic *pertaining to* auto- *self* -nom- *law*	Self-governing visceral motor division of the peripheral nervous system.
axon	ACK-son		Greek *axis*	Single process of a nerve cell carrying nervous impulses away from the cell body
dendrite	DEN-dright		Greek *looking like a tree*	Branched extension of the nerve cell body that receives nervous stimuli
dopamine	DOH-pah-meen		Precursor of norepinephrine	Neurotransmitter in some specific small areas of the brain
efferent (Note: *also called* motor; *opposite of* afferent)	EFF-eh-rent		Latin *to bring away from*	Moving away from a center; for example, conducting nerve impulses away from the brain or spinal cord
glia glial (adj) neuroglia	GLEE-ah GLEE-al nyu-roh-**GLEE**-ah	S/ R/ R/CF	-al *pertaining to* -glia *glue* neur/o- *nerve*	Connective tissue that holds a structure together Pertaining to glia or neuroglia Connective tissue holding nervous tissue together
myelin	MY-eh-lin	S/ R/	-in *substance, chemical compound* myel- *spinal cord*	Material of the sheath around the axon of a nerve
neuron	NYUR-on		Greek *nerve*	Technical term for a nerve cell; consists of cell body with its dendrites and axons
neurotransmitter (Note: Transmit *is a word itself, so the prefix trans is in the middle of the overall word.*)	NYUR-oh-trans-**MIT**-er	S/ R/CF P/ R/	-er *agent* neur/o- *nerve* -trans- *across* -mitt- *send*	Chemical agent that relays messages from one nerve cell to the next
parasympathetic (Note: *This term contains two prefixes.*)	par-ah-sim-pah-**THET**-ik	S/ P/ P/ R/	-ic *pertaining to* para- *beside* -sym- *together* -pathet- *suffering*	Division of the autonomic nervous system; has opposite effects to the sympathetic division
somatic	soh-**MAT**-ik	S/ R/	-ic *pertaining to* somat- *body*	A division of the peripheral nervous system serving the skeletal muscles
sympathetic	sim-pah-**THET**-ik	S/ P/ R/	-ic *pertaining to* sym- *together* -pathet- *suffering*	Division of the autonomic nervous system operating at an unconscious level
synapse	SIN-aps	P/ R/	syn- *together* -apse *clasp*	Junction between two nerve cells, or a nerve fiber and its target cell, where electrical impulses are transmitted between the cells
visceral (adj) viscus viscera (pl)	VISS-er-al VISS-kus VISS-er-ah	S/ R/	-al *pertaining to* viscer- *internal organs* Latin *an internal organ*	Pertaining to the internal organs Any single internal organ

EXERCISE

A. Elements: *Solid knowledge of elements is the key to learning medical terminology. Match each element in column 1 with its correct meaning in column 2.*

___	**1.** ic	**A.** self
___	**2.** sym	**B.** pertaining to
___	**3.** viscer	**C.** suffering
___	**4.** auto	**D.** together
___	**5.** pathet	**E.** internal organ
___	**6.** para	**F.** beside

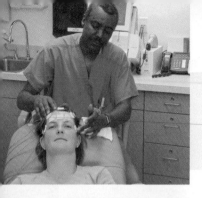

The Brain and Cranial Nerves

OBJECTIVES

The sensations of smelling the roses, seeing them, and touching them are recognized and interpreted in your brain, as are all sensations. The actions of kneeling down, cutting the rose stem, walking into the house, and placing it in a vase originate in your brain, as do all your voluntary actions. The information in this lesson will enable you to use correct medical terminology to:

10.2.1 Describe the essential structures of the brain and spinal cord.

10.2.2 Identify the major sensory and motor areas of the brain.

10.2.3 Explain how the brain and spinal cord are protected and supported.

ABBREVIATION

CSF   cerebrospinal fluid

The Brain (LO 10.1, 10.2, and 10.3)

Your adult brain weighs about 3 pounds. Its size and weight are proportional to your body size, not your intelligence. Your brain is divided into three major regions; the **cerebrum,** the **brain stem,** and the **cerebellum.**

Cerebrum (LO 10.1, 10.2, and 10.3)

The cerebrum makes up about 80% of your brain. It consists of two **cerebral** hemispheres, which are mirror images of each other. These hemispheres are separated by a deep longitudinal fissure, and at the bottom of this, they are connected by a bridge of nerve fibers (the **corpus callosum**).

On the surface of the cerebrum, numerous ridges, **gyri,** are separated by fissures called **sulci** *(Figure 10.4).* The cerebral hemispheres are covered by a thin layer of gray matter (nerve cells and dendrites) called the cerebral **cortex.** It is folded into the gyri, and sulci, and contains 70% of all the neurons in the nervous system. Below the cerebral cortex is a mass of white matter, in which bundles of myelinated nerve fibers connect the neurons of the cortex to the rest of the nervous system.

Functional Cerebral Regions (LO 10.1, 10.2, and 10.3)

Each cerebral hemisphere is divided into four lobes:

1. The **frontal lobe,** located behind the forehead, forms the anterior part of the hemisphere. This lobe is responsible for intellect, planning, problem solving, and the voluntary motor control of muscles.

2. The **parietal lobe** is posterior to the frontal lobe. This lobe receives and interprets sensory information, like spoken words.

3. The **temporal lobe** is below the frontal and parietal lobes. This lobe interprets sensory experiences.

4. The **occipital lobe** forms the posterior part of the hemisphere. This lobe interprets visual images and written words.

Deep inside each cerebral hemisphere are spaces called ventricles, which contain watery **cerebrospinal fluid (CSF).** CSF circulates through the ventricles and around the brain and spinal cord. It helps to protect, cushion, and provide nutrition for the brain and spinal cord.

Located beneath the cerebral hemispheres and ventricles are the:

• **Thalamus** *(Figure 10.4),* which receives all sensory impulses and channels them to the appropriate region of the cortex for interpretation; and

• **Hypothalamus,** which regulates blood pressure, body temperature, water, and electrolyte balance.

Brainstem and Cerebellum (LO 10.1, 10.2, and 10.3)

The **brainstem** relays sensory impulses from peripheral nerves to higher brain centers. It also controls vital cardiovascular and respiratory activities.

The **cerebellum,** the most posterior area of the brain, coordinates skeletal muscle activity to maintain the body's posture and balance.

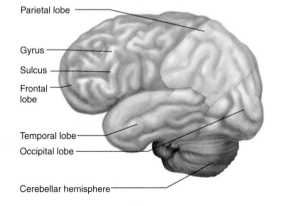

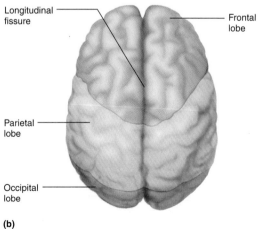

▶ **FIGURE 10.4**
Brain.
(a) View from the left side.
(b) View from above.

Word	Pronunciation	Elements		Definition
cerebellum	ser-eh-**BELL**-um	S/ R/	-um *structure* cerebell- *little brain*	The most posterior area of the brain located between the midbrain and the cerebral hemispheres
cerebrospinal (adj)	SER-ee-broh-**SPY**-nal	S/ R/CF R/	-al *pertaining to* cerebr/o- *brain* -spin- *spinal cord*	Pertaining to the brain and spinal cord
cerebrospinal fluid (CSF)				Fluid formed in the ventricles of the brain; surrounds the brain and spinal cord
cerebrum cerebral (adj)	**SER**-ee-brum **SER**-ee-bral	S/ R/	Latin *brain* -al *pertaining to* cerebr- *brain*	Cerebral hemispheres Pertaining to the cerebral hemispheres or the brain
corpus callosum	**KOR**-pus kah-**LOW**-sum	R/ S/ R/	corpus *body* -um *structure* callos- *thickening*	Bridge of nerve fibers connecting the two cerebral hemispheres
frontal lobe	**FRUNT**-al **LOBE**	S/ R/	-al *pertaining to* front- *front of*	Front area of the cerebral hemisphere
gyrus gyri (pl)	**JI**-rus **JI**-ree		Greek *circle*	Rounded elevation on the surface of the cerebral hemispheres
hypothalamus hypothalamic (adj)	high-poh-**THAL**-ah-muss high-poh-thah-**LAM**-ik	P/ R/ S/ R/	hypo- *below* -thalamus -ic *pertaining to* -thalam- *thalamus*	An endocrine gland in the floor and wall of the third ventricle of the brain Pertaining to the hypothalamus
occipital lobe	ock-**SIP**-it-al **LOBE**	S/ R/	-al *pertaining to* occipit- *back of head*	Posterior area of the cerebral hemisphere
parietal lobe	pah-**RYE**-eh-tal **LOBE**	S/ R/	-al *pertaining to* pariet- *wall*	Area of the brain under the parietal bone
sulcus sulci (pl)	**SUL**-cuss **SUL**-sigh		Latin *furrow, ditch*	Groove on the surface of the cerebral hemispheres that separates gyri
temporal lobe	**TEM**-pore-al **LOBE**	S/ R/	-al *pertaining to* tempor- *time, temple*	Posterior two-thirds of the cerebral hemispheres
thalamus	**THAL**-ah-mus		Greek *inner room*	Mass of gray matter under the ventricle in each cerebral hemisphere

EXERCISES

A. Roots: *The lobes of the brain share the suffix* al, *meaning* pertaining to. *It is the roots that describe their exact location in the brain. Use your knowledge of roots to understand the anatomical location of the lobes. Fill in the blanks.*

1. front/al   root means: _____ ; lobe is located: _____

2. occipit/al   root means: _____ ; lobe is located: _____

3. pariet/al   root means: _____ ; lobe is located: _____

4. tempor/al   root means: _____ ; lobe is located: _____

B. Meet a lesson objective *and use the language of neurology to:*

1. Explain how the brain and spinal cord are protected and supported. _____

_____

_____

2. Identify the major sensory and motor areas of the brain. _____

_____

_____

3. Describe the essential structures of the brain and spinal cord. _____

_____

_____

Cranial Nerves, Spinal Cord, and Meninges
(LO 10.1, 10.2, and 10.3)

Cranial Nerves
(LO 10.1, 10.2, and 10.3)

Your brain communicates with the rest of your body through the cranial nerves and spinal cord. The cranial nerves are part of the peripheral nervous system. They originate on the lower or inferior surface of the brain and are identified by names and numbers, the latter written in Roman numerals *(Figure 10.5)*.

The cranial nerves provide sensory and motor functions for your head and neck areas except for the vagus nerve, which supplies your thorax and abdomen.

Spinal Cord
(LO 10.1, 10.2, and 10.3)

Your spinal cord lies within, and is protected by, the vertebral canal of the spinal column. It has 31 segments, each of which gives rise to a pair of spinal nerves *(Figure 10.6)*. These are the major link between the brain and the peripheral nervous system, and are the pathway for sensory and motor impulses.

Your spinal cord is divided into four regions *(Figure 10.6)*:

1. The **cervical** region is continuous with the brain stem (lower part of the brain). It contains the motor neurons that supply the neck, shoulders, and upper limbs through 8 pairs of cervical spinal nerves (C1–C8);

2. The **thoracic** region contains the motor neurons that supply the thoracic cage, rib movement, vertebral column movement, and postural back muscles through 12 pairs of thoracic spinal nerves (T1–T12);

3. The **lumbar** region supplies the hips and the front of the lower limbs through 5 pairs of lumbar nerves (L1–L5); and

4. The **sacral** region supplies the buttocks, genitalia, and backs of the lower limbs through 5 sacral nerves (S1–S5) and 1 coccygeal nerve, relative to the small bone at the base of the spine.

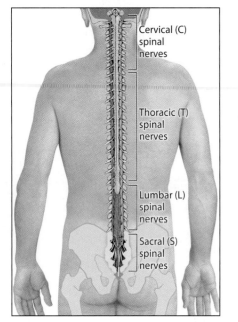

▲ **FIGURE 10.6**
Spinal Cord Regions.

Oh	(olfactory-I)
once	(optic-II)
one	(oculomotor-III)
takes	(trochlear-IV)
the	(trigeminal-V)
anatomy	(abducens-VI)
final	(facial-VII)
very	(vestibulocochlear-VIII)
good	(glossopharyngeal-IX)
vacations	(vagus-X)
are	(accessory-XI)
heavenly!	(hypoglossal-XII)

▲ **FIGURE 10.5** Cranial Nerves
This mnemonic device will help you remember the cranial nerves. Use the sentence in column one (read down) to help you remember the correct order and names of the cranial nerves.

Meninges (LO 10.1, 10.2, and 10.3)

Your brain and spinal cord are protected by the cranium and the vertebrae, cushioned by the CSF, and covered by the **meninges** *(Figure 10.7)*. The meninges have three layers.

1. The **dura mater** is the outermost layer of tough connective tissue attached to the cranium's inner surface, but it is separated from the vertebral canal by the **epidural space,** into which epidural injections are introduced.

2. The **arachnoid mater** is a thin web over the brain and spinal cord. The CSF is contained in the **subarachnoid space** between the arachnoid and pia mater.

3. The **pia mater** is the innermost layer of the meninges, attached to the surface of the brain and spinal cord. It supplies nerves and blood vessels that nourish the outer cells of the brain and spinal cord.

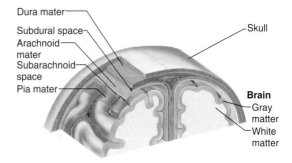

Dura mater
Subdural space
Arachnoid mater
Subarachnoid space
Pia mater
Skull
Brain
Gray matter
White matter

▲ **FIGURE 10.7**
Meninges of Brain.

Word	Pronunciation	Elements		Definition
arachnoid mater	ah-**RACK**-noyd **MAY**-ter	S/ R/ R/	-oid *resembling* arachn- *cobweb, spider* mater *mother*	Weblike middle layer of the three meninges
dura mater (Note: *Both terms are stand-alone roots.*)	**DYU**-rah **MAY**-ter	R/ R/	dura *hard* mater *mother*	Hard, fibrous outer layer of the meninges
epidural	ep-ih-**DYU**-ral	S/ P/ R/	-al *pertaining to* epi- *above* -dur- *dura*	Above the dura
epidural space				Space between the dura mater and the wall of the vertebral canal
meninges	meh-**NIN**-jeez		Greek *membrane*	Three-layered covering of the brain and spinal cord
meningitis	men-in-**JIE**-tis	S/ R/	-itis *inflammation* mening- *meninges*	Inflammation of the meninges
pia mater (*stand-alone roots*)	**PEE**-ah **MAY**-ter	R/ R/	pia *delicate* mater *mother*	Delicate inner layer of the meninges
subarachnoid space	sub-ah-**RACK**-noyd **SPASE**	S/ P/ R/	-oid *resembling* sub- *under* -arachn- *cobweb, spider*	Space between the pia mater and the arachnoid membrane

EXERCISES

A. Construct the following *medical terms by filling in the missing elements. After you have inserted the correct element, circle the word in the statement that was your clue to the missing element. Fill in the blanks.*

1. under the arachnoid mater: _____ /arachn/oid

2. inflammation of the meninges: _____/mening/_____

3. weblike middle layer of meninges: _____/_____/oid   mater

4. pertaining to above the dura: _____ /dur/al

5. hard, fibrous outer layer of meninges: _____/_____/_____

B. Continue to use the WAD *and the text on this spread to find your answers.*

1. Which two prefixes in this WAD denote opposite locations?

_____ means _____.

_____ means _____.

2. Which term is a diagnosis? _____/_____/_____

3. CSF is found in the: sub/ _____ /_____ _____.

4. Describe the location of the spinal cord: _____

_____

5. Name the four regions of the spinal cord: _____ _____

_____ _____

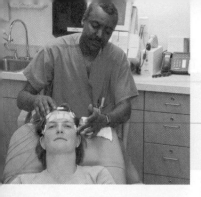

LESSON 10.3

Disorders of the Brain, Cranial Nerves, and Meninges

CASE REPORT 10.2

YOU ARE
. . . a medical assistant working with Dr. Raul Cardenas, a neurologist at Fulwood Medical Center.

YOU ARE COMMUNICATING WITH
. . . Mr. Lester Rood, a 75-year-old man who was diagnosed with **dementia** a year ago. He lives with his daughter, Judy, and she is with him today.

Patient Interview:
Mr. Rood: "How am I feeling? Scared stiff. Sometimes I don't know where I am. I get so messed up. I can't cook anymore. I forget what I'm doing, can't get things straight. I find myself in the street and don't know how I got there. Judy has to help me shower and remind me to go to the bathroom. And it's only going to get worse. I don't want to be a burden. I used to have 100 people working for me. It's so frustrating, so frightening."

Disorders of the Brain (LO 10.1, 10.2, 10.3, and 10.4)

Dementia (LO 10.1, 10.2, 10.3, and 10.4)

Your **empathy** allowed Mr. Rood to talk comfortably without interruption. His situation made clear again the specific symptoms of **dementia.** These include an irreversible short-term memory loss, the inability to solve problems, and confusion. Inappropriate behavior, like wandering away, and impaired intellectual function that interferes with normal activities and relationships are also key signs of dementia. Dementia requires a lot of **sympathy** from family and caregivers.

- **Senile dementia** is not a normal part of aging and is not a specific disease. It is a term used for a collection of symptoms that can be caused by a number of disorders affecting the brain.
- **Alzheimer disease** *(Figure 10.8)*—the most common form of dementia—affects 10% of the population over 65, and 50% of the population over 85. Nerve cells in the areas of the brain associated with memory and **cognition** are replaced by abnormal protein clumps and tangles.
- **Vascular dementia**—the second most common form of dementia—can come on gradually when arteries supplying the brain become arteriosclerotic (narrowed or blocked), depriving the brain of oxygen. It can also occur suddenly after a **stroke** *(see later in this chapter).*

Other conditions causing dementia include reactions to medications, like **sedatives** and antiarthritics; depression in the elderly; and infections, such as AIDS or encephalitis.

Confusion is used to describe people who cannot process information normally. They cannot answer questions appropriately, understand where they are, or remember important facts, like their name and address.

Delirium is an altered mental state **(AMS),** characterized by the sudden onset of disorientation, an inability to think clearly or pay attention. The level of consciousness varies from increased wakefulness to drowsiness. It is not a disease, it is reversible, and it can be part of dementia or a stroke.

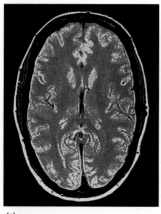
(a)

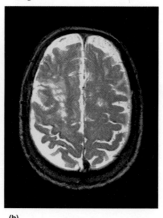
(b)

▲ **FIGURE 10.8**
Brain Sections.
(a) MRI scan, normal brain.
(b) MRI scan of Alzheimer disease, showing cerebral atrophy (yellow).

Word	Pronunciation		Elements	Definition
Alzheimer disease	AWLZ-high-mer DIZ-eez		Dr. Alois Alzheimer, German physician, 1864–1915	Common form of dementia
cognition	kog-NIH-shun		Latin *knowledge*	Process of acquiring knowledge through thinking, learning, and memory
confusion	kon-FEW-zhun	S/ R/	-ion *condition, action* confus- *bewildered*	Mental state in which environmental stimuli are not processed appropriately
delirium	de-LIR-ee-um	S/ R/	-um *structure* deliri- *disorientation, confusion*	Acute altered state of consciousness with agitation and disorientation
dementia	dee-MEN-she-ah	S/ P/ R/	-ia *condition* de- *removal, without* -ment- *mind*	Chronic, progressive, irreversible loss of the mind's cognitive and intellectual functions
empathy sympathy	EM-pah-thee SIM-pah-thee	P/ R/ P/ R/	em- *into* -pathy *emotion, disease* sym- *together* -pathy *emotion, disease*	Ability to place yourself into the feelings, emotions, and reactions of another person Appreciation and concern for another person's mental and emotional state
sedative sedation	SED-ah-tiv seh-DAY-shun	S/ R/ S/	-ive *pertaining to, quality of* sedat- *to calm* -ion *condition, action*	Agent that calms nervous excitement State of being calmed
senile	SEE-nile	S/ R/	-ile *pertaining to* sen- *old age*	Characteristic of old age
stroke (same as cerebrovascular accident, CVA)	STROHK		Old English *to strike*	Acute clinical event caused by impaired cerebral circulation

EXERCISES

A. Review *the Case Report on this spread before answering the questions.*

1. What specific symptoms of dementia does Mr. Rood have? _____

_____

2. How long has Mr. Rood had dementia? _____

3. What is "short term memory"? _____

4. Mr. Rood's short term memory loss is *irreversible.* What does that mean? _____

_____

5. What kind of assistance do people with dementia need? _____

_____

6. List some of the key symptoms of dementia. _____

_____

7. Give an example of "inappropriate behavior." _____

_____

B. Identify *the elements in each medical term, and unlock the meaning of the word. Fill in the chart.*

Medical Term	Meaning of Prefix	Meaning of Root/CF	Meaning of Suffix	Meaning of the Term
dementia	1.	2.	3.	4.
sympathy	5.	6.	7.	8.
delirium	9.	10.	11.	12.
confusion	13.	14.	15.	16.
empathy	17.	18.	19.	20.
sedation	21.	22.	23.	24.

Disorders of the Brain *(continued)*

- Epilepsy affects 1 in 200 people, and 50% of cases develop before age 10.

- Status epilepticus is a medical emergency and requires maintenance of the airway, breathing, and circulation and intravenous administration of anticonvulsant drugs.

- The first-aid treatment during a seizure is to place the person in a reclining position, cushion the head, and turn the person on his or her side. Do not try to hold down the person's arms or legs or restrain the tongue.

- There is no cure for tic disorders, but they can be treated pharmacologically with haloperidol or clonidine.

Epilepsy
(LO 10.1, 10.2, 10.3, and 10.4)

Epilepsy is a chronic disorder in which clusters of neurons (nerve cells) discharge their electrical signals in an abnormal rhythm. This disturbed electrical activity (a **seizure** or a **convulsion**) can cause strange sensations and behavior, convulsions, and loss of consciousness. The causes of epilepsy are numerous, from abnormal brain development to brain damage.

The International League Against Epilepsy created the following classification system for seizures:

1. **Partial seizures** occur when the epileptic activity is in one localized area of the brain only, causing, for example, involuntary jerking movements of a single limb.

2. **Generalized seizures** can be categorized into one of the following three types:

   a. **Absence seizures,** previously known as **"petit mal,"** which begin between ages 5 and 10. The child stares vacantly for a few seconds and may be accused of daydreaming.

   b. **Tonic-clonic seizures,** previously called **"grand mal,"** which are dramatic. The person experiences a **loss of consciousness (LOC),** breathing stops, the eyes roll up, and the jaw is clenched. This "tonic" phase lasts for 30 to 60 seconds. It is followed by the "clonic" phase, in which the whole body shakes with a series of violent, rhythmic jerkings of the limbs. The seizures last for a couple of minutes, and then consciousness returns.

   c. **Febrile seizures,** which are triggered by a fever in infants and toddlers aged 6 months to 5 years. Very few of these children go on to develop epilepsy.

CASE REPORT 10.1

(CONTINUED FROM THE CHAPTER OPENING)

For Ms. Roberta Gaston, who was seen in Dr. Solis' neurosurgery clinic, the EEG did not pinpoint an epileptic source. In order to further investigate the source, Dr. Solis inserted deep brain electrodes into the region of the suspicious mass that showed on the MRI. Seizures were recorded arising in the mass itself. Dr. Solis performed a surgical resection of the mass, which was a glioma. Ms. Gaston has been seizure-free since the surgery a year ago.

Status epilepticus is considered to be a medical emergency. It is defined as having one continuous seizure or recurrent seizures without regaining consciousness for 30 minutes or more.

Any seizure may be followed by a period of diminished function in the area of the brain surrounding the seizure's main origin. This temporary neurologic deficit is called a **postictal** state.

Tourette syndrome and other **tic** disorders are characterized by episodes of involuntary, rapid, repetitive, fixed movements of individual muscle groups in the face or the limbs. They are associated with meaningless vocal sounds or meaningful words and phrases. The tics may be genetic.

Narcolepsy is a chronic disorder in which patients fall asleep during the day—from a few seconds up to an hour. There is no cure.

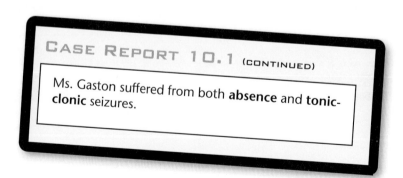

CASE REPORT 10.1 (CONTINUED)

Ms. Gaston suffered from both **absence** and **tonic-clonic** seizures.

Word	Pronunciation	Elements		Definition
grand mal	**GRAHN** MAL	R/ R/	grand *big* mal *bad*	Old name for generalized tonic-clonic seizure
narcolepsy	**NAR**-koh-lep-see	S/ R/CF	-lepsy *seizure* narc/o- *stupor*	Involuntary falling asleep
petit mal	peh-**TEE** MAL	R/ R/	petit *small* mal *bad*	Old name for absence seizures
postictal (adj)	post-**IK**-tal	S/ P/ R/	-al *pertaining to* post- *after* -ict- *seizure*	Transient neurologic deficit after a seizure
ictal (adj)	**ICK**-tal	S/	-al *pertaining to*	Pertaining to, or a condition caused by, a stroke or epilepsy
tic	TIK		French *tic*	Sudden, involuntary, repeated contraction of muscles
tonic	**TON**-ik	S/ R/	-ic *pertaining to* ton- *pressure, tension*	State of muscular contraction
tonic-clonic seizure	**TON**-ik **KLON**-ik **SEE**-zhur	R/ S/ R/	clon- *tumult* -ure *process* seiz- *to grab*	The body alternates between excessive muscular rigidity (tonic) and jerking muscular contractions (clonic)
Tourette syndrome	tur-**ET** **SIN**-drome		Gilles de la Tourette, French neurologist, 1857–1904	Disorder of multiple motor and vocal tics

EXERCISES

A. Review the Case Report *on this spread before answering the questions.*

1. What were the diagnostic findings of the MRI?

_____

2. Since the EEG did not pinpoint an epileptic source, what additional procedure did Dr. Solis perform?

_____

3. Where did Dr. Solis find the source of the seizures? _____

4. What surgical procedure was then performed? _____

5. What type of seizures did Ms. Gaston have? _____

6. How do you know the surgery was successful for Ms. Gaston? _____

7. What is the postoperative diagnosis for Ms. Gaston? _____

B. Critical thinking: *Employ the language of neurology and answer the following questions. Be prepared to answer aloud in class.*

1. Use the root in *narcolepsy* in another medical term which also involves "sleep." _____

2. Why is *status epilepticus* considered to be a medical emergency? _____

_____

3. What is a *postictal state?* Describe and define it. _____

4. What triggers a *febrile* seizure? _____

5. What is the difference between an *absence* seizure and a *tonic-clonic* seizure? _____

_____

Cerebrovascular Accidents (CVAs) or Strokes
(LO 10.1, 10.2, 10.3, and 10.4)

A stroke (also known as a cerebrovascular accident or CVA) occurs when the blood supply to a part of the brain is suddenly interrupted, depriving the brain cells of oxygen. Some cells die; others are badly damaged. With timely treatment, the damaged cells can be saved. There are two types of stroke:

1. **Ischemic strokes** account for 90% of all strokes and are caused by:
   a. **Atherosclerosis:** Plaque in the wall of a cerebral artery *(Figure 10.9a)*; or
   b. **Embolism:** A blood clot in a cerebral artery originating from elsewhere in the body *(Figure 10.9b)*.

Treatment of ischemic strokes is by thrombolysis together with clot busters like **tissue plasminogen activator (tPA).** This must occur within 3½ hours of the stroke, using supportive measures followed by rehabilitation.

2. **Hemorrhagic strokes (intracranial hemorrhage)** occur when a blood vessel in the brain bursts or when a cerebral **aneurysm** ruptures.

Cerebral arteriography can determine the site of bleeding in hemorrhagic stroke. A surgical procedure can be performed to stop the bleed or clip off the aneurysm.

Transient Ischemic Attack (TIA)
(LO 10.1, 10.2, 10.3, and 10.4)

Transient ischemic attacks **(TIAs)** are small, short-term strokes with symptoms lasting for less than 24 hours. If neurologic symptoms persist for more than 24 hours, the condition is a full-blown stroke with brain cell damage and death.

The most frequent cause of TIAs is a small embolus that occludes (blocks) a small artery in the brain. Often, the embolus arises from a clot in the atrium in atrial fibrillation or from an atherosclerotic plaque in a carotid artery. Treatment is directed at the underlying cause. A **carotid endarterectomy** may be necessary if a carotid artery is significantly blocked with plaque.

Atherosclerosis   Residual lumen of artery

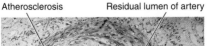
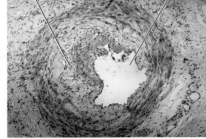

(a)

Embolus

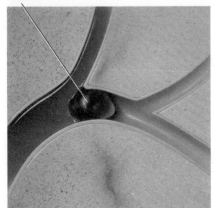

(b)

◀ **FIGURE 10.9**
Causes of Ischemic Strokes.
(a) Atherosclerosis in a cerebral artery, leaving a small, residual lumen. (b) Embolus blocking an artery. Healthy tissue is on the left (pink); blood-starved tissue is on the right (blue).

Other Brain Disorders
(LO 10.1, 10.2, 10.3, and 10.4)

Parkinson disease is caused by the degeneration of neurons in the basic ganglia that produce a neurotransmitter called dopamine. Motor symptoms of abnormal movements, **tremor** of the hands, rigidity, a shuffling gait, and weak voice appear, and gradually become more and more severe. There is no cure.

Creutzfeld-Jakob disease (CJD) produces a rapid deterioration of mental function, with difficulty in muscle movement coordination. Some cases are linked to the consumption of beef from cattle with mad cow disease **(bovine spongiform encephalopathy, BSE).**

Syncope (fainting or passing out) is a temporary loss of consciousness and posture. It is usually due to hypotension and the associated deficient oxygen supply (hypoxia) to the brain.

Migraine produces an intense throbbing, pulsating pain in one area of the head, often with nausea and vomiting. It can be preceded by an aura, visual disturbances like flashing lights, or temporary loss of vision. Prevention is difficult.

Encephalitis, an inflammation of the parenchyma (tissue) of the brain, is often caused by a virus such as HIV, West Nile virus, herpes simplex, or childhood measles, mumps, chickenpox, and rubella.

Brain abscess is usually a direct spread of infection from sinusitis, otitis media (middle ear infection), or mastoiditis (an infection in the skull bone behind the ear). It can also result from blood-borne pathogens arising from lung or dental infections.

Brain tumors are often secondary tumors that have metastasized from cancers in the lung, breast, skin, or kidney. Primary brain tumors arise from any of the glial cells and are called gliomas. In Case Report 10.1, Ms. Gaston has a glioma.

Word	Pronunciation		Elements	Definition
aneurysm	**AN**-yur-izm		Greek *dilation*	Small, circumscribed dilation of an artery or cardiac chamber
arteriography	ar-teer-ee-**OG**-rah-fee	S/ R/	-graphy *recording* arteri/o- *artery*	X-ray visualization of an artery after injection of contrast material
bovine spongiform encephalopathy (BSE)	**BO**-vine **SPON**-jee-form en-sef-ah-**LOP**-ah-thee	S/ R/ S/ R/CF S/ P/ R/CF	-ine *pertaining to* bov- *cattle* -form *appearance of* spong/i- *sponge* -pathy *disease* en- *in* -cephal/o- *head*	Disease of cattle ("mad cow disease") that can be transmitted to humans, causing Creutzfeldt-Jakob disease
carotid endarterectomy	kah-**ROT**-id **END**-ar-ter-**EK**-toe-me	 S/ P/ R/	carotid, Greek *large neck artery* -ectomy *surgical excision* end- *inside* -arter- *artery*	Surgical removal of diseased lining from the carotid artery to leave a smooth lining and restore blood flow
Creutzfeldt-Jakob disease (CJD)	**KROITS**-felt **YAK**-op **DIZ**-eez		Hans Creutzfeldt, 1885–1964, and Alfons Jakob, 1884–1931, German psychiatrists	Progressive, incurable, neurologic disease caused by infectious prions
encephalitis	en-**SEF**-ah-**LIE**-tis	S/ R/	-itis *inflammation* encephal- *brain*	Inflammation of brain cells and tissues
migraine	**MY**-grain	P/ R/	mi- *derived from hemi, half* -graine *head pain*	Paroxysmal severe headache confined to one side of the head
Parkinson disease	**PAR**-kin-son **DIZ**-eez		James Parkinson, British physician, 1755–1824	Disease of muscular rigidity, tremors, and a masklike facial expression
prion	**PREE**-on		Latin *protein*	Small, infectious protein particle
syncope	**SIN**-koh-peh		Greek *cutting short*	Temporary loss of consciousness and postural tone due to diminished cerebral blood flow
tremor	**TREM**-or		Latin *to shake*	Small, shaking, involuntary, repetitive movements of hands, extremities, neck, or jaw

EXERCISES

A. Diagnosis: *Patient documentation is given to you below. Circle the correct language of neurology for the diagnosis.*

1. Patient is experiencing shaking, involuntary movements of her extremities.

    Diagnosis: *syncope*   *prion*   *tremor*

2. Radiologic studies show a small, circumscribed dilation of the cerebral artery.

    Diagnosis: *Parkinson disease*   *aneurysm*   *migraine*

3. The patient's paroxysmal headache is confined to the left temporal region.

    Diagnosis: *syncope*   *tremor*   *migraine*

4. Tests and studies have confirmed inflammation of the brain cells and tissues to make this diagnosis.

    Diagnosis: *meningitis*   *fasciitis*   *encephalitis*

5. This patient has experienced loss of consciousness due to diminished cerebral blood flow.

    Diagnosis: *syncope*   *tremor*   *migraine*

B. Continue working *with the text and the WAD to answer the following questions.*

1. What is another medical term for *intracranial hemorrhage*? _____

2. *Hemorrhage* (noun) and *hemorrhagic* (adjective) both signify the presence of _____.

3. What are the probable causes of a stroke? _____

_____

4. What is an abbreviation used for stroke? _____

Lesson 10.3 Traumatic Brain Injury (TBI) (LO 10.1, 10.2, 10.3, and 10.4)

Keynote

- About 5.3 million Americans (2% of the population) are living with disabilities from TBI.

Traumatic brain injury (TBI) results from any one of many types of injuries to the head, from a bad fall on a hard surface to a car accident to war injuries. Every year, physicians treat over 1 million patients who have experienced TBI; as many as 10% of these have long-term damage affecting their normal **activities of daily living (ADLs).**

Imagine driving your car along the highway at 50 miles per hour. Suddenly, you are hit head-on by another driver. Your brain goes from 50 miles per hour to zero—instantly. Your soft brain is propelled forward and squished against the front of your hard skull **(coup).** Next, you rebound backward, and your brain slams against the back of your skull **(contrecoup).** Your brain now has at least one bruise or **contusion,** if not worse damage.

A mild head injury **(concussion)** may leave you feeling dazed, confused, or unable to recall the event that caused your concussion. Repeated concussions, like those experienced by famous boxer Muhammad Ali, have a cumulative effect, leading to a reduced mental ability and reaction time, and/or trauma-induced Parkinson's disease.

A severe injury may include torn blood vessels that bleed into the brain. The brain may also tear, or swell within the hard, inflexible skull, cutting off important signals and connections.

Shaken baby syndrome (SBS) is a type of TBI produced when a baby is violently shaken. A baby has weak neck muscles and a heavy head. Shaking makes the brain bounce back and forth in the skull, leading to severe brain damage.

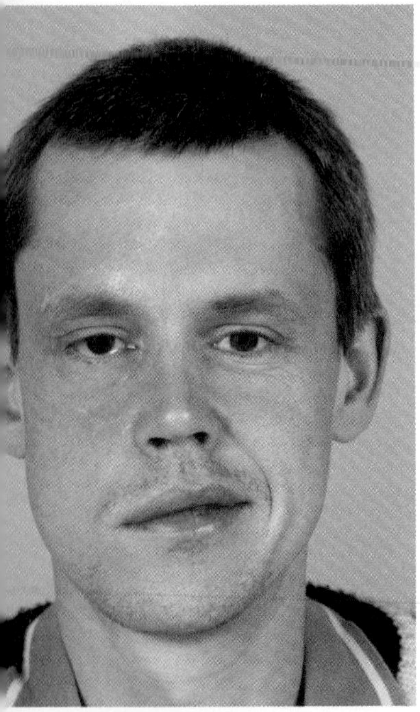

▲ **FIGURE 10.10**
Bell Palsy on the Right Side of His Face.

Disorders of the Meninges (LO 10.1, 10.2, 10.3, and 10.4)

Meningitis is an inflammation of the membranes (meninges) covering the brain and spinal cord. Viral meningitis—the most common form—can occur at any age. Bacterial meningitis predominantly affects the very young or very old. **Meningococcal** meningitis is contagious, transmitted through a simple cough or sneeze. It is most commonly passed among people who live in close quarters—such as students in college dormitories. Vaccines are available to prevent most types of meningitis.

A **subdural hematoma** is bleeding into the subdural space outside the brain, which is frequently associated with closed head injuries and bleeding from broken veins caused by violent head rotations.

An **epidural hematoma** is a pooling of blood in the epidural space outside the brain, often associated with a fractured skull and bleeding from an artery within the meninges.

Disorders of the Cranial Nerves (LO 10.1, 10.2, 10.3, and 10.4)

Bell palsy is a facial nerve disorder characterized by a sudden weakness or paralysis of muscles on one side of the face. The inability to smile or whistle, the uncontrollable drooping of the mouth and drooling of saliva, and an inability to close the eye *(Figure 10.10)* are common symptoms.

Pain Management (LO 10.1, 10.2, 10.3, and 10.4)

It's estimated that more than 6 million Americans are affected by the acute or chronic pain of **fibromyalgia,** 5 million are disabled by back pain, and 40 million suffer from recurrent headaches. Interventional procedures (such as nerve blocks or trigger point injections) can target the tissue or the organ causing pain, and physical medicine and rehabilitation **(physiatry)** can use physical techniques such as heat, electrotherapy, therapeutic exercises, and biofeedback techniques. Pain management practitioners include anesthesiologists, physiatrists, physiotherapists, occupational therapists, and chiropractors.

Medications prescribed based on the severity of the pain include:

- **Analgesics** (such as acetaminophen) and nonsteroidal anti-inflammatory drugs (NSAIDs) for mild pain;
- **Opiates** (codeine, hydrocodone, and oxycodone) in combination with analgesics for moderate pain; and
- Higher doses of opiates for severe pain. These are often used on their own, and include **morphine** and fentanyl.

Abbreviations

ADL	activity of daily living
NSAID	nonsteroidal anti-inflammatory drug
SBS	shaken baby syndrome
TBI	traumatic brain injury

Word	Pronunciation	Elements		Definition
analgesia	an-al-**JEE**-zee-ah	S/ P/ R/	-ia *condition* *an- without* -alges- *sensation of pain*	State in which pain is reduced
analgesic (adj)	an-al-**JEE**-zik	S/	-ic *pertaining to*	Substance that produces analgesia
Bell palsy	BELL **PAWL**-zee		Charles Bell, Scottish -sur-geon, 1774–1842	Paresis, or paralysis, of one side of the face
concussion	kon-**KUSH**-un	S/ R/	-ion *action, condition* concuss- *shake or jar violently*	Mild brain injury
contrecoup	**KON**-treh-koo		French *counterblow*	Injury to the brain at a point directly opposite the point of contact
contusion	kon-**TOO**-zhun	S/ R/	-ion *action, condition* contus- *bruise*	Hemorrhage into a tissue (bruising), including the brain
coup	KOO		French *a blow*	Injury to the brain directly under the skull at the point of contact
fibromyalgia	fie-broh-my-**AL**-jee-ah	S/ R/CF R/	-algia *pain* fibr/o- *fiber* -my- *muscle*	Pain in the muscle fibers
meningococcal	meh-nin-goh-**KOK**-al	S/ R/CF R/	-al *pertaining to* mening/o- *meninges* -cocc- *round bacterium*	Pertaining to the meningococcus bacterium
subdural space	sub-**DYU**-ral SPACE	S/ P/ R/	-al *pertaining to* *sub- below* -dur- *dura, hard*	Space between the arachnoid and dura mater layers of the meninges
trauma traumatic	**TRAW**-mah traw-**MAT**-ik	 S/ R/	Greek *wound* -tic *pertaining to* trauma- *injury*	A physical or mental injury Pertaining to or caused by trauma

EXERCISES

A. Deconstruct the following language of neurology. *First, slash the term in column 1 into its elements. Then write the meaning of each element to see how it will aid you in understanding the meaning of the complete term. Fill in the chart.*

Medical Term	Meaning of Prefix	Meaning of Root/CF	Meaning of Suffix	Meaning of Term
concussion	1.	2.	3.	4.
contusion	5.	6.	7.	8.
fibromyalgia	9.	10.	11.	12.
subdural	13.	14.	15.	16.
meningococcal	17.	18.	19.	20.

Remember: Every term does not need a prefix!

B. Insert medical terms *found in this spread to fill in the answer blanks.*

1. These related neurological injuries occur very often in motor vehicle accidents: _____

2. Medicine given to reduce pain is an _____

3. Hemorrhaging into surrounding brain tissue produces a _____.

4. _____ is a mild brain injury that occurs often in sports.

5. Pain in the muscle fibers is termed _____.

C. Terminology challenge: *Use the language of neurology to describe the difference between a* subdural hematoma *and an* epidural hematoma.

1. _____
_____

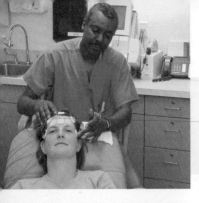

LESSON 10.4

Disorders of the Spinal Cord and Peripheral Nerves

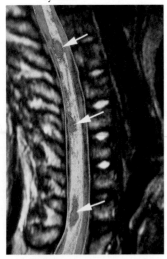

▲ **FIGURE 10.11**
Multiple Sclerosis of the Spinal Cord.
Areas of demyelination are arrowed and shown in red.

CASE REPORT 10.3

YOU ARE

. . . Tanisha Colis, an electroneurodiagnostic technologist working for Raul Cardenas, MD, a neurologist at Fulwood Medical Center.

YOU ARE COMMUNICATING WITH

. . . Mrs. Suzanne Kalish, a 42-year-old social worker employed by the medical center. Mrs. Kalish has recently had an exacerbation of her symptoms due to multiple sclerosis **(MS)**. She is going to have a visual evoked potential **(VEP)** test, followed by an MRI of her brain and spinal cord.

Patient Interview:

Tanisha: "Good morning, Mrs. Kalish. I'm Tanisha Colis, the technologist who'll be performing your visual evoked potential test. How are you feeling?"

Mrs. Kalish: "I've been doing OK for the last 4 or 5 years. Then, a few weeks ago, I started dragging my right foot like a wounded witch. I've got to hang onto the walls to stay vertical. I'm tired out, can't come to work. It's a struggle to walk the few yards just to pick up the mail."

Tanisha: "The MRI you are going to have today will give us a lot of information about what's going on."

Mrs. Kalish: "My mind is going 'wheelchair, wheelchair, wheelchair.' Especially since in the last couple of days the vision in my right eye has gotten all blurred."

Tanisha: "That's the reason you are having the visual evoked potential test."

Mrs. Kalish: "I hate this disease. If I had cancer, I've got a chance. I'd fight it to the end, whatever that would be. Nobody's ever beat MS. You can only lose. It can be kind and leave you for a while, but it's never far away."

Tanisha: "Let me help you up, and we'll go get this test done."

Mrs. Kalish: "I can manage, thank you."

Disorders of the Myelin Sheath of Nerve Fibers

(LO 10.1, 10.2, 10.3, and 10.4)

When the myelin sheath surrounding nerve fibers is damaged, nerves do not conduct impulses normally. In newborns, many of their nerves have immature myelin sheaths, which is why some of their movements are jerky and uncoordinated.

Demyelination, the destruction of an area of the myelin sheath, can occur in the PNS and be caused by inflammation, vitamin B12 deficiency, poisons, and some medications.

Multiple sclerosis (MS), a chronic, progressive disorder, is the most common condition in which demyelination of nerve fibers in the brain, spinal cord, and optic nerves can occur *(Figure 10.11)*. **Intermittent** myelin damage and scarring slows nerve impulses. This leads to muscle weakness, pain, funny sensations **(paresthesias),** numbness, and vision loss. Because different nerve fibers are affected at different times, MS symptoms often worsen **(exacerbations)** or show partial or complete reduction **(remissions).** Suzanne Kalish is now in an exacerbation.

MS, most common in women, has an average age of onset between 18 and 35 years. Its cause is unknown, but it is thought to be an autoimmune disease. There is no known cure for MS.

Word	Pronunciation	Elements		Definition
demyelination	dee-**MY**-eh-lin-**A**-shun	S/ P/ R/	-ation *process* de- *without* -myelin- *myelin*	Process of losing the myelin sheath of a nerve fiber
exacerbation (contrast **remission**)	ek-zas-er-**BAY**-shun	S/ R/	-ation *process* exacerbat- *increase, aggravate*	Period when there is an increase in the severity of a disease
intermittent	**IN**-ter-**MIT**-ent	S/ P/ R/	-ent *end result* inter- *between* -mitt- *send*	Alternately ceasing and beginning again
modify	**MOD**-ih-fie		Latin *to limit*	Change the form or qualities of something; here, the pathology of MS
paresthesia paresthesias (pl)	par-es-**THEE**-ze-ah	S/ P/ R/	-ia *condition* par(a)- *abnormal* -esthes- *sensation*	Abnormal sensation; e.g., tingling, burning, pricking
remission (contrast **exacerbation**)	ree-**MISH**-un	S/ P/ R/	-ion *condition, action* re- *back* -miss- *send*	Period when there is a lessening or absence of the symptoms of a disease
sclerosis	skleh-**ROH**-sis		Greek *hardness*	Thickening and hardening of a tissue; in the nervous system, hardening of nervous tissue by fibrous and glial connective tissue

EXERCISES

A. Review *the Case Report on this spread before answering the questions.*

1. What symptoms made Mrs. Kalish come to see Dr. Cardenas? _____

2. Is the change in her symptoms sudden? _____

3. What diagnostic test is Mrs. Kalish having? _____

4. What type of comments from the patient make her sound depressed about her condition? _____

_____

5. What does it mean if a disease is *chronic* and *progressive*? _____

_____

6. Can this disease be cured? _____

B. Test yourself *on the elements and terms in the above WAD box. Practice pronouncing the terms before you start the exercise. Listen to the pronunciations on the Student Online Learning Center (www.mhhe.com/AllanEss2e). Circle the best answer.*

1. The term *intermittent* contains:

   prefix, root, and suffix   prefix and root   combining form and suffix

2. *Remission* is the opposite of:

   intermittent   exacerbation   demyelination

3. *To modify* something is to:

   dispose of it   change it   renew it

4. In the term *demyelination* the prefix means:

   without   in front of   half

5. If a disease is *exacerbated*, it:

   is more severe   has not changed   is less severe

   Have you pronounced each word correctly?

LESSON 10.4 Disorders of the Spinal Cord (LO 10.1, 10.2, 10.3, and 10.4)

Trauma (LO 10.1, 10.2, 10.3, and 10.4)

The spinal cord can be injured in three ways:

1. **Severed,** by a fractured vertebra *(Figure 10.12a)*;
2. **Contused,** as in a sudden, violent jolt to the spine; and
3. **Compressed,** by a dislocated vertebra, bleeding, or swelling *(Figure 10.12b)*.

Because of its anatomy—with nerve fibers and tracts going up and down, to and from the brain—a spinal cord injury results in a loss of function below the injury site. For example, if the cord is injured in the thoracic region, the arms function normally but the legs can be **paralyzed.** Both muscle control and sensation are lost. **Paresis** is partial paralysis.

If the spinal cord is severed, the loss of function is permanent. Contusions can cause temporary loss, lasting days, weeks, or months.

Compression of the cord can also occur from a tumor in the cord or spine or from a **herniated disc.** Cancer or osteoporosis can cause a vertebra to collapse and also compress the cord.

In **syringomyelia,** fluid-filled cavities form in the spinal cord and compress nerves that detect pain and temperature. There is no specific cure.

Other Disorders of the Spinal Cord (LO 10.1, 10.2, 10.3, and 10.4)

Acute transverse myelitis is a localized spinal cord disorder that blocks the transmission of impulses up and down the spinal cord.

Subacute combined degeneration of the spinal cord is due to a deficiency of vitamin B_{12}. The spinal cord's sensory nerve fibers degenerate, producing weakness, clumsiness, tingling, and a sensory loss as to the position of the limbs. Treatment involves vitamin B_{12} injections.

Poliomyelitis is an acute infectious disease, occurring mostly in children, due to the poliovirus. The virus destroys motor neurons. It is preventable by vaccination and has almost been eradicated worldwide.

Postpolio syndrome (PPS) is when people develop tired, painful, and weak muscles many years after recovery from polio.

Amyotrophic lateral sclerosis (ALS), or "Lou Gehrig's disease," occurs when motor nerves in the spinal cord progressively deteriorate. There is no cure.

Disorders of Peripheral Nerves (LO 10.1, 10.2, 10.3, and 10.4)

Neuropathy is used here as any disorder affecting one or more peripheral nerves. **Mononeuropathy** is damage to a single peripheral nerve. Examples are:

- **Carpal tunnel syndrome,** in which the median nerve at the wrist is compressed between the wrist bones and a strong overlying ligament.
- **Ulnar nerve palsy,** which results from nerve damage as the forearm's ulnar nerve crosses close to the surface over the humerus at the back of the elbow.
- **Peroneal nerve palsy,** which arises from nerve damage as the peroneal or lower leg bone nerve passes close to the surface near the back of the knee. Compression of this nerve occurs in people who are bedridden or strapped in a wheelchair.

Polyneuropathy is damage to, and the simultaneous malfunction of, many motor and/or sensory peripheral nerves throughout the body.

Herpes zoster, or **shingles,** is an infection of peripheral nerves arising from a reactivation of the dormant childhood chickenpox (varicella) virus.

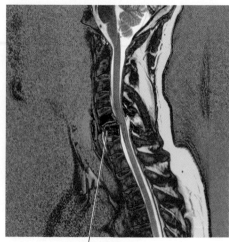

(a) Severed spinal cord / Fracture-dislocation of vertebra

(b) Fractured vertebra

▲ **FIGURE 10.12**
Spinal Cord Injuries.
(a) Severed spinal cord from fracture dislocation of vertebra. (b) Compressed spinal cord with vertebral fracture.

Word	Pronunciation	Elements		Definition
amyotrophic	a-my-oh-**TROH**-fik	S/ P/ R/CF R/	-ic *pertaining to* a- *without* -my/o- *muscle* -troph- *nourishment, development*	Pertaining to muscular atrophy
compression	kom-**PRESH**-un	S/ P/ R/	-ion *action, condition* com- *together* -press- *squeeze*	Squeeze together to increase density and/or decrease a dimension of a structure
herniation hernia (noun) herniate (verb)	**HER**-nee-ay-shun **HER**-nee-ah **HER**-nee-ate	S/ R/ S/	-ation *process* herni- *rupture* -ate *composed of*	Protrusion of an anatomical structure from its normal location Protrusion of a structure through the tissue that normally contains it
myelitis	**MY**-eh-**LIE**-tis	S/ R/	-itis *inflammation* myel- *spinal cord*	Inflammation of the spinal cord
neuropathy mononeuropathy polyneuropathy	nyu-**ROP**-ah-thee **MON**-oh-nyu-**ROP**-ah-thee **POL**-ee-nyu-**ROP**-ah-thee	S/ R/CF P/ P/	-pathy *disease* neur/o- *nerve* mono- *one* poly- *many*	Any disorder of the nervous system Disorder affecting a single nerve Disorder affecting many nerves
paralyze (verb) paralysis (noun) paralytic (adj)	**PAR**-ah-lyze pah-**RAL**-ih-sis par-ah-**LYT**-ik	P/ R/ R/ S/ R/	para- *beside, abnormal* -lyze *destroy* -lysis *destruction* -ic *pertaining to* -lyt- *destroy*	To make incapable of movement Loss of voluntary movement Suffering from paralysis
paresis hemiparesis	par-**EE**-sis **HEM**-ee-pah-**REE**-sis	P/ R/	Greek *weakness* hemi- *half* -paresis *weakness*	Partial paralysis (weakness) Weakness of one side of the body
poliomyelitis polio (abbreviation) postpolio syndrome (PPS)	POE-lee-oh-**MY**-eh-lie-tis post-**POE**-lee-oh **SIN**-drome	S/ R/ R/ P/ R/ P/ R/	-itis *inflammation* polio- *gray matter* -myel- *spinal cord* post- *after* -polio *gray matter* syn- *together* -drome *running*	Inflammation of the gray matter of the spinal cord, leading to paralysis of the limbs and muscles of respiration Progressive muscle weakness in a person previously affected by polio
syringomyelia	sih-**RING**-oh-my-**EE**-lee-ah	S R/ R/CF	-ia *condition* -myel- *spinal cord* syring/o- *tube, pipe*	Abnormal longitudinal cavities in the spinal cord cause paresthesias and muscle weakness
trauma traumatic	**TRAW**-mah traw-**MAT**-ik	S/ R/	Greek *wound* -tic *pertaining to* trauma- *injury*	A physical or mental injury Pertaining to or caused by trauma

EXERCISES

A. Use the language *of neurology to demonstrate your knowledge of the spinal cord.*

1. Name the three ways the spinal cord can be injured: _____

2. Where does loss of function occur in a spinal cord injury? _____

3. What is lost in paralysis? _____

4. What is partial paralysis called? _____

5. What can cause compression of the spinal cord? _____

B. Identify the element, *and give its meaning. Complete the exercise by listing a medical term that contains this element. Review the WAD box above before you start the exercise. Fill in the chart.*

Element	Element Identity (P, R, CF, or S)	Meaning of Element	Medical Term Containing This Element
myo	1.	2.	3.
herni	4.	5.	6.
pathy	7.	8.	9.
troph	10.	11.	12.

Congenital Anomalies of the Nervous System
(LO 10.1, 10.2, 10.3, and 10.4)

- Classification of CP by number of limbs impaired:

  o **Quadriplegia:** All four limbs are affected.

  o **Paraplegia:** Both lower extremities are affected.

  o **Hemiplegia:** The arm and leg of one side of the body are affected.

  o **Monoplegia:** Only one limb is affected, usually an arm.

Some of the most devastating congenital neurologic abnormalities develop in the first 8 to 10 weeks of pregnancy, when the nervous system is in its early stages of formation. These malformations can be detected using ultrasonography and amniocentesis *(see Chapter 15).* Many of these can be prevented by the mother taking 4 mg/day of folic acid before conception and during early pregnancy.

A **teratogen** is an agent that can cause **anomalies** of an embryo or fetus *(see Chapter 15).* It can be a chemical, a virus, or radiation. Some teratogens found in the workplace include textile dyes, photographic chemicals, semiconductor materials, and the metals lead, mercury, and cadmium.

Anencephaly is the absence of the cerebral hemispheres and is incompatible with life. **Microcephaly,** decreased head size, is associated with small cerebral hemispheres and moderate to severe motor and mental retardation.

Hydrocephalus *(Figure 10.13)* is ventricular enlargement in the cerebral hemispheres with excessive CSF; it is usually due to a blockage that prevents the CSF from exiting the ventricles to circulate around the spinal cord. Treatment involves placing a tube (shunt) into the ventricle to divert the excess fluid into the abdominal cavity or a neck vein.

Spina bifida occurs mostly in the lumbar and sacral regions. It is variable in its presentation and symptoms. **Spina bifida occulta** has a small partial defect in the vertebral arch. The spinal cord or meninges do not protrude. Often the only sign is a tuft of hair on the skin overlying the defect.

In **spina bifida cystica** there is no vertebral arch formed. The spinal cord and meninges protrude through the opening and may or may not be covered with a thin layer of skin *(Figure 10.14a and b).* Protrusion of only the meninges is called a **meningocele.** Protrusion of the meninges and spinal cord is called a **meningomyelocele.** The lower limbs may be paralyzed.

Fetal alcohol syndrome (FAS) can occur when a pregnant woman drinks alcohol. A child born with FAS has a small head, narrow eyes, and a flat face and nose. Intellect and growth are impaired. FAS is the third most common cause of mental retardation in newborns.

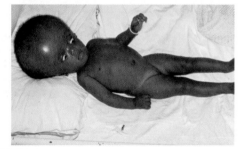

▲ **FIGURE 10.13**
Infant with Hydrocephalus.

FAS   fetal alcohol syndrome
CP   cerebral palsy

Cerebral Palsy
(LO 10.1, 10.2, 10.3, and 10.4)

Cerebral palsy (CP) is the term used to describe the motor impairment resulting from brain damage in an infant or young child. It is not hereditary. In congenital CP, the cause is often unknown but can be a brain malformation or maternal use of cocaine. CP developed at birth or in the neonatal period is usually related to an incident causing hypoxia of the brain.

Cerebral palsy causes delay in the development of normal milestones in infancy and childhood *(see Bonus Chapter).* The affected limbs can be **spastic** (muscles are tight and resistant to stretch) and may show **athetoid** movements, where the limbs involuntarily writhe and constantly move. A poor sense of balance and coordination may also be present, leading to **ataxia.**

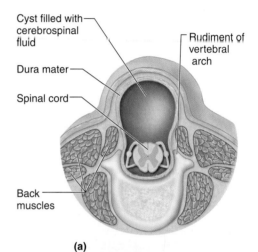

(a)

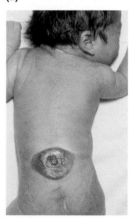

(b)

▲ **FIGURE 10.14**
Spina Bifida Cystica.
(a) Cross section of a spinal meningocele.
(b) Child with spina bifida cystica.

Word	Pronunciation	Elements		Definition
anencephaly	**AN**-en-**SEF**-ah-lee	S/ P/ R/	-aly *condition* an- *without* -enceph- *brain*	Born without cerebral hemispheres
microcephaly	**MY**-kroh-**SEF**-ah-lee	P/ R/	micro- *small* -ceph- *head*	An abnormally small head
ataxia	a-**TAK**-see-ah	S/ P/ R/	-ia *condition* a- *without* -tax- *coordination*	Inability to coordinate muscle activity, leading to jerky movements
ataxic (adj)	a-**TAK**-sik	S/	-ic *pertaining to*	Pertaining to or suffering from ataxia
athetosis	ath-eh-**TOE**-sis	S/ R/	-osis *condition* athet- *without position, uncontrolled*	Slow, writhing involuntary movements
athetoid (adj)	**ATH**-eh-toyd	S/	-oid *resembling*	Resembling or suffering from athetosis
hemiplegia	hem-ee-**PLEE**-jee-ah	S/ P/ R/	-ia *condition* hemi- *half* -pleg- *paralysis*	Paralysis of one side of the body
hemiplegic (adj) hemiparesis	hem-ee-**PLEE**-jik **HEM**-ee-pah-**REE**-sis	S/ R/	-ic *pertaining to* -paresis *weakness*	Pertaining to or suffering from hemiplegia Weakness of one side of the body
meningocele	meh-**NING**-oh-seal	S/ R/CF	-cele *hernia* mening/o-*meninges*	Protrusion of the meninges from the spinal cord or brain through a defect in the vertebral column or cranium
meningomyelocele	meh-nin-goh-**MY**-el-oh-seal	S/ R/CF	-cele *hernia* -myel/o- *spinal cord*	Protrusion of the spinal cord and meninges through a defect in the vertebral arch of one or more vertebrae
monoplegia	**MON**-oh-**PLEE**-jee-ah	S/ P/ R/	-ia *condition* mono- *one* -pleg- *paralysis*	Paralysis of one limb
monoplegic (adj)	**MON**-oh-**PLEE**-jik	S/	-ic *pertaining to*	Pertaining to or suffering from monoplegia
palsy	**PAWL**-zee		Latin *paralysis*	Paralysis or paresis from brain damage
paraplegia	par-ah-**PLEE**-jee-ah	S/ P/ R/	-ia *condition* para- *abnormal* -pleg- *paralysis*	Paralysis of both lower extremities
paraplegic (adj)	par-ah-**PLEE**-jik	S/	-ic *pertaining to*	Pertaining to or suffering from paraplegia
quadriplegia	kwad-rih-**PLEE**-jee-ah	S/ P/ R/	-ia *condition* quadri- *four* -pleg- *paralysis*	Paralysis of all four limbs
quadriplegic (adj)	kwad-rih-**PLEE**-jik	S/	-ic *pertaining to*	Pertaining to or suffering from quadriplegia
spina bifida	**SPY**-nah **BIH**-fih-dah	R/CF P/ R/	spin/a *spine* bi- *two* -fida *split*	Failure of one or more vertebral arches to close during fetal development
spina bifida cystica	**SIS**-tik-ah	S/ R/	-ica *pertaining to* cyst- *cyst*	Meninges and spinal cord protruding through the absent vertebral arch and having the appearance of a cyst
spina bifida occulta	**OH**-kul-tah	R/CF	occult/a *hidden*	The deformity of the vertebral arch is not apparent from the surface
teratogen	**TER**-ah-toe-gen	S/ R/CF	-gen *create, produce* terat/o- *monster, malformed fetus*	Agent that produces fetal deformities

EXERCISE

A. Search and find *the correct term for the element you are given. Circle the best answer.*

1. Find the term with the prefix meaning *without:*

hydrocephalus   anencephaly   bifida

2. Find the term with the suffix meaning *hernia:*

meningocele   cystica   teratogen

3. Find the term with the root meaning *hidden:*

spina bifida   spina bifida cystica   spina bifida occulta

4. Find the term with the root meaning *coordination:*

monoplegia   athetosis   ataxia

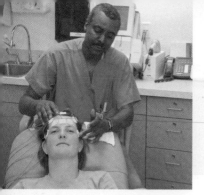

OBJECTIVES

As a health professional, you will find that many of your patients have a mental health problem in addition to their physical ailments. This lesson will enable you to use correct medical terminology to:

10.5.1 Comprehend, analyze, spell, and write the essential terms of psychology and psychiatry to communicate and document accurately and precisely.

10.5.2 Recognize and pronounce the essential terms of psychology and psychiatry to communicate verbally with accuracy and precision.

KEYNOTES

- A licensed specialist in **psychology** is a **psychologist.** Psychologists are not licensed to prescribe medications.

- **Insanity** is a legal term for a severe mental illness that impairs a defendant's ability to understand the moral wrong of the act he or she committed. It is not a medical diagnosis.

ABBREVIATIONS

GAD	generalized anxiety disorder
MPD	multiple-personality disorder
OCD	obsessive-compulsive disorder
PTSD	posttraumatic stress disorder

Mental Health
(LO 10.1, 10.2, 10.3, and 10.4)

Mental health is defined as the emotional, behavioral, and social well-being that enables an individual to cope with internal and external events.

Psychology is the scientific study of behavior—talking, reading, sleeping, interacting with others—and mental processes—thinking, feeling, remembering, and dreaming.

Psychiatry is the medical specialty concerned with the origin, diagnosis, prevention, and treatment of mental, emotional, and behavioral disorders.

Mood Disorders
(LO 10.1, 10.2, 10.3, and 10.4)

Major depression, also called **unipolar disorder** *(Figure 10.15),* occurs when a person is so deeply sad for at least 2 weeks that he or she feels hopeless, sees nothing but sorrow and despair in the future, and may not want to live anymore.

Bipolar disorder, which used to be called **manic-depressive disorder,** is the alternation of episodes of major depression, which include low mood and low energy, with excessive overexcitement and impulsive behavior called **mania.**

Anxiety Disorders
(LO 10.1, 10.2, 10.3, and 10.4)

Anxiety disorders are characterized by unreasonable anxiety or fear that is so intense and chronic that it disrupts the person's life.

- **Generalized anxiety disorder (GAD)** consists of unreasonable anxiety that is not focused on one particular situation or event.
- **Posttraumatic stress disorder (PTSD)** arises after significant trauma like a life-threatening incident, loss of a loved one, abuse, or combat in war.
- **Panic disorder** is characterized by sudden, brief attacks of intense fear.
- **Phobias** differ from generalized anxiety and panic attacks in that a specific situation or object brings on the strong fear response. Examples are **claustrophobia** (fear of being trapped in a confined space), **acrophobia** (fear of heights), and **agoraphobia** (fear of crowded places).

- **Obsessive-compulsive disorder (OCD)** patients have both obsessions and compulsions. The obsessions are recurrent thoughts, fears, doubts, images, or impulses. The compulsions are recurrent, irresistible actions, such as hand washing, counting, and checking. These recurrent actions can also be violent or sexual.

Schizophrenia
(LO 10.1, 10.2, 10.3, and 10.4)

Schizophrenia is a form of **psychosis** in which the patient loses contact with reality. People with schizophrenia do *not* have a split personality, but their words are separated from the meaning, their perceptions are separated from reality, and their behaviors are separated from their thought processes. They perceive things without stimulation (**hallucinations**). They suffer from **delusions** (mistaken beliefs that are contrary to facts). The delusions can be **paranoid** (with pervasive distrust and suspicion of others). Their speech is disorganized and can be incoherent, or they may even refuse to speak or become unable to speak (**mute**).

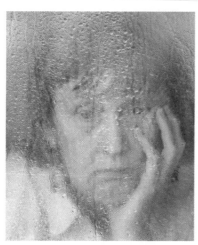

▲ **FIGURE 10.15**
Depressed Woman at Window.

Word	Pronunciation		Elements	Definition
anxiety	ang-**ZI**-eh-tee		Greek *distress, anxiety*	Distress and dread caused by fear
bipolar disorder	bi-**POH**-lar dis-**OR**-der	S/ P/ R/	-ar *pertaining to* bi- *two* -pol- *pole*	A mood disorder with alternating periods of depression and mania
delusion	dee-**LOO**-shun	S/ R/	-ion *action, condition* delus- *deceive*	Fixed, unyielding false belief held despite strong evidence to the contrary
hallucination	hah-loo-sih-**NAY**-shun	S/ R/	-ation *process* hallucin- *imagination*	Perception of an object or event when there is no such thing present
mania	**MAY**-nee-ah		Greek *frenzy*	Mood disorder with hyperactivity, irritability, and rapid speech
manic (adj)	**MAN**-ik	S/ R/	-ic *pertaining to* man- *frenzy*	Pertaining to or suffering from mania
mute	MYUT		Latin *silent*	Unable or unwilling to speak
paranoia	par-ah-**NOY**-ah	P/ R/	para- *abnormal, beside* -noia *to think*	Presence of persecutory delusions
paranoid	**PAR**-ah-noyd	S/	-oid *resembling*	Having delusions of persecution
phobia	**FOH**-bee-ah		Greek *fear*	Pathologic fear or dread
psychiatry	sigh-**KIGH**-ah-tree	S/ R/	-iatry *treatment* psych- *mind*	Diagnosis and treatment of mental disorder
psychiatrist psychiatric (adj)	sigh-**KIGH**-ah-trist sigh-kee-**AH**-trik	S/ S/	-iatrist *one who treats* -ic *pertaining to*	Licensed medical specialist in psychiatry Pertaining to psychiatry
psychology	sigh-**KOL**-oh-jee	S/ R/CF	-logy *study of* psych/o- *mind*	Science concerned with the behavior of the human mind
psychologist	sigh-**KOL**-oh-jisl	S/	-logist *one who studies, specialist*	Licensed specialist in psychology
psychosis	sigh-**KOH**-sis	S/ R/	-osis *condition* psych- *mind*	Disorder causing mental disruption and loss of contact with reality
psychotic (adj)	sigh-**KOT**-ik	S/ R/CF	-tic *pertaining to* psych/o- *mind*	Pertaining to or affected by psychosis
sociopath	**SOH**-see-oh-path	S/ R/CF	-path *disease* soci/o- *society, social*	Person with antisocial personality disorder

EXERCISES

A. Elements *remain your best tool for deconstructing and understanding the meaning of a medical term. Each of the following terms has an element bolded. Identify the type of that element, and write the meaning of the element.*

Medical Term	**Type of Element (P, R, CF, or S)**	**Meaning of the Element**
1. **socio**path	_____	_____
2. **man**ic	_____	_____
3. **psych**osis	_____	_____
4. **para**noia	_____	_____
5. hallucin**ation**	_____	_____

B. Demonstrate *your knowledge of medical terminology for mental health. Fill in the blanks.*

1. What two symptoms do patients with OCD exhibit? _____ and _____

2. Name three different phobias and define them:

    a. _____

    b. _____

    c. _____

3. What characterizes anxiety disorders? _____

4. What is the difference between a psychologist and a psychiatrist? _____

5. What is *bipolar disorder?* _____

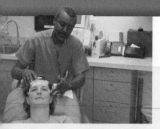

CHAPTER 10 REVIEW THE NERVOUS SYSTEM

CHALLENGE YOUR KNOWLEDGE

A. Prefixes: *This chapter contains a large number of important prefixes that you have also seen in previous chapters and will see again. Knowing these prefixes well will help increase your medical vocabulary. S-T-R-E-T-C-H your memory to recall previous terms with the same prefixes. You must be prepared to define each medical term! Fill in the chart.*

Prefix	Meaning of Prefix	Medical Term in This Chapter	Medical Term from a Previous Chapter
a	1.	2.	3.
anti	4.	5.	6.
auto	7.	8.	9.
de	10.	11.	12.
epi	13.	14.	15.
mono	16.	17.	18.
para	19.	20.	21.
post	22.	23.	24.
re	25.	26.	27.
sub	28.	29.	30.
syn	31.	32.	33.
trans	34.	35.	36.

B. Deconstruct the following medical terms *into their basic elements, and provide a meaning for each element. Remember to answer the final questions.*

Medical Term	Prefix	Meaning of Prefix	Root/CF	Meaning of Root/CF	Suffix	Meaning of Suffix
anesthesiologist	1.	2.	3.	4.	5.	6.
ataxia	7.	8.	9.	10.	11.	12.
endarterectomy	13.	14.	15.	16.	17.	18.
exacerbation	19.	20.	21.	22.	23.	24.
fibromyalgia	25.	26.	27.	28.	29.	30.
neuroglia	31.	32.	33.	34.	35.	36.
postictal	37.	38.	39.	40.	41.	42.
remission	43.	44.	45.	46.	47.	48.
synapse	49.	50.	51.	52.	53.	54.
subdural	55.	56.	57.	58.	59.	60.

61. Which two terms in the table at the bottom of the preceding page are opposites, and what do they mean?

_____ and _____ are opposites.

Term 1 means _____.

Term 2 means _____.

62. Which term in the table is a medical specialty? _____

_____

63. Which term is a surgical procedure? _____

64. Which terms can be a diagnosis? _____

_____

65. Which term refers to the acuteness of an illness? _____

C. Analyze: *Slash the following medical terminology into basic elements. Write the meaning of each element in the space beneath the line. The first one is done for you. Fill in the blanks. Remember: Every term may not have a prefix.*

anencephaly   an   /   enceph   /   aly
                             without   brain   condition

1. somatic _____ / _____ / _____

_____

2. epidural _____ / _____ / _____

_____

3. hydrocephalus _____ / _____ / _____

_____

4. teratogen _____ / _____ / _____

_____

5. meningocele _____ / _____ / _____

_____

6. psychiatrist _____ / _____ / _____

_____

7. synapse _____ / _____ / _____

_____

8. dementia _____ / _____ / _____

_____

9. postictal _____ / _____ / _____

_____

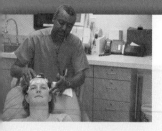

D. Abbreviations: *The following abbreviations could be present in many types of clinical documentation. You must be able to interpret them correctly. The abbreviation is given to you—write out in words the meaning of the abbreviation, and check (✔) whether it is a diagnosis, procedure, test, or "other." If it is "other," assign it a category. The first one is done for you. Fill in the chart.*

Abbreviation	Diagnosis	Procedure/Test	Other	Meaning of Abbreviation
tPA			✔ drug	tissue plasminogen activator
1. CP				**2.**
3. LOC				**4.**
5. CJD				**6.**
7. MRI				**8.**
9. EEG				**10.**
11. MS				**12.**
13. UA				**14.**
15. ALS				**16.**
17. PPS				**18.**
19. OCD				**20.**

E. Pronunciation: *Test yourself on the correct pronunciation of the following terms. Speaking and spelling medical terms correctly is the mark of an educated professional. Circle the correct answer for each pronunciation.*

1. amyotrophic:

   a. **A**-myo-trop-hic

   b. a-my-oh-**TROH**-fik

   c. **A**-my-o-troph-ik

2. hemiparesis:

   a. **HEMI**-par-e-sis

   b. **HEM**-ee-**PAR**-ee-sis

   c. **HEM**-ee-pah-**REE**-sis

3. syncope:

   a. **SINK**-oh-pee

   b. **SIN**-koh-peh

   c. sin-**KOP**-ee

4. meningococcal:

   a. men-**INJ**-oh-coc-al

   b. meh-nin-goh-**KOK**-al

   c. men-ing-oh-**KOK**-al

5. exacerbation:

   a. ek-zas-er-**BAY**-shun

   b. **EX**-ash-er-bay-shun

   c. ex-ash-er-bay-**SHUN**

F. Suffixes *can have more than one meaning, but only one of the meanings will apply to a particular term. In this exercise, practice using the suffix* oma, *and then use it to construct new terms.*

1. The suffix *oma* has two meanings:

   _____ or _____

   Recall from a previous chapter:

2. In the term *hematoma*, the meaning of *oma* is _____.

3. Describe a hematoma: _____

4. In the term *glioma*, the meaning of *oma* is _____.

5. Describe a glioma: _____

   _____

   Construct more terms for the following tumors:

6. A nerve tumor _____/_____/ oma

7. A tumor of the meninges _____/_____/ oma

8. Any tumor implying "cancerous" _____/_____/ oma

9. A tumor arising in a gland _____/_____/ oma

G. Spelling demons: *You choose the 10 most difficult terms to spell in this chapter. Write them below; then dictate them to a fellow student, and see who has more of them spelled correctly. Then have your exercise partner dictate his or her 10 most difficult terms to you. Good luck—the terms you find most difficult will probably be ones that will appear on a test.*

Your 10 Most Difficult Terms	Your Partner's 10 Terms
1.	11.
2.	12.
3.	13.
4.	14.
5.	15.
6.	16.
7.	17.
8.	18.
9.	19.
10.	20.

21. Number of my terms I spelled correctly _____

22. Number of my partner's dictated terms I spelled correctly _____

23. Write here any terms you have spelled incorrectly from either test:_____

   _____

   Can you correctly pronounce each term? Can you define each term?

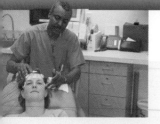

H. Word attack: *Find your clues to the correct answer in the question.*

Question:

Endarterectomy means:

a. surgical excision of an organ   d. surgical excision inside an artery

b. surgical excision inside the skull   e. surgical excision of a bone

c. surgical excision of a gland

1. Slash the term in the question. On the line, write the elements. Below the line, write the meaning of the elements.

_____ / _____ / _____

_____

2. Since all the answers refer to "surgical excision" (which you know is the suffix), use another element for a better clue.

Prefix means: _____

Root means: _____

3. Cross off all the choices that do not have any relation to either the prefix or the root.

I've crossed off choices _____ .

4. My remaining choices are _____

5. What is the *only* choice that contains the meanings of *both* the prefix and the root? _____

6. Therefore, the correct answer is _____ .

I. Elements: *In the following medical terms, one element of the term is capped and bolded. Identify what type of element it is, and give the meaning of the element. Then give the meaning of the term. Fill in the chart.*

Medical Term	Element Identity (P, R, CF, or S)	Meaning of Element	Meaning of Medical Term
arterio**GRAPHY**	1.	2.	3.
CONTUSion	4.	5.	6.
en**CEPHALO**pathy	7.	8.	9.
DEmyelination	10.	11.	12.
MICROcephaly	13.	14.	15.
mi**GRAINE**	16.	17.	18.
BIfida	19.	20.	21.
NEUROtransmitter	22.	23.	24.
ANalgesia	25.	26.	27.
SYRINGOmyelia	28.	29.	30.

J. Greek/Latin *terms cannot be further deconstructed into prefix, root, or suffix. You must know them for what they are. Test your knowledge of these terms with this exercise. Match the meaning in column 1 with the correct medical term in column 2.*

_____ **1.** to bring to

_____ **2.** furrow, ditch

_____ **3.** glue

_____ **4.** to shake

_____ **5.** to bring away from

_____ **6.** hardness

_____ **7.** circle

_____ **8.** membrane

_____ **9.** seizure

_____ **10.** brain

A. gyrus

B. sclerosis

C. efferent

D. cerebrum

E. meninges

F. sulcus

G. epilepsy

H. tremor

I. glia

J. afferent

K. Roots/combining forms *will always be the foundation of every medical term. A solid knowledge of roots can aid you in understanding more medical terms. Match the correct root or combining form in column 1 to its meaning in column 2. Fill in the blanks.*

_____ **1.** myo

_____ **2.** narco

_____ **3.** mut

_____ **4.** myel

_____ **5.** ict

_____ **6.** neuro

_____ **7.** troph

_____ **8.** psycho

_____ **9.** occulta

_____ **10.** herni

A. development

B. mind

C. hidden

D. rupture

E. seizure

F. muscle

G. stupor

H. nerve

I. spinal cord

J. silent

L. Recall and review: *How well do you remember these word elements from a previous chapter? Try to answer without looking back to check. Fill in the chart.*

Element	Type of Element (P, R, CF, or S)	Meaning of Element
tox	1.	2.
attenu	3.	4.
patho	5.	6.
ectomy	7.	8.
emic	9.	10.
megaly	11.	12.
cubit	13.	14.
auto	15.	16.
phylact	17.	18.
anti	19.	20.

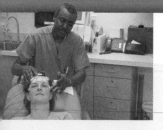

M. Brief answer: *If you really understand the meanings of terms, you can explain the difference between terms to a patient or a fellow student. Explain the difference between:*

1. delusion: _____

   hallucination: _____

2. concussion: _____

   contusion: _____

N. Chapter challenge: *Circle the correct answer.*

1. *Afferent* and *efferent* are opposite terms. Find the pair(s) of opposites below:

   a. acute/chronic   **d.** None of these are opposites.

   b. epidural/subdural   **e.** All of these are opposites.

   c. exacerbation/remission

2. Which of the following abbreviations is *not* a disease?

   a. ALS   **d.** TIA

   b. PID   **e.** ANS

   c. FAS

3. Which term has two prefixes?

   a. myasthenia   **d.** teratogenic

   b. postpolio   **e.** parasympathetic

   c. intermittent

4. Which disease needs treatment by a psychiatrist?

   a. narcolepsy   **d.** monoplegia

   b. status epilepticus   **e.** bovine spongiform encephalopathy

   c. schizophrenia

5. If you are diagnosed with an intracranial hemorrhage, what type of specialist needs to see you?

   a. cardiologist   **d.** hematologist

   b. pathologist   **e.** dermatologist

   c. neurologist

6. What would you take for pain relief?

   a. analgesic   **d.** a and b

   b. NSAID   **e.** a, b, and c

   c. TIA

7. What is the definition of a *spasm?*

   a. paralysis of both lower extremities   **d.** involuntary falling asleep

   b. sudden involuntary contraction of a muscle group   **e.** complete loss of sensation

   c. paralysis of one half of the body

8. Partial *paralysis* is called:

   a. syncope   **d.** paresthesia

   b. tremor   **e.** myelitis

   c. paresis

O. Terminology challenge: *Use your Glossary or dictionary for additional help if you need it. The word febrile has appeared in this chapter but does not appear in a WAD box. Answer the following questions regarding this term and its application in this chapter.*

1. *Febrile* is associated with a certain type of seizure. Who is most prone to a febrile seizure? _____

2. What triggers this seizure? _____

3. What other term, from a previous chapter, is also associated with the answer in question 2? _____

4. Use the term *febrile* in a sentence of your own choice that could be patient documentation. _____

_____

P. Apply your knowledge *of the language of neurology to the following sentences. Complete the sentences by inserting the correct medical terminology in the blanks.*

1. Vascular (irreversible loss of the mind's cognitive function) _____ is the second most common form of (same term) _____ . It can come on gradually when arteries supplying the brain become (narrowed or blocked) _____ . The patient will show signs of (oxygen deprivation) _____ . It can also occur suddenly after a (CVA) _____ .

2. (Squeezing together to increase density) _____ of the spinal cord can occur from a tumor in the cord or spine or from a (ruptured) _____ disc.

3. On the surface of the cerebrum, numerous (ridges) _____ are separated by (fissures) _____ .

Q. Translate: *Rewrite the following sentences in nonmedical language a patient can understand. (Hint: Underline the medical terms first so that you know what you have to translate.)*

1. Other conditions causing dementia include reactions to medications, such as sedatives and antiarthritics; depression in the elderly; and infections, such as AIDS and encephalitis.

_____

_____

_____

2. The EEG shows diffuse epileptic discharges in the left frontal region; her CT is normal, and an MRI shows a 20-mm-diameter mass adjacent to her left ventricle.

_____

_____

_____

3. Demyelination can occur in the PNS and be caused by inflammation, vitamin B_{12} deficiency, toxins, and some medications.

_____

_____

_____

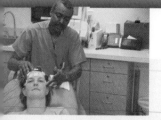

R. Chapter challenge: *Circle the correct answer.*

1. Temporary LOC is a symptom of:

   a. tremor

   b. ataxia

   c. paralysis

   d. syncope

   e. spina bifida

2. What is unusual about the terms *neurotransmitter* and *encephalitis?*

   a. They are both misspelled.

   b. One prefix is not in the usual place.

   c. Neither term contains a prefix.

   d. Neither term contains a suffix.

   e. The only elements in both terms are roots.

3. The dormant primary virus infection in childhood that later manifests as *shingles* is:

   a. prion

   b. varicella

   c. clostridium botulinum

   d. spina bifida cystica

   e. corpus callosum

4. If you are in a *postictal* state, you have had a:

   a. seizure

   b. fainting spell

   c. migraine

   d. hemorrhage

   e. fracture

5. Which term means the process of recording the electrical activity of the brain?

   a. electroneurodiagnostic

   b. electroencephalogram

   c. electroencephalograph

   d. electroencephalography

   e. none of these terms

6. Choose the pair of correctly spelled terms:

   a. parietal/occipital

   b. cerebrospinal/cerebelum

   c. araknoid/menninges

   d. dementia/dellirium

   e. concusion/epilepsy

7. Which of the following could be a sign of child abuse?

   a. PNS

   b. SBS

   c. CSF

   d. ADL

   e. CVA

8. Intense throbbing, pulsating pain in one area of the head, often with nausea and vomiting, can be symptomatic of:

   a. migraine

   b. ataxia

   c. encephalitis

   d. syncope

   e. shingles

9. A short-term, small stroke with symptoms lasting for less than 24 hours is a(n):

   a. TIA

   b. STAT

   c. EEG

   d. CVA

   e. tPA

S. Case Report challenge: *Now that you are more comfortable with the terms in this chapter, you can apply that knowledge and briefly answer the questions about the Case Report. If you read the report through and underline all the medical terminology, this will make it easier to answer the questions.*

CASE REPORT 10.1

YOU ARE

... an **electroneurodiagnostic** technologist working with Gregory Solis, MD, a **neurosurgeon** at Fulwood Medical Center.

YOU ARE COMMUNICATING WITH

... Ms. Roberta Gaston, a 39-year-old woman, who has been referred by Raul Cardenas, MD, a neurologist, for evaluation for possible neurosurgery. Ms. Gaston has had epileptic seizures since the age of 16. She also has daily minor spells in which she stops interacting and blinks rhythmically for about 20 seconds, after which she returns to normal. She is unable to work and is cared for by her parents. Her neurologic examination is normal. Her electroencephalogram (EEG) shows diffuse epileptic discharges in the left frontal region. Her CT scan is normal. An MRI shows a 20-mm-diameter mass adjacent to her left ventricle.

For Ms. Gaston, who was seen in Dr. Solis' neurosurgery clinic, the EEG did not localize an epileptic source. Hence, deep brain electrodes were inserted into the region of the suspicious mass that showed on MRI. Seizures were recorded arising in the mass itself. Dr. Solis performed a surgical resection of the mass, which was a glioma. She has been seizure-free since the surgery a year ago.

Ms. Gaston suffered from both absence and tonic-clonic seizures.

1. What is the difference between a *neurologist* and a *neurosurgeon?* _____

_____

2. Why is Ms. Gaston unable to work? _____

_____

3. What diagnostic tests did Ms. Gaston undergo? _____

_____

4. Define *glioma:* _____

_____

5. What type of surgery did the patient have? _____

_____

6. Explain the difference in the types of seizures Ms. Gaston had: _____

_____

7. What other body system has a *ventricle,* and where is it located? _____

_____

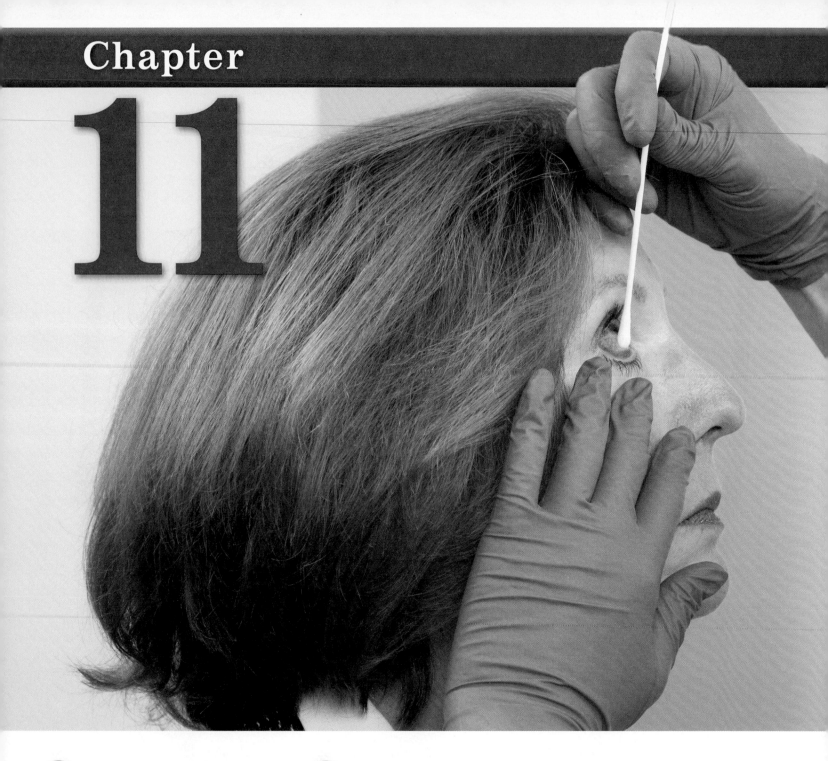

Chapter

11

SPECIAL SENSES OF THE EYE AND EAR

The Essentials of the Languages of Ophthalmology and Otology

CASE REPORT 11.1

YOU ARE

. . . an **ophthalmic** technician (OT) working in the office of **ophthalmologist** Angela Chun, MD, a member of the Fulwood Medical Group.

YOU ARE COMMUNICATING WITH

. . . Mrs. Jenny Hughes, a 30-year-old computer software consultant. She walked into the office with painful, red, swollen eyelids and a sticky, purulent discharge from both eyes. The administrative medical assistant did not hold her in the reception area but brought her directly to you. Mrs. Hughes complains of headache and **photophobia**, and says her eyelids were stuck together when she woke up this morning. She tells you that a couple of days earlier, she had gone into a small business office to install software at the firm's 10 workstations. One of the employees was absent with **pink eye**. Mrs. Hughes wants to know if she could have contracted the disease from that employee's keyboard, and how to prevent her husband and two children from getting it. In your hand, you have a pen and clipboard with the office Notice of Privacy Practices and sign-in sheet for her to sign. How do you proceed?

LEARNING OUTCOMES

In order to make correct decisions in situations like Mrs. Hughes' case, to communicate with Dr. Chun about the patient, to participate in patient education, and to document the patient's care, you need to be able to:

LO 11.1 Comprehend, analyze, spell, and write the medical terms of **ophthalmology.**

LO 11.2 Recognize and pronounce the medical terms of ophthalmology.

LO 11.3 Discuss the cause, diagnosis, and treatment of common disorders of the eye.

NOTE: The sense of smell is discussed as an integral part of the respiratory system; the sense of taste, as an integral part of the digestive system; and the sense of touch, as an integral part of the nervous system.

In your future career, you may work directly and/or indirectly with one or more of the following:

- **Ophthalmologists** are medical specialists in the diagnosis and treatment of diseases of the eye.

- **Optometrists** are professionals skilled in the measurement of vision.

The health professionals listed below perform specific assigned procedures and support ophthalmologists according to the depth of their training:

- Certified ophthalmic medical technicians
- Certified ophthalmic assistants
- Certified ophthalmic technicians
- Certified ophthalmic technologists
- Registered ophthalmic ultrasound biometrists
- Diagnostic ophthalmic sonographers

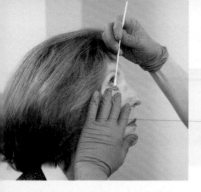

LESSON 11.1

Accessory Structures of the Eye

OBJECTIVES

Mrs. Jenny Hughes' "pink eye" involved her conjunctiva and eyelids—two of the periorbital accessory structures of the eye, located around the orbit and in front of the eyeball. All the accessory structures support and protect the exposed front surface of the eyes.

The information in this lesson will enable you to use correct medical terminology to:

11.1.1 Explain the roles of the accessory structures in protecting the eye.

11.1.2 Describe the accessory structures and their disorders.

11.1.3 Link the structure of the accessory structures of the eye to their functions.

The accessory structures have important functions that support and protect the exposed front surface of the eye.

The **eyebrows** *(Figure 11.1)* keep sweat from running into the eyes and function in nonverbal communication to show how you're feeling in response to certain stimuli.

The **eyelids** protect the eyes from foreign objects. They blink to move tears across the eyes' surface and sweep debris away. They close in sleep to keep out visual stimuli. They are covered in the body's thinnest layer of skin.

The **eyelashes** are strong hairs that help keep debris out of the eyes. They arise from hair follicles with their sebaceous glands on the edge of the lids.

The **conjunctiva** is a transparent mucous membrane that lines the inside of both eyelids. It moves freely over the eyeball and covers the front of the eye but not the central portion (the **cornea**). In the conjunctiva, numerous goblet cells secrete a thin film of mucin (a complex protein) that keeps the eyeball moist. It has numerous small blood vessels and is richly supplied with nerve endings that make it very sensitive to pain.

The **lacrimal apparatus** *(Figure 11.2)* consists of the **lacrimal (tear) gland** located in the superolateral corner of the orbit. This gland secretes tears, and short ducts carry the tears to the conjunctiva's surface. After washing across the conjunctiva, the tears leave the eye at its medial corner by draining into the **lacrimal sac.** They then flow into the **nasolacrimal duct,** which carries the tears into the nose, from where they are swallowed.

The functions of your tears are to:

- **Clean and lubricate** the surface of the eyes;
- **Deliver** nutrients and oxygen to the conjunctiva; and
- **Prevent infection** through bactericidal (bacteria-killing) enzymes.

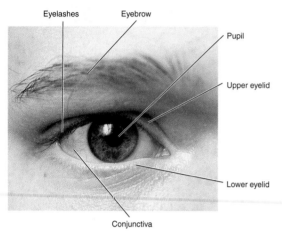

▲ **FIGURE 11.1**
External Anatomy of the Eye.

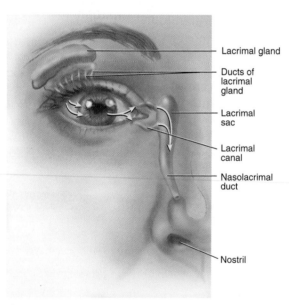

▲ **FIGURE 11.2**
Lacrimal Apparatus.

Word	Pronunciation	Elements		Definition
biometry biometrist	bi-**OH**-meh-tree	R/CF S/ S/	bi/o- *life* -metry *process of measuring* -metrist *skilled In measuring*	The study of numeric data based on biologic observations Skilled in biometry
conjunctiva conjunctival (adj) conjunctivitis "pink eye"	kon-junk-**TIE**-vah kon-junk-**TIE**-val kon-junk-tih-**VI**-tis PINK EYE	 S/ R/ S/	Latin *inner lining of eyelids* -al *pertaining to* conjunctiv- *conjunctiva* -itis *inflammation* Lay term for conjunctivitis	Inner lining of eyelids Pertaining to the conjunctiva Inflammation of the conjunctiva Conjunctivitis
cornea corneal (adj)	**KOR**-nee-ah **KOR**-nee-al		Latin *web, tunic*	The central, transparent part of the outer coat of the eye covering the iris and pupil
lacrimal nasolacrimal duct	**LAK**-rim-al **NAY**-zoh-**LAK**-rim-al DUKT	S/ R/ R/CF R/	-al *pertaining to* lacrim- *tear* nas/o- *nose* duct *to lead*	Pertaining to tears and the tear apparatus Passage from the lacrimal sac to the nose
ophthalmology ophthalmologist ophthalmic (adj)	off-thal-**MALL**-oh-jee off-thal-**MALL**-oh-jist off-**THAL**-mick	S/ R/CF S/ R/ S/	-logy *study of* ophthalm/o- *eye* -logist *one who studies, specialist* ophthalm- *eye* -ic *pertaining to*	Diagnosis and treatment of diseases of the eye Medical specialist in ophthalmology Pertaining to the eye
orbit orbital (adj) periorbital	**OR**-bit **OR**-bit-al per-ee-**OR**-bit-al	 S/ R/ P/	Latin *circle* -al *pertaining to* orbit- *orbit* peri- *around*	The bony socket that holds the eyeball Pertaining to the orbit Pertaining to tissues around the orbit
photophobia photophobic (adj)	foh-toe-**FOH**-bee-ah foh-toe-**FOH**-bik	S/ R/CF R/ S/	-ia *condition* phot/o- *light* -phob- *fear* -ic *pertaining to*	Fear of the light because It hurts the eyes Pertaining to or suffering from photophobia

EXERCISES

A. Build *your medical vocabulary. Many of the prefixes and suffixes you see in this chapter you will meet in later chapters and use to build your knowledge of additional medical terms. Fill in the chart.*

Medical Term	Prefix	Meaning of Prefix	Root(s)/CF(s)	Meaning of R/CF	Suffix	Meaning of Suffix
nasolacrimal	1.	2.	3.	4.	5.	6.
conjunctivitis	7.	8.	9.	10.	11.	12.
periorbital	13.	14.	15.	16.	17.	18.
ophthalmologist	19.	20.	21.	22.	23.	24.
photophobia	25.	26.	27.	28.	29.	30.

B. Continue *working with the terms in the WAD.*

1. Take the term *ophthalmologist,* add two different suffixes to the same root/combining form, and construct two new medical terms:

_____ / _____ means _____

    R/CF   S

_____ / _____ means _____

    R/CF   S

LESSON 11.1 Disorders of the Accessory Glands
(LO 11.1, 11.2, and 11.3)

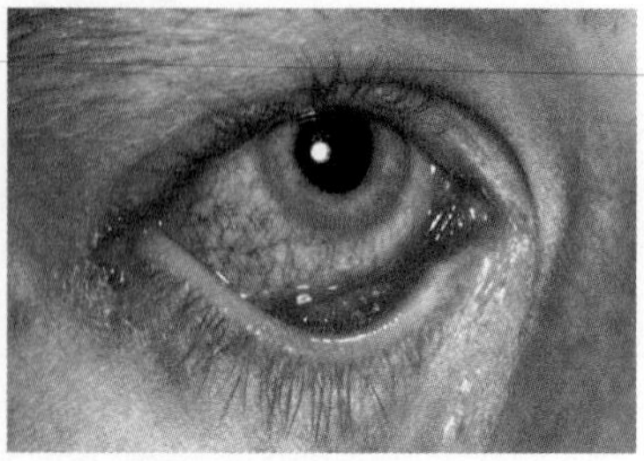

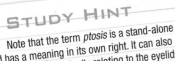

▲ **FIGURE 11.3**
Conjunctivitis.

Stye

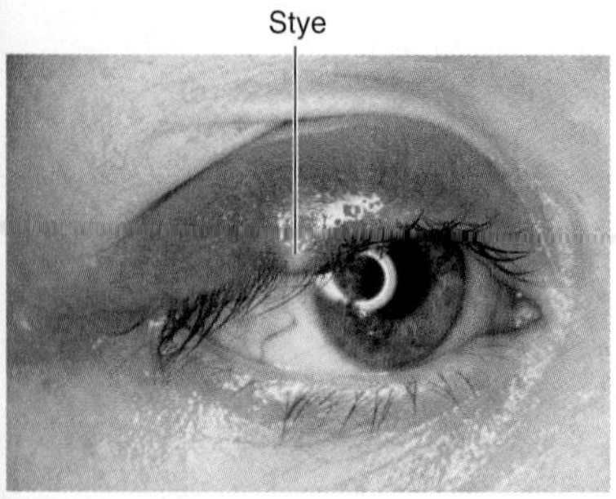

▲ **FIGURE 11.4**
Stye Showing Pus-Filled Cyst.

ABBREVIATION

q4h   Every four hours.

The accessory glands of the eyes can be affected by a number of different disorders, most of which cause noticeable discomfort.

Conjunctivitis *(Figure 11.3)*, an inflammation of the conjunctiva, is more commonly viral than bacterial; it can also be caused by irritants like chlorine, soaps, fumes, and smoke.

Eyelid edema, a generalized swelling of the eyelids, is often produced by an allergic reaction *(see Chapter 8)* from cosmetics, pollen in the air, or insect stings and bites.

A **stye** or **hordeolum** is an infection of an eyelash follicle that produces an abscess *(Figure 11.4)*, with localized pain, swelling, redness, and pus at the edge of the eyelid.

Blepharitis occurs when multiple eyelash follicles become infected. The eyelid's margin shows persistent redness and crusting and may become ulcerated *(Figure 11.5)*.

Ptosis, in which the upper eyelid is constantly drooped over the eye, is due to **paresis** of the muscle that raises the upper lid *(Figure 11.6)*. The term **blepharoptosis** defines the sagging of the eyelids from excess skin. The plastic surgery procedure of **blepharoplasty** is used to repair the eyelid.

CASE REPORT 11.1 (CONTINUED)

Mrs. Hughes' pink eye is called acute **contagious conjunctivitis** *(Figure 11.3)*. It responds well to **antibiotic** eyedrops. Her hands were **contaminated** from the keyboard of the employee who had left work and gone home with pink eye. She transmitted the infection to her eye by touching or rubbing it. Your documentation of Mrs. Hughes' office visit could read:

Progress Note: 04/10/11
Mrs. Jenny Hughes was brought directly into the clinical area at 1030 hrs with what appeared to be conjunctivitis, "pink eye." Both eyelids were red and swollen with a **purulent discharge.** She complained of headache and photophobia. Dr. Chun prescribed three drops q4h of Neosporin eyedrops and sent a swab of the discharge to the laboratory. I instructed and watched Mrs. Hughes wash her hands and use an alcohol-based hand gel. I then had her sign in and sign our Notice of Privacy Practices. I instructed her in the use of the eyedrops and emphasized home care and hand care measures to prevent the infection from spreading to her family. She was given a return appointment in 1 week and told to call the office if the eyedrops do not help.
—Daphne Butras, OT, 1055 hrs.

STUDY HINT
Note that the term *ptosis* is a stand-alone term and has a meaning in its own right. It can also function as a suffix specifically relating to the eyelids when it is added to the combining form *blephar/o*.

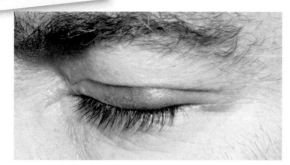

▲ **FIGURE 11.5**
Blepharitis.

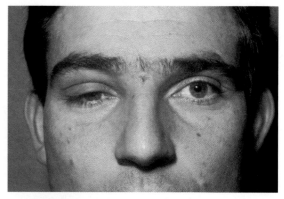

▲ **FIGURE 11.6**
Ptosis of Right Eyelid.

Word	Pronunciation	Elements		Definition
antibiotic	AN-tih-bye-OT-ik	S/ P/ R/	-tic *pertaining to* anti- *against* -bio- *life*	A substance that has the capacity to inhibit the growth of or destroy bacteria and other microorganisms
blepharitis	blef-ah-RYE-tis	S/ R/	-itis *inflammation* blephar- *eyelid*	Inflammation of the eyelid
blepharoptosis	BLEF-ah-ROP-toe-sis	S/ R/CF	-ptosis *drooping* blephar/o- *eyelid*	Drooping of the upper eyelid
blepharoplasty	BLEF-ah-roh-plas-tee	S/	-plasty *surgical repair*	Surgical repair of the eyelid
contagious	kon-TAY-jus		Latin *touch closely*	Infection can be transmitted from person to person or from a person to a surface to a person
contaminate (verb)	kon-TAM-in-ate	S/ P/ R/	-ate *composed of, pertaining to* con- *together* -tamin- *touch*	To cause the presence of an infectious agent to be on any surface
contamination (noun)	KON-tam-ih-NAY-shun	S/	-ation *process*	The presence of an infectious agent on any surface
hordeolum *(also called* stye)	hor-DEE-oh-lum		Latin *stye in the eye*	Abscess in an eyelash follicle
paresis	par-EE-sis		Greek *paralysis*	Partial paralysis
ptosis (Notes: *When a word begins with two consonants, the first is silent.* Ptosis *can also be used as a suffix.*)	TOE-sis		Greek *drooping*	Sinking down of the upper eyelid or an organ
purulent	PURE-you-lent	S/ R/	-ulent *abounding in* pur- *pus*	Showing or containing a lot of pus

EXERCISES

A. Review *the Case Report on this spread before answering the questions.*

1. What are the symptoms Mrs. Hughes was experiencing?_____

2. Explain each of the terms in Mrs. Hughes' diagnosis. _____

_____

3. What was the source of contamination for Mrs. Hughes? _____

4. What is the correct medical term for *pink eye?* _____

5. How can she prevent her family from getting this infection from her? _____

_____

B. The chapter objectives *can be met by inserting the correct medical terminology in the following patient documentation. Use only the terms contained in the WAD box above. Remember to proofread your work for correct spelling! Fill in the blanks.*

1. The patient's drooping left eyelid has been diagnosed as _____, and the surgical procedure

_____ will correct this condition

2. The patient has been advised to wipe down all household surfaces with a disinfectant to reduce the chance of further

_____ in the household.

3. The _____ on the patient's right eyelid has a _____ drainage.

4. Mrs. Hughes' eye infection will be helped by the prescribed _____.

C. Terminology challenge: *Apply your knowledge of the language of ophthalmology and answer the following question.*

1. Which element in the WAD that functions as a suffix is also a medical term in its own right? _____.

- **Amblyopia** is treated with a patch over the stronger eye to develop the vision in the weaker eye.

CASE REPORT 11.2

YOU ARE

... an ophthalmic technician employed by Angela Chun, MD, an ophthalmologist at Fulwood Medical Center.

YOU ARE COMMUNICATING WITH

... Mrs. Jenny Hughes, the mother of Sam Hughes, a 2½-year-old boy, who has been referred by his pediatrician to Dr. Chun. Mrs. Hughes states that for the past couple of months, Sam's right eye has turned in. The only visual difficulty she has noticed is that he sometimes misses a Cheerio when he tries to grab it.
You are responsible for documenting Sam's diagnostic and therapeutic procedures and explaining their significance to his mother.

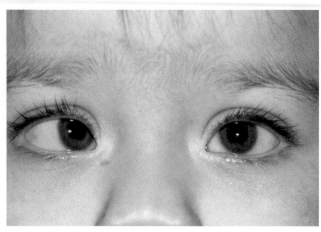

▲ **FIGURE 11.7**
Strabismus.

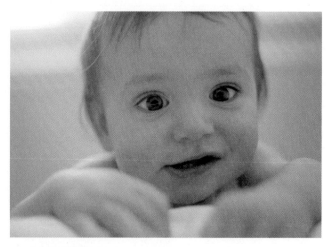

▲ **FIGURE 11.8**
Congenital Esotropia.

Extrinsic Muscles of the Eye
(LO 11.1, 11.2, and 11.3)

Humans have two eyes positioned on the face, one on either side of the nose facing forward, which work closely together. This eye configuration gives us very good three-dimensional perception (**stereopsis**) and hand-eye coordination. Stereopsis depends on an accurate alignment of the two eyes.

Six coordinated **extrinsic** eye muscles in each eye—attached to the inner wall of the orbit and outer surface of the eyeball—keep the eyes properly aligned, and move the eyes in all directions.

When there is a muscle imbalance in one eye, as in Sam Hughes' case, the alignment breaks down and **strabismus** *(Figure 11.7)*, also known as a "cross-eyed" condition, results.

Esotropia is a condition where the eye is turned in toward the nose. In congenital or infantile esotropia, both eyes look in toward the nose—the right eye looks to the left and the left eye looks to the right *(Figure 11.8)*. Children with this condition require surgery.

Accomodative esotropia is an inward eye turn, usually noticed around age 2 in 1% to 2% of children. Sam Hughes had an accommodative esotropia in one eye. Wearing glasses and perhaps a patch over the stronger eye will help to correct Sam's problem.

Exotropia, an outward eye turn, is noticed in children around ages 2 to 4. It will often respond to vision therapy, which includes eye exercises and glasses, from an **optometrist.** Eye muscle surgery can establish good **ocular** alignment.

Strabismus is not the same as **amblyopia,** or "lazy eye," which occurs in children when vision in one eye has not developed as well as vision in the other. Instead, it occurs because the eye and the brain won't cooperate for the affected eye.

S = Suffix   P = Prefix   R = Root   R/CF= Combining Form

Word	Pronunciation	Elements		Definition
accommodation (noun)	ah-kom-oh-**DAY**-shun	S/ P/ R/	-ion *action* ac- *toward* -commodat- *adjust*	The act of adjusting something to make it fit the needs; in this case the lens of the eye adjusts itself
accommodate (verb)	ah-**KOM**-oh-date	S/	-ate *pertaining to, -composed of*	To adapt to meet a need
accommodative (adj)	ah-kom-oh-**DAY**-tiv	S/	-ive *pertaining to*	Pertaining to accommodation
amblyopia	am-blee-**OH**-pee-ah	P/ R/	ambly- *dull* -opia *sight*	Failure or incomplete development of the pathways of vision to the brain
esotropia	es-oh-**TROH**-pee-ah	S/ P/ R/	-ia *condition* eso- *inward* -trop- *turn*	Turning the eye inward toward the nose
exotropia	ek-soh-**TROH**-pee-ah	P/	exo- *outward*	Turning the eye outward away from the nose
extrinsic	eks-**TRIN**-sik		Latin *on the outer side*	Any muscle located entirely on the outside of the structure under consideration; e.g., the eye
intrinsic	in-**TRIN**-sik		Latin *on the inner side*	Any muscle located entirely within (inside) the structure under consideration; e.g., the eye
ocular	**OCK**-you-lar	S/ R/	-ar *pertaining to* ocul- *eye*	Pertaining to the eye
optometrist	op-**TOM**-eh-trist	R/CF S/	opt/o- *vision* -metrist *skilled in measurement*	Someone skilled in the measurement of vision but who cannot treat eye diseases or prescribe medication
optometry	op-**TOM**-eh-tree	S/	-metry *process of measuring*	The profession of the measurement of vision
stereopsis	ster-ee-**OP**-sis	S/ R/	-opsis *vision* stere- *three-dimensional*	Three-dimensional vision
strabismus	strah-**BIZ**-mus	S/ R/	-ismus *take action* strab- *squint*	Turning of an eye away from its normal position

EXERCISES

A. Review *the Case Report on this spread before answering the questions.*

1. What did Mrs. Hughes notice about Sam's right eye? _____

2. Other than #1 above, what other visual difficulty has Mrs. Hughes noticed that Sam has? _____

_____

3. Who referred Sam to the ophthalmologist? _____

4. What is the name of the specialty department where Dr. Chun sees her patients? _____

5. What is Sam's diagnosis? _____

6. How can this condition be corrected in Sam's case? _____

B. Deconstruct *the following medical terms into their elements. Complete the chart. Notice in this exercise that not every medical term needs a prefix and/or a suffix but every medical term does contain one or more roots and/or combining forms.*

Medical Term	Prefix	Root(s)/ Combining Form(s)	Suffix	Meaning of Term
exotropia	1.	2.	3.	4.
optometrist	5.	6.	7.	8.
esotropia	9.	10.	11.	12.
amblyopia	13.	14.	15.	16.
stereopsis	17.	18.	19.	20.
ocular	21.	22.	23.	24.

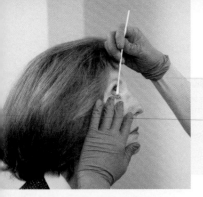

LESSON 11.2

The Eyeball and Seeing

OBJECTIVES

Although your eyeball may appear to be solid, it's actually a hollow sphere that measures around 1 inch in diameter. Knowledge of its terminology, structure, and function allows you to understand how we see and what major problems and disorders can arise with the eye. In this lesson, the information will enable you to use correct medical terminology to:

11.2.1 Identify the principal structures of the eyeball and their functions.

11.2.2 Explain the role of the cornea and the problems that can occur in that structure.

11.2.3 Describe the structures and functions of the lens and its associated structures.

11.2.4 Link the different components of the retina to their functions.

11.2.5 Discuss disorders of the eyeball.

KEYNOTES

• The **cornea** protects the eye and, by changing shape, provides about 60% of the eye's focusing power.

• The **iris** controls the amount of light entering the eye.

• The lens changes its shape to focus rays of light on the retina.

• Medical shorthand for a quick, normal eye examination can be **PERRLA:** pupils equal, round, reactive to light and accommodation.

The Eyeball (Globe)
(LO 11.1, 11.2, and 11.3)

The functions of your eyeball are to continuously:

1. **Adjust** the amount of light it lets in to reach the retina;

2. **Focus** on near and distant objects; and

3. **Produce** images of those objects and instantly transmit them to the brain.

As you learned earlier in this chapter, the front of the eyeball is covered by the conjunctiva. This thin layer of tissue lines the inside of the eyelids and curves over the eyeball to meet the **sclera** *(Figure 11.9)*, the tough, white outer layer of the eye.

At the center of the front of the eye is the **cornea,** a transparent, dome-shaped membrane. The cornea has no blood supply and obtains its nutrients from tears and from fluid in the anterior chamber behind it.

When light rays strike the eye, they pass through the cornea. Because of its dome curvature, those rays striking the edge of the cornea are bent toward its center. The light rays then go through the **pupil,** the black opening in the center of the colored area (the **iris**) in the front of the eye.

The iris controls the amount of light entering the eye. For example, when you're in the dark outside at night the iris opens **(dilates)** to allow more light into the eye. When you're in bright sunlight or in a well-lit room, the iris closes **(constricts)** to allow less light into the eye.

After traveling through the pupil, the light rays pass through the transparent **lens.** This lens can become thicker and thinner, enabling it to bend light rays and focus them on the **retina** at the back of the eye. Accommodation is the process of changing focus, and **refraction** is the process of bending light rays.

The lens does not contain blood vessels **(avascular)** or nerves, and with increasing age, it loses its elasticity. Because of this reduced elasticity, when you reach your forties, your eyes may have difficulty focusing on near objects, a condition called **presbyopia.**

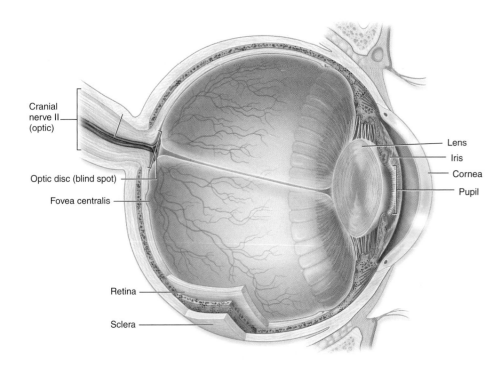

Cranial nerve II (optic)

Optic disc (blind spot)

Fovea centralis

Retina

Sclera

Lens

Iris

Cornea

Pupil

▲ **FIGURE 11.9** Anatomy of the Eyeball.

Word	Pronunciation	Elements		Definition
avascular	a-**VAS**-cue-lar	S/ P/ R/	-ar *pertaining to* a- *without* -vascul- *blood vessel*	Without a blood supply
constrict (verb)	kon-**STRIKT**	P/ R/	con- *with, together* -strict *narrow*	Become or make narrow
constriction (noun)	kon-**STRIK**-shun	S/	-ion *action, condition*	A narrowed portion of a structure
dilate (verb) dilation (noun)	**DIE**-late die-**LAY**-shun	S/ R/	Latin *dilate* -ion *action, condition* dilat- *dilate*	To perform or undergo dilation Stretching or enlarging an opening or a structure
iris	**EYE**-ris		Greek *diaphragm of the eye*	Colored portion of the eye with the pupil in its center
lens	**LENZ**		Latin *lentil shape*	Transparent refractive structure behind the iris
presbyopia	prez-bee-**OH**-pee-ah	S/ R/	-opia *sight* presby- *old man*	Difficulty in nearsighted vision occurring in middle and old age
pupil	**PYU**-pill		Latin *pupil*	The opening in the center of the iris that allows light to reach the lens
pupillary (adj) (Note: *Change to ll.*)	**PYU**-pill-ah-ree	S/ R/	-ary *pertaining to* pupill- *pupil*	Pertaining to the pupil
refract (verb)	ree-**FRACT**		Latin *break up*	Bend or change direction of a ray of light
refraction (noun)	ree-**FRAK**-shun	S/ R/	-ion *condition* refract- *bend*	The bending of light
retina	**RET**-ih-nah		Latin *net*	Light-sensitive innermost layer of the eyeball
retinal (adj)	**RET**-ih-nal	S/ R/	-al *pertaining to* retin- *retina*	Pertaining to the retina
sclera	**SKLAIR**-ah		Greek *hard*	Fibrous outer covering of the eyeball and the white of the eye
scleral (adj)	**SKLAIR**-al	S/ R/	-al *pertaining to* scler- *hardness, white of eye*	Pertaining to the sclera
scleritis	sklair-**RI**-tis	S/	-itis *inflammation*	Inflammation of the sclera

EXERCISES

A. Define *the statements in column 1 using the language of ophthalmology in colum 2. These medical terms all relate to the vision process. Fill in the blanks.*

_____ 1. colored portion of the eye   **A.** lens

_____ 2. bend a ray of light   **B.** retina

_____ 3. opening in the iris   **C.** avascular

_____ 4. transparent, refractive structure   **D.** pupil

_____ 5. difficulty in nearsighted vision   **E.** refract

_____ 6. innermost layer of eyeball   **F.** iris

_____ 7. fibrous, outer covering of the eye **G.** presbyopia

_____ 8. without a blood supply   **H.** sclera

B. The WAD *contains 3 pairs of noun/verb terms. Choose one pair and write a brief sentence for each term that is NOT a definition.*

1. _____

   _____

2. _____

   _____

- Rods of the retina perceive only dim light and not color. Cones of the retina perceive bright light and color.

- Rods and cones are called photoreceptor cells.

The Retina (LO 11.1, 11.2, and 11.3)

Your retina is the size of a postage stamp and has ten layers of cells. Located at the back of your eye *(Figure 11.10a)*, it's the final destination for light rays. The retina has 130 million **rods** *(Figure 11.10b)*, which perceive only light, not color, and function mostly in dim lighting. The retina has 6.5 million light- and color-activated **cones** *(Figure 11.10b)*, which have precise **visual acuity** (sharpness). Different cones respond to red, blue, and green light. Your perception of color is based on the intensity of various color mixtures from the three cone types.

Some people have a hereditary lack of response by one or more of the three cone types and show color blindness. The most common form of this is red-green color blindness. Here, red-green colors and related shades cannot be distinguished from each other.

The rods and cones convert the light rays' energy into electrical impulses. The **optic nerve**—a bundle of more than a million nerve fibers—transmits these impulses to the visual cortex at the back of your brain. The area where the optic nerve leaves the retina is called the **optic disc.** Because it has no rods and cones, the optic disc cannot form images; as a result, it's called the "blind spot."

Just lateral to the optic disc at the back of the retina is a circular, yellowish region called the **macula lutea** *(Figure 11.10a)*. In the center of the macula is a small pit called the **fovea centralis,** which has 4,000 tiny cones but no rods. Each cone has its own nerve fiber, and this gives the fovea area the sharpest vision. As you read this text, the words are precisely focused on your fovea centralis.

Behind the light-sensitive **photoreceptor** layer of the retina is a vascular layer called the **choroid.** This layer, together with the iris and its muscle, is called the **uvea.**

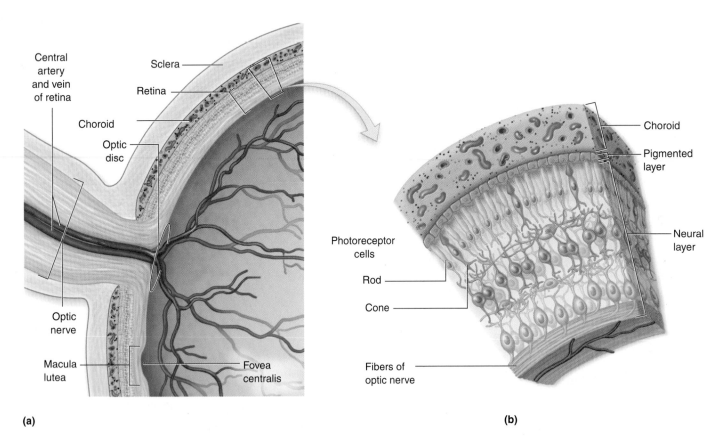

(a)

(b)

▲ **FIGURE 11.10**
Structure of the Retina.
(a) Retina. (b) Rods and cones.

Word	Pronunciation		Elements	Definition
choroid	**KOR**-oid		Greek *membrane*	Region of the retina and uvea
fovea centralis	**FOH**-vee-ah sen-**TRAH**-lis	R/ S/	fovea Latin *a pit* central- *center* -is *pertaining to*	Small pit in the center of the macula that has the highest visual acuity
macula lutea	**MACK**-you-lah **LOO**-tee-ah		macula Latin *small spot* lutea Latin *yellow*	Yellowish spot on the back of the retina; contains the fovea
optic optical (adj)	**OP**-tick **OP**-tih-kal	S/ R/	Greek *eye* -al *pertaining to* optic- *eye*	Pertaining to the eye or vision Pertaining to the eye or vision
photoreceptor	foh-toe-ree-**SEP**-tor	S/ R/CF R/	-or *that which does something* phot/o- *light* -recept- *receive*	A photoreceptor cell receives light and converts it into electrical impulses
uvea uveitis	**YOU**-vee-ah you-vee-**EYE**-tis	 S/ R/	Latin *vascular layer* -itis *inflammation* uve- *uvea*	Middle coat of the eyeball; includes the iris, ciliary body, and choroid Inflammation of the uvea
visual acuity	**VIH**-zhoo-wal ah-**KYU**-ih-tee		acuity Latin *sharpen*	Sharpness and clearness of vision

EXERCISES

A. The language of ophthalmology *will be your answers in this exercise. Review the WAD before you begin the exercise. Circle the best answer.*

1. Sharpness and clearness of vision is called:
   a. optical
   b. acuity
   c. vascular
   d. sclera
   e. choroid

2. Because it has no rods and cones, the optic disc cannot form images and thus is called the:
   a. fovea
   b. blind spot
   c. uvea
   d. visual cortex
   e. optic nerve

3. The term *photoreceptor* has:
   a. two combining forms and a suffix
   b. a prefix, a root, and a suffix
   c. a combining form, a root, and a suffix
   d. two roots and a suffix
   e. a suffix and a root

4. The area of sharpest vision is the:
   a. cornea
   b. rods
   c. macula lutea
   d. fovea centralis
   e. cones

B. Meet chapter *and lesson objectives and apply the language of ophthalmology to answer the questions.*

1. Where is the choroid located? _____

2. What does the term *vascular* mean in *vascular layer*? _____

3. What is the opposite of *vascular*? _____

4. What is the final destination of light rays in the eye? _____

5. What is the pit called that is in the center of the macula? _____

LESSON 11.2 Refraction (LO 11.1, 11.2, and 11.3)

The optic nerves leave each orbit through the optic **foramen.** Light travels at 186,000 miles per second, and even when it hits your eye, this speed remains the same. Light rays that hit the center of your cornea pass straight through the eye, while rays that hit away from the center then bend toward the center. These light rays then hit your lens and bend again, and in normal vision, the image is focused sharply on your retina *(Figure 11.11).*

Farsighted people are said to have **hyperopia** *(Figure 11.12).* Because the eyeball is shortened, objects close to the eye are focused behind the retina and vision is blurred. **Convex** lenses help to correct the problem.

Nearsighted people are said to have **myopia** *(Figure 11.13).* Because the eyeball is elongated, far-away objects are focused in front of the retina. Vision is blurred. **Concave** lenses help to correct the problem.

In **presbyopia,** a condition mentioned earlier in this chapter, the lens loses its flexibility, making it difficult to focus for near vision. This usually occurs when you reach your forties. Convex bifocal or transitional lenses help to correct this problem.

In **astigmatism,** unequal curvatures of the cornea cause unequal focusing and blurred images. This problem can be corrected with cylindrical lenses, which refract light more in one plane than in another.

A surgical procedure, **radial keratotomy,** is used to treat myopia. Radial cuts, like the spokes of a wheel, flatten the cornea so it can refract the light rays to focus on the retina.

Laser surgery can also change the shape of the cornea. It can flatten it to correct myopia, or it can alter the cornea's outer edges to correct hyperopia.

Laser-assisted in situ keratomileusis (LASIK) is used to treat myopia, hyperopia, and astigmatism. LASIK involves a computer-controlled laser that uses a cold beam of ultraviolet light, which alters the shape of the cornea by vaporizing the tissue.

ABBREVIATION

LASIK	laser-assisted in situ keratomileusis

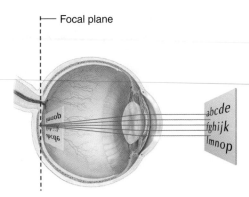

▲ **FIGURE 11.11**
Normal Vision.

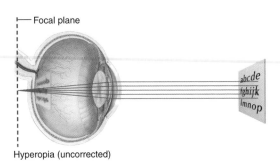

▲ **FIGURE 11.12**
Hyperopia (Farsightedness).

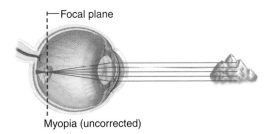

▲ **FIGURE 11.13**
Myopia (Nearsightedness).

Word	Pronunciation	Elements		Definition
astigmatism	ah-**STIG**-mah-tism	P/ S/ R/	a- *without* -ism *process* -stigmat- *focus*	Inability to focus light rays that enter the eye in different planes
concave convex	kon-**KAVE** kon-**VEKS**		Latin concavus *arched* Latin convexus *vaulted*	Having a hollowed surface A surface that is evenly curved outward
foramen foramina (pl)	fo-**RAY**-men fo-**RAM**-ih-nah		Latin *hole*	An opening through a structure
hyperopia	high-per-**OH**-pee-ah	P/ R/	hyper- *beyond* -opia *sight*	Able to see distant objects but unable to see close objects
in situ	IN **SIGH**-tyu		Latin *in its original place*	In the correct place
keratomileusis	ker-ah-**TOE**-mill-oo-sis	R/ R/CF	-mileusis *lathe* kerat/o- *cornea*	Cuts and shapes the cornea
keratotomy	ker-ah-**TOT**-oh-mee	S/ R/CF	-tomy *surgical incision* kerat/o- *cornea*	Incision in the cornea
myopia (Note: *One "op" is removed to allow the term to flow.*)	my-**OH**-pee-ah	R/ R/	myop- *to blink* -opia *sight*	Able to see close objects but unable to see distant objects
radial (adj)	**RAY**-dee-al	S/ R/	-al *pertaining to* radi- *radius*	Diverging in all directions from any given center

EXERCISES

A. Construct *the correct medical term to match the meaning given in column 1. Write each element in the correct column to form the complete term. Fill in the chart.*

Meaning of Medical Term	Prefix	Root(s)/Combining Form(s)	Suffix
inability to focus light rays	1.	2.	3.
able to see distant objects but not close ones	4.	5.	6.
able to see close objects but not distant ones	7.	8.	9.

B. Terminology challenge: *Use the information from this and previous spreads to answer the challenge questions.*

1. What other medical term ending in *opia* means difficulty in nearsighted vision that occurs in middle and old age? _____

2. What is the medical term for "nearsightedness"? _____

3. What eye conditions can laser surgery correct? _____

4. What is a medical term describing the condition that is opposite to the term in question 2? _____

C. Meet lesson objectives *and use the language of opthalmology to answer the following questions.*

1. Name two procedures that correct myopia: _____ and _____.

2. How does LASIK surgery alter the shape of the cornea? _____

3. What corrects astigmatism? _____

4. Why is myopia known as *nearsightedness*? _____

5. What helps to correct *hyperopia*? _____

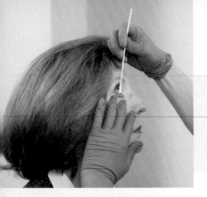

LESSON 11.3
Disorders of the Eye and Ophthalmic Procedures

Many eye disorders can threaten a patient's vision, but if detected early, the majority of these conditions can be cured or treated to slow or prevent the progression of vision loss. Routine eye exams are important for early detection and prevention, and are recommended at different times throughout life. The information in this lesson will enable you to use correct medical terminology to:

11.3.1 Discuss common disorders of the eye and their effects on vision.

11.3.2 Describe common ophthalmic procedures performed in the doctor's office.

Disorders of the Anterior Eyeball (LO 11.1, 11.2, and 11.3)

Conjunctivitis is the infectious, contagious, "bloodshot eyes"-causing condition that Mrs. Jenny Hughes had in the opening Case Report of this chapter. It can be caused by viruses and bacteria, and by organisms that cause sexually transmitted diseases (STDs) *(Chapter 15)*. Three other types of conjunctivitis are:

- **Allergic conjunctivitis,** which can be part of seasonal hay fever or produced by year-round allergens like animal dander and dust mites *(Chapter 8)*;

- **Irritant conjunctivitis,** which can be caused by air **pollutants** (smoke and fumes), chemicals like chlorine, and some ingredients found in soaps and cosmetics; and

- **Neonatal conjunctivitis (ophthalmia neonatorum),** which is specific to babies and can be caused by a blocked tear duct, by the antibiotic eye drops given routinely at birth, or by sexually transmitted bacteria from an infected mother's birth canal.

Corneal abrasions are caused by foreign bodies, by direct trauma (like being poked by a fingernail), or by ill-fitting contact lenses. An abrasion can grow into an ulcer. This ulcer or lesion can be stained with drops of the dye **fluorescein** to make it more easily visible on examination *(Figure 11.14)*.

Scleritis is an inflammation of the sclera (the white outer covering of the eyeball) that can affect one or both eyes.

Glaucoma results if fluid from inside the eyeball cannot escape from the eye into the bloodstream. The fluid continues to be produced and pressure builds up inside the eye. This pressure interferes with the blood supply to the retina, causing retinal cells to die and damage to the optic nerve fibers. Glaucoma is a major cause of blindness *(Figure 11.15)*, and it's treated with a lifelong use of eye drops, which help to prevent the condition from worsening.

A **cataract** is a cloudy or opaque area in the lens *(Figure 11.16)*. It is caused by aging and may be associated with diabetes and cigarette smoke. Symptoms include blurred vision and **photosensitivity.** A cataract may also be discovered during a routine eye exam. It is another major cause of blindness.

Congenital (present at birth) cataracts occur in less than 0.5% of newborns and can be unilateral (present in one eye) or bilateral (present in both eyes). They are treated in the same way as any other cataract.

When a cataract interferes with a patient's vision *(Figure 11.17)*, the lens needs to be removed and replaced with an artificial **intraocular** lens, which becomes a permanent part of the eye.

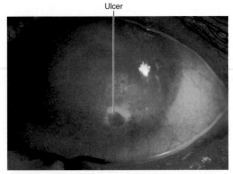

▲ **FIGURE 11.14**
Fluorescein-Stained Corneal Ulcer.

Ulcer

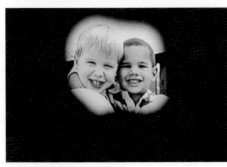

▲ **FIGURE 11.15**
Vision with Glaucoma.

Cataract

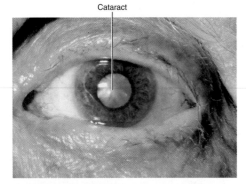

▲ **FIGURE 11.16**
Cataract.

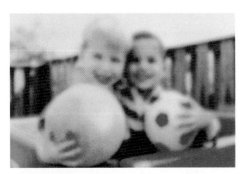

▲ **FIGURE 11.17**
Vision with Cataract.

Word	Pronunciation	Elements		Definition
cataract	**KAT**-ah-ract		Latin *to break down*	Complete or partial opacity of the lens
fluorescein	flor-**ESS**-ee-in	P/ R/	fluo- *fluorine* -rescein *resin*	Dye that produces a vivid green color under a blue light to diagnose corneal abrasions and foreign bodies
glaucoma	glau-**KOH**-mah	S/ R/	-oma *mass, tumor* glauc- *lens opacity*	Increased intraocular pressure
intraocular	in-trah-**OCK**-you-lar	S/ P/ R/	-ar *pertaining to* intra- *inside* -ocul- *eye*	Pertaining to the inside of the eye
ophthalmia neonatorum	off-**THAL**-me-ah ne-oh-nay-**TOR**-um	S/ R/ S/ P/ R/	-ia *condition* ophthalm- *eye* -orum *function of* neo- *new* -nat- *born*	Conjunctivitis of the newborn
photosensitivity	foh-toe-**SEN**-sih-tiv-ih-tee	S/ R/CF	-ity *condition* phot/o- *light*	When light produces pain in the eye
photosensitive (adj)	**FOH**-toe-SEN-sih-tiv	R/	-sensitiv- *feeling*	
pollution	poh-**LOO**-shun		Latin *to defile*	Condition that is unclean, impure, and a danger to health
pollutant	poh-**LOO**-tant	S/ R/	-ant *pertaining to* pollut- *unclean*	Substance that makes an environment unclean or impure

EXERCISES

A. Review *the medical terms contained on the two pages open in front of you. Use these terms to complete the following sentences. You may use a term only one time. Fill in the blanks.*

1. _____ can be the cause of bloodshot eyes.

2. Dust mites and pollen are _____.

3. Scratching your eye with a tree branch can produce a(n) _____.

4. _____ produces increased intraocular pressure.

5. When light causes pain in the eye, this is termed _____.

B. Use critical thinking *and the language of ophthalmology to answer the following questions.*

1. What is a "foreign body"? _____

2. Name two other kinds of foreign bodies that could get into your eye. _____ and _____

3. What type of safety equipment prevents foreign bodies from getting into your eyes? _____

4. What occupations are at greater risk for getting foreign bodies in their eyes? _____

5. Which of the terms in the WAD is a major cause of blindness? _____

6. What is the correct medical term for "conjunctivitis of the newborn"? _____

Disorders of the Retina (LO 11.1, 11.2, and 11.3)

An impaired retina affects your ability to see in the same way that an injured leg affects your ability to walk. In either case, your level of functioning in normal, daily life is limited.

Macular Degeneration (LO 11.1, 11.2, and 11.3)

Degeneration of the central macula results in a loss of visual acuity or sharpness, with a dark blurry area of vision loss in the center of the visual field *(Figure 11.18)*. Photoreceptor cell loss and bleeding with capillary proliferation and scar formation *(Figure 11.19)* also occur. Macular degeneration can progress to blindness. Most cases occur in people over 55. Although there is currently no known cure, laser **photocoagulation** may be used to destroy abnormal capillaries, which slows the pace of vision loss.

Retinal Detachment (LO 11.1, 11.2, and 11.3)

In retinal detachment, the retina may separate partially or completely from its underlying choroid layer, creating a retinal tear or hole. This detachment—visible on an **opthalmoscopic** exam—can happen suddenly, without pain, but is considered a surgical emergency. The patient sees a dark shadow invading his or her peripheral vision. **Laser surgery** is used to treat the small lesions and to "weld" the retina back into place.

Diabetic Retinopathy (LO 11.1, 11.2, and 11.3)

Some 50% of diabetics have **retinopathy.** Patients may experience hemorrhages (bleeding), which can lead to the destruction of the photoreceptor cells (rods and cones) and visual difficulties.

An ophthalmoscopic examination shows the disease *(Figure 11.20)*, and fluorescein **angiography** with pictures taken as the dye passes through the retina reveals more details.

Laser photocoagulation is often effective in controlling the lesions, but once vision is lost from an area of the retina, it usually doesn't return *(Figure 11.21)*.

Cancer of the Eye (LO 11.1, 11.2, and 11.3)

Tumors of the skin of the eyelids include the **squamous cell** and basal cell carcinomas and melanoma described in Chapter 3.

Retinoblastoma is the most common cancer in children and is diagnosed most frequently around 18 months of age. Of those children affected, 20% have the cancer in both eyes. This condition can be hereditary. With early detection and aggressive chemotherapy and laser surgery treatment, 90% of these cases can be cured.

In adults, the most common eye cancers are metastases to the eye from lung cancer in men and breast cancer in women.

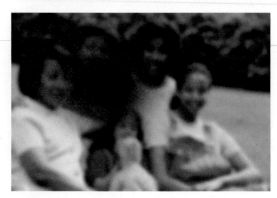

▲ **FIGURE 11.18**
Vision with Macular Degeneration.

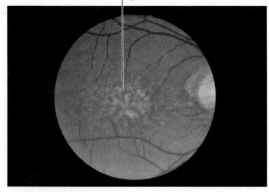

▲ **FIGURE 11.19**
Ophthalmoscopic View of Macular Degeneration.

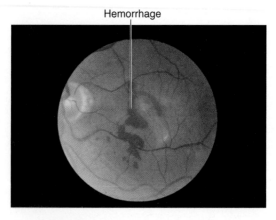

▲ **FIGURE 11.20**
Ophthalmoscopic View of Diabetic Retinopathy.

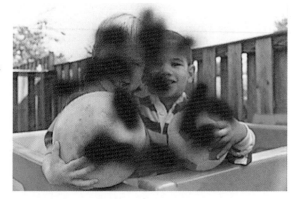

▲ **FIGURE 11.21**
Vision with Diabetic Retinopathy.

Word	Pronunciation		Elements	Definition
angiography	an-jee-**OG**-rah-fee	S/ R/CF	-graphy *process of recording* angi/o- *blood vessel*	Radiography of vessels after injection of contrast material
angiogram	**AN**-jee-oh-gram	S/	-gram *a record*	Radiogram obtained after injection of radiopaque material into blood vessels
laser surgery	**LAY**-zer **SUR**-jer-ee	S/ R/	Light Amplification by Simulated Emission of Radiation -ery *process of* surg- *operate*	Use of a concentrated, intense narrow beam of electromagnetic radiation for surgery
ophthalmoscope	off-**THAL**-moh-skope	S/ R/CF	-scope *instrument for viewing* ophthalm/o- *eye*	Instrument for viewing the retina
ophthalmoscopy ophthalmoscopic (adj)	**OFF**-thal-**MOS**-koh-pee **OFF**-thal-**MOS**-koh-pik	S/ S/	-scopy *to view, examine* -ic *pertaining to*	The process of viewing the retina Pertaining to the use of an ophthalmoscope
photocoagulation	foh-toe-koh-ag-you-**LAY**-shun	S/ R/CF R/	-ation *process* phot/o *light* -coagul- *clotting*	Using light (laser beam) to form a clot
retinoblastoma	**RET**-in-oh-blas-**TOE**-mah	S/ R/CF R/	-oma *tumor, mass* retin/o- *retina* -blast- *immature cell*	Malignant neoplasm of primitive retinal cells
retinopathy	ret-ih-**NOP**-ah-thee	S/	-pathy *disease*	Degenerative disease of the retina

EXERCISES

A. Elements *help build your knowledge of the language of ophthalmology. One element in each of the following medical terms is bolded. Identify the type of element (P, R/CF, S) in column 2, and then write the meaning of the element in column 3. Fill in the chart.*

Medical Term	P, R/CF, S	Meaning of Element
retino**blast**oma	1.	2.
ophthalmo**scope**	3.	4.
angio**graphy**	5.	6.
ophthalmoscopy	7.	8.
photo**coagul**ation	9.	10.
retino**pathy**	11.	12.
angiogram	13.	14.
ophthalmoscop**ic**	15.	16.

B. Apply *the terms in Exercise A to the questions in Exercise B.*

1. List all the terms from the above chart that are medical procedures: _____

2. List all the terms from the above chart that are diagnoses: _____

3. Which term is an adjective? _____

4. Which term is an instrument used in a procedure? _____

5. Which term is a malignant neoplasm of retinal cells? _____

6. Which term contains an element meaning *light?* _____

LESSON 11.3 Ophthalmic Procedures

(LO 11.1, 11.2, and 11.3)

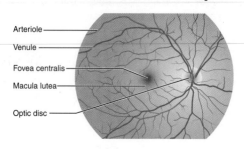

▲ FIGURE 11.22
Anatomy of the Fundus.

Arteriole
Venule
Fovea centralis
Macula lutea
Optic disc

A number of procedures, which are detailed in the following paragraphs, can be used to effectively examine the eye for various purposes.

Examination of the Retina

(LO 11.1, 11.2, and 11.3)

A **fundoscopy** examines the retina with an ophthalmoscope to identify the optic disc *(Figure 11.22)*, where the optic nerve leaves the back of the eye. The optic disc has no receptor cells and, as mentioned earlier in this chapter, it produces a "blind spot" in the visual field of each eye. In the middle of the optic disc, a retinal artery enters to supply the intraocular structures, and a retinal vein leaves the eye.

Color Vision

(LO 11.1, 11.2, and 11.3)

The **Ishihara color system** is used to test color vision. In the example in *Figure 11.23*, people with red-green color blindness would not be able to see the number 16 among the colored dots.

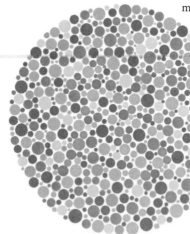

▲ FIGURE 11.23
Test for Color Blindness.
Reproduced with permission from *Ishihara's Tests for Color Deficiency*, published by Kanehara Trading Inc., Tokyo, Japan. Tests for color deficiency cannot be conducted with this figure. For accurate testing, the original plates should be used.

▶ FIGURE 11.24
Visual Acuity Tests.

Distance Vision

(LO 11.1, 11.2, and 11.3)

The **Snellen letter chart** is used to test distance vision *(Figure 11.24a)*. The results are recorded as a fraction. For example, when the chart is viewed from 20 feet, line 8 is the smallest line a person with standard vision can read. This is recorded as 20/20. If the patient using her or his left eye misses two letters on line 8, this is documented as **OS** 20/20 −2. The right eye is documented as **OD,** the left eye as **OS,** and the use of both eyes is noted as **OU.**

Near Vision (LO 11.1, 11.2, and 11.3)

Near vision is measured using handheld charts or **Jaeger reading cards** with printed paragraphs of different sizes of print *(Figure 11.24b)*.

Visual Fields (LO 11.1, 11.2, and 11.3)

Visual fields are tested in the following way: Sit 2 feet in front of your patient, and instruct the patient to cover one eye. Next, cover your own opposite eye. Now, bring a pencil into the horizontal and vertical fields to compare the patient's **peripheral vision** with your own.

Intraocular Pressure

(LO 11.1, 11.2, and 11.3)

Intraocular pressure is measured with a **tonometer,** which determines the eyeball's resistance to indentation or tension. Increased intraocular pressure indicates glaucoma.

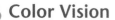

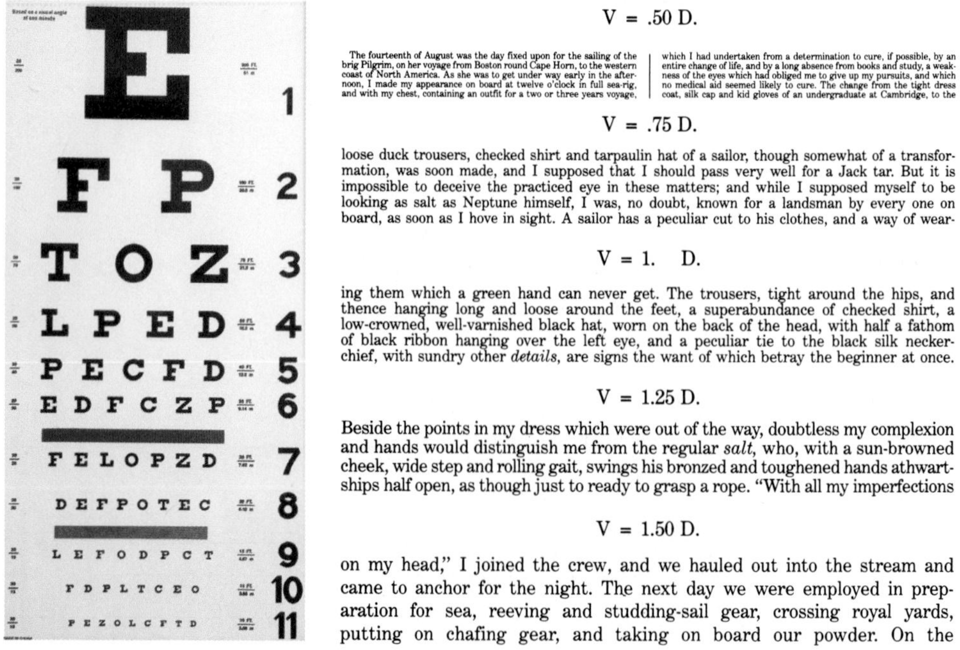

E 1
F P 2
T O Z 3
L P E D 4
P E C F D 5
E D F C Z P 6
F E L O P Z D 7
D E F P O T E C 8
L E F O D P C T 9
F D P L T C E O 10
P E Z O L C F T D 11

(a)

V = .50 D.

The fourteenth of August was the day fixed upon for the sailing of the brig Pilgrim, on her voyage from Boston round Cape Horn, to the western coast of North America. As she was to get under way early in the afternoon, I made my appearance on board at twelve o'clock in full sea-rig, and with my chest, containing an outfit for a two or three years voyage, | which I had undertaken from a determination to cure, if possible, by an entire change of life, and by a long absence from books and study, a weakness of the eyes which had obliged me to give up my pursuits, and which no medical aid seemed likely to cure. The change from the tight dress coat, silk cap and kid gloves of an undergraduate at Cambridge, to the

V = .75 D.

loose duck trousers, checked shirt and tarpaulin hat of a sailor, though somewhat of a transformation, was soon made, and I supposed that I should pass very well for a Jack tar. But it is impossible to deceive the practiced eye in these matters; and while I supposed myself to be looking as salt as Neptune himself, I was, no doubt, known for a landsman by every one on board, as soon as I hove in sight. A sailor has a peculiar cut to his clothes, and a way of wear-

V = 1.   D.

ing them which a green hand can never get. The trousers, tight around the hips, and thence hanging long and loose around the feet, a superabundance of checked shirt, a low-crowned, well-varnished black hat, worn on the back of the head, with half a fathom of black ribbon hanging over the left eye, and a peculiar tie to the black silk neckerchief, with sundry other *details*, are signs the want of which betray the beginner at once.

V = 1.25 D.

Beside the points in my dress which were out of the way, doubtless my complexion and hands would distinguish me from the regular *salt*, who, with a sun-browned cheek, wide step and rolling gait, swings his bronzed and toughened hands athwartships half open, as though just to ready to grasp a rope. "With all my imperfections

V = 1.50 D.

on my head," I joined the crew, and we hauled out into the stream and came to anchor for the night. The next day we were employed in preparation for sea, reeving and studding-sail gear, crossing royal yards, putting on chafing gear, and taking on board our powder. On the

(b)

Word	Pronunciation		Elements	Definition
fundus fundoscopy fundoscopic (adj)	FUN-dus fun-DOS-koh-pee fun-doh-SKOP-ik	S/ R/CF S/	Latin *bottom* -scopy *to examine* fund/o- *fundus* -ic *pertaining to*	Part farthest from the opening of a hollow organ Examination of the fundus (retina) of the eye Pertaining to fundoscopy
Ishihara color system	ish-ee-HAR-ah		Shinobu Ishihara, Japanese ophthalmologist, 1879–1963	Test for color vision defects
Jaeger reading cards	YA-ger		Eduard Jaeger, Austrian ophthalmologist, 1818–1884	Type of different sizes for testing near vision
peripheral peripheral vision	peh-RIF-er-al peh-RIF-er-al VIZH-un	S/ R/ S/ R/	-al *pertaining to* peripher- *external boundary* -ion *action, condition* vis- *sight*	Pertaining to the periphery or external boundary Ability to see objects as they come into the outer edges of the visual field
Snellen letter chart	SNEL-en		Hermann Snellen, Dutch ophthalmologist, 1834–1908	Test for acuity of distant vision
tonometer tonometry	toe-NOM-eh-ter toe-NOM-eh-tree	S/ R/CF S/	-meter *measure* ton/o- *pressure, tension* -metry *process of measuring*	Instrument for determining intraocular pressure The measurement of intraocular pressure

EXERCISES

A. Communication is key. *The OT in Dr. Chun's office needs to be familiar with all the WAD terms in order to communicate with Dr. Chun and her patients. Show your understanding of the language of opthalmology by circling the correct answer.*

1. Which of these instrument(s) can be found in the Eye Clinic?
   a. tonometer
   b. cystoscope
   c. ophthalmoscope
   d. a and b
   e. a and c

2. Which is used to test color vision?
   a. Snellen
   b. Jaeger
   c. Ishihara system
   d. visual fields
   e. otoscope

3. The abbreviation *OD* means:
   a. right eye
   b. both eyes
   c. left eye
   d. does not pertain to the eye
   e. normal eye

4. A test for near vision is:
   a. Snellen chart
   b. ophthalmoscope
   c. Jaeger cards
   d. Ishihara
   e. visual fields

B. Continue using *the language of ophthalmology to answer the following questions.*

1. Explain to your patient the phrase *intraocular pressure.* _____

_____

2. What is the instrument that is used to measure intraocular pressure? _____

3. The instrument named in question #2 above measures the eyeball's resistance to what?

_____

4. What does increased ocular pressure indicate is present? _____

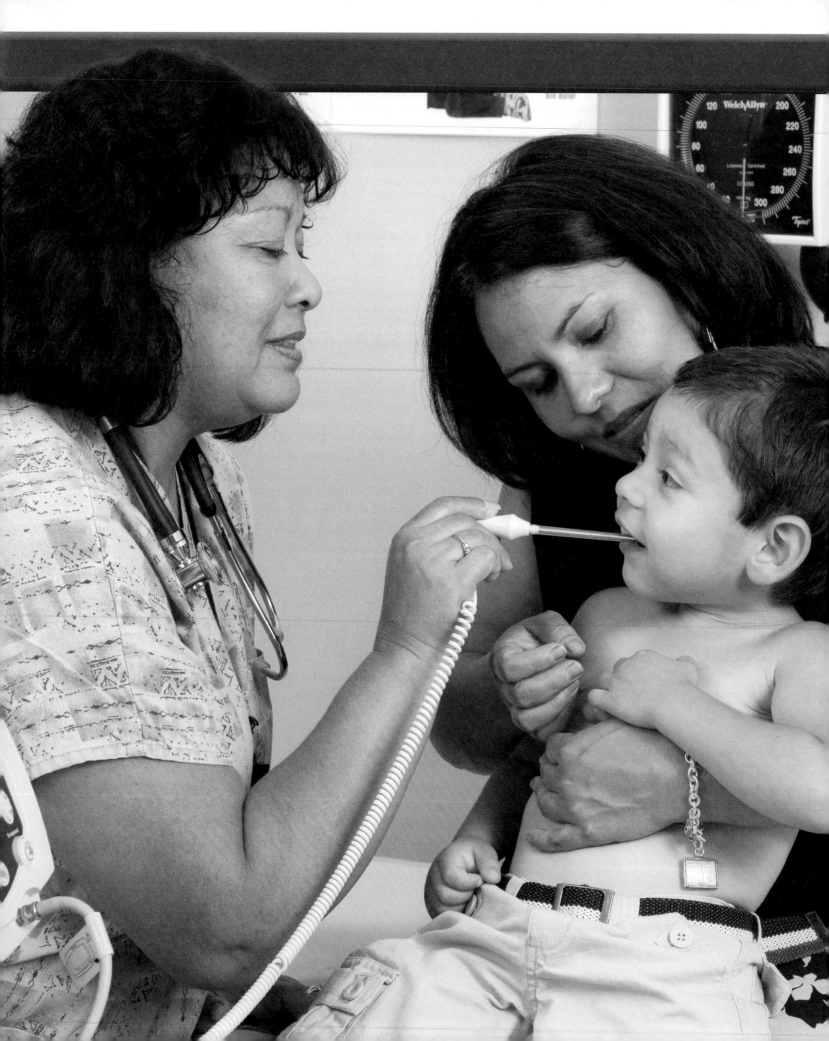

THE EAR AND HEARING

The Language of Otology

CASE REPORT 11.3

YOU ARE

. . . a medical assistant working for primary care physician Susan Lee, MD, of the Fulwood Medical Group.

YOU ARE COMMUNICATING WITH

. . . Mrs. Carmen Cardenas, who has brought in her 3-year-old son, Eddie. She tells you that Eddie has had a cold for a couple of days. Early this morning, he woke up screaming, felt hot, and was tugging his ears. She gave him **acetaminophen** with some orange juice, and he threw up. She also tells you this is the third similar episode in the past year, and, since the last time, she is concerned that he is not hearing normally. You see a worried mother and a restless toddler with a green nasal discharge. His oral temperature taken with an electronic digital thermometer is 102.4°F, and his pulse is 100. You tell Mrs. Cardenas that Dr. Lee will be in to see Eddie as soon as possible.

In your future career, being able to communicate comfortably, accurately, and effectively with the health professionals involved in the diagnosis and treatment of problems of the ear is key. You may work directly and/or indirectly with one or more of the following:

- **Otologists** are medical specialists in diseases of the ear.
- **Otorhinolaryngologists** are medical specialists in diseases of the ear, nose, and throat.
- **Audiologists** are specialists in the evaluation of hearing function.

LEARNING OUTCOMES

In order to understand what is going on with Eddie, to communicate with Dr. Lee about him, to respond to the mother's concerns, and to document this office visit, you need to be able to:

LO 11.4 Comprehend, analyze, spell, and write the medical terms of **otology.**

LO 11.5 Recognize and pronounce the medical terms of otology.

LO 11.6 Discuss the cause, appearance, diagnosis, and treatment of common disorders of the ear.

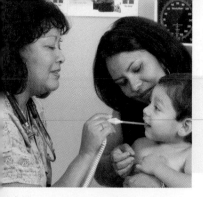

LESSON 11.4

The Ear and Hearing

OBJECTIVES

In order to understand and to address Eddie Cardenas' condition, you must be able to use correct medical terminology to:

11.4.1 Recognize the structures and functions of the three regions of the ear.

11.4.2 Explain how sound waves progress through the ear, are transferred to the brain, and are recognized as sounds.

11.4.3 Identify common diseases of the ear that interfere with the process of hearing.

Your ear has three major sections (*Figure 11.25*):

1. The external ear
2. The middle ear
3. The inner ear

CASE REPORT 11.3 (CONTINUED)

Clinical Note. 05/10/11
Examination by Dr. Lee showed that Eddie has a **bilateral acute otitis media (BOM)** with an upper respiratory infection **(URI)**. Dr. Lee is also concerned that Eddie has a **chronic** otitis media with **effusion (OME)** that is causing a hearing loss. She prescribed Amoxicillin 250 mg **q.i.d.** with acetaminophen 160 **mg p.r.n.** for 10 days, when she will see Eddie again. If, after the acute infection subsides, there remains an effusion with hearing loss, Dr. Lee may need to refer Eddie to an **otologist.** I explained this to Mrs. Cardenas.
—Luis Guittierez, CMA 1115 hrs.

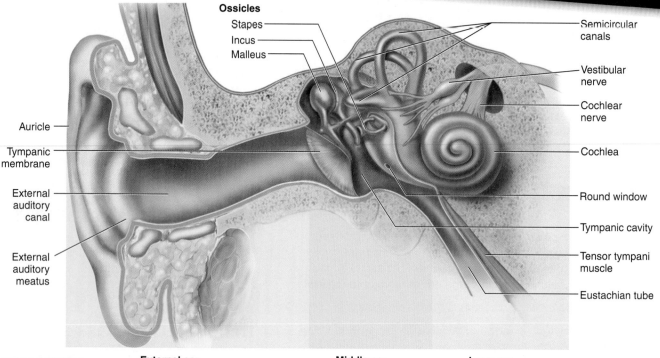

External ear   **Middle ear**   **Inner ear**

▲ **FIGURE 11.25**
Anatomical Regions of the Ear.

ABBREVIATIONS

BOM	bilateral otitis media
mg	milligram
OME	otitis media with effusion
p.r.n.	when necessary
q.i.d.	four times each day
URI	upper respiratory infection

Word	Pronunciation		Elements	Definition
acetaminophen	ah-seat-ah-**MIN**-oh-fen		Generic drug name	Medication that is an analgesic and antipyretic
acute	ah-**KYUT**		Latin *sharp*	Disease of sudden onset
bilateral	by-**LAT**-er-al	S/ P/ R/	-al *pertaining to* bi- *two* -later- *side*	On two sides; e.g., in both ears
chronic	**KRON**-ik		Greek *time*	A persistent, long-term disease
effusion	eh-**FYU**-shun		Latin *pouring out*	Collection of fluid that has escaped from blood vessels into a cavity or tissues
otitis media	oh-**TIE**-tis **ME**-dee-ah	S/ R/ R/	-itis *inflammation* ot- *ear* media *middle*	Inflammation of the middle ear
otologist	oh-**TOL**-oh-jist	S/ R/CF	-logist *specialist* ot/o- *ear*	Medical specialist in diseases of the ear
otology	oh-**TOL**-oh-jee	S/	-logy *study of*	Diagnosis and treatment of disorders of the ear
otorhinolaryngologist	oh-toe-rhino-lah-rin-**GOL**-oh-jist	R/CF R/CF	-rhin/o- *nose* -laryng/o- *larynx*	Ear, nose, and throat medical specialist

EXERCISES

A. Review *the Case Report and Case Report (continued) before you answer the following questions.*

1. What symptoms did Eddie have this morning? _____

2. Is this condition a recurring one for Eddie? _____

3. What two factors in the Case Report indicate that Eddie has an infection? _____

_____

4. What is Mrs. Cardenas' big concern about Eddie now? _____

5. What is Eddie's diagnosis after examination by Dr. Lee? _____

6. Eddie has both an "acute" and a "chronic" condition. What is the difference? _____

_____

7. How often does Eddie take the antibiotic? _____

B. Deconstruct *these medical terms into their basic elements. Complete the chart, and fill in the blanks.*

Medical Term	Prefix	Root(s)/ Combining Form(s)	Suffix	Meaning of Term
otology	1.	2.	3.	4.
otitis media	5.	6.	7.	8.
otologist	9.	10.	11.	12.
otorhinolaryngologist	13.	14.	15.	16.

C. Use the correct *medical term to describe what a medication that is both an analgesic and an antipyretic does.*

1. _____

_____

_____

LESSON 11.4 External Ear

(LO 11.4, 11.5, and 11.6)

Your external ear comprises several structures that keep it functioning effectively.

The **auricle** or **pinna** is a wing-shaped structure that directs sound waves into the ear canal through the external **auditory meatus.** The external auditory canal ends at the very delicate **tympanic** membrane, otherwise known as the eardrum *(Figure 11.26).*

The meatus and canal are lined with skin that contains many modified sweat glands called **ceruminous** glands, which secrete **cerumen.**

If a foreign body, like a small bead, gets into the auditory canal, or if cerumen becomes **impacted** in the canal, the result can be hearing loss.

Disorders of the External Ear

(LO 11.4, 11.5, and 11.6)

Some disorders of the external ear include infections and earwax buildup.

Otitis externa *(Figure 11.27)* is a bacterial or fungal infection of the external auditory canal lining. An **otoscopic** exam shows a painful, red, swollen ear canal, sometimes with a purulent drainage. Treatment entails thorough cleansing of the ear canal, applying a hydrocortisone **topical** solution with 2% acetic acid, and using antibiotic drops. Occasionally, a wick is used to help the topical medications penetrate down the canal.

Swimmer's ear is a form of otitis externa resulting from swimming, particularly if the water is polluted.

Excessive earwax can be removed in your physician's office by ear **irrigation** or with a **curette,** a small metal ring at the end of a handle.

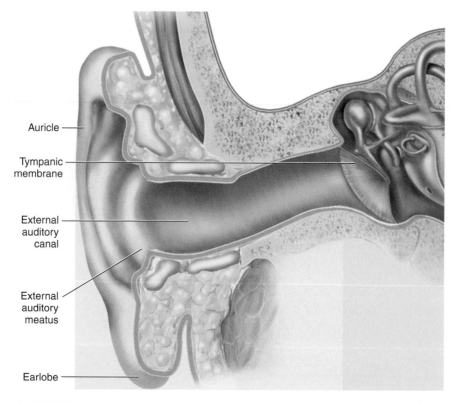

▲ FIGURE 11.26
External Ear.

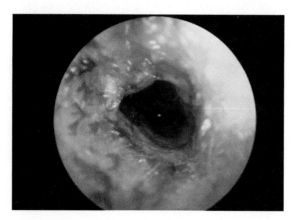

▲ FIGURE 11.27
Otoscopic View of Otitis Externa.

Word	Pronunciation	Elements		Definition
auditory (adj) audiology	AW-dih-tor-ee aw-dee-**OL**-oh-jee	S/ R/CF	Latin *hearing* -logy *study of* audi/o- *hearing*	Relating to hearing or the organs of hearing Study of hearing disorders
audiologist	aw-dee-**OL**-oh-jist	S/	-logist *one who studies, specialist*	Specialist in evaluation of hearing function
auricle (Note: *same as* pinna)	**AW**-ri-kul		Latin *ear*	The shell-like external ear
cerumen ceruminous (adj)	seh-**ROO**-men seh-**ROO**-mih-nus	S/ R/	Latin *wax* -ous *pertaining to* cerumin- *cerumen*	Waxy secretion of glands of the external ear Pertaining to cerumen
curette	kyu-**RET**	S/ R/	-ette *little* cur- *cleanse, cure*	Scoop-shaped instrument for scraping or removal of new growths (or earwax)
curettage (*the final "e" of* curette *is dropped because the suffix* -age *begins with a vowel*)	kyu-reh-**TAHZH**	S/	-age *pertaining to*	The use of a curette
impacted	im-**PAK**-ted		Latin *driven in*	Immovably wedged, as with earwax blocking the external canal
irrigation	ih-rih-**GAY**-shun	S/ R/	-ation *process* irrig- *to water*	Use of water; e.g., to remove wax from the external ear canal
meatus meatal (adj)	me-**AY**-tus me-**AY**-tal		Latin *go through*	Passage or channel; also the external opening of a passage
otoscope	**OH**-toe-skope	S/ R/CF	-scope *instrument for viewing* ot/o- *ear*	Instrument for examining the ear
otoscopy otoscopic (adj)	oh-**TOS**-koh-pee oh-toe-**SKOP**-ik	S/ S/	-scopy *to examine* -ic *pertaining to*	Examination of the ear Pertaining to examination with an otoscope
pinna pinnae (pl)	**PIN**-ah **PIN**-ee		Latin *wing*	Another name for auricle
topical	**TOP**-ih-kal	S/ R/	-al *pertaining to* topic- *local*	Medication applied to the skin to obtain a local effect
tympanic	tim-**PAN**-ik	S/ R/	-ic *pertaining to* tympan- *eardrum*	Pertaining to the tympanic membrane (eardrum) or tympanic cavity

EXERCISES

A. Test *your knowledge of the language of otology by matching correct answers. Every part of the body has its own specialized vocabulary. Fill in the blanks.*

_____ 1. pertaining to the eardrum

_____ 2. external opening of a passage

_____ 3. instrument for examining the ear

_____ 4. procedure for removing ear wax

_____ 5. scoop-shaped instrument

_____ 6. shell-like external ear

A. meatus

B. curette

C. curettage

D. auricle

E. tympanic

F. otoscope

B. Meet *lesson and chapter objectives using the language of otology to answer the questions.*

1. Name the structures in the external ear: _____

2. Explain the keynote: "The external auditory canal is the only skin-lined cul-de-sac in the body." _____
_____

3. What is another name for the auricle? _____

4. Describe the difference between an otoscope and a tonometer. _____
_____
_____

LESSON 11.4 Middle Ear (LO 11.4 and 11.5)

Your middle ear has the following four components (*Figure 11.28*):

1. The **tympanic membrane** (eardrum) rests at the inner end of the external auditory canal. It vibrates freely as sound waves hit it. It has a good nerve supply and is very sensitive to pain. When examined through the otoscope, it is transparent and reflects light (*Figure 11.29*);

2. The **tympanic cavity** is immediately behind the tympanic membrane. It is filled with air that enters through the eustachian tube, and the cavity is continuous with the **mastoid** air cells in the bone behind it. The cavity contains small bones called **ossicles;**

3. The three **ossicles**—the **malleus, incus,** and **stapes**—work to amplify sounds and are attached to the tympanic cavity wall by tiny ligaments. The malleus is attached to the tympanic membrane and vibrates with the membrane when sound waves hit it. The malleus is also attached to the incus, which vibrates, too, and passes the vibrations onto the stapes. The stapes is attached to the oval window, an opening that transmits the vibrations to the inner ear; and

4. The **eustachian (auditory) tube** connects the middle ear with the **nasopharynx** (throat), into which it opens near the pharyngeal **tonsils (adenoids)** (*Figure 11.30*). In children under 5 years of age, this tube is not fully developed. It is short and horizontal, and valve-like flaps in the throat that protect it are not yet developed.

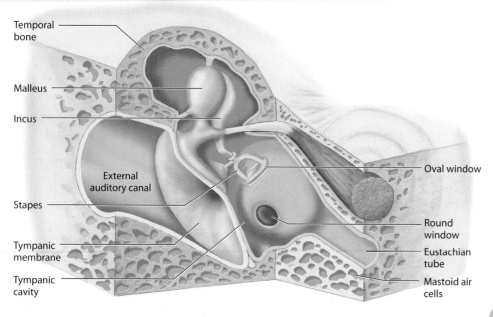

▲ **FIGURE 11.28**
Middle Ear.

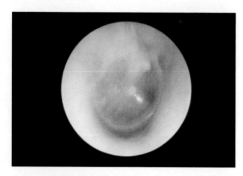

▲ **FIGURE 11.29**
Otoscopic View of Normal Tympanic Membrane.

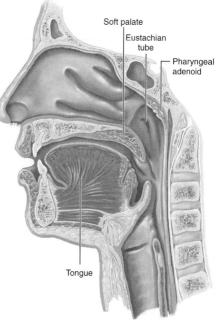

▲ **FIGURE 11.30**
Nasopharynx (Throat).

Word	Pronunciation		Elements	Definition
adenoid	**ADD**-eh-noyd	S/ R/	-oid *resembling* aden- *gland*	Single mass of lymphoid tissue in the midline at the back of the throat
eustachian tube *(syn: auditory tube)*	you-**STAY**-shun TYUB		Bartolomeo Eustachio, Italian anatomist, 1524–1574	Tube that connects the middle ear to the nasopharynx
incus	**IN**-cuss		Latin *anvil*	Middle one of the three ossicles in the middle ear; shaped like an anvil
malleus	**MAL**-ee-us		Latin *hammer*	Outer (lateral) one of the three ossicles in the middle ear; shaped like a hammer
mastoid	**MASS**-toyd	S/ R/	-oid *resembling* mast- *breast*	Small bony protrusion immediately behind the ear
nasopharynx	**NAY**-zoh-fair-inks	R/CF R/	nas/o- *nose* -pharynx *throat*	Region of the pharynx at the back of the nose and above the soft palate
nasopharyngeal (adj)	**NAY**-zoh-fair-**RIN**-jee-al	S/ R/	-eal *pertaining to* -pharyng- *pharynx*	Pertaining to the nasopharynx
ossicle	**OSS**-ih-kel	S/ R/CF	-cle *small* oss/i- *bone*	A small bone, particularly relating to the three bones in the middle ear
stapes	**STAY**-peas		Latin *stirrup*	Inner (medial) one of the three ossicles of the middle ear; shaped like a stirrup

EXERCISES

A. Review *the terms in the WAD box before you start this exercise. Pay special attention to the spelling. Circle the best choice.*

1. In the term *mastoid,* the suffix means:

   condition   resembling   inflammation

2. The element *mast* means:

   throat   breast   ear

3. The element *pharynx* means:

   throat   nose   tongue

4. The term *nasopharynx* is composed of:

   prefix + suffix   root + root   combining form + root

5. Shaped like a hammer:

   malleus   malleolus   maleus

B. Employ *the language of otology and fill in the blanks.*

1. Meet a lesson objective by describing the four componenets of the middle ear.

   _____

   _____

   _____

   _____

2. If the femur is the largest bone in the body, which is the smallest? _____

3. Write a synonym for *eustachian tube.* _____

4. What is the medical term for *eardrum?* _____

5. The pharyngeal tonsils are the _____.

6. What is the medical term for *throat?* _____

LESSON 11.4

CASE REPORT 11.3 (CONTINUED)

Eddie Cardenas' ear problems began with his eustachian tube. His cold (upper respiratory infection, **URI**, and **coryza**) inflamed the mucous membranes of his throat and eustachian tube. Because he is so young, his eustachian tube is short and horizontal and so the inflammation spread easily from his throat into the middle ear, causing his acute otitis media **(AOM)**. The inflammatory process produced fluid (effusion) in the middle ear. His tympanic membrane became inflamed and painful, which you could see through an otoscope *(Figure 11.31)*.

Disorders of the Middle Ear (LO 11.4, 11.5, and 11.6)

The middle ear can be susceptible to the disorders outlined below.

ABBREVIATIONS

AOM	acute otitis media
PE tube	pressure-equalization tube
URI	upper respiratory infection

- **Acute otitis media (AOM)** is the presence of pus in the middle ear with ear pain, fever, and redness of the tympanic membrane. AOM occurs most often in the first 2 to 4 years of age. If the infection is viral, it will go away on its own; if it's bacterial, oral antibiotics may be necessary.

- **Chronic otitis media** occurs when the acute infection subsides but the eustachian tube is blocked. The fluid in the middle ear caused by the infection cannot drain, and it gradually becomes stickier. This is called **chronic otitis media with effusion (OME)** and produces hearing loss because the sticky fluid prevents the ossicles from vibrating. You can see the fluid through the otoscope *(Figure 11.31)*. Dr. Lee was concerned that this had happened to Eddie in his previous ear infection.

- If the sticky fluid persists, a **myringotomy** can be performed, and a small, hollow plastic tube may have to be inserted through the tympanic membrane to allow the effusion to drain. These ear tubes have several names: **tympanostomy** tubes, **pressure-equalization tubes,** and, most commonly, **PE tubes** *(Figure 11.32)*. The tubes are inserted under general anesthesia as outpatient surgery. They remain in the ear for 6 to 18 months before they drop out on their own.

- A **perforated** tympanic membrane *(Figure 11.33)* can occur in acute otitis media **(AOM)** and chronic otitis media when pus in the middle ear cannot escape down the eustachian tube. The pus builds up pressure and punctures the eardrum. Most perforations will heal spontaneously in a month, leaving a small scar. Other perforation causes include a Q-tip puncture, an open-handed slap to the ear, or induced pressure as in scuba diving.

- **Cholesteotoma** is a complication of chronic otitis media with fluid or effusion (OME). Chronically inflamed middle ear cells multiply and collect into a tumor. They damage the ossicles and can spread to the inner ear. Surgical removal is required.

- **Otosclerosis** is a middle-ear disease that usually affects people between 18 and 35 years. It can impair one ear or both and produces a gradual hearing loss for low and soft sounds. Its etiology is unknown. Spongy bone forms around the junction of the oval window and stapes, preventing the stapes from conducting sound vibrations to the inner ear. The only treatment is to replace the stapes with a metal or plastic **prosthesis.**

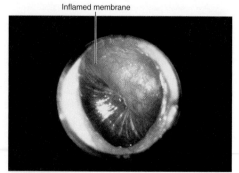

▲ **FIGURE 11.31**
Otoscopic View of Acute Otitis Media.

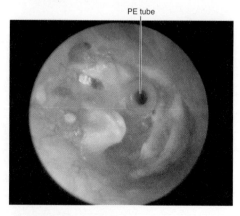

▲ **FIGURE 11.32**
Otoscopic View of a PE Tube in the Tympanic Membrane.

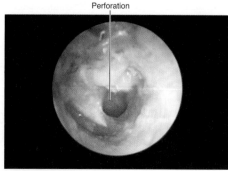

▲ **FIGURE 11.33**
Otoscopic View of Chronic Otitis Media with Perforation.

Word	Pronunciation	Elements		Definition
cholesteatoma	koh-less-tee-ah-**TOE**-mah	S/ R/CF R/	-oma *tumor, mass* chol/e- *bile* -steat- *fat*	Yellow, waxy tumor arising in the middle ear
coryza (syn: *acute rhinitis*)	koh-**RYE**-zah		Greek *catarrh*	Viral inflammation of the mucous membrane of the nose
myringotomy	mir-in-**GOT**-oh-me	S/ R/CF	-tomy *surgical incision* myring/o- *tympanic membrane*	Incision in the tympanic membrane
otosclerosis	oh-toe-sklair-**OH**-sis	S/ R/CF R/CF	-sis *abnormal condition* -scler/o- *hard* ot/o- *ear*	Hardening at the junction of the stapes and oval window that causes loss of hearing
perforated perforation	**PER**-foh-ray-ted per-foh-**RAY**-shun	S/ R/	Latin *to bore through* -ion *action* perforat- *bore through*	Punctured with one or more holes A hole through the wall of a structure
prosthesis	**PROS**-thee-sis		Greek *addition*	Manufactured substitute for a missing or diseased part of the body
tympanostomy	tim-pan-**OS**-toe-me	S/ R/CF	-stomy *new opening* tympan/o- *eardrum*	Surgically created new opening in the tympanic membrane to allow fluid to drain from the middle ear

EXERCISES

A. Review *the Case Report on this spread before answering the questions.*

1. What other terms in the Case Report can be used interchangeably with the word *cold?* _____

2. What is the difference between a *UTI* and a *URI?* _____
_____

3. How did the infection move from Eddie's throat into his middle ear? _____

4. What is the difference between *AOM* and *OME?* _____
_____

5. What is the medical term for the fluid in Eddie's ear? _____

B. Precision in communication *is very important because some terms can look very similar, but have very different meanings. Define the following terms, then answer the challenge questions.*

1. transfusion _____

2. infusion _____

3. effusion _____

4. In what other location in the body can you have *effusion?* _____

5. What body system does this represent? _____

C. Match *the correct element in column 1 to the correct meaning in column 2 below.*

_____ 1. tympan/o   **A.** tumor, mass

_____ 2. myring/o   **B.** fat

_____ 3. oma   **C.** eardrum

_____ 4. steat   **D.** bile

_____ 5. chol/e   **E.** tympanic membrane

LESSON 11.4 Inner Ear for Hearing (LO 11.4, 11.5, and 11.6)

KEYNOTE

• Repeated loud noise causes hearing loss in young people.

Your inner ear is a **labyrinth** of complex, intricate passage systems. The passages in the **cochlea,** a part of the labyrinth *(Figure 11.34),* contain receptors that convert vibrations into electrical nerve impulses so the brain can interpret them as different sounds.

Sound waves cause the tympanic membrane and the ossicles to vibrate *(Figure 11.35).* The stapes moves the oval window's membrane to create pressure waves in the fluid inside the inner ear's cochlea. These pressure waves make the **basilar** membranes in the cochlea vibrate. Hair cells attached to the membrane convert this motion into nerve impulses, which travel via the cochlear nerve to the brain. The excess pressure waves in the cochlea escape to the middle ear through the round window *(Figure 11.35).*

Today, the most common cause of hearing loss is damage to the fine hairs in the cochlea by repeated loud noises—from the work-related use of jackhammers or leaf blowers to the leisure-related exposure to amplified music at concerts, personal listening devices, and motorcycles. This is a **sensorineural hearing loss.**

Hearing aids are becoming more sophisticated and smaller, but they do not help people with cochlear damage. **Cochlear implants** are used to bypass the damaged hair cells and directly stimulate cochlear nerve endings.

A **conductive hearing loss** occurs when sound is not conducted efficiently through the external auditory canal to the tympanic membrane and the ossicles. Causes of this include:

• A middle-ear pathology, like acute otitis media, otitis media with effusion, or a perforated eardrum;

• An infected external auditory canal; or

• The presence of a foreign body in the external canal.

ABBREVIATIONS

AD	right ear
AS	left ear
AU	both ears

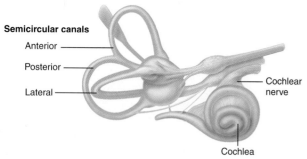

Semicircular canals
- Anterior
- Posterior
- Lateral

Cochlear nerve

Cochlea

Superior view

▲ **FIGURE 11.34**
Labyrinth of Inner Ear.

Hearing Test Procedures (LO 11.4, 11.5, and 11.6)

Hearing tests are available to accurately measure just how much, and at what frequencies, a patient is able to hear. The following test procedures are described below.

• **Whispered speech testing:** Ask the patient to cover one ear. Stand 2 feet away from the uncovered ear, whisper words, and ask the patient to repeat them. If the patient cannot repeat the words, say the words more loudly. This is a simple, but unmeasured, screening method.

• **Weber test:** Place a vibrating tuning fork in the middle of the patient's forehead, and ask whether the tone is louder in one ear or equal on both sides. This determines on which side a hearing loss is located.

• **Rinne test:** Place the vibrating tuning fork on the mastoid process. Then hold it opposite the ear canal. Normally, sound is heard longer by air conduction at the ear canal than by bone conduction at the mastoid process. The reverse indicates a conductive hearing loss.

• **Audiometer:** After proper training, you may use an audiometer to test for hearing loss. The audiometer is an electronic device that generates sounds in different frequencies and intensities and can print out the patient's responses.

In recording the results of hearing testing, **AD** is shorthand for the right ear, **AS** for the left ear, and **AU** for both ears.

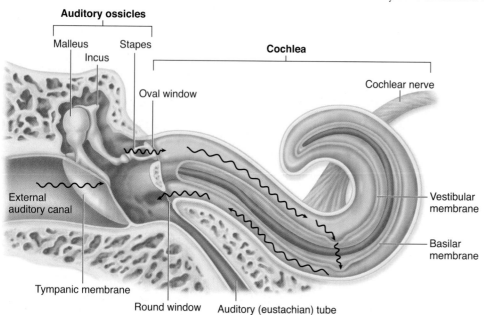

Auditory ossicles
- Malleus
- Incus
- Stapes

Cochlea

Oval window

Cochlear nerve

External auditory canal

Vestibular membrane

Basilar membrane

Tympanic membrane

Round window   Auditory (eustachian) tube

◄ **FIGURE 11.35**
Model of the Hearing Process.

Word	Pronunciation	Elements		Definition
audiometer	aw-dee-**OM**-ee-ter	S/ R/CF	-meter *measure* audi/o- *hearing*	Instrument to measure hearing
audiometric (adj)	**AW**-dee-oh-**MET**-rik	S/	-metric *pertaining to measurement*	Pertaining to the measurement of hearing
basilar	**BAS**-ih-lar	S/ R/	-ar *pertaining to* basil- *base, support*	Pertaining to the base of a structure
cochlea cochlear (adj)	**KOK**-lee-ah **KOK**-lee-ar		Latin *snail shell*	An intricate combination of passages; used to describe the inner ear
conductive hearing loss	kon-**DUK**-tiv		Latin *to lead*	Hearing loss caused by lesions in the outer ear or middle ear
implant	im-**PLANT**		Latin *to plant*	To insert material into tissues; or the material inserted into tissues
labyrinth labyrinthitis	**LAB**-ih-rinth **LAB**-ih-rin-**THI**-tis	S/ R/	Greek *labyrinth* -itis *inflammation* labyrinth -*inner ear*	The inner ear Inflammation of the inner ear
Rinne test	**RIN**-eh TEST		Friedrich Rinne, German otologist, 1819–1868	Test for conductive hearing loss
sensorineural hearing loss	**SEN**-sor-ih-**NYUR**-al	S/ R/CF R/	-al *pertaining to* sensor/i- *sensory* -neur- *nerve*	Hearing loss caused by lesions of the inner ear or the auditory nerve
Weber test	**VA**-ber TEST		Ernst Weber, German physiologist, 1794–1878	Test for sensorineural hearing loss

EXERCISES

A. Match *the meaning of the element in column 1 with the correct element in column 2. Fill in the blanks.*

_____ **1.** hearing

_____ **2.** nerve

_____ **3.** pertaining to

_____ **4.** measure

_____ **5.** inner ear

_____ **6.** sensory

A. meter

B. al

C. sensor/i

D. audi/o

E. neur

F. labyrinth

B. Review *the WAD to find the answers to the questions below.*

1. What are the two eponyms in the WAD? _____ and _____

2. What is the most common cause today of hearing loss? _____

3. What is a *perforated* eardrum? _____

C. Meet lesson *and chapter objectives by using the correct medical language for your answers to the following questions.*

1. Describe the difference between *conductive hearing loss* and *sensorineural hearing loss.*

_____

_____

_____

2. What is the difference between a *transplant* and an *implant?* _____

_____

_____

_____

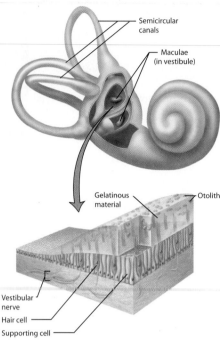

▲ **FIGURE 11.36**
Vestibule of the Inner Ear.

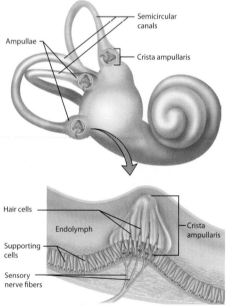

▲ **FIGURE 11.37**
Semicircular Canals.

ABBREVIATION

BPPV   benign paroxysmal positional vertigo

CASE REPORT 11.4

YOU ARE

. . . Sonia Ramos, a medical assistant working with Sylvia Thompson, MD, an otorhinolaryngologist at Fulwood Medical Center.

YOU ARE COMMUNICATING WITH

. . . Mr. Ernesto Santiago, a 44-year-old man who was referred to Dr. Thompson. Mr. Santiago complains of recurrent attacks of nausea, vomiting, a sense of spinning or whirling, and ringing in his ears. The attacks last about 24 hours and are getting more frequent. He has been having trouble hearing quiet speech on his left side. Your role is to document his examination, diagnosis, and care, and to act as translator between Mr. Santiago and Dr. Thompson.

Inner Ear for Equilibrium and Balance
(LO 11.4, 11.5, and 11.6)

Your inner ear contains the organs in your body responsible for maintaining your true sense of balance. The **vestibule** and the three semicircular canals *(Figures 11.36 and 11.37)* in your inner ear maintain your balance. These are your true organs of balance. Inside the fluid-filled vestibule are two raised, flat areas covered with hair cells and a jelly-like material. This gelatinous material contains calcium and protein crystals called **otoliths.** The position of your head alters the amount of pressure this gelatinous mass applies to the hair cells. The hair cells respond to horizontal and vertical changes and send impulses to the brain relating how the head is tilted.

Each of the three fluid-filled semicircular canals has a dilated end called an **ampulla.** The ampulla contains a mound of hair cells set in a gelatinous material that together are called the **crista ampullaris** *(Figure 11.37).* This detects rotational movements of the head that distort the hair cells and lead to stimulation of connected nerve cells. The nerve impulses travel through the vestibular nerve to the brain. From the brain, nerve impulses travel to the muscles to maintain **equilibrium** and balance.

The sensation of spinning or whirling that Mr. Santiago experiences is called **vertigo,** often described by patients as dizziness. The ringing in his ears is called **tinnitus.** Both sensations arise in the inner ear.

Benign paroxysmal positional vertigo (BPPV) is another type of intermittent vertigo caused by fragments of the otoliths in the vestibule migrating into the semicircular canals. The otolith fragments brush against the hair cells, sending conflicting signals to the brain. This produces vertigo.

Acute labyrinthitis is an acute viral infection of the labyrinth producing extreme vertigo, nausea, and vomiting. It usually lasts 1 to 2 weeks.

CASE REPORT 11.4 (CONTINUED)

The recurrent attacks that Mr. Santiago suffered are called **Ménière disease.** The disease involves the destruction of inner-ear hair cells, but the etiology is unknown and there is no cure. Dr. Thompson prescribed medication to control Mr. Santiago's nausea and vomiting.

Word	Pronunciation	Elements		Definition
ampulla	am-**PULL**-ah		Latin *two-handled bottle*	Dilated portion of a canal or duct
crista ampullaris	**KRIS**-tah am-**PULL**-air-is	R/ S/ R/	crista *crest* -aris *pertaining to* ampull- *bottle-shaped*	Mound of hair cells and gelatinous material in the ampulla of a semicircular canal
equilibrium	ee-kwi-**LIB**-ree-um	P/ R/	equi- *equal* -librium *balance*	Being evenly balanced
Ménière disease	men-**YEAR** diz-**EEZ**		Prosper Ménière, French physician, 1799–1862	Disorder of the inner ear with acute attacks of tinnitus, vertigo, and hearing loss
otolith	**OH**-toe-lith	R/ R/CF	-lith *stone* ot/o- *ear*	A calcium particle in the vestibule of the inner ear
paroxysmal	par-ock-**SIZ**-mal	S/ R/	-al *pertaining to* paroxysm- *sudden, sharp attack*	Occurring in sharp, spasmodic episodes
tinnitus	**TIN**-ih-tus		Latin *jingle*	Persistent ringing, whistling, clicking, or booming noise in the ears
vertigo	**VER**-tih-go		Latin *dizziness*	Sensation of spinning or whirling
vestibule vestibular (adj)	**VES**-tih-byul ves-**TIB**-you-lar	S/ R/	Latin *entrance chamber* -ar *pertaining to* vestibul- *vestibule*	Space at the entrance to a canal Pertaining to the vestibule

EXERCISES

A. Review *Case Report 11.4 and the Case Report (continued) before answering the questions.*

1. What are Mr. Santiago's chief complaints? _____

2. What is a *recurrent* attack? _____

3. What shows Mr. Santiago's condition is getting worse? _____

4. Which side of his body is most affected with hearing loss? _____

5. What is Mr. Santiago's final diagnosis? _____

6. What does *its etiology is unknown* mean? _____

7. If there is no cure for this disease, what is the treatment plan? _____

B. Terminology challenge: *Analyze the following challenge questions and employ medical language for your answers.*

1. What other body system has terminology using the element *lith?* _____

2. Can you give an example of a term in this body system? _____

3. How can vertigo affect your equilibrium? _____

4. Define each medical term represented by the abbreviation *BPPV.*

    B_____

    P_____

    P_____

    V_____

C. Use the language *of otology for your answers to the following questions.*

1. Where are the organs located that are responsible for maintaining the body's true sense of balance? _____

2. Name the specific organs in your answer for question 1 above. _____

3. What travels from the brain to the muscles to help the body maintain equilibrium and balance? _____

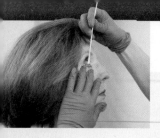

CHAPTER 11 REVIEW SPECIAL SENSES OF THE EYE AND EAR

CHALLENGE YOUR KNOWLEDGE

A. Build terms from the language of otology. *Identify the following elements by placing a check mark (✔) in the appropriate column. Give the meaning of the element, and then give an example of a medical term containing that element. The first one is done for you. Fill in the chart.*

Element	Prefix	Root	CF	Suffix	Meaning of Element	Medical Term
nas		✔			nose	nasal
1. anti					**2.**	**3.**
4. steat					**5.**	**6.**
7. sis					**8.**	**9.**
10. lith					**11.**	**12.**
13. rhino					**14.**	**15.**
16. tympan					**17.**	**18.**
19. sclero					**20.**	**21.**
22. audio					**23.**	**24.**

B. Recall and review: *How well do you remember these word elements from the previous chapters? Try to answer without looking back to check. Fill in the chart.*

Element	Type of Element (P, R, CF, or S)	Meaning of Element
dermato	**1.**	**2.**
logist	**3.**	**4.**
hypo	**5.**	**6.**
cutaneo	**7.**	**8.**
um	**9.**	**10.**

C. Suffixes: *The following terms all have a suffix with a common meaning. Circle the suffix, define each term on the line below, and then answer the question.*

1. periorbital:

_____

2. nasopharyngeal:

_____

3. accommodate:

_____

4. intraocular:

_____

5. antibiotic:

_____

6. optic:

_____

7. pupillary:

_____

8. pollutant:

_____

9. ceruminous:

_____

10. ampullaris:

_____

11. List each of the individual suffixes here:

_____

_____

_____

12. These suffixes all mean _____, and the terms come from the languages of

_____ and _____.

D. Deconstruct the following medical terms. *A portion of the term is bolded—identify that element and give its meaning. The first one is done for you. Fill in the blanks.*

Medical Term	Element	Meaning of Element
1. **ot**itis	root	ear
2. **audio**meter	_____	_____
3. mast**oid**	_____	_____
4. **chole**steatoma	_____	_____
5. **myringo**tomy	_____	_____
6. oto**sclero**sis	_____	_____
7. **neur**al	_____	_____
8. **equi**librium	_____	_____
9. oto**lith**	_____	_____
10. **paroxysm**al	_____	_____

E. Master your documentation—*you are creating a legal record. Circle the most appropriate choice and insert the correct abbreviation where indicated.*

1. Patient complains of sticky eyelids with (purulent/perulent) discharge, both eyes (abbrev. _____). Diagnosis: (scleritis/conjunctivitis)

2. (Refraction/Accommodation) reveals patient's vision now 20-40 in the right eye, (abbrev. _____) with correction.

3. Mr. Baker has continued decreasing vision in his left eye (abbrev. _____). If his diabetes remains uncontrolled, his (retinopathy/retinoblastoma) will worsen.

4. (Opthalmoscopic/Ophthalmoscopic) examination of the left eye reveals (catarracks/cataracts) forming.

5. (Vertigo/Tinnitus) is often described by patients as dizziness.

6. (BPPV/AOM) _____ is another type of intermittent vertigo.

F. Spelling correctly *is the mark of an educated professional. Proofread the following documentation to find the errors. Circle the misspelled terms, and rewrite the correctly spelled terms on the lines below.*

1. The optalmoscopic examination revealed scleriitis and retinopathy.

_____

2. Perulent discharge is coming from both eyes, and the patient also complains of photofobia.

_____

3. The patient's blepharotosis can be remedied surgically. Schedule a blepharopasty as soon as possible.

_____

4. Irigation and curetage have been ordered for the patient with impackted ceruman.

_____

5. The patient suffers from chronick otitis medial with efusion.

_____

G. Roots/combining forms *remain the core foundation of every term.*
Of the three possible answers, circle the correct term related to the question about the root.

1. The R/CF meaning *hearing* appears in the term:

   vestibule   audiometric   auricle

2. The R/CF meaning *fear* appears in the term:

   periorbital   photophobia   nasolacrimal

3. The R/CF meaning *eyelid* appears in the term:

   blepharitis   paresis   ptosis

4. The R/CF meaning *pus* appears in the term:

   extrinsic   stereopsis   purulent

5. The R/CF meaning *cornea* appears in the term:

   myopia   keratotomy   glaucoma

6. The R/CF meaning *blood vessel* appears in the term:

   angiography   fundoscopy   retinopathy

7. The R/CF meaning *side* appears in the term:

   otitis media   periorbital   bilateral

8. The R/CF meaning *nose* appears in the term:

   otorhinolaryngologist   ceruminous   curettage

9. The R/CF meaning *gland* appears in the term:

   adenoid   cornea   tonsil

10. The R/CF meaning *throat* appears in the term:

    tonsillectomy   nasopharynx   myringotomy

STUDY HINT

The term purulent means containing pus. An easy way to remember how to spell it is that the term starts with the same two letters as does the word pus. This term is frequently misspelled "perulent." Remember pus and you will start the term correctly.

H. Match *the Latin and Greek terms in column 1 to their meanings in column 2 to increase your knowledge of the language of ophthalmology. Fill in the blanks.*

	Column 1		Column 2
_____	1. conjunctiva	A.	paralysis
_____	2. lutea	B.	on the outer side
_____	3. hordeolum	C.	circle
_____	4. foramen	D.	hard
_____	5. extrinsic	E.	yellow
_____	6. ptosis	F.	inner lining of eyelids
_____	7. sclera	G.	hole
_____	8. orbit	H.	stye
_____	9. paresis	I.	falling or drooping

Use any one term from column 1 in a sentence of patient documentation.

_____

_____

_____

_____

Word elements *are your most valuable tool for increasing your medical vocabulary. Use your knowledge of word elements to answer the following questions. Circle the correct answer.*

1. Which of the following terms refers to *tears?*

   a. otolith

   b. lacrimal

   c. purulent

   d. uvea

   e. vestibule

2. This term is used to indicate drooping:

   a. parietal

   b. periorbital

   c. paresis

   d. ptosis

   e. presbyopia

3. Based on its suffix, you can tell that a *keratotomy* is:

   a. a body part

   b. a procedure

   c. a diagnosis

   d. a medication

   e. an infection

4. The location of *periorbital* is:

   a. outside the eye

   b. around the eye

   c. beside the eye

   d. within the eye

   e. behind the eye

5. The term *amblyopia* signifies:

   a. sound

   b. light

   c. sight

   d. movement

   e. pain

6. *In situ* is a Latin phrase that means: *(Be precise!)*

   a. in this place

   b. in another place

   c. in the correct place

   d. in the place

   e. in place of

7. The lens of the eye is *avascular* because it has no:

   a. connective tissue

   b. aqueous humor

   c. blood supply

   d. fibrous outer covering

   e. mucous membrane

8. *Angiography* is an x-ray visualization of:

   a. organs

   b. bones

   c. blood vessels

   d. muscles

   e. glands

J. Latin and Greek *terms do not deconstruct into elements like other medical terms. You have to know them for what they are. Match the medical term in column 1 with its meaning in column 2.*

_____ **1.** acute   **A.** time

_____ **2.** cerumen   **B.** ear

_____ **3.** meatus   **C.** snail shell

_____ **4.** effusion   **D.** jingle

_____ **5.** cochlea   **E.** driven in

_____ **6.** vertigo   **F.** sharp

_____ **7.** chronic   **G.** wax

_____ **8.** tinnitus   **H.** dizziness

_____ **9.** impacted   **I.** go through

_____ **10.** auricle   **J.** pouring out

K. Precision in communication: *Using the correct form (noun, verb, adjective) of the term is as important as using the correct term itself. Choose the correct form of the term from the word bank and insert it on the line in the appropriate sentence. After you fill in the term, write under the line what form of the term you have used (noun, verb, adjective).*

> *Remember:*   noun   person, place, or thing
>   verb   action
>   adjective   describes detail

Word Bank:

refract   accommodation   refractive   accommodate   accommodative   refraction

1. The process of bending the light rays by the cornea and lens is called _____.

2. _____ esotropia is an inward eye turn, usually noticed around 2 years of age in 1% to 2% of children.

3. This process of the eye changing focus is called _____.

4. The lens can _____ itself to light rays by becoming thicker or thinner.

5. The cornea and lens work together to _____ light in the vision process.

L. Identify *the following medical terms or abbreviations by specialty; then identify them as either a diagnosis or a procedure. Fill in the chart with a check mark (✓) in the appropriate columns.*

Medical Term	Ophthalmology	Otology	Diagnosis	Procedure
uveitis	1.	2.	3.	4.
BOM	5.	6.	7.	8.
myringotomy	9.	10.	11.	12.
tinnitus	13.	14.	15.	16.
fundoscopy	17.	18.	19.	20.
cholesteatoma	21.	22.	23.	24.
strabismus	25.	26.	27.	28.
otoscopy	29.	30.	31.	32.
photocoagulation	33.	34.	35.	36.

M. Short answers for patient education: *Patients will ask you for clarification of certain terms they do not understand or for more explanation of body processes. Be prepared to answer the following questions for your patients.*

1. Andrew Baker has severe otosclerosis in his left ear. Dr. Lee has recommended replacement of his stapes with a plastic prosthesis. (a) Can you explain to Mr. Baker what a prosthesis is, and compare it to other body part replacements he may already have? _____

   _____

   (b) Look up *prosthesis* in the glossary, a medical dictionary, or online. Define prosthesis: _____

   _____

   (c) Name 3 other types of prostheses that can be inserted into the body.

   Prostheses: _____   _____   _____

   (d) How will this particular prosthesis help Mr. Baker?

   _____

   _____

   _____

2. Caroline Mason has had many ear problems since she was a child. Frequent infections necessitated a myringotomy with PE tubes at a young age. Even after she continued to have frequent URIs, tonsillitis, impacted cerumen, labyrinthitis, and vertigo later in life.

   a. Briefly explain what a myringotomy is: _____

   _____

   Define the following terms and abbreviations that appear on the same line:

   b. PE tubes _____

   c. URI _____

   d. tonsillitis _____

   e. impacted _____

   f. cerumen _____

   g. labyrinthitis _____

   h. vertigo _____

N. Partner exercise: *Ask your study partner to close his or her text. Dictate the following sentences to your partner, and have him or her write them down on a blank sheet of paper. Check your partner's written sentences and the spelling of each word to ensure all are written exactly as shown in the sentences below. The sentence is not correct unless every word is present and everything is spelled correctly. When you have finished checking your partner's answers, close your book, ask your partner to dictate the sentences to you, and then write them down yourself and have your partner check them.*

1. Stye or hordeolum is an infection of an eyelash follicle producing an abscess with localized pain, swelling, redness, and pus formation at the edge of the eyelid.

2. Laser-assisted in situ keratomileusis (LASIK) is being used to treat myopia, hyperopia, and astigmatism.

3. The eustachian tube connects the middle ear with the nasopharynx, into which it opens close to the pharyngeal tonsils.

4. A perforated tympanic membrane can occur in acute otitis media when pus in the middle ear cannot escape down the auditory tube.

O. Patient education: *Your patient is confused by some medical terms the doctor has used. Explain to the patient in simple language the difference between:*

1. *esotropia* and *exotropia*:

_____

2. *amblyopia* and *presbyopia*:

_____

3. *refraction* and *accommodation*:

_____

P. Terminology challenge: *List below all the various medical procedures detailed in this chapter for otology and ophthalmology.*

a. otology _____

_____

b. ophthalmology _____

_____

Q. Chapter challenge: *Circle the best answer.*

1. *Ophthalmia neonatorum* is a type of:

   a. uveitis

   b. retinitis

   c. conjunctivitis

   d. corneal abrasion

   e. scleritis

2. The three terms that are all spelled correctly are:

   a. occular, stereopsis, cornia

   b. blepharoptosis, sty, contagious

   c. pupilary, cornial, avascular

   d. optalmologist, ptosis, paresis

   e. presbyopia, pupil, retinitis

3. A *tonometer* is an instrument used to measure:

   a. peripheral vision

   b. aqueous humor

   c. intraocular pressure

   d. sound waves in the eardrum

   e. fluid in the middle ear

4. The external opening of a passage is:

   a. a pinna

   b. an auricle

   c. a meatus

   d. an adenoid

   e. a labyrinth

5. Which set of three terms is most likely to appear in an otorhinolaryngologist's dictation?

   a. meatus, ceruminous, periorbital

   b. nasopharynx, labyrinth, tonsillectomy

   c. photosensitivity, Ishihara, otitis

   d. foramen, presbyopia, hyperopia

   e. curettage, retina, impacted

6. The term *tympanic* is associated with the:

   a. auricle

   b. eardrum

   c. pinna

   d. ossicles

   e. stapes

CHAPTER 11 REVIEW

Chapter challenge: *Circle the best answer.*

1. Choose the three *ossicles:*

   a. otolith, crista ampullaris, vestibule

   b. malleus, incus, stapes

   c. coryza, cochlea, labyrinth

   d. tonsils, adenoids, mastoids

   e. iris, uvea, sclera

2. The abbreviations *PERRLA*, *OD*, *OU*, and *OS* all relate to:

   a. the nose

   b. therapeutic procedures

   c. the eye

   d. radiology procedures

   e. the ear

3. Name a symptom of *BPPV:*

   a. ringing in the ears

   b. loss of hearing

   c. fever

   d. rash

   e. effusion

4. The term that means the same as "pink eye" is:

   a. blepharitis

   b. conjunctivitis

   c. blepharoptosis

   d. esotropia

   e. scleritis

5. Which term relates to *pus?*

   a. ambylopia

   b. avascular

   c. purulent

   d. aqueous

   e. strabismus

6. What is the medical term for three-dimensional perception?

   a. exotropia

   b. accommodation

   c. presbyopia

   d. stereopsis

   e. refraction

7. What body parts are covered in the body's thinnest layer of skin?:

   a. fingers

   b. nose

   c. scalp

   d. toes

   e. eyelids

8. Turning the eye outward, away from the nose, is:

   a. extrinsic

   b. esotropia

   c. stereopsis

   d. exotropia

   e. external

9. Tympan is a root meaning:

   a. eyeball

   b. retina

   c. eardrum

   d. canal

   e. opening

S. Case Report challenge: *Now that you are more comfortable with the terms in this chapter, you can apply that knowledge and answer the questions about the Case Report. If you read the report through and underline all the medical terminology, this will make it easier to answer the questions.*

1. Which of Eddie's symptoms will be reduced by the *acetaminophen*?

   _____

   _____

2. What does the term *bilateral* mean for Eddie?

   _____

   _____

   _____

3. What is an *effusion*?

   _____

   _____

   _____

4. What are Eddie's symptoms?

CASE REPORT 11.1

YOU ARE

> . . . a medical assistant working for primary care physician Susan Lee, MD, of the Fulwood Medical Group.

YOU ARE COMMUNICATING WITH

> . . . Mrs. Carmen Cardenas, who has brought in her 3-year-old son, Eddie. She tells you that Eddie has had a cold for a couple of days. Early this morning he woke up screaming, felt hot, and was tugging his ears. She gave him acetaminophen with some orange juice, and he threw up. She also tells you this is the third similar episode in the past year, and, since the last time, she is concerned that he is not hearing normally. You see a worried mother and a restless toddler with a green nasal discharge. His oral temperature taken with an electronic digital thermometer is 102.4°F, pulse 100. You tell her that Dr. Lee will be in to see Eddie as soon as possible.
>
> **Clinical Note. 05/10/11**
> Examination by Dr. Lee showed that Eddie has a bilateral acute otitis media (BOM) with an upper respiratory infection (URI). Dr. Lee is also concerned that Eddie has a chronic otitis media with effusion (OME) that is causing a hearing loss. She prescribed amoxicillin 250 mg q.i.d. with acetaminophen 160 mg p.r.n. for 10 days, when she will see Eddie again. If, after the acute infection subsides, there remains an effusion with hearing loss, Dr. Lee may need to refer Eddie to an otologist. I explained this to Mrs. Cardenas.
>   —Luis Guittierez, CMA, 1115 hrs.

_____

_____

_____

5. One medication is to be given q.i.d., while the other is given p.r.n. What is the difference?

   _____

   _____

6. Find the two terms in the Case Report that are opposites, and define them.

   Term: _____

   Means: _____

   Term: _____

   Means: _____

7. What type of specialist will Eddie be referred to if his condition does not improve after medication? _____

   _____

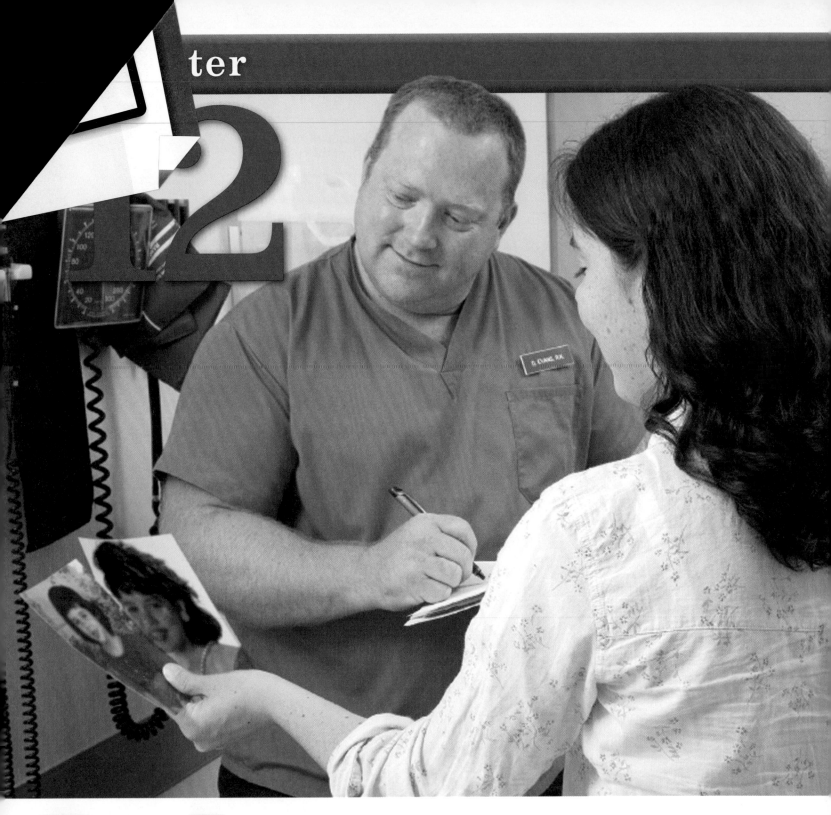

THE ENDOCRINE SYSTEM

The Essentials of the Language of Endocrinology

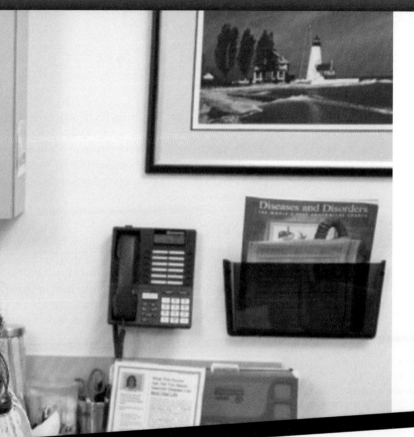

Your **endocrine** system is a communication system. The **hormones** produced by this system are blood-borne messengers secreted by endocrine glands; they circulate in the bloodstream, gaining access to all other body cells. They are distributed anywhere the blood travels, but only affect the target cells that have receptors for them. These hormones alter the metabolism of the target cells. The information in this chapter will enable you to:

LO 12.1   Apply the language of endocrinology to the structures and functions of the endocrine system.

LO 12.2   Comprehend, analyze, spell, and write the medical terms of endocrinology.

LO 12.3   Recognize and pronounce the medical terms of endocrinology.

LO 12.4   Use medical terminology to explain the effects of common endocrine disorders on health.

CASE REPORT 12.1

YOU ARE

. . . a registered nurse working with endocrinologist Sabina Khalid, MD, in the Endocrinology Clinic at Fulwood Medical Center.

YOU ARE COMMUNICATING WITH

. . . Mrs. Gina Tacher, a 33-year-old schoolteacher. She complains of coarsening of her facial features and enlargement of the bones of her hands. Over the past 10 years, Mrs. Tacher's nose and jaw have increased in size and her voice has become husky. She has brought photos of herself at ages 9 and 16. She has no other health problems.

The health professionals involved in the diagnosis and treatment of problems with the endocrine system include:

- **Endocrinologists,** who are medical specialists concerned with the production and effects of hormones.

KEYNOTE

- A hormone is secreted by an endocrine gland or cell and is carried by the bloodstream to act at distant target sites.

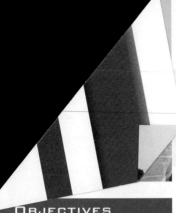

LESSON 12.1

Endocrine System, Hypothalamus, and Pituitary and Pineal Glands

OBJECTIVES

Your endocrine system is a network of ductless glands whose cells secrete hormones directly into your bloodstream. The information in this lesson will enable you to use correct medical terminology to:

12.1.1 Name the glands that make up the endocrine system.

12.1.2 List the hormones produced by the hypothalamus and pituitary gland.

12.1.3 Identify the control that the hypothalamic and pituitary hormones exert over other endocrine glands.

12.1.4 Specify the roles of the pineal gland.

12.1.5 Describe disorders of the hypothalamus, pituitary, and pineal glands.

ABBREVIATIONS

ADH   antidiuretic hormone
SAD   seasonal affective disorder

The Endocrine System

(LO 12.1, 12.2, and 12.3)

Your endocrine system comprises several major organs *(Figures 12.1 and 12.2)*. These organs, with their respective names and numbers in parentheses below, work together to ensure that this system operates smoothly:

- **Pituitary gland (1)** and the nearby **hypothalamus (1).**
- **Pineal gland (1).**
- **Thyroid gland (1).**
- **Parathyroid glands (4).**
- **Thymus gland (1).**
- **Adrenal glands (2).**
- **Pancreas (1).**
- **Gonads: testes (2) in the male; ovaries (2) in the female** (The male gonads are discussed in *Chapter 14* and the female in *Chapter 15.*)

In addition, endocrine cells found in tissues throughout the body secrete particular hormones. For example:

- **Cells in the upper GI tract** secrete hormones that include gastrin, which stimulates gastric secretions.
- **Cells in the kidney** secrete erythropoietin, which stimulates erythrocyte (red blood cell) production.
- **Fat cells** secrete leptin, which helps suppress appetite. Lack of leptin can lead to overeating and obesity.
- **Cells in tissues throughout the body** secrete **prostaglandins,** which act locally to dilate blood vessels, relax airways, stimulate uterine contractions in menstrual cramps or labor, and lower acid secretion in the stomach. When tissues are injured, prostaglandins promote an inflammatory response.

Hypothalamus

(LO 12.1, 12.2, and 12.3)

Your hypothalamus *(Figure 12.1)* forms the floor and walls of your brain's third ventricle *(see Chapter*

10). It produces eight hormones. Six of these hormones are local and regulate the hormones produced by the anterior pituitary gland. The remaining two hormones— **oxytocin** and **antidiuretic hormone (ADH)**—are transported to the posterior pituitary, and stored until needed elsewhere in the body.

Pineal Gland

(LO 12.1, 12.2, 12.3, and 12.4)

Your pineal gland is located on the roof of your brain's third ventricle, posterior to the hypothalamus. It secretes the feel-good hormone **serotonin** by day, and at night, converts it to **melatonin,** which helps to regulate sleep and wake cycles. This gland reaches its maximum size in childhood and may regulate puberty's timing. It may also play a role in **seasonal affective disorder (SAD),** which causes some people to be depressed in the dark days of winter.

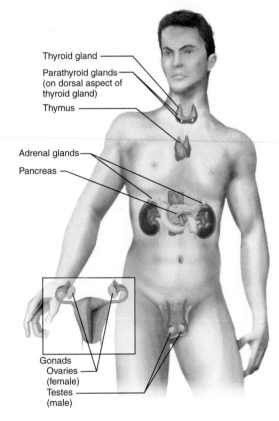

▲ **FIGURE 12.2**
Major Endocrine Glands.

▲ **FIGURE 12.1**
Hypothalamus, Pituitary Gland, and Pineal Gland.

Word	Pronunciation	Elements		Definition
antidiuretic (Note: 2 prefixes)	**AN**-tih-die-you-**RET**-ik	S/ P/ P/ R/	-ic *pertaining to* anti- *against* -di- *complete* -uret- *urination*	An agent that decreases urine production
endocrine	**EN**-doh-krin	P/ R/	endo- *within* -crine *secrete*	A gland that produces an internal or hormonal secretion
endocrinology (Note: *The "e" in* crine *changes to "o" for better flow.*)	**EN**-doh-krih-**NOL**-oh-jee	S/	-logy *study of*	Medical specialty concerned with the production and effects of hormones
endocrinologist	**EN**-doh-krih-**NOL**-oh-jist	S/	-logist *one who studies, specialist*	A medical specialist in endocrinology
hormone	**HOR**-mohn		Greek *to set in motion*	Chemical formed in one tissue or organ and carried by the bloodstream to stimulate or inhibit a function of another tissue or organ
hormonal (adj)	hor-**MOHN**-al	S/ R/	-al *pertaining to* hormon- *hormone*	Pertaining to hormones
hypothalamus	high-poh-**THAL**-ah-muss	P/ R/	hypo- *below* -thalamus	An endocrine gland in the floor and wall of the third ventricle of the brain
hypothalamic (adj)	high-poh-thah-**LAM**-ik	S/ R/	-ic *pertaining to* -thalam- *thalamus*	Pertaining to the hypothalamus
melatonin	mel-ah-**TONE**-in	S/ R/ R/	-in *substance* mela- *black* -ton- *tension, pressure*	Hormone formed by the pineal gland
oxytocin	**OCK**-see-toe-sin	S/ R/ R/	-in *substance* oxy- *oxygen* -toc- *labor and childbirth*	Pituitary hormone that stimulates the uterus to contract
pineal	**PIN**-ee-al		Latin *like a pine cone*	Pertaining to the pineal gland
pituitary	pih-**TYU**-ih-tary	S/ R/	-ary *pertaining to* pituit- *pituitary*	Pertaining to the pituitary gland
prostaglandin	**PROS**-tah-**GLAN**-din	S/ R/ R/	-in *chemical* prosta- *prostate* -gland- *gland*	Hormone present in many tissues, but first isolated from the prostate gland
serotonin	ser-oh-**TOE**-nin	S/ R/CF R/	-in *substance* ser/o- *serum* -ton- *tension, pressure*	Neurotransmitter in central and peripheral nervous systems

EXERCISES

A. Review *the Case Report on the previous spread before answering the questions.*

1. What are Mrs. Tacher's chief complaints? _____

2. What has been happening to Mrs. Tacher's facial features over the past ten years? _____

3. What change has there been in Mrs. Tacher's voice? _____

4. Why was it important for Mrs. Tacher to bring the photos with her? _____

5. Does Mrs. Tacher have any other health problems? _____

B. Elements *remain your best tool for understanding medical terms. The elements are listed in column 1. Identify the type of element in column 2, its meaning in column 3, and an example of a term containing that element in column 4. Fill in the chart.*

Element	Type of Element (P, R, CF, or S)	Meaning of Element	Medical Term Containing This Element
anti	1.	2.	3.
di	4.	5.	6.
endo	7.	8.	9.
hypo	10.	11.	12.
logist	13.	14.	15.
mela	16.	17.	18.

LESSON 12.1 Pituitary Gland

(LO 12.1, 12.2, 12.3, and 12.4)

CASE REPORT 12.1 (CONTINUED)

Dr. Khalid's examination of Mrs. Tacher shows a protruding mandible and an enlarged, deeply-grooved tongue. Her feet and hands are enlarged, her ribs are thickened, and her heart is enlarged. X-rays show a thickened skull and enlarged nasal sinuses. Blood tests display high growth hormone levels. CT and MRI scans show a tumor in the pituitary gland, and as a result, Mrs. Tacher is scheduled for surgery to remove the tumor.

Each hormone plays its part in maintaining your body's homeostasis, but your pituitary gland and hypothalamus work together and often influence hormone production in the other endocrine glands. Your pituitary gland is suspended from your hypothalamus, and it has two components:

- A large anterior lobe; and
- A small posterior lobe.

You have six **anterior-lobe hormones,** which are listed here with their functions:

1. **Follicle-stimulating hormone (FSH)** stimulates target cells in the ovaries to develop eggs, as well as sperm production in the testes.

2. **Luteinizing hormone (LH)** stimulates ovulation. It also encourages a corpus luteum (a yellow tissue mass) to form in the ovary *(see Chapter 15)* to secrete estrogen and progesterone. In the male, LH stimulates testosterone production *(see Chapter 14).*

3. **Thyroid-stimulating hormone (TSH),** or **thyrotropin,** stimulates the growth of the thyroid gland and the production of the chief thyroid hormone, thyroxine.

4. **Adrenocorticotropic hormone (ACTH),** or **corticotropin,** stimulates the adrenal glands to produce hormones called **corticosteroids,** including **hydrocortisone (cortisol)** and **cortisone.**

5. **Prolactin (PRL)** encourages the mammary glands to produce milk after pregnancy. In the male, it sensitizes the testes to LH, which enhances testosterone production.

6. **Growth hormone (GH),** or **somatotropin,** stimulates cells to enlarge and divide. The body produces at least a thousand times more GH than any other pituitary hormone.

An **overproduction of growth hormone** in children produces gigantism. In adults, this overproduction produces **acromegaly** *(Figure 12.4),* the condition that Mrs. Tacher has. An **underproduction of growth hormone,** present at birth, leads to dwarfism.

Tropic hormones are hormones that stimulate other endocrine glands to produce their hormones. FSH and LH are called **gonadotropins** because they stimulate **gonadal** (reproductive organ) functions.

In addition to the six anterior-lobe hormones, you have the **posterior-lobe hormones.** These hormones are produced by nuclei in the hypothalamus and stored and released in the pituitary posterior lobe *(Figure 12.3).* The two types of posterior-lobe hormones and their functions are listed below:

1. **Oxytocin (OT)** in childbirth stimulates uterine contractions, and in lactation, it forces milk to flow down ducts to the nipple. In both sexes, its production increases during sexual intercourse to help give the feelings of satisfaction and emotional bonding.

2. **Antidiuretic hormone (ADH),** also called **vasopressin,** reduces the volume of urine produced by the kidneys.

Diabetes insipidus (DI) (not diabetes mellitus) results from a decreased production of ADH. Symptoms of DI are excessive urine production leading to excessive thirst.

ABBREVIATIONS

ACTH	adrenocorticotropic hormone
ADH	antidiuretic hormone
DI	diabetes insipidus
FSH	follicle-stimulating hormone
GH	growth hormone
LH	luteinizing hormone
OT	oxytocin
PRL	prolactin
TSH	thyroid-stimulating hormone

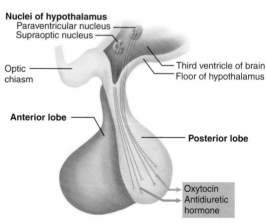

Nuclei of hypothalamus
Paraventricular nucleus
Supraoptic nucleus
Optic chiasm
Third ventricle of brain
Floor of hypothalamus
Anterior lobe
Posterior lobe
Oxytocin
Antidiuretic hormone

▲ **FIGURE 12.3**
Hormones of the Posterior Lobe
of the Pituitary Gland.

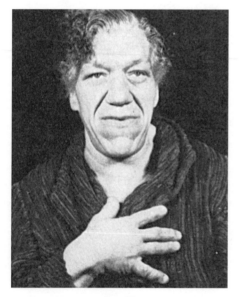

Age 52

▲ **FIGURE 12.4**
Woman with
Acromegaly, Age 52.

Word	Pronunciation	Elements		Definition
acromegaly	ak-roe-**MEG**-ah-lee	S/ R/CF	-megaly *enlargement* acr/o- *peak, highest point*	Enlargement of head, face, hands, and feet due to excess growth hormone in an adult
adrenocorticotropic	ah-**DREE**-noh-**KOR**-tih-koh-**TROH**-pik	S/ R/CF R/CF	-tropic *a turning, change* adren/o- *adrenal gland* -cortic/o- *from the cortex*	Hormone of the anterior pituitary that stimulates the cortex of the adrenal gland to produce its own hormones
corticosteroid	**KOR**-tih-koh-**STEHR**-oyd	S/ R/CF	-steroid *steroid* cortic/o- *from the cortex*	A hormone produced by the adrenal cortex
corticotropin	**KOR**-tih-koh-**TROH**-pin	S/ R/CF	-tropin *stimulation* cortic/o- *from the cortex, cortex*	Pituitary hormone that stimulates the cortex of the adrenal gland to secrete cortisone
cortisone	**KOR**-tih-sohn	S/ R/	-one *hormone* cortis- *from the cortex*	A corticosteroid produced in small amounts by the adrenal cortex
diabetes insipidus (DI)	dye-ah-**BEE**-teez in-**SIP**-ih-dus	S/ P/ R/	diabetes, Greek *siphon* -us *pertaining to* in- *not* -sipid- *flavor*	Excretion of large amounts of dilute urine as a result of inadequate antidiuretic hormone production
gonadotropin gonad	GO-nad-oh-**TROH**-pin GO-nad	S/ R/CF	-tropin *stimulation* gonad/o- *testis, ovary* gonad, Latin *seed*	Any hormone that stimulates gonadal function An organ that produces sex cells; a testis or an ovary
hydrocortisone (also called **cortisol**)	high-droh-**KOR**-tih-sohn	S/ R/CF R/	-one *hormone* hydr/o- *water* -cortis- *from the cortex*	Potent glucocorticoid with antiinflammatory properties
prolactin	pro-**LAK**-tin	S/ P/ R/	-in *substance* pro- *before* -lact- *milk*	Pituitary hormone that stimulates the production of milk
somatotropin (also called **growth hormone, GH**)	SO-mah-toh-**TROH**-pin	S/ R/CF	-tropin *stimulation* somat/o- *the body*	Hormone of the anterior pituitary that stimulates the growth of body tissues
thyrotropin	thigh-roe-**TROH**-pin	S/ R/CF	-tropin *stimulation* thyr/o- *thyroid*	Hormone from the anterior pituitary gland that stimulates function of the thyroid gland

EXERCISES

A. Review *the Case Report on this spread before answering the questions.*

1. What does Dr. Khalid learn from his physical examination of Mrs. Tacher? _____

2. List below one of the diagnostic tests Mrs. Tacher had, and the results of that test.

_____

3. Which test(s) pinpointed the source of Mrs. Tacher's problems? _____

4. What is the next step in her treatment plan? _____

B. Abbreviations *will be your answers in this matching exercise. Match the correct abbreviation to its description.*

_____ 1. stimulates ovulation   **A.** LH

_____ 2. stimulates production of corticosteroids   **B.** ADH

_____ 3. stimulates uterine contractions   **C.** ACTH

_____ 4. stimulates ovaries to develop eggs   **D.** TSH

_____ 5. reduces volume of urine   **E.** OT

_____ 6. stimulates production of thyroxin   **F.** FSH

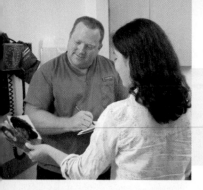

LESSON 12.2

Thyroid, Parathyroid, and Thymus Glands

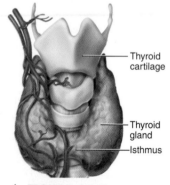

▲ **FIGURE 12.5**
Anatomy of the Thyroid Gland.

ABBREVIATIONS

PTH	parathyroid hormone
T3	triiodothyronine
T4	tetraiodothyronine (thyroxine)
VS	vital signs: measurement of temperature (T), pulse (P), respiration (R), and blood pressure (BP)

CASE REPORT 12.2

YOU ARE

. . . an EMT working in the Emergency Department at Fulwood Medical Center at 0200 hours in the morning.

YOU ARE COMMUNICATING WITH

. . . the parents of Ms. Norma Leary, a 22-year-old college student who is living with her parents for the summer. Ms. Leary is **emaciated,** extremely agitated, and at times disoriented and confused. Her parents tell you that in the past 3 or 4 days she has been coughing and not feeling well. In the past 12 hours, she has become feverish and been complaining of a left-sided chest pain. Upon questioning, the parents reveal that prior to this acute illness, Ms. Leary had lost about 20 pounds in weight, although she was eating voraciously. Her **VS** are T 105.2, P 180 and irregular, R 24, BP 160/85. You call for Dr. Hilinski, an emergency physician, STAT. On his initial examination, he believes that the patient is in thyroid storm, which is a medical emergency. There are no immediate laboratory tests that can confirm this diagnosis.

Thyroid Gland
(LO 12.1, 12.2, and 12.3)

Shaped like a bow tie and measuring about 2 inches wide, your **thyroid** gland lies just beneath the skin of your neck and below the thyroid cartilage ("Adam's apple"). Two lobes extend up on either side of the trachea (or windpipe) and are joined by an isthmus *(Figure 12.5).*

Cells in your thyroid gland secrete the two thyroid hormones **T3** and **T4.** The latter is known as **thyroxine.** The term **thyroid hormone** refers to T3 and T4 collectively, and it performs the following functions:

- **Stimulates** almost every tissue in the body to produce proteins;

- **Increases** the amount of oxygen that cells use; and

- **Controls** the speed of the body's chemical functions, known as the **metabolic rate.**

The thyroid also produces the hormone **calcitonin,** which promotes calcium deposition and bone formation.

Parathyroid Glands
(LO 12.1, 12.2, and 12.3)

Most people have four **parathyroid** glands, and these are partially embedded in the posterior surface of your thyroid gland. The parathyroid glands secrete **parathyroid hormone (PTH).** PTH stimulates bone resorption to bring calcium back into the blood, and calcitonin takes calcium from the blood to stimulate bone deposition *(see Chapter 4).*

Thymus Gland
(LO 12.1, 12.2, and 12.3)

Your **thymus** gland is located in the mediastinum *(Figure 12.6).* This gland is large in children and over time, it decreases in size until it is mostly fibrous tissue in the elderly. It secretes a group of hormones that stimulate the production of T lymphocytes *(see Chapter 7).*

▲ **FIGURE 12.6**
Position of the Thymus Gland.

Word	Pronunciation	Elements		Definition
calcitonin	kal-sih-**TONE**-in	S/ R/CF R/	-in *substance* calc/i- *calcium* -ton- *tension, pressure*	Hormone produced by the thyroid gland that moves calcium from blood to bones
emaciation	ee-may-see-**AY**-shun	S/ R/CF	-ation *process* emac/i- *make thin*	Abnormal thinness
emaciated (adj)	ee-may-see-**AY**-ted	S/	-ated *pertaining to a condition*	Pertaining to or suffering from emaciation
parathyroid	par-ah-**THIGH**-royd	S/ P/ R/	-oid *resembling* para- *adjacent, beside* -thyr- *thyroid*	Endocrine glands embedded in the back of the thyroid gland
thymus	**THIGH**-mus		Greek *sweetbread*	Endocrine gland located in the mediastinum
thyroid	**THIGH**-royd		Greek *an oblong shield*	Endocrine gland in the neck; or a cartilage of the larynx
thyroxine	thigh-**ROCK**-sin	S/ R/ R/	-ine *pertaining to* thyr- *thyroid gland* -ox- *oxygen*	Thyroid hormone T4, tetraiodothyronine

EXERCISES

A. Review *the Case Report on this spread before answering the questions.*

1. What are the outward signs Ms. Leary presents with in the ED? _____

2. What were her symptoms 4 days ago? _____

3. What additional symptoms has she developed in the last 12 hours? _____

4. Name one vital sign that shows Ms. Leary is now a medical emergency _____

5. What does Dr. Hilinski believe is Ms. Leary's diagnosis? _____

B. Critical thinking: *Apply your knowledge of the language of endocrinology and answer these additional questions about the Case Report.*

1. Why was Dr. Hilinski called to the ED STAT? _____

2. What information about Ms. Leary's weight is surprising, based on her eating pattern? _____

3. Will Dr. Hilinski order diagnostic tests for Ms. Leary? _____

C. Meet lesson *and chapter objectives and use the language of endocrinology to answer the following questions.*

1. What is the *speed of the body's chemical functions* known as? _____

2. What is *bone resorption?* _____

3. What is the role of calcitonin in bone deposition? _____

4. The processes in questions 2 and 3 are *antagonistic.* What does that mean? _____

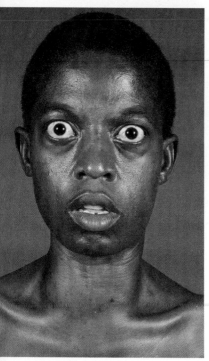

► FIGURE 12.7
Hyperthyroidism May
Cause the Eyes to Protrude
(Exophthalmos).

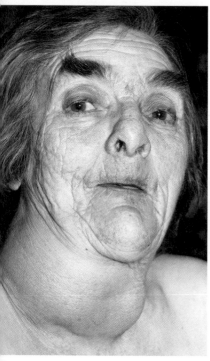

► FIGURE 12.8
Elderly Woman with
Hypothyroidism and
Goiter.

LESSON **12.2** Disorders of the Thyroid and Parathyroid Glands
(LO 12.1, 12.2, 12.3, and 12.4)

Hyperthyroidism (Thyrotoxicosis)
(LO 12.1, 12.2, 12.3, and 12.4)

The symptoms of **hyperthyroidism** (excessive thyroid hormone production) are those of an increased body metabolism. These include tachycardia (rapid heart rate), hypertension, sweating, shakiness, anxiety, weight loss despite increased appetite, and diarrhea.

Graves disease is an autoimmune disorder *(see Chapter 7)* in which an antibody stimulates the thyroid to produce and secrete excessive amounts of thyroid hormone into the blood. It presents with **exophthalmos** (bulging of the eyes) *(Figure 12.7)*, a **goiter** (an enlarged thyroid gland) *(Figure 12.8)*, and a nonpitting, waxy edema of the lower leg.

Hypothyroidism
(LO 12.1, 12.2, 12.3, and 12.4)

Hypothyroidism is the opposite of hyperthyroidism and results from an inadequate production of thyroid hormone. This decreases the body's metabolism. Primary hypothyroidism affects 10% of older women. Symptoms develop gradually and include: hair loss; dry, scaly skin; a puffy face and eyes; slow, hoarse speech; weight gain; constipation; and a high sensitivity to cold temperatures. No specific cause has been found,

Severe hypothyroidism is called **myxedema.** In developing countries, a common cause of this is a lack of **iodine** in the diet. In the United States, iodine is added to table salt to prevent hypothyroidism. Iodine is also found in dairy products and seafood.

Thyroiditis is an inflammation of the thyroid gland. It presents most commonly as **Hashimoto thyroiditis,** an autoimmune disease with lymphocytic infiltration of the gland. Hypothyroidism results, necessitating lifelong thyroid hormone replacement therapy.

Cretinism *(Figure 12.9)* is a congenital form of thyroid deficiency that severely retards mental and physical growth. If diagnosed and treated early with thyroid hormones, the patient can achieve significant improvement.

Thyroid cancer usually presents as a symptomless nodule in the thyroid gland. It can metastasize (spread) to cervical and mediastinal lymph nodes, and to the liver, lungs, and bones. A total **thyroidectomy** with local lymph node dissection is the first step in treating thyroid cancer.

CASE REPORT 12.2 (CONTINUED)

Thyroid storm is the condition Ms. Norma Leary presented with in the Emergency Department. It is the most extreme state of **hyperthyroidism,** with severely exaggerated effects of the thyroid hormones causing **hyperpyrexia,** tachycardia, agitation, and delirium. The weight loss prior to her illness becoming acute was part of her undiagnosed hyperthyroidism.

Disorders of the Parathyroid Glands (LO 12.1, 12.2, 12.3, and 12.4)

Hypoparathyroidism is a deficiency of parathyroid hormone (PTH) that lowers levels of blood calcium. Most symptoms of this are neuromuscular (in nerve and muscle tissue), ranging from tingling in the fingers, to muscle cramps, to the painful muscle spasms of **tetany** (not **tetanus,** which is caused by a toxin acting on the central nervous system).

Hyperparathyroidism is an excess of PTH and is more common than hypoparathyroidism. It is usually caused by one of the four glands enlarging and working out of pituitary control. It leads to calcium depletion in bones (making bones brittle), high blood calcium levels, and kidney stones.

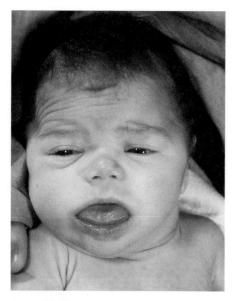

► FIGURE 12.9
Infant with
Cretinism.

Word	Pronunciation	Elements		Definition
cretin cretinism	**KREH**-tin **KREH**-tin-izm	 S/ R/	 -ism *condition, process* cretin- *cretin*	Severe congenital hypothyroidism Condition of severe congenital hypothyroidism
exophthalmos	ek-sof-**THAL**-mos	P/ R/	ex- *out* -ophthalmos *eye*	Protrusion of the eyeball
goiter	**GOY**-ter		Latin *throat*	Enlargement of the thyroid gland
Graves disease	**GRAVZ** diz-**EEZ**		Robert Graves, Irish physician, 1796–1853	Hyperthyroidism with toxic goiter
Hashimoto disease	hah-shee-**MOH**-toe diz-**EEZ**		Hakaru Hashimoto, Japanese surgeon, 1881–1934	Autoimmune disease of the thyroid gland
hyperparathyroidism (Note: *2 suffixes and 2 prefixes*)	**HIGH**-per-par-ah-**THIGH**-royd-izm	S/ S/ P/ P/ R/	-ism *condition* -oid- *resembling* hyper- *excessive* -para- *adjacent* -thyr- *thyroid*	Excessive levels of parathyroid hormone
hypoparathyroidism	**HIGH**-poh-par-ah-**THIGH**-royd-izm	P/	hypo- *deficient, below*	Deficient levels of parathyroid hormone
hyperpyrexia	**HIGH**-per-pie-**REK**-see-ah	S/ P/ R/	-ia *condition* hyper- *excessive* -pyrex- *fever*	Extremely high body temperature or fever
hyperthyroidism (Note: *2 suffixes*) (Also called thyrotoxicosis.)	high-per-**THIGH**-royd-izm	S/ S/ P/ R/	-ism *condition* -oid- *resembling* hyper- *excessive* -thyr- *thyroid*	Excessive production of thyroid hormones
hypothyroidism (Note: *2 suffixes*)	high-poh-**THIGH**-royd-izm	S/ S/ P/ R/	-ism *condition* -oid- *resembling* hypo- *deficient, below* -thyr- *thyroid*	Deficient production of thyroid hormones
iodine	**EYE**-oh-dine or **EYE**-oh-deen	S/ R/	-ine *pertaining to* iod- *violet*	Chemical element, the lack of which causes thyroid disease
myxedema	miks-eh-**DEE**-muh	P/ R/	myx- *mucus* -edema *swelling*	Nonpitting, waxy edema of the skin in hypothyroidism
tetany	**TET**-ah-nee		Greek *convulsive tension*	Severe muscle twitches, cramps, and spasms
thyroidectomy	thigh-roy-**DEK**-toe-me	S/ S/ R/	-ectomy *surgical excision* -oid- *resembling* thyr- *thyroid*	Surgical removal of the thyroid gland
thyroiditis	thigh-roy-**DIE**-tis	S/	-itis *inflammation*	Inflammation of the thyroid gland
thyrotoxicosis *(also called hyperthyroidism)*	**THIGH**-roe-toks-ih-**KOH**-sis	S/ R/CF R/CF	-sis *condition* thyr/o- *thyroid* -toxic/o- *poison*	Disorder produced by excessive thyroid hormone production

EXERCISES

A. Review *the Case Report on this spread before answering the questions.*

1. What is the most extreme state of hyperthyroidism called? _____

2. What is the difference between hyperthyroidism and hyperpyrexia? _____

_____

3. What three terms in the Case Report (continued) signify body processes that have speeded up or are in an excessive state?

_____, _____ and _____.

4. What condition did Ms. Leary have that had been undiagnosed until it reached an acute state? _____

_____

B. Meet lesson objectives *and apply the language of endocrinology to answer the following questions.*

1. Describe the difference between *tetany* and *tetanus*. _____

_____

2. List some of the common disorders of the thyroid gland. _____

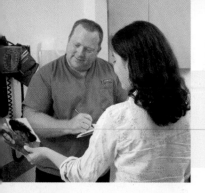

LESSON 12.3

Adrenal Glands and Hormones

CASE REPORT 12.3

OBJECTIVES

Your adrenal glands produce several key hormones that help to maintain homeostasis. The information in this lesson will enable you to use correct medical terminology to:

12.3.1 Locate the adrenal glands.

12.3.2 Differentiate between the adrenal cortex and the medulla.

12.3.3 Identify the functions of the hormones produced by the cortex and medulla.

12.3.4 Detail how the body adapts to stress.

12.3.5 Explain common disorders of the adrenal glands.

Adrenal Glands

(LO 12.1, 12.2, 12.3, and 12.4)

An **adrenal (suprarenal)** gland is anchored like a cap on the upper pole of each kidney *(Figure 12.11 inset).* The outer layer of the gland—the adrenal cortex *(Figure 12.11)*—synthesizes more than 25 **steroid** hormones known collectively as **adrenocortical** hormones, or corticosteroids. These hormones include:

1. **Glucocorticoids,** mainly **hydrocortisone (cortisol),** which help regulate blood glucose levels, particularly in response to stress. They also have an anti-inflammatory effect, and are often found in dermatologic lotions and ointments;

2. **Mineralocorticoids,** mostly **aldosterone,** which promote sodium retention and potassium secretion by the kidneys; and

3. **Sex steroids,** which include a weak androgen that is converted to testosterone *(see Chapter 14)* and estrogen *(see Chapter 15).*

The inner layer of the adrenal gland, the adrenal medulla *(Figure 12.11),* also secretes hormones. These hormones are called **catecholamines,** and principally include **epinephrine (adrenaline)** and **norepinephrine (noradrenaline).** These hormones prepare the body for physical activity and are responsible for the "flight or fight" response.

Disorders of the Adrenal Glands

(LO 12.1, 12.2, 12.3, and 12.4)

Adrenocortical hypofunction, most commonly seen as **Addison disease,** is caused by the **idiopathic** atrophy (wasting away) of the adrenal cortex. Symptoms are weakness, fatigue, increased susceptibility to infection, and diminished resistance to stress. This disorder is treated with hormone replacement therapy, which John F. Kennedy received until he died.

Adrenocortical hyperfunction most commonly appears as **Cushing syndrome.** Excess production of the steroid hormones produces "moon" **facies** (facial features and expressions), muscle wasting and weak-

CASE REPORT 12.3

John Fitzgerald Kennedy (JFK) (1917–1963) was elected President of the United States of America in 1960 at the age of 43 *(Figure 12.10).* He had health problems from the age of 13, when he was first diagnosed as having colitis. At age 27, he had lower back pain that necessitated lower back surgery. He was then diagnosed as having adrenal gland insufficiency (Addison disease) with osteoporosis of his lumbar spine. This required lower back surgery on three more occasions. JFK received adrenal hormone replacement therapy for the rest of his life, together with pain medication for his lower back pain, until his assassination in Dallas, Texas, in 1963. In medical retrospect, instead of colitis, JFK probably had celiac disease *(see Chapter 9),* which has strong associations with Addison disease.

ness, kidney stones, and reduced resistance to infection. Most cases are due to a pituitary tumor secreting too much ACTH, causing the adrenal glands to produce an excess of steroids. Sometimes, Cushing syndrome can be produced by the administration of excess steroid medications.

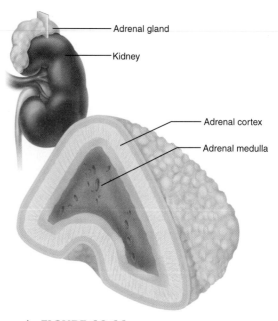

▲ **FIGURE 12.11**
Adrenal Gland.

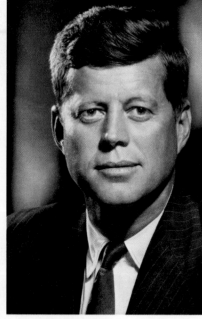

▲ **FIGURE 12.10**
John F. Kennedy.

Word	Pronunciation	Elements		Definition
Addison disease	**ADD**-ih-son diz-**EEZ**		Thomas Addison, English physician, 1793–1860	An autoimmune disease leading to decreased production of adrenocortical steroids
adrenal *(same as* **suprarenal***)*	ah-**DREE**-nal	S/ P/ R/ P/	-al *pertaining to* ad- *to, toward* -ren- *kidney* supra- *above*	Endocrine gland on the upper pole of each kidney
adrenaline *(also called* **epinephrine***)*	ah-**DREN**-ah-lin ep-ih-**NEF**-rin	S/ P/ R/	-ine *pertaining to* epi- *above* -nephr- *kidney*	Main catecholamine produced by the adrenal medulla
adrenocortical	ah-dree-noh-**KOR**-tih-kal	S/ R/CF R/	-al *pertaining to* adren/o- *adrenal* -cortic- *cortex*	Pertaining to the cortex of the adrenal gland
aldosterone	al-**DOS**-ter-own	S/ R/CF R/	-one *hormone* ald/o- *organic compound* -ster- *steroid*	Mineralocorticoid hormone of the adrenal cortex
catecholamine	kat-eh-**COAL**-ah-meen	S/ R/	-amine *nitrogen-containing substance* catechol- *tyrosine containing*	Major elements produced by the adrenal cortex in the stress response; include epinephrine and norepinephrine
Cushing syndrome	**KUSH**-ing **SIN**-drohm		Harvey Cushing, U.S. neurosurgeon, 1869–1939	Hypersecretion of cortisol (hydrocortisone) by the adrenal gland
facies	**FASH**-eez		Latin *appearance*	Facial features and expressions
glucocorticoid	glu-co-**KOR**-tih-koyd	S/ R/ R/CF	-oid *resembling* -cortic- *cortisone* gluc/o- *glucose*	Hormone of the adrenal cortex that helps regulate glucose metabolism
hydrocortisone *(also called* **cortisol***)*	high-droh-**KOR**-tih-sohn	S/ R/CF R/	-one *hormone* hydr/o- *water* -cortis- *cortisone*	Potent glucocorticoid with anti-inflammatory properties
idiopathic	id-ih-oh-**PATH**-ik	S/ R/CF R/	-ic *pertaining to* idi/o- *unknown* -path- *disease*	Pertaining to a disease of unknown etiology
mineralocorticoid	**MIN**-er-al-oh-**KOR**-tih-koyd	S/ R/ R/CF	-oid *resemble* -cortic- *cortex* mineral/o- *inorganic material*	Hormone of the adrenal cortex that influences sodium and potassium metabolism
norepinephrine *(Note: 2 prefixes) (also called* **noradrenaline***)*	**NOR**-ep-ih-**NEFF**-rin	S/ P/ P/ R/	-ine *pertaining to* nor- *normal* -epi- *above* -nephr- *kidney*	Catecholamine hormone of the adrenal gland that is a parasympathetic neurotransmitter
steroid	**STER**-oyd	S/ R/	-oid *resembling* ster- *solid*	Large family of chemical substances found in many drugs, hormones, and body components

EXERCISE

A. Review *the Case Report on this spread before answering the questions.*

1. What is *colitis* and what body system does it affect?

   Definition _____

   Body system _____

2. *Adrenal gland insufficiency* is also known as _____

3. What lumbar spine problem did John Kennedy also have? _____

4. What two conditions did John Kennedy treat with medications?

   _____ and _____

5. What other disease has a *strong association* with Addison disease? _____

6. What does *strong association with* mean in this case? _____

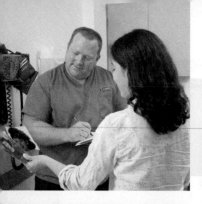

OBJECTIVES

Your pancreas measures approximately 6 inches in length, rests across the back of your abdomen, and has many important functions, including the secretion of digestive juices and the production of hormones. The information provided in this lesson will enable you to use correct medical terminology to:

12.4.1 Distinguish between the different cells of the pancreas and their secretions.

12.4.2 Identify the functions of the hormones produced by the pancreas.

12.4.3 Explain common disorders of the pancreatic hormones.

KEYNOTES

- Glucagon is not the only hormone that raises blood glucose; epinephrine, hydrocortisone, and growth hormone do as well.

- Insulin is the only hormone that lowers blood glucose.

CASE REPORT 12.4

YOU ARE

. . . a certified medical assistant working with Susan Lee, MD, in her Primary Care Clinic at Fulwood Medical Center.

YOU ARE COMMUNICATING WITH

. . . Mrs. Martha Jones, who is here for her monthly checkup. She is a 53-year-old type 2 diabetic on insulin. Mrs. Jones has diabetic retinopathy and diabetic neuropathy of her feet. Bariatric surgery has enabled her to reduce her weight from 275 to 156 pounds. The time is 0930 hrs. She is complaining of having a cold and cough for the past few days. Now, she is feeling drowsy and nauseous and has a dry mouth. As you talk with her, you notice that her speech is slurred. She cannot remember if she gave herself her morning insulin. Examination of her lungs reveals rales (wet, crackly lung noises) at her right base.

Her VS: T 97.8, P 120, R 20, BP 100/50. You perform her blood **glucose** measurement. The reading is 600 milligrams per deciliter (mg/dL). A recommended value 2 hours after breakfast is < 145 mg/dL.

The Pancreas (LO 12.1, 12.2, and 12.3)

The location and structure of the pancreas are further detailed in *Chapter 9.* Most of your pancreas is an **exocrine** gland (external secretion gland) that secretes digestive juices through a duct *(Figure 12.12a).* Scattered throughout the pancreas are clusters of endocrine cells grouped around blood vessels. These clusters are called **pancreatic islets (islets of Langerhans).** Within the islets are three distinct cell types *(Figure 12.12b):*

1. **Alpha cells:** Secrete the hormone **glucagon** in response to low a blood **glucose.** Glucagon's actions are:

   a. In the liver, to stimulate **gluconeogenesis, glycogenolysis,** and the release of glucose into the bloodstream; and

   b. In adipose tissue, to stimulate fat catabolism and the release of free fatty acids.

2. **Beta cells:** Secrete **insulin** in response to a high blood glucose level. Insulin has the opposite effects to those of glucagon, and its actions are:

   a. In muscle and fat cells, to enable them to absorb glucose, and to store glycogen and fat; and

   b. In the liver, to stimulate the conversion of glucose to glycogen.

3. **Delta cells:** Secrete **somatostatin,** which acts within the pancreas to prevent the secretion of glucagon and insulin.

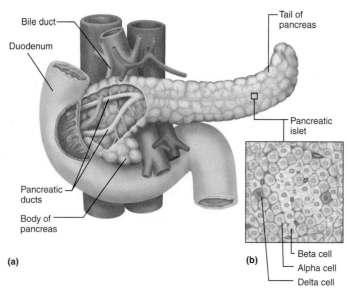

(a)

(b)

◀ **FIGURE 12.12**
Pancreas.
(a) Anatomy of the pancreas. (b) Alpha, beta, and delta cells.

Word	Pronunciation	Elements		Definition
exocrine	**EK**-soh-krin	P/ R/	exo- *outward* -crine *secrete*	A gland that secretes outwardly through excretory ducts
glucagon	**GLU**-kah-gon	S/ R/	-agon *to fight* gluc- *sugar, glucose*	Pancreatic hormone that supports blood glucose levels
gluconeogenesis	**GLU**-koh-nee-oh-**JEN**-eh-sis	S/ P/ R/CF	-genesis *creation* -neo- *new* gluc/o- *sugar, glucose*	Formation of glucose from noncarbohydrate sources
glucose	**GLU**-kose	S/ R/	-ose *full of* gluc- *sugar, glucose*	The final product of carbohydrate digestion and the main sugar in the blood
glycogenolysis	**GLYE**-koh-jen-oh-**LYE**-sis	S/ R/CF R/CF	-lysis *separate, dissolve* glyc/o- *glycogen* -gen/o- *create*	Conversion of glycogen to glucose
insulin	**IN**-syu-lin	S/ R/	-in *a substance* insul- *an island*	Hormone produced by the islet cells of the pancreas
islets of Langerhans	**EYE**-lets of **LAHNG**-er-hahnz		Paul Langerhans, German anatomist, 1847–1888	Areas of pancreatic cells that produce insulin and glucagon
somatostatin	**SOH**-mah-toh-**STAT**-in	S/ R/CF	-statin *inhibit* somat/o- *body*	Hormone that inhibits release of growth hormone and insulin

EXERCISES

A. Review *the Case Report on this spread before answering the questions.*

1. What body system is affected by diabetic retinopathy? _____

2. What type of surgery has Mrs. Jones had to help reduce her weight? _____

3. What are her complaints that caused her to see Dr. Lee? _____

4. Explain what *rales* are and how you detect them. _____
_____

5. In which body system would you have the term *neuropathy?* _____

6. What symptoms is Mrs. Jones experiencing now? _____
_____

7. What outward signs does the CMA notice in Mrs. Jones? _____

8. Why is it important for Mrs. Jones to go for monthly checkups? _____
_____

9. Is Mrs. Jones' blood glucose measurement too high or too low? _____

10. Which other specialists might Mrs. Jones have to consult for her other conditions? _____ and _____.

B. Build the correct medical term *that matches the definition. Insert each missing element on the line, and label what type of element it is under the line. Then answer question 5.*

1. Conversion of glycogen to glucose: _____ / _____ /lysis

2. Main sugar in the blood: _____ / _____ /ose

3. Hormone that inhibits release of GH and insulin: _____ / _____ /statin

4. The formation of glucose from noncarbohydrate sources: gluco/ _____ /genesis

5. What is unusual about the elements in the term in question 4 above? _____

Diabetes Mellitus (DM)
(LO 12.1, 12.2, 12.3, and 12.4)

Diabetes mellitus is a condition characterized by hyperglycemia, resulting from an impairment of insulin secretion and/or insulin action. Diabetes affects the body's ability to make use of the energy found in food, disrupting the normal process of carbohydrate, fat, and protein metabolism. It is the world's most prevalent metabolic disease and the leading cause of blindness, renal failure, and gangrene of the lower extremities. There are four categories of diabetes mellitus:

1. **Type 1 diabetes,** also called **insulin-dependent diabetes mellitus (IDDM),** accounts for 10% to 15% of all cases of DM. It is the predominant type of DM found in patients under the age of 30. When symptoms become apparent, 90% of the pancreatic insulin-producing cells have already been destroyed by **autoantibodies** (antibodies that attack the patient's own system).

2. **Type 2 diabetes,** also called **non-insulin-dependent diabetes mellitus (NIDDM),** accounts for 85% to 90% of all DM cases. Nearly 18 million people in the U.S. have been diagnosed with type 2 DM. Not only is there an impairment of insulin response, but there is also a decreased glucose uptake by tissues due to insulin resistance. In addition to contributing to type 2 DM, insulin resistance leads to other common disorders like hypertension, hyperlipidemia, and coronary artery disease.

3. **Gestational diabetes** occurs in about 5% of pregnancies. While most cases of gestational diabetes resolve after the pregnancy, a woman who has this complication of pregnancy has a 30% chance of developing type 2 DM within 10 years.

4. **Mature-onset diabetes of the young (MODY)** is genetically inherited, occurs in thin individuals in their teens and twenties, and is comparable to type 2 DM in its severity.

Hypoglycemia
(LO 12.1, 12.2, 12.3, and 12.4)

Hypoglycemia is present when blood glucose is below 70 mg/dL. Because brain metabolism depends primarily on glucose, the brain is the first organ affected by hypoglycemia. This disorder presents clinically as an impaired mental efficiency, followed by shakiness, anxiety, confusion, tremor, seizures, and, if untreated, loss of consciousness. Symptomatic hypoglycemia is sometimes called **insulin shock.** Low blood glucose can be raised to normal in minutes by taking 10 to 20 grams of carbohydrate (3 to 4 ounces), such as orange, apple, or grape juice, or a sugar-containing soft drink.

Hyperglycemia
(LO 12.1, 12.2, 12.3, and 12.4)

In **hyperglycemia,** the classic symptoms are **polyuria** (excessive urination), **polydipsia** (excessive thirst) and **polyphagia** (excessive hunger), with unexplained weight loss.

Symptomatic hyperglycemia is how type 1 DM usually presents. Type 2 DM can be symptomatic or asymptomatic, and is often found during a routine health exam.

Because of high glucose levels, hyperglycemia damages capillary endothelial cells in the retina, renal glomerulus *(see Chapter 13),* and neurons and Schwann cells in peripheral nerves *(see Chapter 10).* Of all diabetics, 85% develop some degree of **diabetic retinopathy;** 30% develop diabetic nephropathy, which can progress to end-stage renal disease *(see Chapter 13).* Diabetic neuropathy causes sensory defects with numbness, tingling, and **paresthesias** (abnormal skin sensations) in the feet and/or hands.

In larger blood vessels, the hyperglycemia contributes to endothelial cell-lining damage and atherosclerosis. Coronary artery disease and peripheral vascular disease with claudication *(see Chapter 6)* are complications. Hyperglycemia is the most common cause of foot ulcers and gangrene of the lower extremity, sometimes requiring **amputation.** The risk of infection is increased by the cellular hyperglycemia and the circulatory deficits.

The complications of hyperglycemia can be kept at bay by stringent control of blood glucose levels.

Word	Pronunciation	Elements		Definition
amputation	am-pyu-**TAY**-shun	S/ R/	-ation *a process* amput- *to prune, lop off*	Process of removing a limb, part of a limb, a breast, or other projecting part
autoantibody (Note: 2 prefixes)	awe-toe-**AN**-tee-bod-ee	P/ P/ R/	auto- *self, same* -anti- *against* -body *body*	Antibody produced in response to an antigen from the host's own tissue
coma comatose (adj)	**KOH**-mah **KOH**-mah-toes	 S/ R/	Greek *deep sleep* -ose *full of* comat- *coma*	State of deep unconsciousness In a state of coma
diabetes mellitus diabetic (adj)	dye-ah-**BEE**-teez **MEL**-ih-tus dye-ah-**BET**-ik	 S/ R/	diabetes, Greek *a siphon* mellitus, Latin *sweetened with honey* -ic *pertaining to* diabet- *diabetes*	Metabolic syndrome caused by absolute or relative insulin deficiency and/or ineffectiveness Pertaining to or suffering from diabetes
hyperglycemia hyperglycemic (adj)	**HIGH**-per-gly-**SEE**-me-ah **HIGH**-per-gly-**SEE**-mik	S/ P/ R/ S/	-emia *a blood condition* hyper- *above* -glyc- *glucose* -emic *pertaining to a blood condition*	High level of glucose (sugar) in the blood Pertaining to or having hyperglycemia
hypoglycemia hypoglycemic (adj)	**HIGH**-poh-gly-**SEE**-me-ah **HIGH**-poh-gly-**SEE**-mik	S/ P/ R/ S/	-emia *a blood condition* hypo- *below, deficient* -glyc- *glucose* -emic *pertaining to a blood condition*	Low level of glucose (sugar) in the blood Pertaining to or suffering from low blood sugar
paresthesia paresthesias (pl)	par-es-**THEE**-ze-ah	S/ P/ R/	-ia *condition* par- *abnormal* -esthes- *sensation*	An abnormal sensation; e.g., tingling, burning, pricking
polydipsia	pol-ee-**DIP**-see-ah	S/ P/ R/	-ia *condition* poly- *many, excessive* -dips- *thirst*	Excessive thirst
polyphagia	pol-ee-**FAY**-jee-ah	S/ P/ R/	-ia *condition* poly- *many, excessive* -phag- *eat*	Excessive eating
polyuria	pol-ee-**YOU**-ree-ah	S/ P/ R/	-ia *condition* poly- *many, excessive* -ur- *urine*	Excessive production of urine
retinopathy	ret-ih-**NOP**-ah-thee	S/ R/CF	-pathy *disease* retin/o- *retina of the eye*	Degenerative disease of the retina

EXERCISES

A. Diabetes *is the world's most prevalent metabolic disease. Many patients have diabetes as a concurrent condition with other health problems, which always makes it a consideration in treatment and the prescribing of medications. Test your knowledge of this disease by answering the following questions. Circle the correct choice.*

1. Diabetes is the leading cause of:

blindness   renal failure   gangrene   all of these   none of these

2. The first organ affected by hypoglycemia is the:

kidney   heart   pancreas   brain   liver

3. Impairment of insulin response and decreased insulin effectiveness is termed insulin:

production   resistance   autoantibodies   control   conversion

4. Most cases of gestational diabetes resolve after:

medication   treatment   testing   pregnancy   surgery

B. Apply *your knowledge of the endocrine system and the correct medical terminology to answer the following questions.*

1. What are the three classic symptoms of diabetes? _____, _____, and _____.

2. Hyperglycemia can result in _____.

3. What is the correct medical term for abnormal skin sensations? _____

Diabetes Mellitus

(continued)

(LO 12.1, 12.2, 12.3, and 12.4)

- Diabetic ketoacidosis is a medical emergency.

- Maintaining normal plasma glucose levels is the basis for good management of DM.

- Many insulin-dependent diabetics need multiple subcutaneous insulin injections each day.

Diabetic ketoacidosis (DKA) is a state of marked hyperglycemia with dehydration, **metabolic acidosis** (abnormal increase in blood acidity), and **ketone** formation. This is seen mostly in type 1 DM and usually results from a lapse in insulin treatment, an acute infection, or a trauma that makes the usual insulin treatment inadequate.

DKA presents with polyuria, vomiting, and lethargy and can progress to coma. The ketone **acetone** can be smelled on the breath. DKA is a medical emergency. There is a 2% to 5% mortality rate from circulatory collapse if the DKA is not promptly controlled.

Diabetic coma is a severe medical emergency, caused by hyperglycemia.

Insulin shock is another severe medical emergency, caused by hypoglycemia.

A blood glucose test will differentiate hypoglycemia from hyperglycemia.

Treatment of Diabetes Mellitus

(LO 12.1, 12.2, 12.3, and 12.4)

The basic principle of diabetes treatment is to avoid hyperglycemia and hypoglycemia. The areas of treatment are as follows:

- **Diet and exercise** to achieve weight reduction of 2 pounds per week in overweight type 2 DM patients is essential.

- **Patient education** is necessary so that the patient understands the disease process, can recognize the indications for seeking immediate medical care, and will follow a foot care regimen.

- **Plasma glucose monitoring** is an essential skill that all diabetics must learn. Patients on insulin must learn to adjust their insulin doses. Home glucose analyzers use a drop of blood obtained from the fingertip or forearm by a spring-powered lancet. The frequency of testing varies individually.

BUN	blood urea nitrogen
DKA	diabetic ketoacidosis
Hb A1c	glycosylated hemo-globin, hemoglobin A one-C

CASE REPORT 12.4 (CONTINUED)

Mrs. Martha Jones is in the early stages of a diabetic ketoacidosis coma, probably initiated by a right lower-lobe pneumonia. A urine specimen was obtained. Dr. Lee was notified. Blood was taken for a full chemistry panel, and arterial blood gases were drawn. Dr. Lee treated Mrs. Jones immediately with an IV infusion of **saline** solution and IV insulin. She was admitted to the hospital.

- **Assessment of the patient** should be performed on routine physician visits for symptoms or signs of complications.

- **Periodic laboratory evaluation** includes **BUN** and serum creatinine (kidney function), lipid profile, ECG, and an annual complete ophthalmologic evaluation.

Glycosylated hemoglobin (Hb A1c) is used to monitor plasma glucose control during the preceding 1 to 3 months.

Oral antidiabetic drugs are used for type 2 DM but not type 1 DM. There are numerous drugs available, and they produce their effect in three main ways:

- Stimulate the beta cells of the pancreas to produce more insulin.

- Decrease glucose production by the liver.

- Block the breakdown of starches in the intestine.

Combinations of these different-acting drugs are often used.

Injectable insulin preparations are used in type 1 DM and sometimes in type 2 DM. They are classified by their speed of action.

For some patients requiring frequent doses of insulin, continuous subcutaneous insulin infusion is given by an implanted battery-powered, programmable pump. This pump provides continuous insulin through a small needle in the abdominal wall.

Word	Pronunciation	Elements		Definition
acetone	**ASS**-eh-tone		Latin *vinegar*	Ketone that is found in blood, urine, and breath when diabetes mellitus is out of control
ketoacidosis	**KEY**-toe-ass-ih-**DOE**-sis	S/ R/ R/CF	-osis *condition* -acid- *acid* ket/o- *ketone*	Excessive ketones in the blood, making it acid
ketone	**KEY**-tone		Greek *acetone*	Chemical formed in uncontrolled diabetes or in starvation
ketosis	key-**TOE**-sis	S/ R/	-osis *condition* ket- *ketone*	Excessive production of ketones
metabolic acidosis	met-ah-**BOL**-ik ass-ih-**DOE**-sis	S/ R/ S/ R/	-ic *pertaining to* metabol- *change* -osis *condition* acid- *acid*	Decreased pH in blood and body tissues as a result of an upset in metabolism
saline	**SAY**-leen		Latin *salt*	Salt solution, usually sodium chloride

EXERCISES

A. Case Report *(continued): Read aloud the Case Report on the opposite page. Read it a second time, and highlight or underline the medical terms. Answer the following questions based on this Case Report.*

1. "Diabetic ketoacidosis is a state of marked hyperglycemia with dehydration." Explain this in layperson's language. _____
_____
_____

2. Mrs. Jones' pneumonia is in her right lower lobe. How many lobes are in the right lung? _____

3. Define pneumonia: _____

4. Name an abbreviation that could have been used in this Case Report: _____, which stands for
_____.

5. What chemical is contained in a *saline* solution? _____

6. Name three possible causes of DKA: _____, _____, and _____.

7. If DKA is not promptly controlled, _____ and _____ can result, which can cause death.

B. Terminology challenge *on the Case Report and Case Report (continued). Challenge yourself to use all the correct medical terminology in your answers.*

1. What was the probable cause of Mrs. Jones' coma? _____

2. What diagnostic tests did Mrs. Jones have? _____

3. Why did Mrs. Jones have an *infusion* and not a *transfusion?* _____

4. Diabetic coma is caused by _____. Conversely, insulin shock is caused by _____.

5. What is the chemical produced in uncontrolled diabetes or starvation? _____

6. Define *metabolic acidosis.* _____
_____

7. Which specific ketone can be smelled on the breath? _____

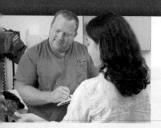

CHALLENGE YOUR KNOWLEDGE

A. Build your knowledge *of the language of endocrinology by analyzing the elements in the following terms. Then write a sentence of your choice for any one term in the chart.*

Medical Term	Meaning of Prefix	Meaning of Root/CF	Meaning of Suffix	Meaning of Term
acromegaly	1.	2.	3.	4.
endocrinology	5.	6.	7.	8.
glycogenolysis	9.	10.	11.	12.
hypoglycemia	13.	14.	15.	16.
neuropathy	17.	18.	19.	20.
paresthesia	21.	22.	23.	24.
polyphagia	25.	26.	27.	28.
serotonin	29.	30.	31.	32.

Sentence: _____

_____ _____ _____

B. Deconstruct *the following terms into the meanings of their elements. First, slash the term into elements. Then write the appropriate elements on the line, and the meaning of each element under the line. Fill in the blanks.*

1. endocrinology _____ / _____ / _____

2. acromegaly _____ / _____ / _____

3. oxytocin _____ / _____ / _____

4. polydipsia _____ / _____ / _____

5. exophthalmos _____ / _____ / _____

C. Roots *are the fundamental core of every term. Test yourself on the roots below, found in the language of endocrinology. Write the root on the line, and write the meaning of just the root under the line. Based on the elements, you will not have to fill in every blank. Don't forget to answer the questions at the end of the exercise.*

1. an agent that increases urine production   di/ _____ /ic

2. medical specialty concerned with hormones   endo/ _____ /logy

3. neurotransmitter in CNS   _____ / _____ /in

4. enlargement of extremities due to excess GH   acro/ _____ / _____

5. pituitary hormone that stimulates uterus to contract   _____ / _____ /in

6. hormone that stimulates secretion of milk   pro/ _____ /in

7. protrusion of the eyeball   ex/ _____ / _____

8. extremely high fever   hyper/ _____ / _____

9. severe hypothyroidism   myx/ _____ / _____

10. disorder produced by excessive thyroid hormone production   _____ / _____ /osis

11. Based on what you see in the empty blanks above, notice that not every term needs a _____.

12. Sometimes, a _____ will start the term.

D. Prefixes: *The following prefixes appear in this chapter and have also appeared in previous chapters. Give the meaning of the prefix, and list two different terms in which the prefix appears. Fill in the blanks.*

1. *anti* means _____

    Term from this chapter: _____ Term from a previous chapter: _____

2. *endo* means _____

    Term from this chapter: _____ Term from a previous chapter: _____

3. *hyper* means _____

    Term from this chapter: _____ Term from a previous chapter: _____

4. *ex* means _____

    Term from this chapter: _____ Term from a previous chapter: _____

5. *ad* means _____

    Term from this chapter: _____ Term from a previous chapter: _____

6. *epi* means _____

    Term from this chapter: _____ Term from a previous chapter: _____

7. *neo* means _____

    Term from this chapter: _____ Term from a previous chapter: _____

8. *poly* means _____

    Term from this chapter: _____ Term from a previous chapter: _____

9. *supra* means _____

    Term from this chapter: _____ Term from a previous chapter: _____

E. Elements are your clues in the following terms. *You do not necessarily have to know what an entire term means, but if you recognize an element in the term, it will help you answer the questions. Choose the correct terms from among this group to fit the descriptions. Some blanks may need more than one term, and there are extra terms you will not use. Fill in the blanks.*

nephropathy	comatose	adrenalectomy	retinopathy	polyuria	saline	hypoglycemia
serotonin	antidiuretic	endocrine	nephrectomy	prolactin	ketoacidosis	thyroidectomy

1. term(s) connected to the kidney: _____

2. term(s) for blood conditions: _____

3. terms that are procedures: _____

4. term(s) connected to milk _____

5. terms describing a disease or condition: _____

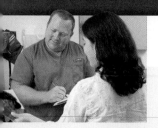

F. Recall and review: *This exercise on word elements contains elements from a previous chapter. Try to recall the previous elements without turning back in your book. Check (✔) the type of element; then write its meaning. Fill in the chart.*

Element	Type of Element			Meaning of Element
	Prefix	Root/CF	Suffix	
1. a				2.
3. ad				4.
5. ambulat				6.
7. centesis				8.
9. glut				10.
11. later				12.
13. menisc				14.
15. necrot				16.
17. quadri				18.
19. vascul				20.

G. Spelling demons: *The following terms from this chapter are particularly difficult to spell and pronounce. Correct pronunciation and spelling of medical terms is the mark of an educated professional. Circle the correct spelling, and then check (✔) that you have practiced the pronunciation. Remember: Pronunciations are on the Student Online Learning Center (www.mhhe.com/AllanEss2e).*

Pronunciation

1.	emaciation	emmaciation	emacciation	_____
2.	cretenism	creitenism	cretinism	_____
3.	epinephrine	epineprine	epinephrin	_____
4.	exofthalmos	exophalmus	exophthalmos	_____
5.	thyrotoxicosis	tyrotoxicosis	thyrotoxicossis	_____
6.	hyperpexia	hyperprexia	hyperpyrexia	_____
7.	paresthesia	peresthesia	parestia	_____
8.	facies	fascies	feces	_____
9.	misedema	mixedema	myxedema	_____

H. Latin and Greek *terms cannot be further deconstructed into prefix, root, or suffix. You must know them for what they are. Test your knowledge of these terms in this exercise. Match the meaning in column l with the correct medical term in column 2.*

_____ 1. gland located in the mediastinum

_____ 2. facial features and expression

_____ 3. salt solution

_____ 4. severe muscle twitches

_____ 5. person with severe hypothyroidism

_____ 6. gland and cartilage in neck

_____ 7. hormone produced by pancreas

_____ 8. deeply unconscious

_____ 9. ketone found in blood

_____ 10. enlargement of thyroid gland

A. thyroid

B. acetone

C. facies

D. goiter

E. insulin

F. coma

G. tetany

H. saline

I. thymus

J. cretin

I. Symptoms: *Each of the documentations below presents a classic symptom of hyperglycemia. Write the correct medical terms for the symptoms on the blanks.*

1. Patient reports he needs to urinate many times during the day and even gets up three or four times at night to urinate.

   Symptom: _____

2. Patient states she has to carry water with her at all times because she is always very thirsty.

   Symptom: _____

3. Patient says he is always hungry, despite eating three big meals and several smaller ones each day.

   Symptom: _____

J. Terminology challenge: *There can be two medical terms that each mean the same thing. Test your knowledge of endocrine terminology and fill in the blanks.*

1. hydrocortisone: _____

2. somatotropin: _____

3. hyperthyroidism: _____

4. adrenal: _____

5. adrenaline: _____

6. norepinephrine: _____

K. Word attack. *Follow the instructions below the question.*

Question: Which is the only term that contains two prefixes?

a. endocrine

b. antidiuretic

c. hypothalamus

d. diabetic

e. neuropathy

Read the question and possible answers twice.

Notice that the question is asking for the term with two prefixes, not just one.

Slash each term into elements first. Since the question is asking about prefixes, analyze the answer choices starting at the beginning of the term, where the prefix would usually occur. *Remember that not every element at the beginning of a term has to be a prefix. Some roots or combining forms can start a term.*

1. Which term(s) can be eliminated because there is no prefix? _____

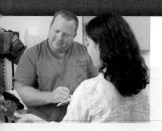

Remember to cross out answer choices after you have eliminated them as possible correct answers.

2. Which terms among the remaining choices have a single prefix? _____

3. Therefore, the only term that has two prefixes is _____.

L. Precision in communication: *Because of an error in communication, this patient was sent to the wrong specialist! Find the error.*
Underline the incorrect medical terminology in each sentence:

1. Because of this patient's neuropathy, I am referring him to a kidney specialist.

This sentence *should* have read:

Because of _____.

2. Because of this patient's nephropathy, I am referring her to an immunologist.

This sentence *should* have read:

Because of _____.

You are ultimately responsible for everything you communicate regarding patient care!

M. Patient education: *Briefly explain to your patient the difference between* tetany *and* tetanus. *Be sure to use nonmedical language the patient can understand. Consult the Glossary or a dictionary if you need to. Fill in the blanks.*

1. *tetany:* _____

_____

_____

2. *tetanus:* _____

_____

_____

N. Rewrite *the following sentences in language a patient can understand. Review any terms you need to in the Glossary or a dictionary before you start writing.*

1. "Hyperglycemia can contribute to cell lining damage and atherosclerosis; coronary artery disease and peripheral vascular disease with claudication are complications."

_____

_____

2. "Thyroid cancer usually presents as a symptomless nodule in the thyroid gland, but it can metastasize to cervical and mediastinal lymph nodes and to liver, lungs, and bones."

_____

_____

O. Short answer: *Write a brief description of each of the three terms below in language a patient can understand. Check your writing for correct spelling, and be ready to read your answers aloud in class. Fill in the blanks.*

1. *insulin-dependent:* _____

_____

2. *insulin shock:* _____

_____

3. *insulin resistance:* _____

_____

P. Brain teasers.

1. In the term *thyrotoxicosis*, the element *toxic/o* means _____

What, then, is a toxicologist? _____

Where might this occupation be employed, and why? _____

2. "Most diabetics develop some degree of *retinopathy, nephropathy,* and *neuropathy.*"

Which body systems are affected by each of these diagnoses?

retinopathy _____   nephropathy _____

neuropathy _____

Name the specialist a patient would consult for each of these conditions:

retinopathy _____   nephropathy _____

neuropathy _____

Q. Chapter challenge: *Circle the correct answer.*

1. Which term has an element that means *black?*

   a. oxytocin   **d.** pineal

   b. melatonin   **e.** acromegaly

   c. serotonin

2. *Hyperpyrexia, tetany,* and *edema* can all be considered:

   a. diseases   **d.** a, b, and c

   b. symptoms   **e.** only b and c

   c. diagnoses

3. In the abbreviation *BUN,* the "B" stands for:

   a. blood   **d.** bariatric

   b. bile   **e.** bone

   c. bilirubin

4. What is *serotonin* converted to at night?

   a. antidiuretic   **d.** prolactin

   b. prostaglandin   **e.** melatonin

   c. oxytocin

5. Mrs. Tacher had an *enlarged heart;* the medical term for this is:

   a. cardiopulmonary   **d.** cardiography

   b. cardiomyopathy   **e.** carditis

   c. cardiomegaly

6. This hormone reduces the volume of urine produced by the kidneys and is also called *vasopressin:*

   a. FSH   **d.** PRL

   b. LH   **e.** ADH

   c. ACTH

7. Find the incorrectly spelled term:

   a. cretenism   **d.** aldosterone

   b. antagonist   **e.** norepinephrine

   c. myxedema

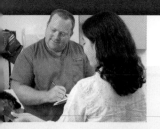

R. Specialists: *This chapter introduced you to an endocrinologist. Write below the names of five other specialists you have met in previous chapters, and give one disease or condition each would treat. Fill in the blanks.*

    Specialist   **Disease/Condition**

1. _____   _____

2. _____   _____

3. _____   _____

4. _____   _____

5. _____   _____

Have you checked your spelling?

S. Chapter challenge: *Circle the correct answer.*

1. Two symptoms of hyperthyroidism are *tachycardia* and *hypertension*. These are the same as:

    a. increased heart rate and high blood pressure   **d.** increased heart rate and low blood pressure

    b. decreased heart rate and low blood pressure   **e.** none of these

    c. decreased heart rate and high blood pressure

2. Identify the only pair of terms that is spelled correctly:

    a. aldostirone/facies   **d.** glycogenolisis/gluconeogenesis

    b. hydrocortison/mineralocorticoid   **e.** mellitus/paresthesia

    c. epinephrin/somatostatin

3. What is the only hormone that can lower blood glucose?

    a. GH   **d.** glucagon

    b. insulin   **e.** ADH

    c. oxytocin

4. In the term *hypothalamus,* the element hypo means:

    a. excessive   **d.** beside

    b. deficient   **e.** between

    c. below

5. A term that contains a prefix in the middle of the word is:

    a. gluconeogenesis   **d.** adrenocorticotropic

    b. somatostatin   **e.** thyrotoxicosis

    c. epinephrine

6. *Idiopathic* means that a disease:

    a. is just starting   **d.** is contagious

    b. has no known cause   **e.** has no known cure

    c. is in the acute stage

T. Case Report challenge: *Now that you are more comfortable with the terms in this chapter, you can apply that knowledge and briefly answer the questions about the Case Report. If you read the report through and underline all the medical terminology, this will make it easier to answer the questions.*

YOU ARE COMMUNICATING WITH

The parents of Ms. Norma Leary, a 22-year-old college student living with her parents for the summer. Ms. Leary is emaciated, extremely agitated, and at times disoriented and confused. Her parents tell you that in the past 3 or 4 days she has been coughing and not feeling well. In the past 12 hours she has become feverish and been complaining of a left-sided chest pain. With questioning, the parents reveal that prior to this acute illness Ms. Leary had lost about 20 pounds in weight, although she was eating voraciously. Her VS are T 105.2, P 180 and irregular, R 24, BP 160/85.

You call for Dr. Hilinski STAT. On his initial examination he believes that the patient is in thyroid storm. This is a medical emergency. There are no immediate laboratory tests that can confirm this diagnosis. Thyroid storm is the condition Ms. Leary presented with in the Emergency Department. It is the most extreme state of hyperthyroidism, with severely exaggerated effects of the thyroid hormones causing hyperpyrexia, tachycardia, agitation, and delirium. The weight loss prior to her illness becoming acute was part of her undiagnosed hyperthyroidism.

1. Ms. Leary is described as "emaciated"—how would she look? _____

_____

2. What is the significance of her elevated vital signs relative to her body's homeostasis? _____

_____

_____

3. Use a dictionary to look up the word *voraciously*. Define it here: _____

_____

4. After looking up the term above, what does *not* make sense about the patient's weight loss?

_____

_____

5. What is the opposite of an *acute* illness? _____

6. What other specialist might be called in to consult regarding this patient's tachycardia? _____

7. Does this patient have an overactive or underactive thyroid condition? _____

_____

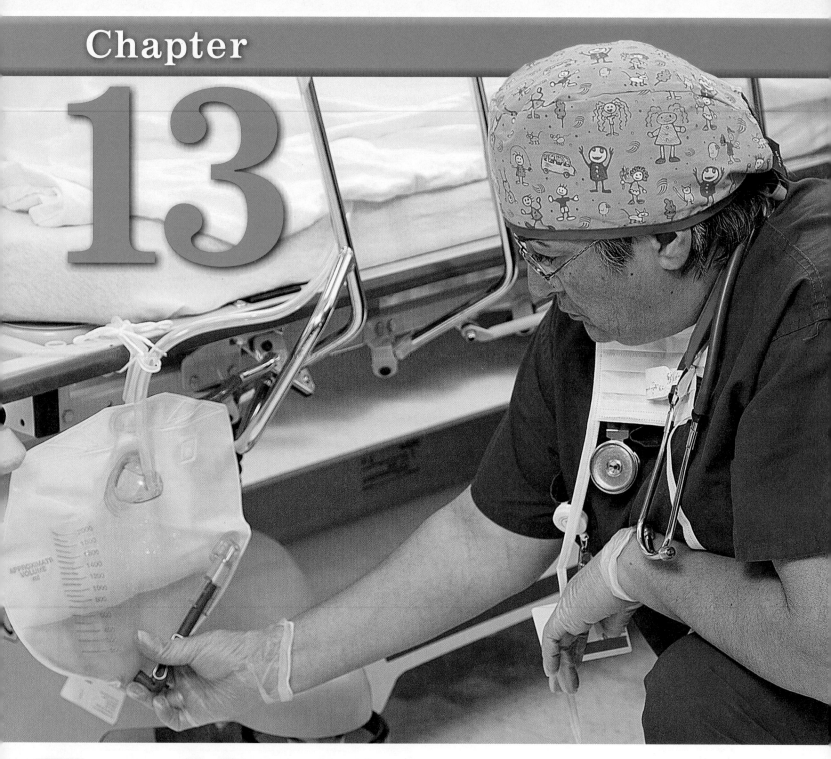

Chapter
13

THE URINARY SYSTEM
The Essentials of the Language of Urology

CASE REPORT 13.1

YOU ARE

. . . a surgical physician assistant working with **urologist** Phillip Johnson, MD, at Fulwood Medical Center.

YOU ARE COMMUNICATING WITH

. . . Mr. Nelson Hughes, a 58-year-old school principal. You are making your afternoon hospital visits to Dr. Johnson's patients. Earlier today, you assisted at Mr. Hughes' surgery. A laparoscopic radical nephrectomy (kidney removal) for a **TNM** Stage II **renal** cell carcinoma (cancer) with no evidence of local invasion or lymph node involvement (metastasis) was performed. Your job is to assess Mr. Hughes' postoperative state and determine whether postoperative complications exist.

In your future career, being able to communicate comfortably, accurately, and effectively with the health professionals involved in the diagnosis and treatment of problems with the urologic system is key. You may work directly and/or indirectly with one or more of the following:

- **Urologists** are specialists in the diagnosis and treatment of diseases of the urinary system.

- **Nephrologists** are specialists in the diagnosis and treatment of diseases of the kidney.

- **Urologic nurses** and **nurse practitioners** are registered nurses with advanced academic and clinical experience in urology.

LEARNING OUTCOMES

In order to understand and to assess Mr. Hughes' situation, define and recognize the areas of concern, communicate with Dr. Johnson and the patient, and document the patient's progress, you need to be able to:

LO 13.1 Apply the language of urology to the structures and functions of the urinary system.

LO 13.2 Comprehend, analyze, spell, and write the medical terms of urology.

LO 13.3 Recognize and pronounce the medical terms of urology.

LO 13.4 Explain the effects of common urinary disorders on health.

ABBREVIATION

TNM	tumor, node, metastasis (tumor staging method)

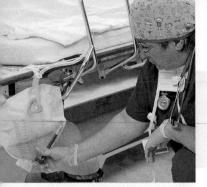

LESSON 13.1

Urinary System, Kidneys, and Ureters

*Your body's metabolism continually produces metabolic waste products. If these wastes are not eliminated, they will poison your body. Your **urinary** system carries the major burden of excreting these wastes, and within this system, the kidney is the organ that does the actual eliminating. So, the kidney is a vital organ to understand, and it brings with it a whole new set of terminology.*

In this lesson, the information will enable you to use correct medical terminology to:

13.1.1 Name and locate the organs of the urinary system.

13.1.2 Identify the structures and functions of the kidneys and ureters.

13.1.3 Describe disorders of the kidneys and ureters.

• The kidney removes waste products from the blood by a process of **filtration.**

• Each renal cortex contains about 1 million **nephrons**, the functional filtration unit of the kidney.

• The filtrate from the kidney's filtration process is urine. It consists of excess water, electrolytes, and urea.

Urinary System
(LO 13.1, 13.2, and 13.3)

Your **urinary system** *(Figure 13.1)* consists of **six organs:**

• Two **kidneys**

• Two **ureters**

• A single **urinary bladder**

• A single **urethra**

The process of removing metabolic wastes is called excretion, and it's essential in maintaining your body's homeostasis *(see Chapter 2)*. Metabolic wastes include carbon dioxide, excess water and electrolytes, **nitrogenous** compounds including **ammonia** (from the breakdown of proteins), and **urea.** If these wastes are not eliminated, they will poison the entire body.

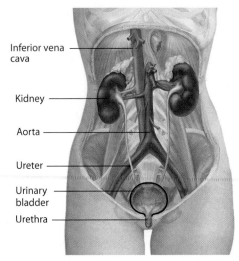

▲ **FIGURE 13.1**
Urinary System.

The Kidneys
(LO 13.1, 13.2, and 13.3)

Each of your kidneys is a bean-shaped organ about the size of your clenched fist. One kidney is located on each side of the vertebral column and lies against the deep muscles of your back *(Figure 13.1)*.

Waste-laden blood enters your kidney at its **hilum** (an opening for nerves and vessels) *(Figure 13.2)* through the **renal** artery. Excess water, urea, and other waste products are **filtered** from the blood by the **nephrons** in your kidney's cortex. The ureters carry the **filtrate,** now called **urine,** from the kidneys to the urinary **bladder.**

The **excretion functions of the kidneys** are to:

• **Filter** blood to eliminate wastes;

• **Regulate** blood volume and pressure by eliminating or conserving water; and

• **Maintain homeostasis** by controlling the amounts of water and electrolytes that are eliminated.

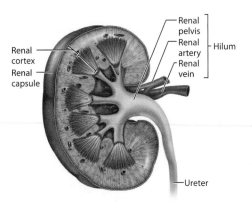

▲ **FIGURE 13.2**
Urinary System.

Word	Pronunciation	Elements		Definition
ammonia	ah-**MOAN**-ih-ah	S/ R/	-ia *condition* ammon- *ammonia*	Toxic breakdown product of amino acids (proteins)
bladder	**BLAD**-er		Old English *bladder*	Hollow sac that holds fluid; e.g., urine or bile
filter (noun or verb)	**FIL**-ter		Latin *strain through material*	Porous substance used to separate liquids and gases from particulate matter; or to subject a substance to the action of a filter
filtrate	**FIL**-trate	S/ R/	-ate *composed of, pertaining to* filtr- *strain through*	Liquid that has passed through a filter
filtration	fil-**TRAY**-shun	S/	-ation *process*	Process of passing liquid through a filter
hilum hila (pl)	**HIGH**-lum **HIGH**-lah		Latin *small bit*	The part where the nerves and blood vessels enter and leave an organ
kidney	**KID**-nee		Old English *kidney*	Organ of excretion
nephron nephrology	**NEF**-ron neh-**FROL**-oh-jee	 S/ R/CF	Greek *kidney* -logy *study of* nephr/o- *kidney*	Filtration unit of the kidney; glomerulus + renal tubule Medical specialty of diseases of the kidney
nephrologist	neh-**FROL**-oh-jist	S/	-logist *one who studies, specialist*	Medical specialist in disorders of the kidney
nitrogenous (adj)	ni-**TROJ**-en-us	S/ R/CF R/	-ous *pertaining to* nitr/o- *nitrogen* -gen- *create*	Containing or generating nitrogen
renal (adj)	**REE**-nal	S/ R/	-al *pertaining to* ren- *kidney*	Pertaining to the kidney
urea	you-**REE**-ah		Greek *urine*	End product of nitrogen metabolism
ureter (Note: *Two "es" = two tubes.*) ureteral (adj)	you-**REE**-ter you-ree-**TER**-al	 S/ R/	Greek *urinary canal* -al *pertaining to* ureter- *ureter*	Tube that connects each kidney to the urinary bladder Pertaining to a ureter
urine urinary (adj)	**YUR**-in **YUR**-in-ary	 S/ R/	Latin *urine* -ary *pertaining to* urin- *urine*	Fluid and dissolved substances excreted by kidney Pertaining to urine
urinate (verb)	**YUR**-in-ate	S/	-ate *composed of, pertaining to*	To pass urine
urination	yur-ih-**NAY**-shun	S/	-ation *process*	Process of passing urine
urology	yur-**ROL**-oh-jee	S/ R/CF	-logy *study of* ur/o- *urinary system*	Medical specialty that studies the urinary system
urologist	yur-**ROL**-oh-jist	S/	-logist *one who studies, specialist*	Specialist in urology
urological (adj)	yur-roh-**LOJ**-ik-al	S/	-ical *pertaining to*	Pertaining to urology

EXERCISE

A. Construct *the following terms by inserting the correct elements. After you insert an element, write the identity (P, R, CF, or S) of the element below the line. Review the terms in the WAD box first. Fill in the blanks.*

1. specialist in the urinary system: _____/_____/_____

2. containing or generating nitrogen: _____/_____/_____

3. pertaining to the ureter: _____/_____/_____

4. study of diseases of the kidney: _____/_____/_____

5. pertaining to the kidney: _____/_____/_____

6. liquid that has passed through a filter: _____/_____/_____

- 25% to 30% of all renal cancers relate directly to smoking.

- As little as 1 milliliter of blood will turn the urine red.

- The acute form of glomerulonephritis has a 100% recovery rate.

Renal cell carcinoma, the most common form of kidney cancer, occurs twice as often in men as in women. The cancer develops in the lining cells of the renal tubules, which is why Mr. Hughes had hematuria. Radical **nephrectomy** is the most common treatment for renal cell carcinoma.

Wilms tumor, or **nephroblastoma,** is a malignant childhood kidney tumor, usually occurring between the ages of 3 and 8. It is treated effectively with a combination of surgery and chemotherapy.

Renal adenomas (benign kidney tumors) are usually asymptomatic (produce no symptoms), are discovered by chance, and are not life threatening.

Hematuria (blood in the urine) can be caused by lesions anywhere in the urinary system. These lesions may result from trauma, infections, and congenital diseases like sickle cell anemia. In microscopic hematuria, the urine is not red, and red blood cells can be seen only under a microscope or identified by a urine dipstick.

Acute glomerulonephritis is an inflammation of the kidney's filtration unit (the nephron). It damages the glomerular capillaries and allows protein and red blood cells to leak into the urine. It can develop rapidly after a strep throat infection, especially in children.

Chronic glomerulonephritis can occur with no history of kidney disease and present as kidney failure. It also occurs in **diabetic nephropathy** and can be associated with autoimmune diseases like lupus erythematosus (a disease of the connective tissues).

Nephrotic syndrome causes large amounts of protein to leak into the urine, so the level of protein in the blood drops. In children, this condition almost always responds to steroid treatment. The most obvious symptom is fluid retention, with edema of the ankles and legs. This is treated with **diuretics,** by restricting salt in the diet, and by reducing fluid intake.

CASE REPORT 13.1 (CONTINUED)

Mr. Nelson Hughes had been well until a few months before his surgery, when he noticed a vague, aching pain in the left side of his abdomen. One week prior to his surgery, he suddenly passed bright red urine. A urinalysis showed red blood cells **(hematuria)** and a physical examination revealed an enlarged left kidney. **Intravenous pyelogram (IVP)** and other imaging tests showed a tumor 3 inches in diameter in the center of his left kidney. His bone scan was normal, indicating no metastases to the bones.

ABBREVIATION

IVP	intravenous pyelogram

Word	Pronunciation	Elements		Definition
diuretic (adj) (Note: The "a" is dropped from dia to enable the word to flow.)	die-you-RET-ik	S/ P/ R/	-etic *pertaining to* di(a)- *complete* -ur- *urine*	Agent that increases urine output
diuresis (noun)	die-you-REE-sis	S/	-esis *condition*	Excretion of large volume of urine
glomerulonephritis	glo-MER-you-low-nef-RYE-tis	S/ R/CF R/	-itis *inflammation* glomerul/o- *glomerulus* -nephr- *kidney*	Infection of the glomeruli of the kidney
hematuria	he-mah-TYU-ree-ah	S/ R/	-uria *urine* hemat- *blood*	Blood in the urine
nephrectomy	neh-FREK-toe-me	S/ R/	-ectomy *surgical excision* nephr- *kidney*	Surgical removal of a kidney
nephroblastoma (Wilms tumor) Wilms tumor	NEF-roh-blas-TOE-mah WILMZ TOO-mor	S/ R/CF R/	-oma *tumor, mass* nephr/o- *kidney* -blast- *immature cell* Max Wilms, German surgeon, 1867–1918	Cancerous kidney tumor of childhood
nephropathy	neh-FROP-ah-thee	S/ R/CF	-pathy *disease* nephr/o- *kidney*	Any disease of the kidney
nephrotic syndrome nephrosis (*same as* nephrotic syndrome)	neh-FROT-ik SIN-drohm neh-FROH-sis	S/ R/CF S/ R/	-tic *pertaining to* nephr/o- *kidney* -osis *condition* nephr- *kidney*	Glomerular disease with marked loss of protein
pyelogram	PIE-el-oh gram	S/ R/CF	-gram *record, recording* pyel/o- *renal pelvis*	X-ray image of renal pelvis and ureters

EXERCISES

A. Review *the Case Report on this spread before answering the questions.*

1. What are Mr. Hughes' chief complaints? _____

2. What does the doctor find on physical examination of Mr. Hughes? _____

3. Define the two medical terms in the abbreviation *IVP.* _____

4. What does a "normal bone scan" mean for Mr. Hughes? _____

B. Unscramble the terms on the right to match them with their definitions. Check the correct spelling in the WAD box. Fill in the blanks.

1. infection of the glomeruli of the kidney: eeopilrnrtohisugml   _____
2. also known as Wilms tumor: hbsaelmoanprto   _____
3. any disease of the kidney: teopyahnprh   _____
4. excretion of large volume of urine: iessudri   _____
5. X-ray image of renal pelvis and ureters: lrgeyoapm   _____
6. blood in the urine: arameithu   _____

Interstitial nephritis is an inflammation (often acute and temporary) of the kidney tissue between the renal tubules. It can be an allergic reaction to or a side effect of drugs like penicillin or ampicillin, **NSAIDs,** and diuretics.

Pyelonephritis is an infection of the renal pelvis. This usually occurs as part of a total urinary tract infection **(UTI),** beginning in the urinary bladder *(see the next lesson in this chapter)*. It has a high mortality rate in the elderly and in people with a compromised immune system.

Polycystic kidney disease (PKD) is an inherited disease. Large fluid-filled cysts grow within the kidneys and press against the kidney tissue. Eventually, the kidneys cannot function effectively.

Acute renal failure (ARF) makes the kidneys suddenly stop filtering waste products from the blood. Initially, **oliguria** and then **anuria** are associated with confusion, seizures, and coma.

The causes of acute renal failure include: severe burns; trauma; septicemia; toxins like mercury and excess alcohol; excessive amounts of drugs like aspirin and ibuprofen; and antibiotics like streptomycin and gentamycin.

When caring for a patient who has ARF, the goal is to treat the underlying disease. **Dialysis** may be necessary while the kidneys are healing.

Chronic renal failure (CRF), or **chronic kidney disease (CKD),** is a gradual loss of renal function. Symptoms and signs may not appear until the kidney's level of functioning is less than 25% of normal. The causes of chronic renal failure are diabetes, hypertension, kidney disease (including chronic glomerulonephritis, nephrotic syndrome), and lead poisoning.

Uremia is the complex of symptoms resulting from excess nitrogenous waste products in the blood, as seen in renal failure.

End-stage renal disease (ESRD) means the kidneys are functioning at less than 10% of their normal capacity. At this point, life cannot be maintained, and either dialysis or a kidney transplant is needed.

Dialysis is an artificial method of removing waste materials and excess fluid from the blood. It is not a cure but can prolong life. There are several types of kidney dialysis:

- **Hemodialysis** *(Figure 13.3)* filters the blood through an artificial kidney machine **(dialyzer).** Most patients require 12 hours of hemodialysis a week, usually in three sessions.

- **Peritoneal dialysis** uses a dialysis solution that is infused into and drained out of your abdominal cavity through a small, flexible, **implanted** catheter. The dialysis solution extracts wastes and excess fluid from the network of capillaries in the peritoneal lining of the abdominal cavity.

- **Continuous ambulatory peritoneal dialysis (CAPD)** is performed by the patient at home through an implanted abdominal catheter *(Figure 13.4)*, usually four times a day, 7 days a week.

- **Continuous cycling peritoneal dialysis** uses a machine to automatically infuse dialysis solution into and out of the abdominal cavity during sleep.

Kidney transplant provides a better quality of life than dialysis—if a suitable donor can be found. The donor has to match the recipient's blood type, cell surface proteins, and antibodies. A **sibling** or a blood relative can often qualify as a donor. If not, tissue banks across the country can search for a kidney from an accident victim or a donor who has died.

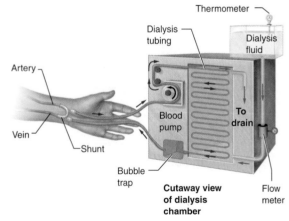

▲ **FIGURE 13.3**
Hemodialysis.

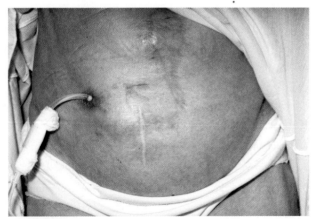

▲ **FIGURE 13.4**
Continuous Ambulatory Peritoneal Dialysis.

Word	Pronunciation		Elements	Definition
anuria	an-**YOU**-ree-ah	S/ P/ R/	-ia *condition* an- *a lack of, no* -ur- *urine*	Absence of urine production
dialysis	die-**AL**-ih-sis	P/ R/	dia- *complete* -lysis *destruction*	An artificial method of filtration to remove excess waste materials and water from the body
hemodialysis	**HE**-moh-die-**AL**-ih-sis	R/CF	hem/o- *blood*	An artificial method of filtration to remove excess waste materials and water directly from the blood
nephritis	neh-**FRY**-tis	S/ R/	-itis *inflammation* nephr- *kidney*	Inflammation of the kidney
oliguria	ol-ih-**GYUR**-ee-ah	S/ R/ R/	-ia *condition* olig- *scanty* -ur- *urine*	Scanty production of urine
polycystic	pol-ee-**SIS**-tik	S/ P/ R/	-ic *pertaining to* poly- *many* -cyst- *sac, bladder, cyst*	Composed of many cysts
pyelonephritis	**PIE**-eh-loh-neh-**FRY**-tis	S/ R/CF R/	-itis *inflammation* pyel/o- *renal pelvis* -nephr- *kidney*	Inflammation of the kidney and renal pelvis
sibling	**SIB**-ling	S/ R/	-ling *small* sib- *relative*	Brother or sister
transplant	**TRANZ**-plant	P/ R/	trans- *across* -plant *insert, plant*	The act of transferring tissue from one person to another
uremia	you-**REE**-me-ah	S/ R/	-emia *a blood condition* ur- *urine*	The complex of symptoms arising from renal failure

EXERCISES

A. Build your knowledge *of the elements contained in the language of urology. First slash the term into elements. A specific element in each term is bolded. Write the identity (P, R, CF, or S) of the bolded element under it, and write the meaning of that element on the line next to the term.*

1. **hemo**dialysis _____

2. **poly**cystic _____

3. **an**uria _____

4. ur**emia** _____

5. **olig**uria _____

6. **pyelo**nephritis _____

Remember: Every element at the beginning of a medical term is not necessarily a prefix!

7. Give an example from this exercise: _____

B. Meet chapter and lesson objectives *and use the language of urology for your answers.*

1. What is the difference between ARF and CRF?

   ARF _____

   CRF _____

2. Which specific kidney disease is inherited? _____

3. Which type of RF has no cure? _____

4. Which diagnosis has a high mortality rate in the elderly? _____

- The muscle wall of the bladder acts as a sphincter around the ureters to prevent reflux of urine.

- The presence of urine in the renal pelvis initiates peristalsis of the ureters.

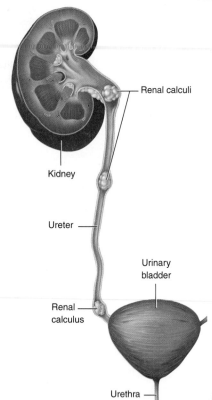

▲ **FIGURE 13.5**
Renal Calculi.
Calculi can become lodged at sites along the urinary tract.

ABBREVIATIONS

ESWL	extracorporeal shock wave lithotripsy
IV	intravenous
KUB	X-ray of abdomen to show **K**idneys, **U**reters, and **B**ladder

---

CASE REPORT 13.2

Clinical Note   **Emergency Department, Fulwood Medical Center** 9/12/11

Mr. Justin Leandro, a 37-year-old construction worker, presented at 1520 hrs. He complained of a sudden onset of excruciating pain in his right abdomen and back an hour previously, while at work. The pain is spasmodic and radiates down into his **groin**. He has vomited once, and keeps having the urge to urinate. He has no previous medical history of significance.

VS: T 99.4°F, P 92, R 20, BP 130/86.

Patient's abdomen is slightly distended, with tenderness in the right upper and lower quadrants and **flank**. A dipstick test showed blood in his urine.

Provisional diagnosis by Mark Eagle, MD: stone in the right ureter.

An IV line was started, and 2 mg of morphine sulfate was given by IV push at 1540 hrs. He is going to X-ray STAT for KUB and IVP.

—Andrea Facundo, EMT-P, 1555 hrs.

The Ureters (LO 13.1, 13.2, and 13.3)

Each of your ureters is a muscular tube, about 10 inches long and ¼ inch wide. The ureters carry urine from your renal pelvis to your urinary bladder. Each ureter lies on the posterior abdominal wall. This is why Mr. Leandro had pain in his back.

Your ureters pass obliquely through your bladder's muscle wall. As pressure builds in your filling bladder, the muscle wall compresses the ureters and prevents urine from being forced back up the ureters to your kidneys (**reflux**).

In addition to gravity, muscular **peristaltic** waves, originating in the renal pelvis, squeeze urine down the ureters and squirt it into the bladder. The peristaltic waves are intermittent (come and go), which is why Mr. Leandro's pain was spasmodic.

Kidney and Ureteral Stones (Nephrolithiasis)

(LO 13.1, 13.2, 13.3, and 13.4)

Stones (**calculi**) begin in the pelvis of the kidney as a tiny grain of undissolved material, usually a mineral called calcium oxalate *(Figure 13.5)*. When the urine flows out of the kidney, this grain of material is left behind. Over time, more material is deposited and a stone is formed. Most stones enter one of the ureters while they are still small enough to pass down the ureter into the bladder and out of the body in urine.

CASE REPORT 13.2 (CONTINUED)

Mr. Leandro's KUB (X-ray of **k**idney, **u**reter and **b**ladder) showed a suspicious lesion halfway down his right ureter. IVP confirmed that this was a stone (renal **calculus**) blocking the ureter and showed the pelvis of the right kidney to be slightly dilated. Mr. Leandro's stone was large enough to be lodged in the ureter, blocking the flow of urine, with the backflow pressure leading to **hydronephrosis** of the kidney. Mr. Leandro was kept in the hospital overnight with IV pain medication but did not pass the stone. **Extracorporeal shock wave lithotripsy (ESWL)** was successful in crumbling the stone. He urinated through a strainer so that the stone fragments could be recovered and chemically analyzed.

Word	Pronunciation		Elements	Definition
calculus calculi (pl)	**KAL**-kyu-lus **KAL**-kyu-lie		Latin *pebble*	Small stone
extracorporeal	**EKS**-tra-kor-**POH**- ree-al	S/ P/ R/CF	-al *pertaining to* extra- *outside* -corpor/e- *body*	Outside the body
flank	FLANK		Latin *broad*	Side of the body between the pelvis and the ribs
groin	GROYN		Old English *groin*	Crease where the thigh joins the abdomen
hydronephrosis	**HIGH**-droh-neh-**FRO**-sis	S/ R/CF R/CF	-osis *condition* hydr/o- *water* -nephr/o- *kidney*	Dilation of the pelvis and calyces of a kidney
hydronephrotic (adj)	**HIGH**-droh-neh-**FROT**-ik	S/	-tic *pertaining to*	Pertaining to or suffering from the dilation of the pelvis and calyces of the kidney
lithotripsy	**LITH**-oh-trip-see	S/ R/CF	-tripsy *crushing* lith/o- *stone*	Crushing stones by sound waves
lithotripter	**LITH**-oh-trip-ter	S/	-tripter *crusher*	Instrument that generates sound waves
nephrolithiasis	**NEF**-roe-lih-**THIGH**-ah-sis	S/ R/CF R/	-iasis *condition, state of* nephr/o- *kidney* -lith- *stone*	Presence of a kidney stone
peristalsis	per-ih-**STAL**-sis	P/ R/	peri- *around* -stalsis *constrict*	Waves of alternate contraction and relaxation of the muscle wall of a tube

EXERCISES

A. Review *the Case Report on this spread before answering the questions.*

1. Where in the Case Report can abbreviations be substituted for medical terms? _____

2. Where is Mr. Leandro's stone lodged, and what is it blocking? _____

3. What are his diagnoses? _____

4. What procedure will he have as part of his treatment plan? _____

5. What is the medical term for *blood in the urine?* _____

6. Why was Mr. Leandro given morphine? _____

7. What is the medical term for a kidney stone? _____   _____

8. What diagnostic tests were ordered for Mr. Leandro? _____

9. What is *urinary reflux?* _____

B. Match *the element in column 1 with the correct meaning in column 2.*

_____ **1.** extra   **A.** body

_____ **2.** lith   **B.** crushing

_____ **3.** corpore   **C.** water

_____ **4.** tripsy   **D.** stone

_____ **5.** hydro   **E.** outside

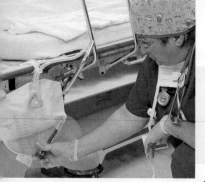

LESSON 13.2

Urinary Bladder and Urethra

*Your urinary bladder is a temporary storage place for urine before it is **voided** through the **urethra**. A moderately full bladder contains about 500 mL (1 pint) of urine. The maximum capacity of the bladder is around 750 to 800 mL (1½ pints). **Urination,** or emptying of the bladder, is also called **micturition.** The information in this lesson will enable you to use correct medical terminology to:*

13.2.1 Describe the structure and functions of the urinary bladder.

13.2.2 Contrast the differences in structure of the male and female urethras and the incidence of urinary tract infections in the two sexes.

13.2.3 Discuss common disorders of the bladder and urethra.

CASE REPORT 13.3

YOU ARE

. . . a medical assistant working in the office of Dr. Susan Lee, a primary care physician, at Fulwood Medical Center.

YOU ARE COMMUNICATING WITH

. . . Mrs. Caroline Dobson, a 32-year-old housewife. You have asked her the reason for her visit to the office today.

Mrs. Dobson: "Since yesterday afternoon, I've had a lot of pain low down in my belly and in my lower back. I keep having to go to the bathroom every hour or so to pee. It's often difficult to start, and it burns as it comes out. I've had this problem twice before when I was pregnant with my two kids, so I've started drinking cranberry juice. I've been shivering since I woke up this morning, and the last urine I passed was pink. Was that due to the cranberry juice?"

The Urinary Bladder and Urethra (LO 13.1, 13.2, and 13.3)

Urinary Bladder (LO 13.1, 13.2, and 13.3)

The urinary bladder is a hollow, muscular organ on the floor of your pelvic cavity, posterior to the pubic symphysis *(Figure 13.6).*

Urethra (LO 13.1, 13.2, and 13.3)

Your urethra, a thin-walled tube, transports urine from the floor of your bladder to the outside. The base of your bladder's muscular wall is thickened to form the **internal urethral sphincter.** As the urethra passes through the skeletal muscles of the pelvic floor, the **external urethral sphincter** provides voluntary control of urination.

In the male *(Figure 13.6a),* the urethra is 7 to 8 inches long and passes through the penis. In the female *(Figure 13.6b),* the urethra is only about 1½ inches long, and it opens to the outside just above the vagina.

In both the male and female, the opening of the urethra to the outside is called the **external urinary meatus.**

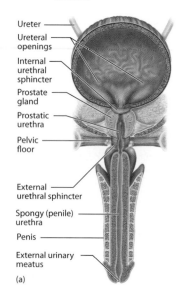

Ureter
Ureteral openings
Internal urethral sphincter
Prostate gland
Prostatic urethra
Pelvic floor
External urethral sphincter
Spongy (penile) urethra
Penis
External urinary meatus
(a)

▲ **FIGURE 13.6**
Urinary Bladder.
(a) Male anatomy.
(b) Female anatomy.

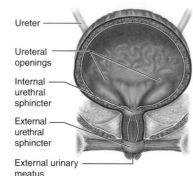

Ureter
Ureteral openings
Internal urethral sphincter
External urethral sphincter
External urinary meatus
(b)

Micturition
(LO 13.1, 13.2, 13.3, and 13.4)

When your bladder contains about 200 mL or 7 fluid ounces (just less than a cup) of urine, stretch receptors in its wall trigger the **micturition reflex.** Parasympathetic nerves stimulate the bladder's muscle wall to contract and the internal sphincter to relax, and the need to urinate feels urgent. However, voluntary control of the external sphincter can keep that sphincter contracted and can hold urine in the bladder until you decide to urinate. Involuntary micturition during sleep in older children or adults is called **enuresis.**

Word	Pronunciation	Elements		Definition
enuresis	en-you-**REE**-sis	S/ R/	-esis *condition* enur- *urinate*	Involuntary bedwetting
meatus	me-**AY**-tus		Latin *a passage*	The external opening of a passage
micturition (noun)	mik-choo-**RISH**-un	S/ R/	-ition *process* mictur- *pass urine*	Act of passing urine
micturate (verb)	**MIK**-choo-rate	S/	-ate *pertaining to*	Pass urine
reflex	**REE**-fleks		Latin *to bend back*	An involuntary response to a stimulus
sphincter	**SFINK**-ter		Greek *a band*	A band of muscle that encircles an opening; when it contracts, the opening squeezes closed
urethra (Note: *One "e" = one tube.*)	you-**REE**-thra		Greek *passage for urine*	Tube that carries urine from bladder to outside
urethral		R/ S/	-urethr- *urethra* -al *pertaining to*	Pertaining to the urethra
void (verb)	VOYD		Latin *to empty*	To evacuate urine or feces

EXERCISES

A. Reread *the Case Report on the opposite page and review all the terms and elements in the WAD box above. Fill in the blanks.*

1. List all of Mrs. Dobson's symptoms:

2. Has Mrs. Dobson ever had this condition before?

3. If Dr. Lee feels that Mrs. Dobson might need a referral to a specialist, what kind of specialist would she recommend?

4. According to the terms in the WAD, what symptom does Mrs. Dobson not have?

5. What substance may be in Mrs. Dobson's urine, as indicated by the urine's pink color?

B. Apply your knowledge *of the language of urology to answer the following questions relating to chapter and lesson objectives.*

1. Describe the location, structure and function of the urinary bladder:

2. What is the function of a sphincter?

3. Voiding and micturition can both be used to mean which body function?

4. What is the function of a meatus?

Disorders of the Urinary Bladder and Urethra
(LO 13.1, 13.2, 13.3, and 13.4)

Urinary Tract Infection (UTI) (LO 13.1, 13.2, 13.3, and 13.4)

A urinary tract infection occurs when bacteria invade and multiply in the urinary tract. The bacteria's point of entry is through the urethra. Because the female urethra is shorter than that of the male and opens to the surface near the anus *(Figure 13.7)*, bacteria from the GI tract, like *E. coli,* can more easily invade the female urethra. This is why women are more prone to UTIs than men. Once UTIs have occurred, they often recur.

An infection of the urethra is called **urethritis; cystitis** is an infection of the urinary bladder. If cystitis is untreated, infection can spread up the ureters to the renal pelvis, causing **pyelitis.** The infection can then travel to the renal cortex and nephrons, causing pyelonephritis.

CASE REPORT 13.3 (CONTINUED)

Mrs. Dobson described many of the symptoms of cystitis. She had **suprapubic** and lower back pain. She had increased frequency of micturition with **dysuria** (difficulty with and pain or burning on urination). Her pink urine is probably hematuria.

The diagnosis of a UTI can be made through a urinalysis. A culture of the infection-causing organism and testing of its sensitivity to different antibiotics allows the appropriate antibiotic therapy to be prescribed. Cranberry juice can make the urine more acidic and resistant to infection.

Urinary Incontinence
(LO 13.1, 13.2, 13.3, and 13.4)

Urinary incontinence is a loss of bladder control, which results in wet clothes and bedding. About 12 million adults in America have this condition. Urinary incontinence is most common in women over the age of 50, and it's also seen frequently in elderly men. However, aging alone is not a cause of urinary incontinence.

Urinary Retention
(LO 13.1, 13.2, 13.3, and 13.4)

Urinary retention is the abnormal, involuntary holding of urine in the bladder. **Acute retention** can be caused by an obstruction in the urinary system, like an enlarged prostate in the male. Neurologic problems, like multiple sclerosis, can also be responsible. **Chronic retention** can be caused by an untreated obstruction in the urinary tract, like an enlarged prostate gland.

Bladder Cancer
(LO 13.1, 13.2, 13.3, and 13.4)

Bladder cancer is more common in men than in women. In fact, it's the fourth most common cancer in men and the eighth most common in women.

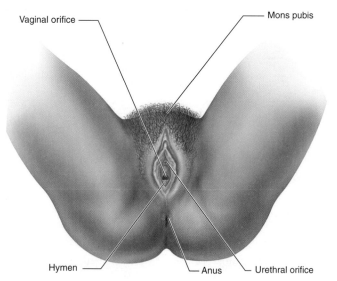

▲ **FIGURE 13.7**
Female External Genitalia.

Word	Pronunciation	Elements		Definition
cystitis	sis-**TIE**-tis	S/ R/	-itis *inflammation* cyst- *bladder*	Inflammation of the urinary bladder
dysuria	dis-**YOU**-ree-ah	S/ P/ R/	-ia *condition* dys- *bad, difficult* -ur- *urine*	Difficulty or pain with urination
incontinence	In-**KON**-tin-ence	S/ P/ R/	-ence *state of* in- *not* -contin- *hold together*	Inability to prevent discharge of urine or feces
incontinent	in-**KON**-tin-ent	S/	-ent *pertaining to*	Denoting incontinence
pyelitis	pie-eh-**LYE**-tis	S/ R/	-itis *inflammation* pyel- *renal pelvis*	Inflammation of the renal pelvis
retention	ree-**TEN**-shun		Latin *hold back*	Holding back in the body what should normally be discharged (e.g., urine)
suprapubic	**SOO**-prah-pyu-bik	S/ P/ R/	-ic *pertaining to* supra- *above* -pub- *pubis*	Above the symphysis pubis
urethritis	you-ree-**THRI**-tis	S/ R/	-itis *inflammation* urethr- *urethra*	Inflammation of the urethra

EXERCISES

A. Review *the Case Report on this spread before answering the questions.*

1. Mrs. Dobson was diagnosed with dysuria and hematuria. Explain to Mrs. Dobson, in language she can understand, the difference in the medical terms.

   Dysuria _____

   Hematuria _____

2. Describe on the body the location of *suprapubic* pain. _____

3. What is the diagnosis for Mrs. Dobson? _____

4. Define the diagnosis in question 3 above. _____

B. Deconstruct *the language of urology found in the WAD above. Knowledge of elements is your best key to understanding the meaning of a term. Slash the terms in column 1 into elements, and fill in the chart. Then fill in the blanks.*

Medical Term	Meaning of Root/CF	Meaning of Suffix	Meaning of Term
pyelitis	1.	2.	3.
urethritis	4.	5.	6.
cystitis	7.	8.	9.

10. How are the terms in the chart the same? _____

11. How are they different? _____

12. What, then, is *pyelonephritis?* _____

- Random urine collection is taken with no precautions regarding contamination. It is often used for collecting drug testing samples.

- Early morning urine collection is used to determine the ability of the kidneys to concentrate urine following overnight dehydration.

- Clean-catch, midstream urine specimen is collected after the external urethral meatus is cleaned. The first part of the urine is passed, and the sterile collecting vessel is introduced into the urinary stream to collect the last part.

- Twenty-four-hour urine collection is used to determine the amount of protein being excreted and to estimate the kidneys' filtration ability.

- Suprapubic transabdominal needle aspiration of the bladder is used in newborns and small infants to obtain a pure sample of urine.

- Catheterization of the bladder can be used as a last resort to obtain a urine specimen. A soft plastic or rubber tube (catheter) is inserted through the urethra into the bladder to drain and collect urine.

Diagnostic Procedures
(LO 13.1, 13.2, 13.3, and 13.4)

Urinalysis (LO 13.1, 13.2, 13.3, and 13.4)

A **dipstick** (a plastic strip bearing paper squares of reagent) is the most cost-effective method of screening urine *(Figure 13.8)*. After the stick is dipped into the urine specimen, the color change in each segment of the dipstick is compared to a color chart on the container. Dipsticks can screen for pH, specific gravity, protein, blood, glucose, ketones, bilirubin, **nitrite,** and leukocyte esterase *(see below)*.

A **routine urinalysis (UA)** in the lab can include the following tests:

- **Visual observation** examines color and clarity. Normal, healthy urine is pale yellow or amber in color and clear. Cloudiness indicates excess cells or cellular material. Red and cloudy indicates red blood cells.

- **Odor** of normal urine has a slight "nutty" scent. Infected urine has a foul odor. **Ketosis** gives urine a fruity odor.

- **pH** measures how acidic or alkaline urine is.

- **Specific gravity (SG)** measures how dilute or concentrated the urine is.

- **Protein** is not normally detected in urine; its presence (**proteinuria**) indicates infection or urinary tract disease.

- **Glucose** in the urine (**glycosuria**) is a spill over of sugar into the urine when the nephrons are damaged or diseased, or blood sugar is high in uncontrolled diabetes.

- **Ketones** are present in the urine in diabetic **ketoacidosis** *(see Chapter 12)* or in starvation.

- **Leukocyte esterase** indicates the presence of white blood cells in the urine, which can point to a UTI.

- **Urine culture** from a clean-catch specimen *(see box)* is the definitive test for a UTI.

A **microscopic urinalysis** is performed on the solids deposited by centrifuging a specimen of urine. It can reveal:

- **Red blood cells (RBCs), white blood cells (WBCs),** and renal tubular epithelial cells stuck together to form **casts,** WBCs stuck together to form casts, and bacteria.

Other Diagnostic Procedures
(LO 13.1, 13.2, 13.3, and 13.4)

Other diagnostic procedures used to test for urinary bladder and urethra infections include:

- **KUB.** An X-ray of the abdomen shows the kidneys, ureters, and bladder.

- **Intravenous pyelogram (IVP).** A contrast material containing iodine is injected intravenously, and its progress through the urinary tract is recorded on a series of rapid X-ray images.

- **Retrograde pyelogram.** Contrast material is injected through a urinary catheter into the ureters to locate stones and other obstructions.

- **Voiding cystourethrogram (VCUG).** Contrast material is inserted into the bladder through a catheter and X-rays are taken as the patient voids.

- **CT scan.** X-ray images show cross-sectional views of the kidneys and bladder.

- **MRI.** Magnetic fields are used to generate cross-sectional images of the urinary tract.

- **Ultrasound imaging.** High-frequency sound waves and a computer generate non-invasive images of the kidneys.

- **Renal angiogram.** X-rays with contrast material are used to assess blood flow to the kidneys.

- **Cystoscopy.** A pencil-thin, flexible, tube-like optical instrument is inserted through the urethra into the bladder to examine the bladder's lining and to take a biopsy if needed *(Figure 13.9)*.

RBC	red blood cell
SG	specific gravity
UA	urinalysis
VCUG	voiding cystourethrogram
WBC	white blood cell

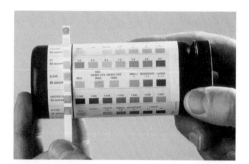

▲ **FIGURE 13.8**
Urinalysis Dipstick Being Compared Against Color Chart on Container.

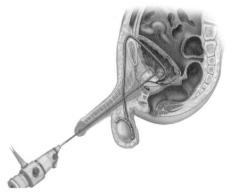

▲ **FIGURE 13.9**
Cystoscopy.

Word	Pronunciation		Elements	Definition
cast	KAST		Latin *pure*	A cylindrical mold formed by materials in kidney tubules
cystoscope	**SIS**-toh-skope	S/	-scope *instrument for viewing*	An endoscope inserted to view the inside of the bladder
		R/CF	cyst/o- *bladder*	
cystoscopy	sis-**TOS**-koh-pee	S/	-scopy *to examine*	The process of using a cystoscope
cystourethrogram	sis-toh-you-**REETH**-roe-gram	S/	-gram *a record*	X-ray image during voiding to show structure and function of bladder and urethra
		R/CF	cyst/o- *bladder*	
		R/CF	-urethr/o- *urethra*	
glycosuria (Note: *The "s" is added to make the word flow.*)	**GLYE**-koh-**SYU**-ree-ah	S/	-la *condition*	Presence of glucose in urine
		R/CF	glyc/o- *glucose*	
		R/	-ur- *urinary system*	
ketone	**KEY**-tone		Greek *acetone*	Chemical formed in uncontrolled diabetes or in starvation
ketosis	key-**TOE**-sis	S/	-sis *abnormal condition*	Excess production of ketones
ketoacidosis	**KEY**-toe-as-ih-**DOE**-sis	R/CF	ket/o- *ketones*	Excessive production of ketones, making the blood acid
		R/CF	-acid/o- *acid, low pH*	
nitrite	**NI**-trite		Greek *niter, saltpeter*	Chemical formed in urine by E. coli and other microorganisms
proteinuria	pro-tee-**NYU**-ree-ah	R/	-uria *urine*	Presence of protein in urine
		R/	protein- *protein*	
retrograde	**RET**-roh-grade	P/	retro- *backward*	Reversal of a normal flow; for example, back from the bladder into the ureters
		R/	-grade *going*	
urinalysis	you-rih-**NAL**-ih-sis	S/	-lysis *to separate*	Examination of urine to separate it into its elements and define their kind and/or quantity
		R/CF	urin/a- *urine*	

EXERCISES

A. Apply your knowledge *of medical language to this exercise. All the questions can be answered using terms from this spread. Circle the best answer.*

1. An X-ray image taken during voiding: retrograde pyelogram   angiogram   cystourethrogram

2. Presence of glucose in urine: hematuria   polyuria   glycosuria

3. Urine collection method to test for proteinuria: catheterization   24 hour   clean catch

4. Reversal of normal flow: reflex   retrograde   regenerate

5. Excessive ketones in the blood, making it acid: ketosis   ketoacidosis   ketone

6. Separate urine into its elements: urinalysis   cystourethrogram   retrograde pyelogram

B. Demonstrate your knowledge *of abbreviations and the medical terms they represent. Write out in medical terms what each abbreviation represents.*

1. KUB _____

2. UA _____

3. IVP _____

4. VCUG _____

C. Employ *the language of urology and match the correct diagnostic procedure in column 1 with the correct statement in column 2.*

_____ 1. KUB   **A.** uses contrast material

_____ 2. cystoscopy   **B.** X-ray

_____ 3. renal angiogram   **C.** invasive procedure

_____ 4. CT scan   **D.** cross-sectional views

_____ 5. ultrasound imaging   **E.** noninvasive procedure

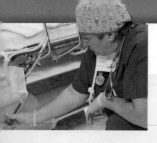

CHAPTER **13** REVIEW THE URINARY SYSTEM

CHALLENGE YOUR KNOWLEDGE

A. Elements *remain your best clue to understanding the medical term. Write the meaning of the element in the second column, give an example of a medical term containing this element in the third column, and give the meaning of the medical term in the fourth column.*

Element	Meaning of Element	Medical Term Containing This Element	Meaning of the Medical Term
supra	1.	2.	3.
cyst	4.	5.	6.
emia	7.	8.	9.
tomy	10.	11.	12.
lith	13.	14.	15.

B. Prefixes: *The following terms all end with* uria, *but the prefix makes each term different. First match the prefix in columns 1 and 2 with its meaning in columns 3 and 4. Then construct the new terms to match the definitions in the rest of the exercise. Fill in the blanks.*

_____	1. dys	_____	4. an	**A.** blood	**D.** lack of
_____	2. olig	_____	5. noct	**B.** bad, difficult	**E.** scanty
_____	3. hemat			**C.** night	

6. blood in the urine _____ / _____ / _____

7. lack of urine production _____ / _____ / _____

8. scanty production of urine _____ / _____ / _____

9. difficulty or pain with urination _____ / _____ / _____

10. excessive urination at night _____ / _____ / _____

C. Roots/combining forms: *The root/combining form nephr/o will be the basis for each of the defined terms below. Use the appropriate suffix to construct the correct term. Elements you have seen in previous chapters will aid you in constructing the appropriate term. Fill in the blanks.*

logist   iasis   osis   pathy   scope   itis   tomy   scopy   ectomy   logy   tic

1. study of the kidney and its diseases: _____ / _____ / _____

2. instrument used to examine the kidney: _____ / _____ / _____

3. surgical removal of a kidney: _____ / _____ / _____

4. any disease of the kidney: _____ / _____ / _____

5. examination of the kidney with a scope: _____ / _____ / _____

6. specialist in the study of the kidney: _____ / _____ / _____

7. inflammation of a kidney: _____ / _____ / _____

8. incision into the kidney: _____ / _____ / _____

9. a kidney condition: _____ / _____ / _____

10. incision for removal of a kidney stone: _____ / _____ / _____

D. Spelling demons: *The following terms from this chapter are particularly difficult to spell and pronounce. Correct pronunciation and spelling of medical terms is the mark of an educated professional. Circle the correct spelling, and then check (✔) that you have practiced the pronunciation. Remember that pronunciations are on the Student Online Learning Center (www.mhhe.com/AllanEss2e).*

Pronunciation

1.	nefotic	nephrotic	nefrotic	_____
2.	micturition	mastication	mikturition	_____
3.	urulogical	uralogical	urological	_____
4.	extracorpureal	extracorporeal	extracorporal	_____
5.	pyelogram	pilogram	pylogram	_____
6.	dyalisis	dialysis	dialisis	_____
7.	dyuretic	diuretic	dyoretic	_____
8.	hydronephrosis	hydranephrosis	hydronephrhosis	_____
9.	hylum	hilam	hilum	_____
10.	bladdar	bladder	blader	_____

E. Latin and Greek terms *cannot be further deconstructed into prefix, root, or suffix. You must know them for what they are. Test your knowledge of these terms with this exercise. Match the meaning in column l with the correct medical term in column 2.*

_____ 1. small stone   **A.** void

_____ 2. external opening of a passage   **B.** urea

_____ 3. to empty   **C.** groin

_____ 4. end product of nitrogen metabolism   **D.** meatus

_____ 5. involuntary response to stimulus   **E.** calculus

_____ 6. to evacuate urine or feces   **F.** void

_____ 7. crease where thigh joins abdomen   **G.** reflex

F. Abbreviations: *Test your knowledge of this chapter's abbreviations by circling the correct answer.*

1. A nephrologist would be consulted for:	NSAID	ARF	PKD
2. Which of the following is not a diagnosis?	UTI	CRF	CAPD
3. TNM is a:	diagnosis	tumor staging method	procedure
4. Which of the following is a procedure?	ESWL	ESRD	PKD
5. Which one is not a radiological procedure?	KUB	IVP	UA
6. IVP is a:	diagnostic test	sexually transmitted disease	diagnosis

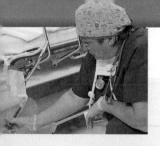

G. Recall and review: *How well do you remember these word elements from previous chapters? Try to answer without looking back to check. Fill in the chart.*

Element	Type of Element (P, R, CF, or S)	Meaning of Element	Example of a Medical Term with This Element
arachn	1.	2.	3.
cerebell	4.	5.	6.
encephalo	7.	8.	9.
myelo	10.	11.	12.
occipit	13.	14.	15.
para	16.	17.	18.
pleg	19.	20.	21.
extra	22.	23.	24.
peri	25.	26.	27.
ary	28.	29.	30.

H. Proofread *the following sentences for errors in fact or spelling. If a sentence is incorrect, rewrite it correctly on the lines below. There is only one sentence that is entirely correct.*

1. At the base of the bladder, the muscular wall of the bladder is thickened to form the external ureteral spinchter.

_____

_____

2. The urinary bladder is a hollow, muscular organ on the floor of the abdominal cavity, anterior to the public symphysis.

_____

_____

3. Involuntary micturition during sleep in older children or adults is called enuresis.

_____

_____

4. Loss of control of the kidney is called urinary retention.

_____

_____

5. Most stones enter the uretter while they are still small enough to pass down the urethra into the bladder and out of the body in urea.

_____

_____

I. Seek and find: *Below is a sample of terms and definitions that have appeared in this chapter. Challenge yourself to define these terms without turning back to check in the book. Fill in the blanks.*

1. Wilms tumor _____

2. nephrosis _____

3. small kidney or gallstone _____

4. voiding _____

J. Difference between: *If you really understand a term, you can explain it to someone else. Write an explanation to a classmate of the difference between:*

1. ureter:

_____

_____

2. urethra:

_____

_____

K. Scope/scopy: *Change the root, and you have the name of a different "scope" and a different procedure ("scopy"). Recall the roots/combining forms from previous chapters to complete the table. Don't forget to answer the question at the end.*

Root/CF	Meaning of Root	R/CF	Term for Instrument Used for This Examination	Term for Process of Examining with This Scope	Name of Specialist Who Performs This Procedure
arthro	1.	2.	3.	4.	5.
broncho	6.	7.	8.	9.	10.
cysto	11.	12.	13.	14.	15.
gastro	16.	17.	18.	19.	20.
nephro	21.	22.	23.	24.	25.
oto	26.	27.	28.	29.	30.

Generally speaking, any scope inserted within the body can be called an _____. (Clue: "within")

L. Patient education: *Your patient has just been told by the doctor that he has nephrolithiasis and has the option of ESWL for a procedure. Explain this in language your patient can understand.*

1. _____

_____

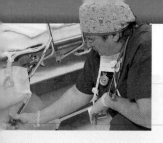

M. Study hint: *Keep a list in the back of your book of various elements like* nephr/o *and* ren *that both have the same meaning but generate their own vocabulary.*

1. Nephr/o means _____ .

   Example of a term using this element: _____

   Ren means _____ .

   Example of a term using this element: _____

   Recall other elements from previous chapters that both have the same meaning.

2. In the language of ophthalmology there are two examples. Write them here:

   _____ means _____ .

   Example of a term using this element: _____

   _____ means _____ .

   Example of a term using this element: _____

3. In the language of pulmonology there are two examples. Write them here:

   _____ means _____ .

   Example of a term using this element: _____

   _____ means _____ .

   Example of a term using this element: _____

N. This word bank *contains ten medical terms. Pick any three terms and write a sentence of patient documentation for each term.*

urinary	renal	nephrectomy	nephrosis	uremia
polycystic	calculus	enuresis	void	proteinuria

1. _____

   _____

2. _____

   _____

3. _____

   _____

O. Chapter challenge: *Circle the correct answer.*

1. A suprapubic, transabdominal needle aspiration is:

   a. below the pubis, through the abdomen

   b. above the pelvis, below the pubis

   c. above the pubis, through the abdomen

   d. inside the pelvis, below the abdomen

   e. below the pelvis, through the abdomen

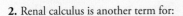

STUDY HINT
Immediately cross off any answer you know is not correct. In your remaining choices, there is only one best answer.

2. Renal calculus is another term for:

   a. kidney stone

   b. vas deferens

   c. tunica vaginalis

   d. seminiferous tubules

   e. malignant kidney tumor

3. An agent that increases urine output is:

   a. diuresis

   b. dysuria

   c. polyuria

   d. diuretic

   e. anuria

4. Within the urinary system, which organ is the agent that filters the metabolic waste products?

   a. ureter

   b. kidney

   c. urethra

   d. penis

   e. pancreas

5. Inflammation of the kidney and renal pelvis would be:

   a. cystitis

   b. pyelitis

   c. urethritis

   d. pyelonephritis

   e. nephritis

6. In both the male and the female, the opening of the urethra to the outside is called the:

   a. internal urethral sphincter

   b. external urethral sphincter

   c. external urinary meatus

   d. vas deferens

   e. pubic symphysis

7. Which of these is an inherited disease?

   a. PKD

   b. ESRD

   c. BPH

   d. CRF

   e. ARF

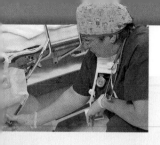

P. Consider *the following terms as a group. Analyze the elements in the terms, and answer the questions.*

anuria	polyuria	urination	diuresis	hematuria	diuretic
dysuria	oliguria	uremia	enuresis	micturation	urinalysis

1. Which terms are a diagnosis? _____

2. Which terms relate to blood? _____

3. Which term involves lab work? _____

4. What common element do all the terms contain? _____

5. Which two terms are opposites? _____ and _____

6. Which two terms are similar in meaning? _____ and _____

7. Which term concerns bedwetting? _____

8. Which term contains an element meaning "scanty"? _____

9. Which terms have prefixes? _____

10. These terms all relate to: _____

Q. Translate *the following documentation into layperson's language your patient can understand. Rewrite each sentence, and do not use any abbreviations.*

1. "The IVP and KUB confirmed a renal calculus occluding the ureter, and a dilated pelvis of the right kidney, leading to hydronephrosis."

_____

_____

_____

2. "Mrs. Dobson described many of the symptoms of cystitis: suprapubic and low-back pain and increased frequency of micturition with dysuria and hematuria."

_____

_____

_____

R. Critical thinking: *Analyze the following medical terminology and be prepared to discuss the difference in the terms.*

1. Incontinence

_____

_____

2. Retention

_____

_____

S. Case Report challenge: *Now that you are more comfortable with the terms in this chapter, you can apply that knowledge and briefly answer the questions about the Case Report. If you read the report through and underline all the medical terminology, this will make it easier to answer the questions.*

CASE REPORT 13.2

Emergency Department, Fulwood Medical Center 9/12/11

Clinical Note

Mr. Justin Leandro, a 37-year-old construction worker, presented at 1520 hrs. He complained of a sudden onset of excruciating pain in his right abdomen and back an hour previously, while at work. The pain is spasmodic and radiates down into his groin. He has vomited once, and keeps having the urge to urinate. He has no previous medical history of significance. VS: T 99.4°F, P 92, R 20, BP 130/86.

Patient's abdomen is slightly distended, with tenderness in the right upper and lower quadrants and flank. A dipstick test showed blood in his urine.

Provisional diagnosis by Mark Eagle, MD: stone in the right ureter.

An IV line was started, and 2 mg of morphine sulfate was given by IV push at 1540 hrs. He is going to X-ray STAT for KUB and IVP.

Andrea Facundo, EMT-P, 1555 hrs.

1. In your own words, describe "excruciating" pain. _____

2. Does Mr. Leandro have any past medical history of significance relating to this episode?

   _____

3. What does it mean when pain radiates? _____

4. What is the difference between Mr. Leandro's flank and his groin?

   Flank: _____

   Groin: _____

5. Mr. Leandro has a stone in his right ureter. What is the medical term for this? _____ _____

6. What kind of test is a dipstick test? _____

7. What did Mr. Leandro's dipstick test confirm? _____

8. Use the Glossary or a medical dictionary to define the term *distended*, which is used to describe Mr. Leandro's abdomen. _____

   _____

   _____

9. What is a *provisional* diagnosis? _____

   _____

10. How does a *provisional* diagnosis differ from a *postoperative* diagnosis? _____

    _____

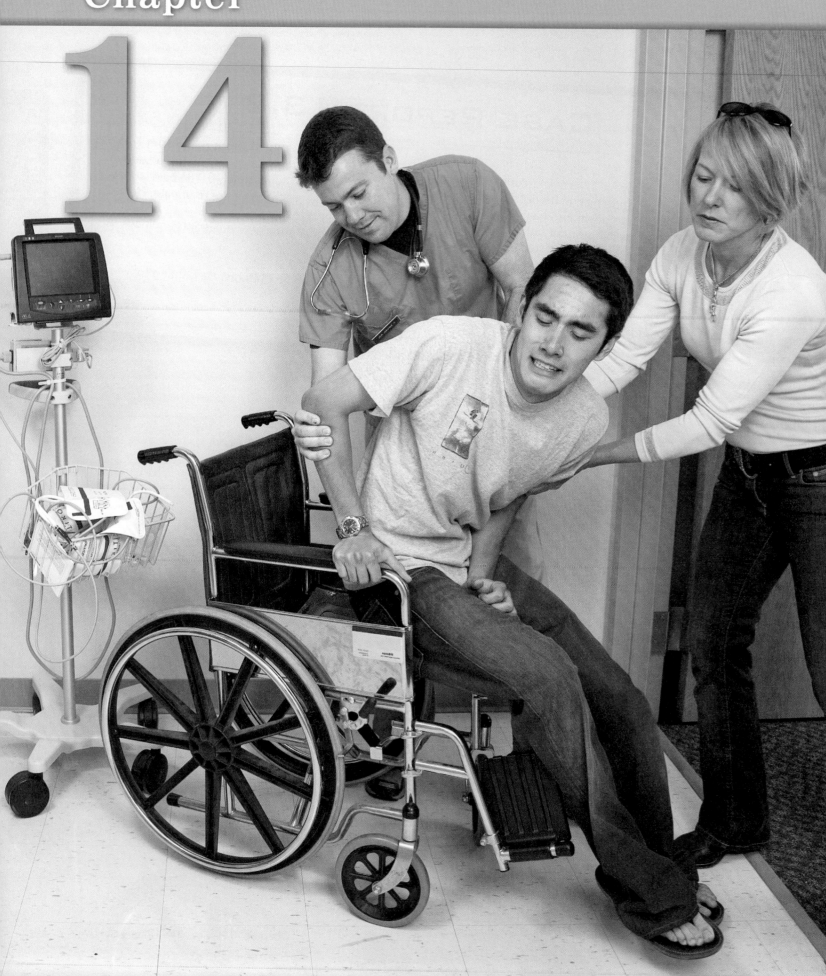

YOU ARE

> . . . an EMT-P working in the Emergency Department at Fulwood Medical Center.

YOU ARE COMMUNICATING WITH

> . . . Joseph Davis, a 17-year-old high school senior, who has been brought in by his mother at 0400 hrs. Joseph is complaining of (c/o) a sudden onset of pain in his left **testicle**, which began 3 hours earlier and woke him up. The pain is intense and has made him vomit. VS: T 99.2°F, P 88, R 15, BP 130/70. An examination reveals his left testicle to be enlarged, warm, and tender. His abdomen is normal to palpation. At your request, Dr. Helinski, the emergency physician on duty, examines Joseph immediately. He diagnoses a **torsion** (twisting) of the patient's left testicle.

LEARNING OUTCOMES

As you set up the next stage of Joseph's treatment, immediate clinical decisions will need to be made. You will have to communicate clearly with Dr. Helinski, other health professionals, the patient, and the patient's family. You will also need to document the patient's care. In order to participate effectively in this process, you must be able to:

LO 14.1 Apply the language of urology to the structure and functions of the male reproductive system.

LO 14.2 Discuss the medical terminology for the process of spermatogenesis.

LO 14.3 Recognize and pronounce the medical terms of urology as they relate to the male reproductive system.

LO 14.4 Identify the medical terminology of common disorders of the male reproductive system.

THE MALE REPRODUCTIVE SYSTEM

The Essentials of the Language of the Male Reproductive System

The health professionals involved in the diagnosis and treatment of problems with the male reproductive system include:

- Urologists, who are specialists in the diagnosis and treatment of diseases of the urinary system.

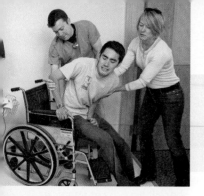

LESSON 14.1

The Male Reproductive System

Unlike every other organ system, the reproductive system is not essential for an individual human to survive. However, without the reproductive system, the human species could not survive. The information in this lesson will enable you to use correct medical terminology to:

14.1.1 Identify the components of the male reproductive system.

14.1.2 Describe the male external genitalia.

14.1.3 Explain the structure and functions of the testes.

14.1.4 Outline the process of **spermatogenesis** and the structure of a sperm.

14.1.5 Distinguish common disorders of the testes.

ABBREVIATION

c/o   complaining of

Male Reproductive System (LO 14.1)

The **male reproductive organ system** *(Figure 14.1)* consists of the primary and secondary sex organs, and the accessory glands. These are categorized as follows:

1. The **primary sex organs,** or **gonads,** are the two **testes.**

2. The **secondary sex organs** include:

   a. The **penis;**

   b. The **scrotum;** and

   c. A system of ducts, including the **epididymis, ductus (vas) deferens,** and **urethra.**

3. The accessory glands include:

   a. The **prostate;**

   b. The **seminal vesicles;** and

   c. The **bulbourethral glands.**

Perineum (LO 14.1)

The external **genitalia** (the penis, scrotum, and testes) occupy the **perineum,** a diamond-shaped region between the thighs. The perineum borders the pubic symphysis anteriorly and the coccyx posteriorly *(Figure 14.2).* The anus is also in the perineum.

Scrotum (LO 14.1)

The scrotum is a skin-covered sac between the upper thighs, which is divided into two compartments. Each compartment contains a testis. The scrotum's function is to provide a cooler environment for the testes than the one inside the body. **Sperm** are best produced and stored at a few degrees cooler than that of the male's internal body temperature.

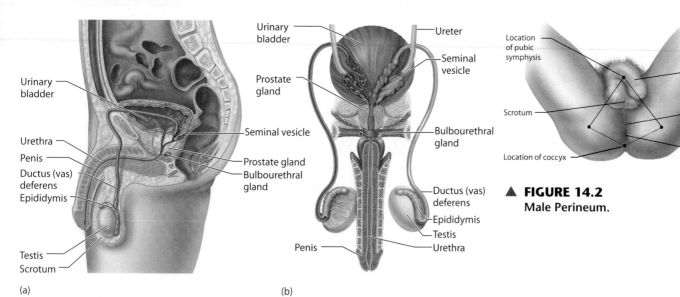

(a)

(b)

▲ **FIGURE 14.1**
Male Reproductive System.
(a) Male pelvic cavity, midsagittal section.
(b) Male reproductive organs.

▲ **FIGURE 14.2**
Male Perineum.

S = Suffix   P = Prefix   R = Root   R/CF= Combining Form

Word	Pronunciation	Elements		Definition
bulbourethral	**BUL**-boh-you-**REE**-thral	S/ R/CF R/	-al *pertaining to* bulb/o- *bulb* -urethr- *urethra*	Pertaining to the bulbous penis and urethra
ductus deferens (same as **vas deferens**)	**DUK**-tus **DEH**-fuh-renz VAS		ductus, Latin *to lead* deferens, Latin *carry away* vas, Latin *vessel, canal*	Tube that receives sperm from the epididymis
epididymis	**EP**-ih-**DID**-ih-miss	P/ R/	epi- *above* -didymis *testis*	Coiled tube attached to testis
genitalia (Note: 2 suffixes) genital (adj)	**JEN**-ih-**TAY**-lee-ah **JEN**-ih-tal	S/ R/ S/	-ia *condition* genit- *primary male or female sex organs* -al- *pertaining to*	External and internal organs of reproduction Pertaining to reproduction or to the male or female sex organs
gonad gonads (pl)	**GO**-nad **GO**-nads		Greek *seed*	Testis or ovary
penis penile (adj)	**PEE**-nis **PEE**-nile	S/ R/	Latin *tail* -ile *pertaining to* pen- *penis*	Conveys urine and semen to the outside Pertaining to the penis
perineum perineal (adj)	**PER**-ih-**NEE**-um **PER**-ih-**NEE**-al	S/ R/	Greek *perineum* -al *pertaining to* perine- *perineum*	Area between the thighs, extending from the coccyx to the pubis Pertaining to the perineum
scrotum scrotal (adj)	**SKRO**-tum **SKRO**-tal	S/ R/	Latin *scrotum* -al *pertaining to* scrot- *scrotum*	Sac containing the testes Pertaining to the scrotum
seminal vesicle	**SEM**-in-al **VES**-ih-kull	S/ R/ S/ R/	Greek *seed* -al *pertaining to* semin- *semen* -le *small* vesic- *sac containing fluid*	Sac of the ductus deferens that produces seminal fluid
sperm spermatozoa (pl) spermatic (adj) spermatogenesis	SPERM **SPER**-mat-oh-**ZOH**-ah **SPER**-mat-ik **SPER**-mat-oh-**JEN**-eh-sis	S/ R/CF S/ S/	Greek *seed* -zoa *animal* spermat/o- *sperm* -ic *pertaining to* -genesis *creation, formation*	Mature male sex cell Sperm (plural) Pertaining to sperm The process by which male germ cells differentiate into sperm
testicle testicular (adj) testis testes (pl)	**TES**-tih-kul tes-**TICK**-you-lar **TES**-tis **TES**-tez	S/ R/	Latin *small testis* -ar *pertaining to* testicul- *testicle* Latin *testis*	One of the male reproductive glands Pertaining to the testicle Same as testicle
torsion	**TOR**-shun		Latin *to twist*	The act or result of twisting

EXERCISES

A. Review *the Case Report on the opening spread before answering the questions.*

1. What is the site of Joseph Davis' intense pain? _____

2. What is *palpation?* _____

3. What does *torsion* mean? _____

B. Documentation: *You could be working in the Emergency Department when this patient comes in. Take the information presented in Case Report 14.1, and document the case in the patient's record. Use the following terms to fill in the blanks.*

    testicular   **testes**   **testis**   **testicle**   **torsion**

1. This patient presented to the ED because of pain in his left _____.

2. Both _____ were examined, but the left _____ was enlarged, warm, and tender.

3. The emergency physician on duty diagnosed _____ ; patient will be scheduled for emergency surgery.

LESSON **14.1** Testes and Spermatic Cord (LO 14.1)

Testes (LO 14.1)

In the adult male, each testis is a small, oval organ that measures about 2 inches long and ¾ of an inch wide *(Figure 14.3)*. Each testis is covered by a serous membrane—the **tunica vaginalis**—which has outer and inner layers that are separated by serous fluid.

Inside the testis are some 250 lobules (small lobes); each contains three or four **seminiferous tubules,** which produce **semen.** Within these tubules are several layers of germ cells that are in the process of developing into sperm. Between the seminiferous tubules are the interstitial (occurring between tissues) cells. These cells produce hormones called **androgens.**

Testosterone is the major androgen produced by the interstitial cells of the testes. Its effects include the stimulation of the following activities:

1. **Spermatogenesis,** which is responsible for testosterone levels peaking at age 20, then declining steadily to one-fifth of that level at age 80.

2. The development of the male secondary sex characteristics at puberty, which include:

   a. The enlargement of the testes, scrotum, and penis.

   b. The development of the pubic, axillary, body, and facial hair.

   c. The secretion of sebum in skin, which can result in acne *(Chapter 3)*.

3. A burst of growth at puberty, including an increased muscle mass, a higher basal metabolic rate **(BMR)**, and a larger larynx (which deepens the voice).

4. Stimulating the brain to increase the male's **libido** (sex drive).

Spermatic Cord (LO 14.1)

The blood vessels and nerves to the testes— which arise in the abdominal cavity—pass through the inguinal, or groin, canal, where they join with connective tissue. This forms the **spermatic cord** that suspends each testis in the scrotum *(Figure 14.3)*. The left testis is suspended lower than the right. Within the cord exist:

- an artery

- a **plexus** of veins

- nerves

- a thin muscle

- the ductus (vas) deferens into which sperm are deposited when they leave the testis

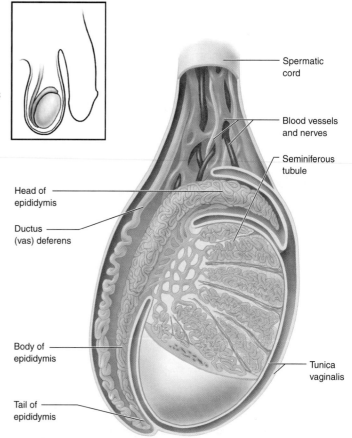

Spermatic cord

Blood vessels and nerves

Seminiferous tubule

Head of epididymis

Ductus (vas) deferens

Body of epididymis

Tunica vaginalis

Tail of epididymis

▲ **FIGURE 14.3**
The Testis and Associated Structures.

KEYNOTES

- The sperm count of a 65-year-old man is approximately one-third of the count when he was 20.

- The spermatic cord can be palpated through the skin of the scrotum.

ABBREVIATION

BMR   basal metabolic rate

Word	Pronunciation	Elements		Definition
androgen	**AN**-droh-jen	S/ R/CF	-gen *create, produce* andr/o- *masculine*	Hormone that promotes masculine characteristics
libido	lih-**BEE**-doh		Latin *lust*	Sexual desire
plexus plexuses (pl)	**PLEK**-sus **PLEK**-sus-ez		Latin *braid*	A weblike network of joined nerves
semen	**SEE**-men		Latin *seed*	Penile ejaculate containing sperm and seminal fluid
seminiferous (adj)	sem-ih-**NIF**-er-us	S/ R/ R/	-ous *pertaining to* semin/i- *semen* -fer- *to bear, carry*	Pertaining to carrying semen
testosterone	tes-**TOSS**-ter-own	S/ R/CF	-sterone *steroid* test/o- *testis*	Powerful androgen produced by testes
tunica vaginalis	**TYU**-nih-kah vaj-ih-**NAHL**-iss	 S/ R/	tunica, Latin *coat* -alis *pertaining to* vagin- *sheath, vagina*	Covering, particularly of a tubular structure The tunica vaginalis is the sheath of the testis and epididymis

EXERCISES

A. Write *the correct medical term to answer the question.*

1. What is the name of the serous membrane that covers the testis? _____

2. The term *seminiferous* pertains to: _____

3. What is another medical term for sex drive? _____

4. What does the abbreviation BMR mean? _____

5. What structure supports the testes? _____

B. Continue *using the language of the male reproductive system to complete the questions.*

1. Which part of the male reproductive system produces semen? _____

2. What does *interstitial* mean? _____

3. What are the male hormones called? _____

4. What is the major male hormone, and where is it produced? _____ is produced in the _____.

5. What is another name for the "inguinal area"? _____

C. Meet lesson *and chapter objectives using the language of medicine to answer the following questions.*

1. What does having a larger larynx do to the voice? _____

2. In the growing process, when does muscle mass begin to appear? _____

3. What separates the outer and inner layer of the tunica vaginalis? _____

4. Name the secondary sex characteristics in the male:

a. _____

b. _____

c. _____

LESSON 14.1 Testes and Spermatic Cord (continued)

- The testis in testicular torsion will die in approximately 6 hours unless the blood supply is restored.

- Self-examination of the testes (SET) for swelling or tenderness should be performed monthly by all men.

Sperm (LO 14.1)

A mature sperm has a pear-shaped head and a long tail. The sperm's head contains these three segments *(Figure 14.4):*

- The **nucleus,** which contains 23 chromosomes;
- The **cap,** which contains enzymes used to penetrate the egg if the sperm is successful; and
- The **basal body** of the tail.

The tail is further divided into three segments and is responsible for movement as the sperm swims up the female reproductive tract.

> **CASE REPORT 14.1** (CONTINUED)
>
> Joseph Davis presented with typical symptoms and signs of testicular torsion. The affected testis rapidly became painful, tender, swollen, and inflamed. Emergency surgery was performed, and the testis and cord were manually untwisted through an incision in the scrotum. The testis was stitched to surrounding tissues to prevent a recurrence of the torsion.

ABBREVIATIONS

SET	self-examination of the testis
STD	sexually transmitted disease

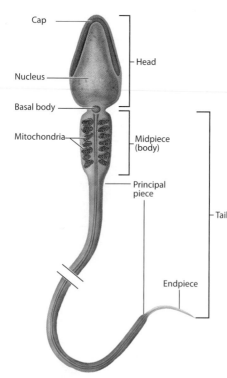

▲ **FIGURE 14.4**
Mature Sperm.

Disorders of the Testes (LO 14.1 and 14.4)

Testicular torsion is the twisting of a testis on its spermatic cord. The testicular artery in the twisted cord becomes blocked, and the blood supply to the testis is cut off. The condition occurs in men between puberty and age 25. In half the cases, it starts in bed at night.

Varicocele is a condition in which the veins in the spermatic cord become dilated and painful as varicose veins. If it is uncomfortable, it can be treated by surgically tying off the affected veins.

Hydrocele is a collection of excess fluid in the space between the visceral and parietal layers of the tunica vaginalis of the testis. It is most common after age 40.

Spermatocele is a collection of sperm in a sac formed in the epididymis, which is the sperm-containing tube attached to a testicle. It occurs in about 30% of men, is benign, and rarely causes symptoms. It does not require treatment unless it becomes uncomfortable.

Cryptorchism occurs when a testis fails to descend from the abdomen into the scrotum before a boy is 12 months old. As undescended testicles have a higher risk of infertility and cancer, an **orchiopexy** is performed to bring the testis into the scrotum.

Epididymitis is an inflammation of the epididymis; **epididymoorchitis (orchitis)** is an inflammation of the epididymis and testis. Orchitis, an inflammation of the testis, is usually a consequence of epididymitis. In each of these cases, the inflammation is most commonly caused by a bacterial infection spreading from an infection in the urinary tract or prostate. These infections can also be caused by sexually transmitted diseases **(STDs),** like gonorrhea or chlamydia.

A viral cause of orchitis is **mumps.** In males past puberty who develop mumps, 30% will develop orchitis, and 30% of those will develop resulting testicular atrophy. A bilateral infection can result in **infertility.** Mumps is avoidable by immunization in childhood.

Testicular cancer usually develops in men under 40.

> **CASE REPORT 14.2**
>
> Lance Armstrong, the world-renowned cyclist, presented with **hemoptysis** (coughing up blood). He had ignored a slight swelling of one testis, and the cancer in that testis had already metastasized to his lungs and brain. He required extensive chemotherapy, with brain surgery to remove several metastases. The initial treatment for testicular cancer is surgical removal of the affected testis **(orchiectomy),** followed by chemotherapy and sometimes radiation therapy.

Word	Pronunciation	Elements		Definition
cryptorchism	krip-**TOR**-kizm	S/ P/ R/	-ism *condition* crypt- *hidden* -orch- *testicle*	Failure of one or both testes to descend into the scrotum
epididymitis	**EP**-ih-did-ih-**MY**-tis	S/ P/ R/	-itis *inflammation* epi- *above* -didym- *testis*	Inflammation of the epididymis
epididymoorchitis (same as **orchitis**) (one of the two consecutive "i"s is not used)	ep-ih-**DID**-ih-moh-or-**KIE**-tis	S/ P/ R/CF R/	-itis *inflammation* epi- *above* -didym/o- *testis* -orchi- *testicle*	Inflammation of the epididymis and testicle
hydrocele	**HIGH**-droh-seal	S/ R/CF	-cele *swelling* hydr/o- *water*	Collection of fluid in the space of the tunica vaginalis
orchiectomy	or-key-**ECK**-toe-me	S/ R/	-ectomy *surgical excision* orchi- *testicle*	Removal of one or both testes
orchiopexy	**OR**-key-oh-**PEK**-see	S/ R/CF	-pexy *surgical fixation* orchi/o- *testicle*	Surgical fixation of a testis in the scrotum
orchitis (one of the two consecutive "i"s is not used)	or-**KIE**-tis	S/ R/	-itis *inflammation* orchi- *testicle*	Inflammation of the testis
spermatocele	**SPER**-mat-oh-seal	S/ R/CF	-cele *swelling* spermat/o- *sperm*	Cyst of the epididymis that contains sperm
varicocele	**VAIR**-ih-koh-seal	S/ R/CF	-cele *swelling* varic/o- *varicosity*	Varicose veins of the spermatic cord

EXERCISES

A. Review *the Case Report 14.1 (continued) before answering the questions.*

1. What is the difference between a "symptom" and a "sign"?

   Symptom:_____

   Sign: _____

2. Name one symptom Joseph had when he presented to the Emergency Department. _____

3. Why was emergency surgery necessary for Joseph? _____

4. What is the medical term for the surgery that Joseph had? _____

5. Describe what the surgeon did to repair Joseph's condition. _____

_____

B. Build your knowledge *of the language of the male reproductive system by correctly answering the questions regarding the elements in the following terms. Circle the best answer.*

1. In the term *hydrocele,* the R/CF means:

   testis   water   sperm

2. In the term *cryptorchism,* the prefix means:

   outside of   behind   hidden

3. In the term *orchiopexy,* the suffix means:

   removal   incision   fixation

4. In the term *epididymitis,* which element means *above?*

   epi   didym   itis

5. In the term *epididymoorchitis,* the element *orch* means:

   threadlike   testicle   hidden

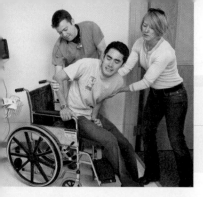

LESSON 14.2

Spermatic Ducts, Accessory Glands, and Penis

CASE REPORT 14.3

YOU ARE

. . . a surgical technologist (LCC-ST) working for urologist Phillip Johnson, MD, in the Urology Clinic at Fulwood Medical Center.

YOU ARE COMMUNICATING WITH

. . . Mr. Ronald Detrick, a 60-year-old man, who has been referred to the Urology Clinic.

Patient Interview
Mr. Detrick complains of having to get out of bed to urinate four or five times at night. He has difficulty starting urination, has a weak stream, and feels he is not emptying his bladder completely. He has lost interest in sex. His physical examination is unremarkable except that a digital rectal examination (DRE) reveals a diffusely enlarged **prostate** with no nodules.

Spermatic Ducts (LO 14.1)

As the sperm cells mature in the testes over a 60-day period, they move down the seminiferous tubules into the epididymis for storage. The epididymis adheres to the posterior side of the testis. It is a single-coiled duct or tube in which the sperm are stored for 12 to 20 days until they mature and become **motile** (capable of movement).

To be ejaculated, the sperm move into the ductus (vas) deferens, the **ejaculatory** duct, and finally the urethra to reach the outside of the body.

The ductus (vas) deferens is a muscular duct that travels up from the epididymis in the scrotum, passes behind the urinary bladder, and joins with the duct of the seminal vesicle to form the ejaculatory duct, which empties sperm and semen into the urethra.

Accessory Glands (LO 14.1)

The five accessory glands are:

1. The two **seminal vesicles,** located on the posterior surface of the urinary bladder;

2. The single **prostate gland** is close in size and shape to the average walnut. The prostate gland is located immediately below the bladder and anterior to the rectum. It surrounds the urethra and the ejaculatory duct. It is composed of 30 to 50 glands that open directly into the urethra; and

3. The two **bulbourethral glands,** located one on either side of the membranous urethra. Each gland has a short duct leading into the spongy (penile) urethra.

Word	Pronunciation	Elements		Definition
ejaculate (Note: *can be a verb or a noun*)	ee-**JACK**-you-late	S/ R/	-ate *composed of, pertaining to* ejacul- *shoot out*	To expel suddenly; *or* the semen expelled in ejaculation
ejaculation (noun)	ee-**JACK**-you-**LAY**-shun	S/	-ation *process*	Process of expelling semen suddenly
ejaculatory (adj)	ee-**JACK**-you-lay-**TOR**-ee	S/	-atory *pertaining to*	Pertaining to ejaculation
motile	**MOH**-til	S/ R/	-ile *pertaining to* mot- *to move*	Capable of spontaneous movement
motility	moh-**TILL**-ih-tee	R/ S/	motil- *to move* -ity *condition, state*	The ability for spontaneous movement
prostate	**PROS**-tate (Note: *not PROS-trate, which means exhausted*)		Greek *one standing before*	Organ surrounding the beginning of the urethra
prostatic (adj)	pros-**TAT**-ik	S/ R/	-tic *pertaining to* prosta- *prostate*	Pertaining to the prostate

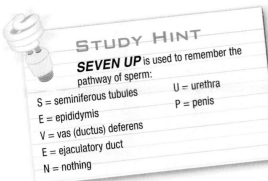

STUDY HINT

SEVEN UP is used to remember the pathway of sperm:

S = seminiferous tubules
E = epididymis
V = vas (ductus) deferens
E = ejaculatory duct
N = nothing
U = urethra
P = penis

EXERCISES

A. Review *the Case Report on this spread before answering the questions.*

1. What are Mr. Detrick's complaints? _____

_____

2. What does the abbreviation *DRE* mean? _____

3. What did Mr. Detrick's DRE reveal? _____

4. What is a *nodule?* _____

5. What is responsible for Mr. Detrick's symptoms? _____

B. Writing practice: *Write a sentence that is not a definition for each of the following terms. Be sure to employ the correct form of the term in your sentence. Fill in the blanks.*

1. *ejaculate* (as a noun—thing):

2. *ejaculate* (as a verb—action):

3. *ejaculatory* (adjective):

LESSON 14.2 Disorders of the Prostate Gland
(LO 14.1 and 14.4)

KEYNOTES

• Survival from prostate cancer is up to 80% if it is detected before it spreads outside the gland.

• Male infertility is involved in 40% of the 2.6 million infertile married couples in the United States. [Source: National Institutes of Health (NIH)]

• Vasectomy is almost 100% successful in producing male sterility.

Benign prostatic hyperplasia (BPH), also known as benign prostatic hypertrophy or **benign enlargement of the prostate (BEP)**—a noncancerous enlargement of the prostate—can cause symptoms starting around age 45; by age 80, some 90% of men have symptoms. This enlargement is one of **hyperplasia** rather than **hypertrophy,** and it compresses the prostatic urethra to produce symptoms including:

• Difficulty starting and stopping the urine stream.

• **Nocturia** (excessive nighttime urination), **polyuria** (excessive urine production), and dysuria (difficulty or pain in urination).

> **CASE REPORT 14.3**
> (CONTINUED)
>
> Ronald Detrick was describing the symptoms listed above when he was referred to the Urology Clinic.

In some patients, surgical treatment by **transurethral resection (TURP)** relieves the symptoms. An endoscope called a **resectoscope** is inserted into the urethra and used to remove the tissue surrounding and compressing the urethra.

Prostatic cancer affects 10% of men over the age of 50, and its incidence is increasing. It forms hard nodules in the periphery of the gland and is often asymptomatic (produces no symptoms) in its early stages, as it does not compress the urethra.

Screening for prostatic cancer is performed using the following procedures:

• A **digital rectal exam (DRE),** which involves palpating the size and texture of the prostate by inserting a finger into the rectum;

• A **prostate-specific antigen (PSA)** test, which measures the PSA level in the blood. Even though cancer can be present when the level is zero, the benefit of this test is that it can show whether levels rise rapidly over time; and

• An **early prostate cancer antigen (EPCA-2)** test. This is more accurate than the PSA and is now in clinical trials.

Several treatment options involving radiotherapy are available for prostate cancer. **Brachytherapy** involves the insertion of small radioactive rods directly into the tumor. Sometimes, a **radical prostatectomy** is performed. This involves complete surgical removal of the prostate and surrounding tissues. A vaccine has been introduced that provides some extension of life in men with advanced prostate cancer.

Prostatitis is an inflammation of the prostate gland that causes groin pain and difficulty and discomfort when urinating.

Male Infertility (LO 14.1 and 14.4)

Male infertility is the inability to conceive after at least one year of unprotected intercourse. The primary causes of infertility are:

• Impaired sperm production, due to cryptorchidism, anorchism (absence of one or both testes), testicular trauma, testicular cancer, or orchitis after puberty;

• Impaired sperm delivery, due to infections and blockage of spermatic ducts; and

• Testosterone deficiency **(hypogonadism).** Phthalates in plastics and dioxins in paper are examples of environmental endocrine disrupters that can contribute to testosterone deficiency.

Each year, in the United States, half a million men choose to be made infertile **(sterile)** by having a **vasectomy.** Under local anesthesia, the ductus deferens is cut in two places, a 1-centimeter segment is removed, and the ends of the ductus deferens are cauterized and tied. The site of the surgery makes the man infertile but still able to produce and ejaculate seminal fluid.

Should a man choose to reverse his vasectomy, he can undergo a **vasovasostomy.** This is a microsurgical procedure, which reverses a vasectomy by suturing back together the cut ends of the ductus deferens.

ABBREVIATIONS

BEP	benign enlargement of the prostate
BPH	benign prostatic hyperplasia
EPCA-2	early prostate cancer antigen-2
TURP	transurethral resection of the prostate
PSA	prostate-specific antigen
NIH	National Institutes of Health

Word	Pronunciation	Elements		Definition
brachytherapy	brah-kee-**THAIR**-ah-pee	P/ R/	brachy- *short* -therapy *treatment*	Radiation therapy in which the source of radiation is implanted in the tissue to be treated
hyperplasia	**HIGH**-per-**PLAY**-zee-ah	S/ P/ R/	-ia *condition* hyper- *excessive* -plas- *molding, formation*	Increase in the *number* of the cells in a tissue or organ
hypertrophy (Note: *See Study Hint below.*)	high-**PER**-troh-fee	R/	-trophy *development*	Increase in the *size* of the cells in a tissue or organ
hypogonadism	**HIGH**-poh-**GOH**-nad-izm	S/ P/ R/	-ism *condition* hypo- *deficient* -gonad- *testis or ovary*	Deficient gonad production of sperm or eggs or hormones
infertility	in-fer-**TIL**-ih-tee	S/ P/ R/	-ity *condition* in- *not* -fertil- *able to conceive*	Failure to conceive
nocturia	nok-**TYU**-ree-ah	S/ P/ R/	-ia *condition* noct- *night* -ur- *urine*	Excessive urination at night
polyuria	pol-ee-**YOU**-ree-ah	S/ P/ R/	-ia *condition* poly- *excessive* -ur- *urine*	Excessive production of urine
prostatectomy	pros-tah-**TEK**-toe-me	S/ R/	-ectomy *surgical excision* prostat- *prostate*	Surgical removal of the prostate
prostatitis	pros-tah-**TIE**-tis	S/	-itis *inflammation*	Inflammation of the prostate
resectoscope	ree-**SEK**-toe-skope	R/ R/CF	-scope *instrument for viewing* resect/o- *cut off*	Endoscope for the transurethral removal of lesions
transurethral	**TRANS**-you-**REE**-thral	S/ P/ R/	-al *pertaining to* trans- *across, through* -urethr- *urethra*	Procedure performed through the urethra
vasectomy	vah-**SEK**-toe-me	S/ R/	-ectomy *surgical excision* vas- *duct*	Excision of a segment of the ductus deferens
vasovasostomy (vasectomy reversal)	**VAY**-soh-vay-**SOS**-toe-me	S/ R/CF	-stomy *new opening* vas/o- *duct*	Reanastomosis of the ductus deferens to restore the flow of sperm

EXERCISES

A. Review *the Case Report on this spread before answering the questions.*

1. Mr. Detrick presented to the Urology Clinic with nocturia, polyuria, and dysuria. Briefly define each term for your patient.

   nocturia: _____

   polyuria: _____

   dysuria: _____

2. Building on the suffix "uria", what is "hematuria" ? _____

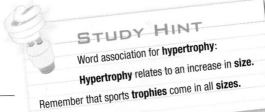

STUDY HINT

Word association for **hypertrophy**:
Hypertrophy relates to an increase in **size**.
Remember that sports **trophies** come in all **sizes**.

B. Recognition: *As you become more familiar with elements (especially suffixes), you will be able to recognize medical terms that are procedures and diagnoses. Practice with the terms in the WAD box above. Fill in the blanks.*

1. List all the terms in the WAD that could be a possible diagnosis for a patient:

   _____

2. List all the terms in the WAD that are procedures:

   _____

3. What surgical procedure is the reversal of a vasectomy? _____

4. What is the medical term for testosterone deficiency? _____

5. What is another term for *infertile?* _____

LESSON 14.2

Penis (LO 14.1)

KEYNOTES

- Erectile dysfunction occurs in some 20 million American men.

- Erectile dysfunction can be associated with diabetes, stroke, multiple sclerosis, hypertension, cigarette smoking, radiation therapy, drugs such as anti-depressants and cholesterol-lowering medications, and loss of interest in one's sexual partner.

The **penis** *(Figure 14.5)* is an important male external body structure, which is specifically designed to meet its two main functions:

- To enable urine to flow to the outside.

- To deposit semen in the female vagina around the cervix.

The external, visible part of the penis is composed of the **shaft** and the **glans.** The external urethral meatus is located at the tip of the glans. The skin of the penis continues over the glans as the **prepuce,** otherwise known as the foreskin. A ventral fold of tissue called the **frenulum** attaches the foreskin to the glans.

The shaft of the penis contains these three **erectile** vascular bodies *(Figure 14.5a):*

- The paired **corpora cavernosa** (columns of erectile tissue found in the penis) are located dorsolaterally.

- The single **corpus spongiosum** is located inferiorly. It contains the urethra and goes on to form the glans.

Erection occurs when the corpora cavernosa fill with blood, causing the erectile bodies to distend and become rigid. It is a parasympathetic nervous system response to stimulation.

Ejaculation occurs when the sympathetic nervous system stimulates the smooth muscle of the ductus deferens, ejaculatory ducts, and the glands in the prostate to contract.

The Prepuce (Foreskin) and Urethra (LO 14.1)

The functions of the **prepuce** (fore-skin) are to cover and protect the glans *(Figure 14.5b),* and to produce smegma. **Smegma** is a lubricant containing lipids, cell debris, and some natural antibiotics. Removal of the foreskin is called **circumcision** *(Figure 14.6).*

Disorders of the Penis
(LO 14.1 and 14.4)

Disorders involving the penis range from minor injuries to STDs to cancer. These conditions are outlined below.

Trauma to the penis can vary from being caught in a pants' zipper to being fractured while erect during vigorous sexual intercourse.

Priapism is a persistent, painful erection that occurs when blood cannot escape from the erectile tissue. It can be caused by drugs like epinephrine, by blood clots, or by spinal cord injury.

Cancer of the penis occurs most commonly on the glans and is rare in circumcised men.

Sexually transmitted diseases (STDs) are discussed in detail in Chapter 15.

Erectile dysfunction (ED), or impotence, is the inability to have a satisfactory erection. Treatment is aimed at addressing any underlying disease.

Premature ejaculation is more common than erectile dysfunction. It occurs when a man ejaculates so quickly during intercourse that it causes distress or embarrassment to one or both partners.

Disorders of the Prepuce
(LO 14.1 and 14.4)

- **Balanitis** is an infection of the glans and foreskin with bacteria or yeast.

- **Phimosis** is a condition in which the foreskin is tight because of a small opening and cannot be retracted over the glans for cleaning. It can lead to balanitis.

- **Paraphimosis** is a condition in which the retracted foreskin cannot be pulled forward to cover the glans.

Disorders of the Penile Urethra
(LO 14.1 and 14.4)

Urethritis is an inflammation of the urethra. It can be caused by bacteria, STDs, viruses, and chemical irritants from **spermicides** and contraceptive gels.

Urethral stricture is scarring that narrows the urethra. It results from infection or injury.

Hypospadias is a congenital defect in which the opening of the urethra is on the undersurface of the penis instead of at the head of the glans. It can be corrected surgically.

Epispadias is a congenital defect in which the opening of the urethra is on the dorsum of the penis.

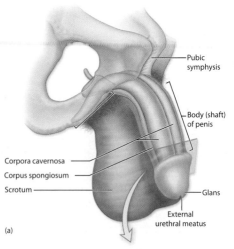

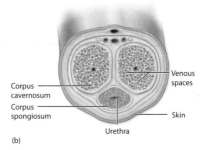

▲ **FIGURE 14.5**
Anatomy of the Penis.
(a) External anatomy.
(b) Cross-sectional view.

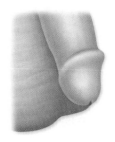
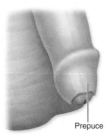

▲ **FIGURE 14.6**
Prepuce.
(a) Circumcised penis. (b) Uncircumcised penis.

ABBREVIATIONS

ED   erectile dysfunction
STD   sexually transmitted disease

Figure labels (a): Pubic symphysis, Body (shaft) of penis, Corpora cavernosa, Corpus spongiosum, Scrotum, Glans, External urethral meatus

Figure labels (b): Venous spaces, Corpus cavernosum, Corpus spongiosum, Skin, Urethra

Figure 14.6 labels: Prepuce

Word	Pronunciation		Elements	Definition
balanitis	bal-ah-**NIE**-tis	S/ R/	-itis *inflammation* balan- *glans penis*	Inflammation of the glans and prepuce of the penis
cavernosa	kav-er-**NOH**-sah	S/ R/	-osa *like* cavern- *cave*	Resembling a cave
circumcision	ser-kum-**SIZH**-un	S/ P/ R/	-ion *action, condition* circum- *around* -cis- *to cut*	To remove part or all of the prepuce
corpus corpora (pl)	**KOR**-pus kor-**POR**-ah		Latin *body*	Major part of a structure
epispadias	ep-ih-**SPAY**-dee-as	S/ P/ R/	-ias *condition* epi- *above* -spad- *tear or cut*	Condition in which the urethral opening is on the dorsum of the penis
erectile	ee-**REK**-tile	S/ R/	-ile *pertaining to* erect- *to set up, straight*	Capable of erection or being distended with blood
erection	ee-**REK**-shun	S/	-ion *action, condition*	Distended and rigid state of an organ
frenulum	**FREN**-you-lum		Latin *small bridle*	Fold of mucous membrane between the glans and the prepuce
glans	GLANZ		Latin *acorn*	Head of the penis or clitoris
hypospadias	high-poh-**SPAY**-dee-as	S/ P/ R/	-ias *condition* hypo- *below* -spad- *tear or cut*	Urethral opening is more proximal than normal on the ventral surface of the penis
impotence	**IM**-poh-tence		Latin *inability*	Inability to achieve an erection
paraphimosis	**PAR**-ah-fih-**MOH**-sis	S/ P/ R/	-osis *condition* para- *abnormal* -phim- *muzzle*	Condition in which a retracted prepuce cannot be pulled forward to cover the glans
phimosis	fih-**MOH**-sis	S/ R/	-osis *condition* phim- *muzzle*	A condition where the prepuce cannot be retracted
prepuce (same as foreskin)	**PREE**-puce		Latin *foreskin*	Fold of skin that covers the glans penis
priapism	**PRY**-ah-pizm		Priapus, mythical Roman god of procreation	Persistent erection of the penis
smegma	**SMEG**-mah		Greek *ointment*	Oily material produced by the glans and prepuce
spermicide	**SPER**-mih-side	S/ R/CF	-cide *destroy* sperm/i- *sperm*	Agent that destroys sperm
spermicidal (adj)	sper-mih-**SIGH**-dal	S/	-al *pertaining to*	Pertaining to the killing of sperm; *or* destructive to sperm
spongiosum	spun-jee-**OH**-sum	S/ R/	-um *tissue* spongios- *sponge*	Spongelike tissue

EXERCISES

A. Language of urology: *Refine your knowledge of urological terminology by choosing the correct term to complete the statement. Circle the best choice. Be precise, and watch the spelling!*

1. Condition in which a retracted prepuce cannot be pulled forward to cover the glans:

   hypospadias   phimosis   spongiosum   paraphimosis

2. To remove all or part of the prepuce:

   circumcision   circumscion   circummcision   circumsion

3. Skin that covers the glans penis:

   forskin   fourskin   forksin   foreskin

4. Fold of mucous membrane:

   frennulum   freeulum   freenulum   frenulum

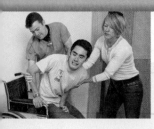

CHAPTER **14** REVIEW MALE REPRODUCTIVE SYSTEM

CHALLENGE YOUR KNOWLEDGE

A. Elements *remain your best clue to understanding the medical term. Write the meaning of the element in the second column, give an example of a medical term containing this element in the third column, and give the meaning of the medical term in the fourth column.*

Element	Meaning of Element	Medical Term Containing This Element	Meaning of the Medical Term
genit	1.	2.	3.
vesic	4.	5.	6.
genesis	7.	8.	9.
andro	10.	11.	12.
didym	13.	14.	15.
testo	16.	17.	18.
pexy	19.	20.	21.
orchi	22.	23.	24.
cele	25.	26.	27.

B. Deconstruct *the following terms into their basic elements. First slash the term; then write the meaning of each element under the line. Know the elements—know the term:*

1. *vaginalis* _____/_____/_____

Definition: _____

2. *cryptorchism* _____/_____/_____

Definition: _____

3. *hydrocele* _____/_____/_____

Definition: _____

4. *transurethral* _____/_____/_____

Definition: _____

5. *vasovasostomy* _____/_____/_____

Definition: _____

6. *hypospadias* _____/_____/_____

Definition: _____

7. *hematuria* _____/_____/_____

Definition: _____

C. Prefixes: *The following terms all have prefixes, which provide additional information about the term. First match the prefix in column 1 with its meaning in column 2. Then construct the new terms to match the definitions in the rest of the exercise. Fill in the blanks.*

_____	**1.** epi	**A.** hidden
_____	**2.** brachy	**B.** excessive
_____	**3.** trans	**C.** across
_____	**4.** crypt	**D.** above
_____	**5.** hyper	**E.** short

6. procedure performed through the urethra _____ / _____ / _____

7. increased number of cells _____ / _____ / _____

8. coiled tube attached to the testis _____ / _____ / _____

9. radiation treatment implanted in tissue _____ / _____ / _____

10. failure of one or both testes to descend _____ / _____ / _____

D. Latin and Greek terms *cannot be further deconstructed into prefix, root, or suffix. You must know them for what they are. Test your knowledge of these terms with this exercise. Match the meaning in column l with the correct medical term in column 2.*

_____	**1.** head of the penis or the clitoris	**A.** prostate
_____	**2.** inability to achieve an erection	**B.** impotence
_____	**3.** major part of a structure	**C.** corpus
_____	**4.** to twist	**D.** gonad
_____	**5.** fold of skin that covers the glans penis	**E.** scrotum
_____	**6.** conveys urine and semen to the outside	**F.** glans
_____	**7.** mature male sex cell	**G.** penis
_____	**8.** organ surrounding the beginning of the urethra	**H.** prepuce
_____	**9.** testis or ovary	**I.** sperm
_____	**10.** sac containing the testes	**J.** torsion

E. Recall and review: *How well do you remember these word elements from a previous chapter? Try to answer without looking back to check. Fill in the chart.*

Element	Type of Element (P, R, CF, or S)	Meaning of Element
con	1.	2.
trophy	3.	4.
myo	5.	6.
pector	7.	8.
ambulat	9.	10.
dys	11.	12.
brachio	13.	14.
lysis	15.	16.
ventr	17.	18.
teno	19.	20.

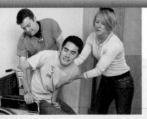

F. Abbreviations: *Test your knowledge of abbreviations in this and previous chapters by circling the correct answer.*

1. A burst of growth at puberty increases:

   RUL   BMR   TTN

2. Which of the following is a diagnosis?

   STD   CT   CXR

3. What should be performed monthly by all men?

   SET   PSA   EPCA-2

4. Increase in the number of cells in an organ:

   TURP   BPH   ED

5. An inability to have an erection is called:

   OME   EMT   ED

6. Which abbreviation would be found in medication orders?

   mL   BEP   NIH

7. A blood test for the prostate:

   PKD   PAP   PSA

8. Used to diagnose an enlarged prostate:

   PKD   CKD   DRE

9. A noncancerous enlargement of the prostate:

   BRCA   BPH   BEP

10. A surgical treatment for prostatic hypertrophy:

    ESWL   TURP   CABG

G. Spelling demons: *The following terms from this and a previous chapter are particularly difficult to spell and pronounce. Correct pronunciation and spelling of medical terms is the mark of an educated professional. Circle the correct spelling, and then check (✓) that you have practiced the pronunciation. Remember that pronunciations are on the Student Online Learning Center (www.mhhe.com/AllanEss2e).*

Pronunciation ✓

1. genitallia   genitalea   genitalia   _____

2. perineal   pereneal   parineal   _____

3. libydo   lybido   libido   _____

4. incontienence   incontinence   incontenance   _____

5. epidydymis   epididymis   epidydimis   _____

6. beenign   benine   benign   _____

7. gomerulonephritis   glomerulonephritis   glomerulonepritis   _____

8. circumcision   cercumcision   cirrcumsion   _____

9. parapymosis   paraphimosis   parapimosis   _____

10. priaprism   preaprism   priapism   _____

H. Critical thinking: *Name and define the two medical terms in this chapter that are applicable to both male and female bodies.*

1. The term is _____ and the definition is _____

_____

2. The term is _____ and the definition is _____

_____

I. Plurals: *You are given the singular form of a term in the first column. Change the term to the plural form in the second column and write a brief definition of the plural term in the third column.*

Term	Plural Form	Definition
sperm	1.	2.
testis	3.	4.
testicle	5.	6.
plexus	7.	8.
varicocele	9.	10.
corpus	11.	12.

J. Translate *the following documentation into layperson's language your patient can understand. Rewrite each sentence, and do not use any abbreviations.*

1. "The IVP and KUB confirmed a renal calculus occluding the ureter, and a dilated pelvis of the right kidney, leading to hydronephrosis."

_____

_____

2. "Mrs. Dobson described many of the symptoms of cystitis: suprapubic and low-back pain and increased frequency of micturition with dysuria and hematuria."

_____

_____

K. Seek and find: *Some terms in this book are defined in context and do not appear in a WAD. Below is a sample of terms and definitions that have appeared in this chapter. Challenge yourself to answer without turning back to check in the book. Fill in the blanks.*

What is another name for:

1. produces no symptoms _____

2. coughing up blood _____

3. vas deferens _____

4. infertile _____

5. foreskin _____

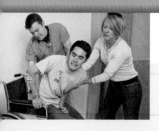

L. Terminology challenge: *This exercise requires recall and analysis. Try to answer the questions without turning back in the book. Fill in the blanks.*

1. Recall this term from a previous chapter: *occult.*

Meaning of occult: _____

Use this term in a sentence: _____

2. What element from this chapter means the same thing?

_____

3. List a term with this element: _____

Use this term in a sentence: _____

_____

Recall other elements from previous chapters that both have the same meaning.

4. In the *language of ophthalmology* there are two examples. Write them here:

_____ means _____.

Example of a term using this element: _____

_____ means _____.

Example of a term using this element: _____

5. In the *language of pulmonology* there are two examples. Write them here:

_____ means _____.

Example of a term using this element: _____

_____ means _____.

Example of a term using this element: _____

M. Terminology challenge: *Use your knowledge of medical language learned in this chapter to answer the following questions.*

1. There are two surgical procedures mentioned in this chapter. The second term reverses the procedure performed in the first term. Can you name them?

The original surgery is:

_____

The surgical procedure that reverses the original surgery is:

_____

2. Name the terms that constitute the pathway of sperm: _____

_____

_____

3. What are some of the classic symptoms of an enlarged prostate? _____

_____

4. Hypogonadism is a deficiency of _____.

N. Chapter challenge: *Circle the correct answer.*

1. What surgical procedure reverses sterility?

   a. vasectomy

   b. orchiopexy

   c. vasovasostomy

   d. prostatectomy

   e. cystectomy

2. Which pair of terms is spelled correctly?

   a. hypogonadism   vassovasostomy

   b. segma   prepuce

   c. frennulum   forskin

   d. errectile   dysfunction

   e. paraphimosis   priapism

STUDY HINT

Immediately cross off any answer you know is not correct. In your remaining choices, there is only one best answer.

3. Undescended testicles present a higher risk for:

   a. infertility

   b. cancer

   c. spermatocele

   d. a and b

   e. a, b, and c

4. What is true of the abbreviations *BPH* and *BEP*?

   a. Both pertain to the male.

   b. Neither one is malignant.

   c. Both can be a diagnosis.

   d. Answers a, b, and c are true.

   e. Only a and c are true.

5. The area between the thighs, extending from the coccyx to the pubis, is the:

   a. periosteum

   b. perineum

   c. symphis pubis

   d. vas deferens

   e. scrotum

6. What can repair *cryptorchism?*

   a. micturition

   b. ochitis

   c. orchiectomy

   d. orchiopexy

   e. spermatogenesis

O. Meet lesson *and chapter objectives and use the medical language of the male reproductive system to answer the following questions.*

1. What body parts comprise the external male genitalia? _____

2. What is the difference between sperm and semen?

   Sperm

   _____

   Semen

   _____

3. What is the function of the _____ _____

4. A viral cause of orchitis is the childhood disease _____.

5. Where are the testes located at birth, and where should they finally be located by age 12 months?

   Birth _____

   Age 12 months _____

6. If a testicular torsion is not quickly repaired, what happens to the testis? _____

   _____

   _____

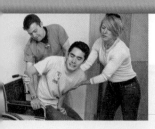

P. **Case Report challenge:** *Now that you are more comfortable with the terms in this chapter, you can apply that knowledge and briefly answer the questions about the Case Report. If you read the report through and underline all the medical terminology, this will make it easier to answer the questions.*

CASE REPORT 14.1

YOU ARE an EMT-P working in the Emergency Department at Fulwood Medical Center.

YOU ARE COMMUNICATING WITH

Joseph Davis, a 17-year-old high school senior, who has been brought in by his mother at 0400 hrs. He is complaining of (c/o) sudden onset of pain in his left testicle, which began 3 hours earlier and woke him up. The pain is intense and has made him vomit. VS: T 99.2°F, P 88, R 15, BP 130/70. An examination reveals his left testicle to be enlarged, warm, and tender. His abdomen is normal to palpation.

At your request, Dr. Helinski, the emergency physician on duty, examines Joseph immediately. He diagnoses a torsion of the patient's left testicle. Joseph is healthy otherwise. Joseph Davis presented with typical symptoms and signs of testicular torsion. The affected testis rapidly became painful, tender, swollen, and inflamed.

Dr. Helinski has referred Joseph Davis to a surgeon to repair his condition, and it is your duty to obtain preapproval for the surgery from the patient's insurance company. You must be prepared to furnish answers to the questions the insurance company will ask.

You make the telephone call to the 800 number listed on the patient's insurance card for preauthorization of hospitalization or surgery. You have answered all the usual insurance questions regarding the patient's subscriber ID number, group number, name of policyholder, and so on. The insurance company needs answers to the following clinical questions in order to preapprove the surgery.

Use your knowledge of the male reproductive system to answer the following questions for the insurance company representative.

1. What is the patient's diagnosis? _____

2. Is this condition the result of an accident? _____

3. What are Joseph's vital signs? _____

4. Will the surgeon operate on one or both testicles? _____

5. Has Joseph ever been treated for this condition in the past? _____

6. Does Joseph have any other current health problems? _____

Emergency surgery was performed, and the testis and cord were manually untwisted through an incision in the scrotum.
The testis was stitched to surrounding tissues to prevent a recurrence.

On the basis of your answers, the insurance company representative has preapproved the surgery and one overnight stay in the hospital for the patient. Be sure to write down in the patient's chart the preapproval reference number, the name of the person who gave it to you, and the date and time of your conversation.

These questions pertain to the clinical (as opposed to the insurance) aspects of the Case Report.

7. What does *sudden onset* mean? _____

_____

8. Is Joseph in the Emergency Department at 4 a.m. or 4 p.m.? _____

9. What part of Joseph's physical examination is normal? _____

10. What is the medical term for the procedure that was performed to alleviate the patient's pain? _____

11. Briefly describe how this procedure was performed. _____

_____

12. What was done during the surgery to prevent a recurrence of this condition for Joseph? _____

_____

CHAPTER 14 REVIEW

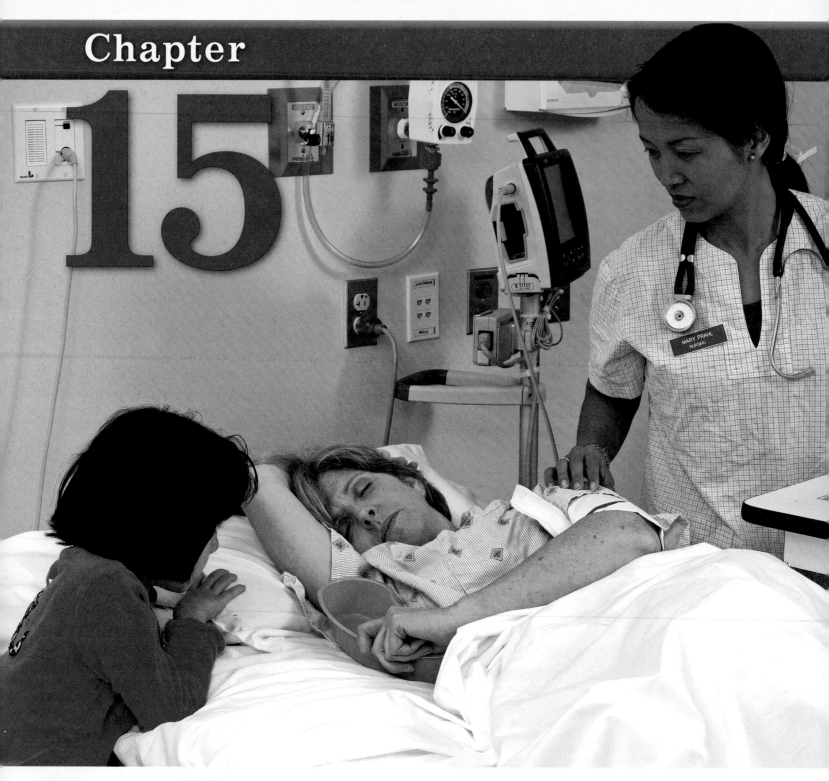

Chapter 15

THE FEMALE REPRODUCTIVE SYSTEM

The Essentials of the Languages of Gynecology and Obstetrics

YOU ARE

> . . . a licensed practical nurse (LPN) working in the Emergency Department at Fulwood Medical Center.

YOU ARE COMMUNICATING WITH

> . . . Ms. Lara Baker, a 32-year-old single mother who works in the billing department of the medical center. You have been asked to take her vital signs. For the past couple of days, she has had muscle aches and a feeling of general uneasiness that she thought were due to her heavy menstrual period. In the past 3 hours, she has developed a severe headache with nausea and vomiting. A diffuse rash over her trunk that looks like sunburn is now spreading to her upper arms and thighs. VS: T 104.2°F, P 120 and irregular, R 20, BP 86/50. As you took her VS, you noted that she did not seem to understand where she was. She was unable to pass a urine specimen. For this patient, the treatment she receives in the next few minutes is vital for her survival. You have your supervising nurse and the emergency physician come to see her immediately. As you participate in this patient's care, clear communication among the team members is essential.

The health professionals involved in the diagnosis and treatment of problems with the female reproductive system include:

- **Gynecologists** are physicians who are specialists in diseases of the female reproductive tract.

- **Obstetricians** are physicians who are specialists in the care of women during pregnancy and childbirth.

- **Neonatologists** are physicians who are pediatric subspecialists in disorders of the newborn, particularly ill or premature infants.

- **Perinatologists** are physicians who are obstetric subspecialists in the care of the mother and fetus who are at higher-than-normal risk for complications.

- **Certified midwives/nurse-midwives** are independent practitioners who provide care to mothers during pregnancy, delivery, and birth, and to mothers and newborn infants for 6 weeks after birth.

- **Obstetrical–gynecological nurse practitioners** are registered nurses who have acquired skills in the management of health and illness for women throughout their life cycle.

LEARNING OUTCOMES

As a health care professional in the area of gynecology and obstetrics, it's essential that you become familiar with not only the functions and structures of the female reproductive system, but also with its associated medical terminology. In order to provide patients with the best possible care, you will need to be able to:

LO 15.1 Apply the languages of gynecology and obstetrics to the structures and functions of the female reproductive system.

LO 15.2 Comprehend, analyze, spell, and write the medical terms of gynecology and obstetrics as they relate to the female reproductive system.

LO 15.3 Recognize and pronounce the medical terms of gynecology and obstetrics as they relate to the female reproductive system.

LO 15.4 Use correct medical terminology to describe common disorders of the female reproductive system.

LO 15.5 Specify the correct medical terminology for the stages of embryonic development, the implantation of the embryo in the uterus, and fetal development.

LO 15.6 Recognize and use appropriately the medical terminology for the functions of the placenta and for childbirth.

LO 15.7 Discuss some of the most common problems of fetal development and childbirth using correct medical terminology.

LO 15.8 Apply correct medical terminology to the structure and functions of the breast and its common disorders.

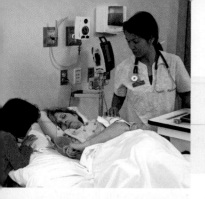

LESSON 15.1

External Genitalia and Vagina

*The female reproductive system is dormant or undeveloped until puberty, when the **ovaries** begin to secrete significant amounts of the sex hormones **estrogen** and **progesterone**. Then, the external genitalia become more prominent, pubic hair develops, the **vagina** becomes lubricated, and the breasts begin to enlarge. The information in this lesson will enable you to use correct medical terminology to:*

15.1.1 Describe the essential structures and functions of the external genitalia, vagina, and accessory glands.

15.1.2 Describe common disorders of the external genitalia and vagina.

▶ **FIGURE 15.1**
Female Perineum and Vulva.
(a) Surface anatomy.
(b) Subcutaneous structures.

External Genitalia (LO 15.1, 15.2, and 15.3)

The female external genitalia occupy most of the perineum and are collectively called the **vulva.** The structures of the vulva *(Figure 15.1a)* include the:

- **Mons pubis,** a mound of skin and adipose or fatty tissue overlying the symphysis pubis.
- **Labia majora,** a pair of thick folds of skin, connective tissue, and adipose tissue.
- **Labia minora,** a pair of thin folds of hairless skin immediately internal to the labia majora. Anteriorly, the labia minora join together to form the prepuce (hood) of the **clitoris**. The clitoris is a small erectile body capped with a glans. Posteriorly, these structures merge with the labia majora.
- **Vestibule,** the area enclosed by the labia minora. It contains the urinary and vaginal openings.

Deep into the labia majora on each side of the vaginal orifice (opening) is a pea-sized greater vestibular **(Bartholin)** gland *(Figure 15.1b)*. These glands secrete mucus to lubricate the vulva and vagina, and this secretion increases during sexual intercourse.

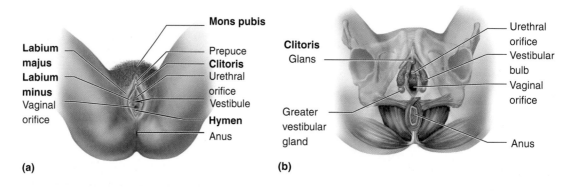

(a)   (b)

Vagina (LO 15.1, 15.2, and 15.3)

The **vagina,** or birth canal, is a fibromuscular tube that measures 4 to 5 inches long. It connects the vulva with the uterus *(Figure 15.2)* and has three main functions:

- To discharge menstrual fluid;
- To receive the penis and semen; and
- To deliver a baby.

The vagina is located between the rectum and the urethra. The urethra is embedded in the anterior wall of the vagina.

At its posterior end, the vagina extends beyond the **cervix** of the uterus and forms arch-shaped blind spaces called the anterior and posterior **fornices.** The lower end of the vagina contains numerous crosswise folds. These folds project into the vaginal opening to form the **hymen,** which stretches across the opening. The hymen contains one or two openings to allow menstrual fluid to escape.

▶ **FIGURE 15.2**
Female Reproductive Organs.

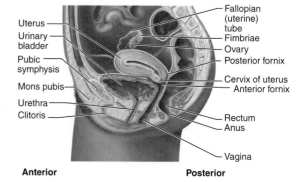

Word	Pronunciation		Elements	Definition
cervix cervical (adj) (Note: This term also means pertaining to the neck region.)	**SER**-viks **SER**-vih-kal	S/ R/	Latin *neck* -al *pertaining to* cervic- *neck*	Lower part of the uterus Pertaining to the cervix
clitoris	**KLIT**-oh-ris		Greek *clitoris*	Erectile organ of the vulva
estrogen	**ES**-troh-jen	S/ R/CF	-gen *produce* estr/o *woman*	Generic term for hormones that stimulate female secondary sex characteristics
fornix fornices (pl)	**FOR**-niks **FOR** nih-seez		Latin *a vault*	Arch-shaped, blind-ended part of the vagina behind and around the cervix
gynecology (GYN) gynecologist gynecologic (adj)	guy-nih-**KOL**-oh-jee guy-nih-**KOL**-oh-jist **GUY**-nih-koh-**LOJ**-ik	S/ R/CF S/ S/ R/CF R/	-logy *study of* gynec/o- *woman, female* -logist *one who studies, specialist* -ic *pertaining to* gynec/o- *woman, female* -log- *to study*	Medical specialty of diseases of the female reproductive tract Specialist in gynecology Pertaining to gynecology
hymen	**HIGH**-men		Greek *membrane*	Thin membrane partly occluding the vaginal orifice
labium labia (pl)	**LAY**-bee-um **LAY**-bee-ah		Greek *lip*	Fold of the vulva
majus majora (pl)	**MAY**-jus **MAY**-jora		Latin *greater*	Bigger or greater; e.g., the labia majora
minus minora (pl)	**MY**-nus **MY**-nora		Latin *smaller*	Smaller or lesser; e.g., the labia minora
mons pubis	MONZ **PYU**-bis		mons, Latin *mountain* pubis, Latin *pubic bone*	Fleshy pad with pubic hair, overlying the pubic bone
ovary ovaries (pl) ovarian (adj)	**OH**-vah-ree **OH**-vah-rees oh-**VAIR**-ee-an	S/ R/	Latin *egg* -an *pertaining to* ovari- *ovary*	One of the paired female reproductive glands Pertaining to the ovary(ies)
progesterone (Note: 2 suffixes)	pro-**JESS**-ter-own	S/ S/ P/ R/	-one *hormone, chemical substance* -er- *agent, one who does* pro- *before* -gest- *pregnancy*	Hormone that prepares the uterus for pregnancy
vagina vaginal (adj)	vah-**JIE**-nah **VAJ**-ih-nal	S/ R/	Latin *sheath* -al *pertaining to* vagin- *vagina*	The female genital canal extending from the uterus to the vulva Pertaining to the vagina
vulva vulvar (adj)	**VUL**-vah **VUL**-var	S/ R/	Latin *a wrapper or covering* -ar *pertaining to* vulv- *vulva*	Female external genitalia Pertaining to the vulva

EXERCISE

A. Review *the Case Report on the opening spread before answering the questions.*

1. When Ms. Baker presented to the ED, what was her temperature? _____

2. What indicates that Ms. Baker was in a confused state of mind? _____

3. What is a "diffuse" rash? _____

4. What urinary symptom was Ms. Baker having? _____

5. List the rest of Ms. Baker's symptoms. _____

6. Is this a life-threatening emergency? _____

7. Which symptoms did Ms. Baker believe were caused by her heavy menstrual period? _____

_____

Disorders of the Vulva and Vagina (LO 15.1, 15.2, 15.3, and 15.4)

- Bacterial vaginosis is associated with increased risk of gonorrhea and HIV infection.

- Of all adult women, 75% have at least one genital yeast infection in their lifetimes.

- Ten million office visits annually are for vulvodynia.

Bacterial vaginosis is the most common cause of **vaginitis** in women of childbearing age. The main symptom is an abnormal vaginal discharge with a fishlike odor. With bacterial vaginosis, different types of invading bacteria outnumber the vagina's normal bacteria. This disorder is diagnosed by a lab exam of a vaginal swab specimen, and it is treated with antibiotics.

Toxic shock syndrome is a life-threatening illness caused by toxins (poisons) circulating in the bloodstream. Bacteria in the vagina are encouraged to grow by the presence of a superabsorbent **tampon** that is not changed frequently *(see Case Report 15.1)*. These bacteria produce toxins that are absorbed into the bloodstream. Other risk factors for toxic shock syndrome include skin wounds and surgery.

CASE REPORT 15.1 (CONTINUED)

Ms. Lara Baker presented to the Emergency Department with toxic shock syndrome. Because of her heavy period, she was using a superabsorbent tampon. She was admitted to intensive care. The tampon was removed and cultured. IV fluids and antibiotics were administered. Her kidney and liver functions were monitored. The causative organism was *Staphylococcus aureus*. She recovered well but had a second episode 6 months later.

Vulvovaginal candidiasis is a common cause of genital itching or burning with a "cottage-cheese" vaginal discharge. It is caused by an overgrowth of the yeast fungus ***Candida*** and can occur after taking antibiotics. Treatment is with antifungal drugs.

Vulvovaginitis can be caused by allergic and irritative agents found in vaginal hygiene products, spermicides, detergents, and synthetic underwear.

Vulvodynia is a chronic, severe pain around the vaginal orifice, which feels raw. Painful intercourse (**dyspareunia**) is common. The vulva may look normal or be slightly swollen. The etiology (cause) is unknown. Treatment varies from local anesthetics and creams to biofeedback therapy with exercises for the pelvic floor muscles. Surgical removal of the affected area (**vestibulectomy**) has been tried with variable results.

Vaginal cancers are uncommon, comprising only 1% to 2% of gynecologic malignancies. They can be effectively treated with surgery and radiation therapy.

Word	Pronunciation	Elements		Definition
dyspareunia	dis-pah-**RUE**-nee-ah	S/ P/ R/	-ia *condition* dys- *painful* -pareun- *lying beside, sexual intercourse*	Pain during sexual intercourse
tampon	**TAM**-pon		French *plug*	Plug or pack in a cavity to absorb or stop bleeding
vaginosis	vah-jih-**NOH**-sis	S/ R/	-osis *condition* vagin- *vagina*	A disease of the vagina
vaginitis	vah-jih-**NIE**-tis	S/	-itis *inflammation*	Inflammation of the vagina
vestibulectomy	ves tib-you-**LEK**-toe-me	S/ R/	-ectomy *surgical excision* vestibul- *entrance*	Surgical excision of the vulva
vulvodynia	vul-voh-**DIN**-ee-uh	S/ R/CF	-dynia *pain* vulv/o- *vulva*	Chronic vulvar pain
vulvovaginal	**VUL**-voh-**VAJ**-ih-nal	S/ R/CF R/	-al *pertaining to* vulv/o- *vulva* -vagin- *vagina*	Pertaining to the vulva and vagina
vulvovaginitis	**VUL**-voh-vaj-ih-**NIE**-tis	S/	-itis *inflammation*	Inflammation of the vulva and vagina

EXERCISES

A. Review *the Case Report on this spread before answering the questions.*

1. What term in the diagnosis means *poison?* _____

2. Why was Ms. Baker admitted to the ICU? _____

3. Which other body systems could be affected by her toxic shock syndrome? _____

_____

4. Is *Staphylococcus aureus* a viral or bacterial infection? _____

5. What term in the Case Report is your clue to the answer in #4? _____

6. What specific type of drug was administered by IV? _____

7. Did Ms. Baker have a transfusion or an infusion? _____

8. What harbored the staph infection? _____

9. How can toxic shock syndrome be prevented? _____

B. Suffixes in this WAD *box have appeared in many terms in previous chapters. Slash the medical term in the first column into elements to isolate the suffix. Define the meaning of the suffix, define the term in which it appears, write another term with a similar ending, and define that term. Fill in the chart.*

Medical Term from WAD Above	Meaning of Suffix	Meaning of this Medical Term	Term from a Previous Chapter, with the Same Suffix	Meaning of that Medical Term
dyspareunia	1	2	3.	4.
vaginosis	5.	6.	7.	8.
vestibulectomy	9.	10.	11.	12.
vulvovaginal	13.	14.	15.	16.
vulvovaginitis	17.	18.	19.	20.

LESSON 15.1 Sexually Transmitted Diseases (STDs) (LO 15.1, 15.2, 15.3, and 15.4)

According to the Centers for Disease Control (**CDC**), 15 million new cases of sexually transmitted diseases (**STDs**) are reported annually in the United States. Adolescents and young adults have the greatest risk of contracting STDs.

Chlamydia is known as the "silent" disease because up to 75% of infected women and men have no symptoms. When there are signs, a vaginal or penile discharge and irritation with dysuria (difficult or painful urination) are common. Highly accurate urine tests and DNA probes are available for diagnosis. Treatment is with oral antibiotics. If left untreated, chlamydia can spread higher into the female reproductive tract and cause **pelvic inflammatory disease (PID)**. It can also be passed on to a newborn during childbirth and cause eye infections or pneumonia. For this reason, newborns receive antibiotic eyedrops.

Trichomoniasis ("trich") is caused by the parasite *Trichomonas vaginalis*. In women, it can produce a frothy yellow-green vaginal discharge with irritation and itching of the vulva. Because it is a "ping-pong" infection that goes back and forth between partners, both individuals should be treated.

Gonorrhea is spread by unprotected sex and can be passed on to a baby in childbirth, causing a serious eye infection. As with chlamydia, newborns receive antibiotic eyedrops to prevent eye infections from gonorrhea. Symptoms include a vaginal discharge, bleeding, and dysuria. Lab testing on a swab taken from the surface of the infected area can confirm the diagnosis. DNA probes are also available. Gonorrhea can be treated with a single dose of an antibiotic. However, it is developing resistance to antibiotics.

Syphilis is transmitted sexually and can spread through the bloodstream to every organ in the body. **Primary syphilis** begins 10 to 90 days after infection as an ulcer or **chancre** at the infection site. Four to ten weeks later, if the primary syphilis is not treated, **secondary syphilis** appears as a rash on the palms of the hands and the soles of the feet. Swollen glands and muscle and joint pain accompany the rash. **Tertiary syphilis** can occur years after the primary infection and cause permanent damage to the brain, with dementia.

Genital herpes simplex is a disease caused by the virus herpes simplex (**HSV2**). It manifests with painful genital sores, which can recur throughout life. There is no cure for genital herpes. Antiviral medications can provide a clinical benefit by limiting the **replication** of the virus.

Human papilloma virus (HPV) causes genital warts in both men and women *(Figure 15.3)*. HPV can also cause changes to the cells in the cervix. Some strains of the virus can increase a woman's risk for cervical cancer. More than 90% of abnormal **Pap** smears are caused by HPV infections. A vaccine is available that can prevent lasting infections with strains that cause cervical cancers and genital warts. The vaccine can be given to females aged 9 to 26, before they are sexually active. The vaccine can be given to males aged 9 to 26 years to reduce the likelihood of acquiring genital warts.

Molluscum contagiosum is a virus that can be sexually transmitted and produces small, shiny bumps that contain a milky-white fluid *(Figure 15.4)*. They can disappear and reappear anywhere on the body.

Human immunodeficiency virus (HIV) is a virus that attacks the immune system and usually leads to **acquired immune deficiency syndrome (AIDS)**. HIV is carried in body fluids and transmitted during unprotected sex. Sharing needles can spread the virus. The virus can also pass from an infected pregnant woman to her unborn child, so she must take medications to protect the baby.

There is no cure for HIV or AIDS, but combinations of anti-HIV medications can be taken to stop the **replication** of the virus in the cells of the body, and to stop the progression of the disease. However, the development of resistance to the drugs is a problem.

HIV damages the immune system, allowing infections to develop that the body would normally cope with easily. These are **opportunistic infections** and include herpes simplex, candidiasis, syphilis, and tuberculosis (**TB**).

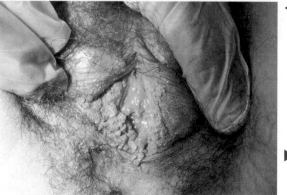

◀ **FIGURE 15.3**
HPV in the Female Vulva.

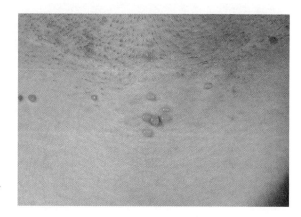

▶ **FIGURE 15.4**
Molluscum Contagiosum.

S = Suffix   P = Prefix   R = Root   R/CF= Combining Form

Word	Pronunciation	Elements		Definition
acquired immunodeficiency syndrome (AIDS)	ah-KWIRED IM-you-noh-dee-FISH-en-see	S/ R/CF R/	acquired, Latin *obtain* -ency *condition* immun/o- *immune response* -defici- *lacking, inadequate*	Infection with the HIV virus
	SIN-drohm	P/ R/	syn- *together* -drome *running*	Combination of signs and symptoms associated with a particular disease process
chancre	SHAN-ker		Latin *cancer*	Primary lesion of syphilis
chlamydia	klah-MID-ee-ah		Latin *cloak*	An STD caused by infection with *Chlamydia*, a species of bacteria
condom	KON-dom		Old English *sheath or cover*	A sheath or cover for the penis or vagina to prevent conception and infection
gonorrhea	gon-oh-REE-ah	R/ R/CF	-rrhea *flow, discharge* gon/o- *seed*	Specific contagious sexually transmitted infection
human immunodeficiency virus (HIV)	HYU-man IM-you-noh-dee-FISH-en-see VIE-rus	R/ S/ R/CF R/	human *human being* -ency *condition* immun/o- *immune response* -defici- *lacking, inadequate* virus, Latin *poison*	Etiologic agent of acquired immunodeficiency syndrome (AIDS)
human papilloma virus (HPV)	HYU-man pap-ih-LOW-mah VIE-rus	R/ S/ R/	human *human being* -oma *tumor* papill- *pimple* virus, Latin *poison*	Causes warts on the skin and genitalia and can increase the risk for cervical cancer
molluscum contagiosum (Note: "s" in "sum" added to enable word to flow) (modern word contagious)	moh LUS kum kon-TAY-jee-oh-sum	S/ R/ R/CF	-um *structure* mollusc- *soft* contagi/o- *transmissible by contact*	STD caused by a virus
opportunistic infection (Note: 2 suffixes)	OP-or-tyu-NIS-tik in-FEK-shun	S/ S/ R/	-ic *pertaining to* -ist- *agent, specialist* opportun- *take advantage of*	An infection that causes disease when the immune system is compromised for other reasons
replication	rep-lih-KAY-shun	S/ R/	-ation *process of* replic- *reply*	Reproduction to produce an exact copy
syphilis	SIF-ih-lis		Principal character in a Latin poem	Sexually transmitted disease caused by a spirochete
Trichomonas	trik-oh-MOH-nas	R/CF R/	trich/o- *hair* -monas *single unit*	A parasite causing an STD
trichomoniasis	TRIK-oh-moh-NIE-ah-sis	S/ R/	-iasis *condition* -mon- *single*	Infection with *Trichomonas vaginalis*

EXERCISE

A. Construct *the correct medical term to match the definition that is given. Write the appropriate* **element on** *the line and the* **meaning** *of the element* **below** *the line.*

1. Infection with *Trichomonas* _____ / _____ / _____

2. Reproduction of an exact copy _____ / _____ / _____

3. Infection that takes advantage of a compromised immune system

_____ / _____ / _____

4. Contagious STD infection _____ / _____ / _____

5. Combination of signs and symptoms associated with a particular disease process

_____ / _____ / _____

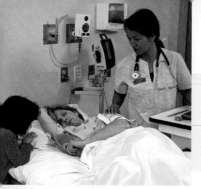

LESSON 15.2

Ovaries, Fallopian (Uterine) Tubes, and Uterus

CASE REPORT 15.2

YOU ARE

. . . a certified health education specialist **(CHES)** employed by Fulwood Medical Center.

YOU ARE COMMUNICATING WITH

. . . Ms. Claire Marcos, a 21-year-old student referred to you by Anna Rusak, MD, a gynecologist. Ms. Marcos has been diagnosed with polycystic ovarian syndrome **(PCOS)**, and your task is to develop a program of self-care as part of her overall plan of therapy. From her medical record, you see that she presented with irregular, often missed **menstrual** periods since the beginning of puberty, persistent acne, a loss of hair from the front of her scalp, and an inability to control her weight. She is 5 feet 4 inches tall and weighs 150 pounds. You are expected to counsel her about her self-care program involving exercise, diet, and the use of birth control medications.

Anatomy of the Female Reproductive Tract
(LO 15.1, 15.2, and 15.3)

Ovaries (LO 15.1, 15.2, and 15.3)

Each **ovary** is an almond-shaped organ about 1 inch long and ½ inch in diameter. The ovaries are held in place by ligaments that attach them to the pelvic wall and uterus. The ovaries' main functions are to:

- produce and release eggs; and
- secrete hormones that affect puberty, menstruation, and pregnancy.

S = Suffix   P = Prefix   R = Root   R/CF= Combining Form

Word	Pronunciation		Elements	Definition
fallopian tubes (also called *uterine tubes*)	fah-**LOW**-pee-an		Gabrielle Fallopio, Italian anatomist, 1523–1562	Uterine tubes connected to the fundus of the uterus
menses (noun) **menstruation** (noun)	**MEN**-seez men-stru-**AY**-shun	S/ R/CF	Latin *month* -ation *process* menstr/u- *menses*	Monthly uterine bleeding Same as *menses*
menstruate (verb)	**MEN**-stru-ate	S/	-ate *composed of, pertaining to*	Act of menstruation
menstrual (adj)	**MEN**-stru-al	S/	-al *pertaining to*	Pertaining to menstruation
ovum **ova** (pl)	**OH**-vum **OH**-vah		Latin *egg*	Egg

EXERCISES

A. Review *the Case Report on this spread before answering the questions.*

1. In her past medical history, what symptom did Ms. Marcos have relating to her menstrual period? _____

2. What other symptoms does she have now? _____

3. What is Ms. Marcos being counseled about in relation to her condition? _____

4. What has been prescribed for Ms. Marcos? _____

5. What is the diagnosis for this patient? _____

B. Demonstrate *your knowledge of this chapter's medical vocabulary and circle the correct answer.*

1. Which term in the WAD has an element meaning *menses?*

   menstruate   fallopian   ova

2. Which term in the WAD refers to *egg?*

   menses   fallopian   ova

3. What other term means the same thing as *menses?*

   uterine   fallopian   menstruation

4. The plural of ovum is

   oval   oveas   ova

5. What is another name for the fallopian tubes?

   urinary tubes   uterine tubes   ureteral tubes

C. Meet lesson *and chapter objectives by describing the structure and functions of an ovary in the following questions.*

1. Structure:
_____
_____

2. Functions:
_____
_____

Anatomy of the Female Reproductive Tract *(continued)*

Fallopian (Uterine) Tubes
(LO 15.1, 15.2, and 15.3)

Each **fallopian tube** is a canal about 4 inches long that extends from the uterus and opens to the abdominal cavity near an ovary. At the ovarian end, the outer third of the tube flares out into finger-like folds, each of which is called a **fimbria.** At ovulation, the **fimbriae** enclose the ovary *(Figure 15.5).* The tubes' main functions are to enable sperm and eggs to meet and fertilize.

Uterus (LO 15.1, 15.2, and 15.3)

The **uterus** is a thick-walled, muscular organ in the pelvic cavity. The main functions of the uterus are to cradle and nourish the fetus from conception to birth, and to produce a woman's monthly menstrual flow (period). Anatomically, the uterus is divided into these three regions:

- The **fundus** is the broad, curved upper region between the lateral attachments of the fallopian (uterine) tubes;

- The **body** is the midportion; and

- The **cervix** is the cylindrical inferior portion that projects into the vagina.

The inner lining of the uterus is called the **endometrium;** the muscular layer is called the **myometrium.** The lower end of the uterine cavity communicates with the vagina through the cervical canal that has an external **os** (opening) into the vagina.

Ovarian Hormones
(LO 15.1, 15.2, and 15.3)

The ovaries of the sexually mature female secrete the hormones estrogen and progesterone.

Estrogens are produced in the ovarian follicles and their sexual functions are to:

1. Convert girls into sexually mature women through **thelarche, pubarche,** and **menarche;**

2. Regulate the menstrual cycle; and

3. Be involved in pregnancy when it occurs.

Progesterone is produced by the ovary's corpus luteum and also by the adrenal glands *(see Chapter 12).* Its sexual functions are to:

1. Prepare the lining (endometrium) of the uterus for implantation of the egg *(Figure 15.5);*

2. Inhibit lactation during pregnancy; and

3. Produce menstrual bleeding if pregnancy does not occur.

The ovaries also secrete small amounts of androgens, which are male hormones.

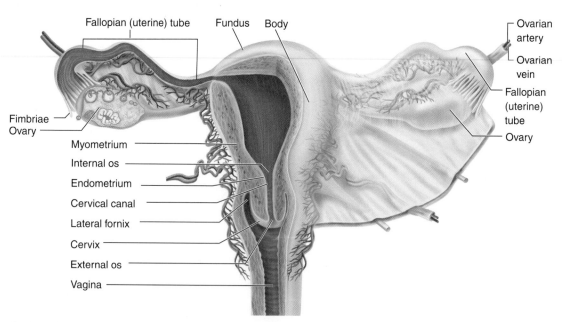

▲ **FIGURE 15.5**
Female Reproductive Tract.

Word	Pronunciation	Elements		Definition
endometrium	en-doh-**ME**-tree-um	S/ P/ R/CF	-um *tissue* endo- *within, inside* -metr/i- *uterus*	Inner lining of the uterus
endometrial (adj)	en-doh-**ME**-tree-al	S/	-al *pertaining to*	Pertaining to the inner lining of the uterus
fallopian tubes (also called *uterine tubes*)	fah-**LOW**-pee-an		Gabrielle Fallopio, Italian anatomist, 1523–1562	Uterine tubes connected to the fundus of the uterus
fimbria fimbriae (pl)	**FIM**-bree-ah **FIM**-bree-ee		Latin *fringe*	Fringelike structure
fundus	**FUN**-dus		Latin *bottom*	The upper, rounded top of the uterus above the openings of the fallopian tubes
menarche	meh-**NAR**-key	S/ R/	-arche *beginning* men- *month*	First menstrual period
myometrium	my-oh-**MEE**-tree-um	S/ R/CF R/CF	-um *tissue* my/o- *muscle* -metr/i- *uterus*	Muscle wall of the uterus
os	OS		Latin *mouth*	Opening into a canal; e.g., the cervix
pubarche	pyu-**BAR**-key	S/ R/	-arche *beginning* pub- *pubis*	Onset of development of pubic and axillary hair
thelarche	thee-**LAR**-key	S/ R/	-arche *beginning* thel- *breast, nipple*	Onset of breast development
uterus uterine (adj)	**YOU**-ter-us **YOU**-ter-ine	S/ R/	Latin *womb* -ine *pertaining to* uter- *uterus*	Organ in which an egg develops into a fetus Pertaining to the uterus

EXERCISES

A. Meet lesson and chapter objectives *with the language of the female reproductive system. Fill in the blanks.*

1. Which body cavity contains the uterus? _____

2. What is the main function of the fallopian tubes? _____

3. What two functions does the uterus have? _____

_____

4. What does the os open into? _____

5. Where are estrogens produced? _____

6. Name one function of progesterone. _____

B. Choose *the correct pair of terms related to the question. Circle the correct answer.*

1. Which two terms are structures inside the uterus?

    a. myocardium and pericardium   **d.** myometrium and endometrium

    b. perineum and periosteum   **e.** sphincter and meatus

    c. endocardium and myocardium

2. Name the regions of the uterus:

    a. fundus and os   **d.** hypogastric, cervical and fundus

    b. fundus, os and body   **e.** none of these is correct

    c. fundus, cervix and body

3. Which pair of terms is associated with the production of progesterone?

    a. pubarche and menarche   **d.** fornix and myometrium

    b. fundus and cervix   **e.** fimbriae and urethra

    c. adrenal glands and corpus luteum

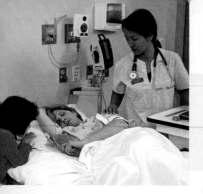

Disorders of the Female Reproductive Tract

OBJECTIVES

In order to care for a female patient who is experiencing reproductive tract disorders, you will need to effectively communicate with the patient, and with any of the other health care professionals involved in her case. The information provided in this lesson will enable you to use correct medical terminology to:

15.3.1 Describe common disorders of the ovaries, fallopian tubes, and uterus.

15.3.2 Identify the causes of and treatments for infertility.

15.3.3 Discuss different methods of contraception and their failure rates.

KEYNOTES

- The peak incidence of ovarian cancer is in the 50- and 60-year age groups.

- Oral contraceptives are 80% to 90% effective in relieving symptoms of PMS.

ABBREVIATIONS

GYN — gynecology

PCOS — polycystic ovarian syndrome

PMS — premenstrual syndrome

CASE REPORT 15.2 (CONTINUED)

When Ms. Claire Marcos first presented in the gynecology clinic, Dr. Rusak examined her abdomen and pelvis. The doctor was able to palpate both enlarged ovaries on vaginal examination. A vaginal ultrasound scan showed multiple small cysts in each ovary. Dr. Rusack diagnosed Ms. Marcos with polycystic ovarian syndrome, and prescribed birth control pills because they contain estrogen and progesterone. The pills can correct the hormone imbalance, regulate Ms. Marcos' menses, and lower the level of testosterone to diminish her acne and hair loss problems.

Disorders of the Ovaries (LO 15.1, 15.2, 15.3, and 15.4)

Ovarian Cysts (LO 15.1, 15.2, 15.3, and 15.4)

Polycystic ovarian syndrome (PCOS), in which multiple follicular cysts form in both ovaries *(Figure 15.6),* is the disorder Ms. Marcos presented with. The repeated cyst formation prevents any eggs from maturing or being released, so ovulation does not occur and progesterone is not produced. Without progesterone, a female's menstrual cycle is irregular or absent.

Ovarian cysts produce androgens, which prevent ovulation and produce acne, the male-pattern hair loss from the front of the scalp, and weight gain. Women with PCOS are also at increased risk for endometrial cancer, type 2 diabetes, high blood cholesterol, hypertension, and heart disease.

Ovarian cancer is the second most common gynecologic cancer after endometrial cancer. However, ovarian cancer accounts for more deaths than any other gynecologic cancer. Symptoms develop late in the disease process and are usually vague. Treatment is to surgically remove the tumor and administer chemotherapy. The five-year survival rate is below 20%.

Primary amenorrhea occurs when a girl has not menstruated by age 16. This can occur with or without other signs of puberty.

Causes of primary amenorrhea include: drastic weight loss from malnutrition, dieting, bulimia, or anorexia nervosa; extreme exercise, as in some young gymnasts.; extreme obesity; and chronic illness. Treatment is directed at the basic cause.

Secondary amenorrhea occurs when a woman who has menstruated normally misses three or more periods in a row and she is not pregnant or in her **menopause.**

The causes of secondary amenorrhea include: ovarian disorders, such as polycystic ovarian syndrome; excessive weight loss, low body fat percentage (e.g., as in gymnasts), or excessive exercise (e.g., as in marathon runners); and certain drugs, including antidepressants.

Primary dysmenorrhea, or **premenstrual syndrome (PMS)** refers to pain or discomfort associated with menstruation. The pain often begins 1 or 2 days before menses, peaks on the first day, and then slowly subsides.

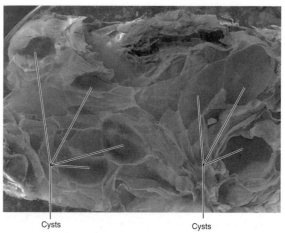

Cysts   Cysts

▲ **FIGURE 15.6**
Polycystic Ovary.

S = Suffix   P = Prefix   R = Root   R/CF= Combining Form

Word	Pronunciation	Elements		Definition
amenorrhea	a-men-oh-**REE**-ah	R/ P/ R/CF	-rrhea *flow, discharge* a- *without* -men/o- *menses*	Absence or abnormal cessation of menstrual flow
dysmenorrhea	dis-men-oh-**REE**-ah	R/ P/ R/CF	-rrhea *flow, discharge* dys- *painful or difficult* men/o- *menses*	Painful and difficult menstruation
menopause (Note: *This term has no suffix, only a combining form and root.*)	**MEN**-oh-paws	R/ R/CF	-pause *cessation* men/o- *menses*	Permanent ending of menstrual periods
menopausal (adj)	**MEN**-oh-paws-al	S/	-al *pertaining to*	Pertaining to the menopause
premenstrual	pree-**MEN**-stru-al	S/ P/ R/	-al *pertaining to* pre- *before* -menstru- *menses*	Pertaining to the time immediately before the menses
primary	**PRY**-mah-ree		Latin *first*	The first disease or symptom, after which others may occur as complications
secondary	**SEK**-ond-ah-ree		Latin *following or second*	Diseases or symptoms following a primary disease or symptom

EXERCISES

A. Review *the Case Report on this spread before answering the questions.*

1. What body cavity is formed by the abdomen and pelvis? _____

2. Explain the phrase *able to palpate*. _____

3. What was found on physical examination by the doctor? _____

4. What is the hormone content in Ms. Marcos' birth control pills? _____

5. What will her prescribed pills correct? _____

6. What is the final diagnosis for Ms. Marcos? _____

B. Apply your knowledge *of the medical terminology for the female reproductive system by choosing the correct answer to each of the following questions. Circle the best choice.*

1. The permanent ending of menstrual periods is:

   menopause   dysmenorrhea   amenorrhea

2. *Premenstrual* happens:

   before menses   after menses   in the middle of menses

3. The gynecologic malignancy that accounts for the most deaths is:

   cervical cancer   breast cancer   ovarian cancer

4. Pick the term that contains a prefix, root, and suffix:

   menopause   secondary   premenstrual

5. In the medical term *dysmenorrhea,* the prefix *dys* means:

   without   first   painful

• Residual scarring of the fallopian tube from salpingitis is a common cause of infertility.

ABBREVIATION

FUS   focused ultrasound surgery

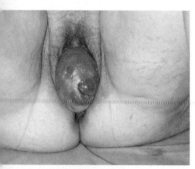

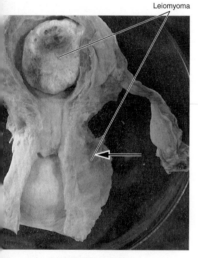

▲ **FIGURE 15.7**
Prolapsed Uterus Protruding from the Vagina.

Leiomyoma

▲ **FIGURE 15.8**
Leiomyomas (Fibroids). In this sectioned uterus a smaller, rounded leiomyoma is present, causing a bulge in the posterior uterine wall. The larger mass at the top is another leiomyoma projecting into the uterine cavity.

CASE REPORT 15.3

YOU ARE

. . . a women's health nurse practitioner working with Anna Rusak, MD, a gynecologist at Fulwood Medical Center.

YOU ARE COMMUNICATING WITH

. . . Mrs. Carol Isbell, a 29-year-old woman c/o severe dysmenorrhea since the age of 15. Mrs. Isbell has been unable to conceive after 2 years of unprotected intercourse. She experiences severe, cramping lower abdominal pain for 2 days before, during, and 2 days after her periods, which are very heavy. She also has lower abdominal pain on intercourse. Her physical examination is unremarkable except that her pelvic examination shows several tender masses on each side of a normal-sized uterus. Dr. Rusak has also examined her and agreed with your diagnosis of endometriosis. Mrs. Isbell is to have an ultrasound examination.

Disorders of the Female Reproductive Tract (continued)

Disorders of the Uterus and Fallopian (Uterine) Tubes
(LO 15.1, 15.2, 15.3, and 15.4)

Endometriosis is said to affect 1 in 10 American women of childbearing age. Here, the endometrium becomes implanted outside the uterus on the fallopian tubes, the ovaries, and the pelvic peritoneum. The displaced endometrium continues to go through its monthly cycle. It thickens and bleeds, leads to cysts and scar tissue, and produces pain. The cause of endometriosis is unknown. Treatment involves removing the abnormal tissue through laparoscopy.

Salpingitis is an inflammation of the fallopian (uterine) tubes and is part of pelvic inflammatory disease (**PID**). A bacterial infection, often from an **STD,** spreads from the vagina through the cervix and uterus. Symptoms are lower abdominal pain, fever, and a vaginal discharge. Treatment is with antibiotics.

Uterine Prolapse
(LO 15.1, 15.2, 15.3, and 15.4)

The uterus is normally supported by the pelvic floor's muscles, ligaments, and connective tissue. However, a difficult childbirth, aging, obesity, lack of exercise, chronic coughing, and chronic constipation can weaken these tissues, causing the uterus to descend into the vaginal canal (*Figure 15.7*). Uterine prolapse can be accompanied by prolapse of the bladder and anterior vaginal wall (**cystocele**), or by prolapse of the rectum and posterior wall of the vagina (**rectocele**).

Treatment for uterine prolapse can be an individually-fitted vaginal **pessary,** which is inserted into the vagina to support the uterus. Surgical procedures like sacral **colpopexy** (where a mesh patch is inserted into the pelvic floor), or vaginal **hysterectomy** (where the uterus is removed through the vagina) achieve good results.

Retroversion of the uterus is a normal variation, found in 20% of women. In retroversion, the body of the uterus is tipped backward instead of forward (**anteversion**). It can also be caused by lax pelvic muscles and ligaments, pelvic adhesions (scar tissue in the pelvis following salpingitis), or pelvic inflammatory disease (PID). Retroversion by itself does not cause symptoms, and treatment is not usually necessary.

Uterine Fibroids
(LO 15.1, 15.2, 15.3, and 15.4)

Uterine **fibroids** are noncancerous growths that appear during childbearing years. Three out of four women have them, but only one out of four women experiences their symptoms, which include **menorrhagia, metrorrhagia, polymenorrhea,** lower back pain, and pelvic pain.

Fibroids are also called **fibromyomas, leiomyomas,** or **myomas** (*Figure 15.8*). They arise in the **myometrium** and produce a pale, firm, rubbery mass separate from the surrounding tissue. They vary in size from seedlings to large masses that distort the uterus. They can protrude into the uterine cavity, causing menorrhagia, or project outside the uterus and press on the bladder or rectum, thereby producing symptoms.

Treatment options are numerous and include watchful waiting, a **myomectomy,** and **focused ultrasound surgery (FUS)**. **Hysterectomy** is a major surgery and is considered by many gynecologists as a last resort.

Word	Pronunciation	Elements		Definition
anteversion	an-teh-**VER**-shun	S/ P/ R/	-ion *action, condition* ante- *forward* -vers- *turn*	Forward displacement or tilting of a structure (in this case, the uterus)
colpopexy	**KOL**-poh-peck-see	S/ R/CF	-pexy *surgical fixation* colp/o- *vagina*	Surgical fixation of the vaginal walls
cystocele	**SIS**-toh-seal	S/ R/CF	-cele *hernia* cyst/o- *bladder*	Hernia of the bladder into the vagina
endometriosis	**EN**-doh-me-tree-**OH**-sis	S/ P/ R/CF	-osis *condition* endo- *within, inside* -metr/i- *uterus*	Endometrial tissue outside the uterus
fibroid	**FIE**-broyd	S/ R/	-oid *resembling* fibr- *fiber*	Uterine tumor resembling fibrous tissue
fibromyoma	**FIE**-broh-my-**OH**-mah	S/ R/CF R/	-oma *tumor, mass* fibr/o- *fiber* -my- *muscle*	Benign neoplasm derived from smooth muscle and containing fibrous tissue
hysterectomy	his-ter-**EK**-toe-me	S/ R/	-ectomy *surgical excision* hyster- *uterus*	Surgical removal of the uterus
leiomyoma (also called fibroid)	**LIE**-oh-my-**OH**-mah	S/ R/ R/CF	-oma *tumor, mass* -my- *muscle* lei/o- *smooth*	Benign neoplasm derived from smooth muscle
menorrhagia	men-oh-**RAY**-jee-ah	S/ R/CF	-rrhagia *flow, discharge* men/o- *menses*	Excessive menstrual bleeding
metrorrhagia	**MEH**-troh-**RAY**-jee-ah	S/ R/CF	-rrhagia *flow, discharge* metr/o- *uterus*	Irregular uterine bleeding between menses
myoma	my-**OH**-mah	S/ R/	-oma *tumor, mass* my- *muscle*	Benign tumor of muscle
myomectomy	my-oh-**MEK**-toe-me	S/ R/ R/	-ectomy *surgical excision* my- *muscle* -om- *tumor*	Surgical removal of a myoma
pessary	**PES**-ah-ree		Greek *an oval stone*	Appliance inserted into the vagina to support the uterus
polymenorrhea	**POL**-ee-men-oh-**REE**-ah	R/ P/ R/CF	-rrhea *flow* poly- *many, excessive* men/o- *menses*	More than normal frequency of menses
rectocele	**REK**-toe-seal	S/ R/CF	-cele *hernia* rect/o- *rectum*	Hernia of the rectum into the vagina
retroversion	reh-troh-**VER**-shun	S/ P/ R/	-ion *action, condition* retro- *backward* -vers- *turn*	Tipping backward of the uterus
salpingitis	sal-pin-**JIE**-tis	S/ R/	-itis *inflammation* salping- *tube*	Inflammation of the fallopian (uterine) tube
salpingectomy	sal-pin-**JEK**-toe-me	S/	-ectomy *surgical excision*	Surgical removal of a fallopian tube

EXERCISES

A. Review the Case Report on this spread before answering the questions.

1. What is *dysmenorrhea* in layman's language? _____

2. Describe the symptoms Mrs. Isbell had with her monthly periods. _____
_____

3. What is shown on pelvic examination by Dr. Rusak? _____

4. What is the treatment for endometriosis? _____

- More than 600,000 hysterectomies are performed each year in the United States.

- In postmenopausal women, the risk of heart disease becomes almost the same as that of men.

ABBREVIATIONS

Pap   Papanicolaou (Pap test, Pap smear)

D & C   dilation and curettage

Endometrial Cancer (LO 15.1, 15.2, 15.3, and 15.4)

Endometrial cancer is the fourth most common cancer in women, after lung, breast, and colon cancer. Each year, 40,000 new cases are diagnosed in the United States, mostly in women between ages 60 and 70. The most frequent symptom is vaginal bleeding after menopause. Surgery is the most prescribed treatment, which can involve a **total hysterectomy** (where the uterus and cervix are removed), or a **radical hysterectomy** (where the fallopian tubes and ovaries are removed along with the uterus). If the cancer has spread to other parts of the body, progesterone therapy, radiation therapy, and chemotherapy are used.

    Cervical cancer is less common than endometrial cancer, but 50% of cervical cancer cases occur between ages 35 and 55. Some 10,000 new cases are diagnosed in the United States each year. Early cervical cancer produces no symptoms but may be found on a routine **Pap test.** In the **precancerous** stage, abnormal cells **(dysplasia)** are found only in the outer layer of the cervix. Thirteen types of human papilloma virus (HPV) can convert these **dysplastic** cells to cancer cells *(Figure 15.9)*. A vaccine has been developed that appears to make people immune to two of the most common types of HPV. It has been licensed by the FDA for use in females aged 9 to 26.

    Treatment depends on the stage of the cancer. In **preinvasive** cancer, when the cancer is only in the outer layer of the lining, the abnormal cells can be removed with a scalpel **(conization),** electrical current, or laser beam. In an **invasive** stage, when the cancer has invaded the cervix and beyond, treatment can include a simple or radical hysterectomy, chemotherapy, and radiation therapy.

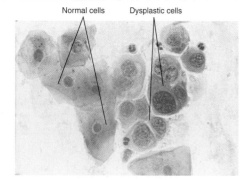

Normal cells   Dysplastic cells

LM 160×

▲ **FIGURE 15.9**
Abnormal Pap Smear with Dysplastic Cells.

Pap Test (LO 15.1, 15.2, 15.3, and 15.4)

In a Pap test, the doctor brushes cells from the cervix *(Figure 15.10)*. These cells are smeared onto a slide or rinsed into a special liquid and sent to the laboratory for examination. The Pap test enables abnormal cells, precancerous or cancerous, to be detected. It is the most successful and accurate test for early detection of cervical abnormalities.

Other Causes of Uterine Bleeding
(LO 15.1, 15.2, 15.3, and 15.4)

Dysfunctional uterine bleeding is a term that's used when no cause can be found for a patient's menorrhagia. Treatment is with oral contraceptives. If that fails, **dilation and curettage (D & C)** may be effective. This procedure involves dilating the entrance to the uterus through the cervix so that a thin instrument can be inserted to scrape or suction away the lining of the uterus and take tissue samples. An alternative is endometrial **ablation,** in which a heat-generating tool or a laser removes or destroys the lining of the uterus and prevents or reduces menstruation. An endometrial ablation and hysterectomy can be used in women who have finished childbearing.

Menopause (LO 15.1, 15.2, 15.3, and 15.4)

Menopause occurs when a woman has not menstruated for a year and is not **pregnant;** she is in the "change of life." For most women, menstruation ceases between the ages of 45 and 55.

    Without estrogen and progesterone, the uterus, vagina, and breasts atrophy, and more bone is lost than is replaced. Blood vessels constrict and dilate in response to changing hormone levels and can cause the characteristic menopausal "hot flashes."

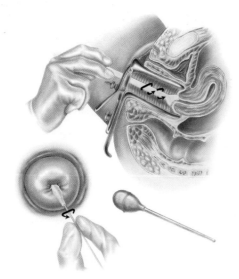

▲ **FIGURE 15.10**
Pap Smear Being Performed.

Word	Pronunciation	Elements		Definition
ablation	ab-**LAY**-shun	S/ P/ R/	-ion *action, condition* ab- *away from* -lat- *to take*	Removal of tissue to destroy its function
conization	koh-ni-**ZAY**-shun	S/ R/	-ation *process* coniz- *cone*	Surgical excision of a cone-shaped piece of tissue
curettage	kyu-reh-**TAHZH**	S/ R/	-age *pertaining to* curett- *to cleanse*	Scraping the interior of a cavity
dysfunctional	dis-**FUNK**-shun-al	S/ P/ R/	-al *pertaining to* dys- *painful, difficult* -function- *perform*	Difficulty in performing
dysplasia	dis-**PLAY**-zee-ah	S/ P/ R/	-ia *condition* dys- *painful, difficult* -plas- *development, formation*	Abnormal tissue formation
dysplastic (adj)	dis-**PLAS**-tik	S/	-tic *pertaining to*	Pertaining to or showing abnormal tissue formation
Pap test	PAP TEST		George Papanicolaou, Greek-U.S. physician, 1883–1962	Examination of cells taken from the cervix

EXERCISES

A. Deconstruct *the following medical terms into their elements with slashes. Be sure to write the identity of the element (P, R, CF, or S) under the line. Remember: Every element may not be present in every term. Space is provided for you to briefly define the term. Fill in the blanks.*

1. *ablation* _____ / _____ / _____

   Definition: _____

2. *dysfunctional* _____ / _____ / _____

   Definition: _____

3. *curettage* _____ / _____ / _____

   Definition: _____

4. *conization* _____ / _____ / _____

   Definition: _____

B. Patient education: *In language your patient can understand, explain to her the difference between:*

1. A total hysterectomy and a radical hysterectomy

   Total: _____

   Radical: _____

2. Explain to your patient the various treatment options available for endometrial cancer. _____

   _____

3. Your patient is asking you to explain what causes her "hot flashes." _____

   _____

LESSON 15.3 Female Infertility and Contraception (LO 15.1, 15.2, 15.3, and 15.4)

- In women, fertility begins to decrease as early as age 30, and **pregnancy** rates are very low after age 44.

- Approximately 20% of women now have their first child at age 35 or older.

- In 20% to 30% of female infertility problems, no identifiable cause is found.

- The success rate for IVF is approximately 30% for each egg retrieval.

- Unprotected sex has a failure rate of 85%, with resulting pregnancy.

Female Infertility (LO 15.1, 15.2, 15.3, and 15.4)

Infertility is the inability to become pregnant after 1 year of unprotected intercourse. It affects 10% to 15% of all couples. The causes of infertility include:

- The female factor alone in 35% of cases.
- The male factor alone in 30% of cases.
- Male and female factors in 20% of cases.
- Unknown factors in 15% of cases.

Causes of female infertility include scarring of the fallopian tubes, structural abnormalities of the uterus, and infrequent ovulation, all of which were addressed earlier in this chapter. Treatment is applied to any underlying cause arising from the results of the infertility evaluation.

Surgical procedures performed to initiate pregnancy include:

- **Intrauterine insemination,** in which sperm are inserted directly into the uterus via a special catheter.
- **In vitro fertilization (IVF),** in which eggs and sperm are combined in a laboratory dish and two to four resulting embryos are placed inside the uterus. This can result in twins or triplets.

Contraception (LO 15.1, 15.2, 15.3, and 15.4)

Contraception is the prevention of pregnancy. There are several common methods of contraception, including the approaches outlined below.

- **Behavioral methods:** These include **abstinence, coitus interruptus,** and the **rhythm method.** The latter two methods have a 20% failure rate.

- **Barrier methods:**
  - **Condoms** are available for males and females *(Figure 15.11)*. They have a 5% to 10% failure rate.
  - **Diaphragms** *(Figure 15.12)* and **cervical caps** consist of a latex or rubber dome that is inserted into the vagina and placed over the cervix. When used with a spermicide, they have a 5% to 10% failure rate.
  - **Spermicidal foams and gels** are inserted into the vagina. Used on their own, they have a 25% failure rate.

- **Intrauterine devices (IUDs):** These are T-shaped flexible plastic or copper devices inserted into the uterus and left in place for 1 to 4 years. The failure rate is less than 3%.

- **Hormonal methods:**
  - **Oral contraceptives** (birth control pills) utilize a mixture of estrogen and progesterone to prevent follicular development and ovulation. They have a 5% failure rate, usually due to inconsistent pill taking.

- **Estrogen/progestin patches** deliver the hormones transdermally (through the skin). Their failure rate is below 1%.
  - **Injected progestins,** like Depo-Provera, are given by injection every 3 months. Their failure rate is below 1%.
  - **Implanted progestins,** like Norplant, are contained in porous silicone tubes that are inserted under the skin and slowly release the progestin for up to 5 years. Their failure rate is below 1%.
  - **Morning-after pills,** like Plan B, contain large doses of progestins to inhibit or delay ovulation. They are a backup when taken within 72 hours of unprotected intercourse. Their failure rate is around 10%.
  - **Mifepristone (RU486),** when taken with a prostaglandin, induces a miscarriage. It has an 8% failure rate.

Surgical Methods
(LO 15.1, 15.2, 15.3, and 15.4)

- **Tubal ligation** ("getting your tubes tied") is performed with laparoscopy. Both fallopian tubes are cut, a segment is removed, and the ends are tied off and cauterized shut. The contraception failure rate is below 1%.

▲ **FIGURE 15.11**
Male and Female Condoms.

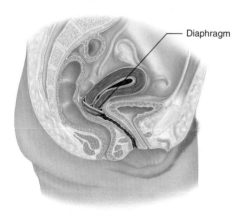

Diaphragm

▲ **FIGURE 15.12**
Diaphragm.

Word	Pronunciation		Elements	Definition
coitus postcoital (adj)	KOH-it-us post-KOH-ih-tal	S/ P/ R/	Latin *come together* -al *pertaining to* post- *after* -coit- *sexual intercourse*	Sexual intercourse After sexual intercourse
contraception	kon-trah-SEP-shun	S/ R/ R/	-ion *action, condition* contra- *against* -cept- *receive*	Prevention of pregnancy
contraceptive	kon-trah-SEP-tiv	S/	-ive *quality of*	An agent that prevents conception
diaphragm (Note: *also the term for the muscle that separates the thoracic and abdominal cavities*)	DIE-ah-fram		Greek *partition or wall*	A ring and dome-shaped material inserted into the vagina to prevent pregnancy
insemination	in-sem-ih-NAY-shun	S/ P/ R/	-ation *process* in- *in* -semin- *semen*	Introduction of semen into the vagina
inseminate (verb)	in-SEM-ih-nate	S/	-ate *pertaining to*	To introduce semen into the vagina
in vitro fertilization (IVF)	IN VEE-troh FER-til-ih-ZAY-shun	P/ S/ R/	in- *in* vitro, Latin *glass* -ization *process of creating* fertil- *able to conceive*	Process of combining sperm and egg in a laboratory dish and placing resulting embryos inside the uterus
progestin	pro-JESS-tin	S/ P/ R/	-in *substance* pro- *before* -gest- *produce, gestation*	A synthetic form of progesterone

EXERCISES

A. Match *the definitions in column 1 with the correct medical term in column 2.* **Hint:** *Be sure to use the correct form (noun, verb, adjective) of the term.*
Fill in the blanks.

_____ **1.** synthetic form of progesterone	**A.** diaphragm
_____ **2.** agent that prevents conception	**B.** pregnant
_____ **3.** sexual intercourse	**C.** insemination
_____ **4.** introduction of semen into vagina	**D.** coitus
_____ **5.** having conceived	**E.** progestin
_____ **6.** egg and sperm in a lab dish	**F.** contraceptive
_____ **7.** ring and dome-shaped contraceptive device	**G.** IVF

B. *The following terms in the language of gynecology all appear in the text on contraception. Briefly define the following terms.*

1. injected _____

2. intrauterine _____

3. oral _____

4. implanted _____

5. spermicidal _____

6. transdermal _____

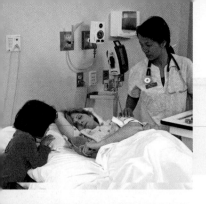

LESSON 15.4

Pregnancy

OBJECTIVES

For any health care professional involved in the care of a patient who is pregnant, it's necessary to be aware and informed of all aspects concerning pregnancy, childbirth and their related conditions. The information in this lesson will enable you to use correct medical terminology to:

15.4.1 Describe conception and implantation.

15.4.2 Identify the characteristics of an embryo and **fetus.**

15.4.3 List the functions of the placenta.

15.4.4 Discuss the mechanisms of pregnancy (**PGY**) and childbirth and their common disorders.

CASE REPORT 15.4

YOU ARE

. . . an obstetric assistant (**OA**) employed by Garry Joiner, MD, an obstetrician at Fulwood Medical Center.

YOU ARE COMMUNICATING WITH

Mrs. Gloria Maggay, a 29-year-old housekeeper. Her last menstrual period was 8 weeks ago, and she has a positive home pregnancy test. This is her first pregnancy. She has breast tenderness and mild nausea. For the past 2 days, she has had some cramping, right-sided, lower abdominal pain and this morning had vaginal spotting. Her VS are T 99°F, P 80, R 14, BP 130/70. While you are waiting for Dr. Joiner to come and examine her, Mrs. Maggay complains of feeling faint and has a sharp, severe pain in the right side of her lower abdomen. Her pulse rate has increased to 92. You need to recognize what is happening and to use the correct medical terminology as you talk with Dr. Joiner.

Conception and Development (LO 15.5 and 15.6)

Conception (LO 15.5 and 15.6)

When released from the ovary, an egg takes 72 hours to travel to the uterus—but it must be **fertilized** within 12 to 24 hours to survive. Therefore, **fertilization** must take place in the distal third of the fallopian tube.

During unprotected intercourse, with male ejaculation, between 200 million and 600 million sperm are deposited in the vagina near the cervix. The journey through the uterus into the fallopian tube takes about an hour. Some 2,000 to 3,000 sperm reach the egg. Several of these sperm penetrate the outer layers of the egg to clear the path for the one sperm that will penetrate all the way into the egg to **fertilize** it *(Figure 15.13).* Once fertilized, the egg becomes a zygote.

Implantation (LO 15.5 and 15.6)

While still in the fallopian tube, the zygote divides; a fluid-filled cavity develops, and the zygote becomes a **blastocyst** (its first two weeks as a developing **embryo**). A week after fertilization, the blastocyst enters the uterine cavity and burrows into the endometrium, and **implantation** occurs. A group of cells in the blastocyst differentiate into the embryo. Other cells from the blastocyst, together with endometrial cells, form the **placenta.**

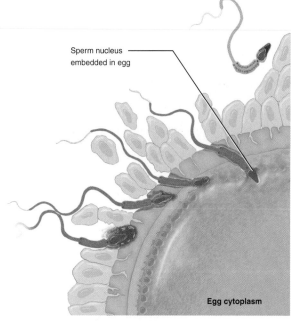

Sperm nucleus embedded in egg

Egg cytoplasm

▲ **FIGURE 15.13**
Fertilization.

Word	Pronunciation	Elements		Definition
blastocyst	**BLAS**-toe-sist	S/ R/CF	-cyst *cyst, bladder* blast/o- *germ or immature-* *cell*	First 2 weeks of the developing embryo
embryo	**EM**-bree-oh		Greek *a young one*	Developing organism from conception until the end of the second month
embryonic (adj)	em-bree-**ON**-ic	S/ R/	-ic *pertaining to* embryon- *embryo*	Pertaining to the embryo
fetus	**FEE**-tus		Latin *offspring*	Human organism from the end of the eighth week after conception to birth
fetal (adj)	**FEE**-tal	S/ R/	-al *pertaining to* fet- *fetus*	Pertaining to the fetus
fertilize (verb) fertilization (noun)	**FER**-til-ize **FER**-til-eye-**ZAY**-shun	S/ R/	Latin *make fruitful* -ation *process* fertiliz- *make fruitful*	Penetration of the oocyte by sperm Union of a male sperm and a female egg
implantation	im-plan-**TAY**-shun	S/ P/ R/	-ation *process* im- *in* -plant- *to plant, insert*	Attachment of a fertilized egg to the endometrium
placenta	plah-**SEN**-tah		Latin *a cake*	Organ that allows metabolic exchange between the mother and the fetus

EXERCISES

A. Review *the Case Report on this spread before answering the questions.*

1. When was Mrs. Maggay's last menstrual period? _____

2. What are her presenting symptoms? _____

3. What has happened to her in the past two days? _____

4. What occurs while she is waiting for Dr. Joiner to examine her? _____

5. Which vital sign has increased? _____

6. Where is her sharp, severe pain now? _____

B. Meet lesson and chapter objectives *using the language of obstetrics.*

1. Where does fertilization actually take place in the body? _____

2. Once fertilized, what is the new term for the egg and sperm? _____

3. During its first two weeks of development, the embryo is called the _____ .

4. The entity in question #3 undergoes division into two separate entities called the _____ and the _____ .

5. Attachment of the fertilized egg to the endometrium is called the _____ .

C. Critical thinking: *What do you think could be happening to Mrs. Maggay based on her sudden, severe pain and the fact that she feels faint?*

1. _____

   _____

Placenta (LO 15.5 and 15.6)

The placenta is a disc of tissue that increases in size as pregnancy proceeds *(Figure 15.14)*. The surface facing the fetus is smooth and gives rise to the **umbilical cord.** The surface attached to the uterine wall consists of treelike structures called **chorionic villi.** The cells of the villi keep the maternal and fetal circulations separate, but they are very thin and allow the exchange of gases, nutrients, and waste products.

The functions of the placenta are to:

* **Transport** nutrients and oxygen from the mother to the fetus;

* **Transport** nitrogenous wastes and carbon dioxide from the fetus to the mother, who can excrete them;

* **Transport** maternal antibodies and hormones to the fetus; and

* **Secrete** hormones like estrogen and progesterone.

Unfortunately, some undesirable matter and many medications can cross the placenta. These include: the HIV and rubella viruses; bacteria that cause syphilis; alcohol; nicotine and carbon monoxide from smoking; and drugs ranging from aspirin to heroin and cocaine. All of these can have detrimental effects on the fetus.

There are currently two common procedures that are performed during pregnancy to check the health of the fetus. Both **amniocentesis** (removal of amniotic fluid) and **chorionic villus sampling (CVS)** (where a sample of the chorionic villus cells is removed for a biopsy) test for chromosomal abnormalities and genetic birth defects.

ABBREVIATION

CVS   chorionic villus sampling

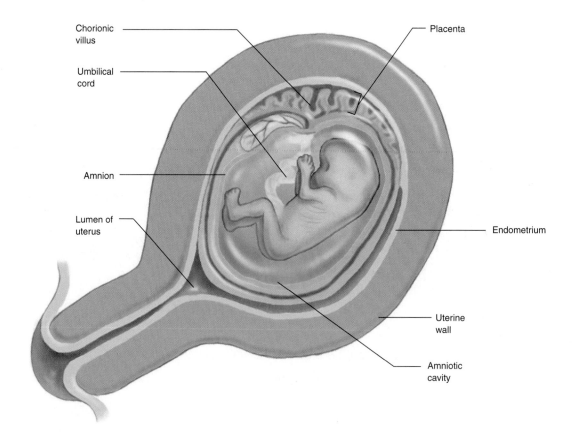

▲ **FIGURE 15.14**
Embryo and Placenta at 13 Weeks.

Word	Pronunciation	Elements		Definition
amniocentesis	AM-nee-oh-sen-tee-sis	S/ R/CF	-centesis *to puncture* amni/o- *amnion, fetal* *membrane*	Removal of amniotic fluid for diagnostic purposes
chorion chorionic (adj)	KOH-ree-on koh-ree-ON-ick	S/ R/	Greek *membrane* -ic *pertaining to* chorion- *chorion*	The fetal membrane that forms the placenta Pertaining to the chorion
chorionic villus	VILL-us		villus, Latin *shaggy hair*	Vascular process of the embryonic chorion to form the placenta
conception	kon-SEP-shun		Latin *something received*	Fertilization of the egg by sperm to form a zygote

EXERCISES

A. Precision in documentation *includes using the correct form (noun, verb, adjective) of the medical term.*

Practice precision in this written language of obstetrics. Fill in the blanks.

1. embryo   embryonic

In the _____ stage of gestation, the _____ forms in the first 8 weeks of human development.

2. chorionic   chorion

The _____ villi keep the maternal and fetal circulations separate. The _____ is the fetal membrane that forms the placenta.

Practice your precision in pronunciation, please!

B. Meet lesson objectives *and name the four functions of the placenta.*

1. _____

2. _____

3. _____

4. _____

C. Challenge your knowledge *of the language of obstetrics by answering the following questions.*

1. Where does the umbilical cord originate? _____

2. To what structure are the chorionic villi attached in the reproductive system? _____

3. What are the main functions of the villi? _____

_____

4. Name all the undesirable matter that can cross the placenta: _____

_____

5. Which two procedures can be performed during pregnancy to check the health of the fetus?

a. _____

b. _____

6. What two fetal problems are the procedures listed in question #5 looking for?

a. _____

b. _____

7. Why is the information gained in question #6 important to know early in pregnancy? _____

_____

WORD ANALYSIS AND DEFINITION

Conception and Development *(continued)*

Embryo (LO 15.5 and 15.6)

The **embryonic period** occurs from week 2 until week 8. During this time, most of the embryo's external structures and internal organs are formed, together with the placenta, umbilical cord, **amnion** (the amniotic fluid-filled membrane around the fetus), and **chorion.** The amnion grows to envelop the embryo. At the eighth week, all the embryo's organ systems are present. The embryo is just over 1 inch long and is now officially a **fetus.**

Fetus (LO 15.5 and 15.6)

The fetal period lasts from the eighth week until birth. At the eighth week, the heart is beating. By the twelfth week, the bones have begun to calcify, and the external genitalia can be differentiated as male or female. In the fourth month, downy hair called **lanugo** appears on the body. In the fifth month, skeletal muscles become active, and the baby's movements are felt between 16 and 22 weeks of **gestation** *(Figure 15.15)*. A protective substance called **vernix caseosa** covers the skin. In the sixth and seventh months, there is an increase in weight gain and body fat is deposited.

At 38 weeks, the baby is at full-term and ready for birth.

Gestation is divided into **trimesters:** The first trimester is up to week 12; the second from weeks 13 to 24; and the third from week 25 to birth.

Disorders of Pregnancy (LO 15.5, 15.6, and 15.7)

The paragraphs below explain the disorders in pregnancy that you will need to be familiar with when caring for a pregnant patient.

Ectopic Pregnancy (LO 15.5, 15.6, and 15.7)

In an **ectopic pregnancy,** there is an obstruction in the fallopian tube. As a result, the fertilized egg will be prevented from moving into the uterus. Instead, the egg will continue its development in the fallopian tube. Tubal disorders that cause ectopic pregnancy include previous salpingitis, pelvic inflammatory disease (PID), and endometriosis.

Preeclampsia and Eclampsia (LO 15.5, 15.6, and 15.7)

Preeclampsia is a sudden, abnormal increase in maternal blood pressure after the 20th week of pregnancy, with edema (swelling) of the face, hands, and feet. It is also accompanied by proteinuria (protein in the urine). Severe preeclampsia can lead to stroke, bleeding disorders, and death of the mother and fetus.

Eclampsia is a life-threatening condition, characterized by the signs and symptoms of preeclampsia, with the addition of convulsions. Management involves immediate admission to the hospital and control of the mother's blood pressure. The baby is delivered as soon as the mother is stabilized, regardless of its maturity.

Amniotic Fluid Abnormalities (LO 15.5, 15.6, and 15.7)

Amniotic fluid abnormalities occur in the second trimester, when the fetus breathes in and swallows amniotic fluid. This promotes development of the gastrointestinal tract and lungs. In the third trimester, the total amount of amniotic fluid is about 1 quart and is mostly fetal urine.

Oligohydramnios is a condition involving too little amniotic fluid. It is associated with an increase in the risk of birth defects and poor fetal growth. Its etiology is unknown.

Polyhydramnios is the opposite of oligohydramnios, and involves too much amniotic fluid. It causes abdominal discomfort and breathing difficulties for the mother. It is associated with **preterm delivery,** placental problems, and poor fetal growth.

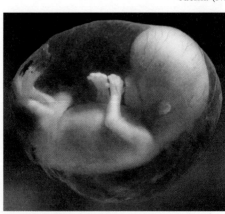

▲ **FIGURE 15.15**
Developing Fetus at 20 Weeks.

S = Suffix   P = Prefix   R = Root   R/CF= Combining Form

Word	Pronunciation		Elements	Definition
amnion	AM-nee-on		Greek *membrane around fetus*	Membrane around the fetus that contains amniotic fluid
amniotic (adj)	am-nee-OT-ic	S/ R/CF	-tic *pertaining to* amni/o- *amnion, fetal membrane*	Pertaining to the amnion
ectopic	ek-TOP-ik	S/ R/	-ic *pertaining to* ectop- *on the outside, displaced*	Out of place, not in a normal position
gestation	jes-TAY-shun	S/ R/	-ion *action, condition* gestat- *pregnancy*	From conception to birth
gestational (adj)	jes-TAY-shun-al	S/	-al *pertaining to*	Pertaining to gestation
lanugo	la-NYU-go		Latin *wool*	Fine, soft hair on the fetal body
oligohydramnios	OL-ih-goh-high-DRAM-nee-os	P/ R/ R/	oligo- *scanty, too little* -hydr- *water* -amnios *amnion*	Too little amniotic fluid
polyhydramnios	POL-ee-high-DRAM-nee-os	P/	poly- *many, excessive*	Too much amniotic fluid
preeclampsia	pree-eh-KLAMP-see-uh	S/ P/ R/	-ia *condition* pre- *before* -eclamps- *shining forth*	Hypertension, edema, and proteinuria during pregnancy
preterm *(same as premature)*	pree-TERM	P/ R/	pre- *before* -term *limit, end*	Baby delivered before 37 weeks of gestation
trimester	TRY-mes-ter		Latin *of 3 months' duration*	One-third of the length of a full-term pregnancy
vernix caseosa	VER-nicks kay-see-OH-sah		vernix, Latin *varnish* caseosa, Latin *cheese*	Cheesy substance covering the skin of the fetus

EXERCISES

A. Review *the Case Report on the opposite page before answering the questions.*

1. "Mrs. Maggay has symptoms indicative of an ectopic pregnancy." What does that mean? _____

_____

2. Which two severe and sudden symptoms and signs may signal that her fallopian tube has ruptured? _____

_____

3. What is the treatment for Mrs. Maggay now? _____

_____

4. Name one tubal disorder that can cause an ectopic pregnancy._____

B. Prefixes: *The WAD box contains prefixes that have appeared in previous chapters. In the chart below, the meaning of the prefix is given to you in the first column. List a term with that prefix from the WAD above, and give the meaning of the term. Then add another term with the same prefix from any previous chapter, and be sure to write its meaning as well. Fill in the chart.*

Meaning of Prefix	WAD Term with this Prefix	Meaning of this Term	Term from Previous Chapter	Meaning of Term from Previous Chapter
before	1.	2.	3.	4.
excessive	5.	6.	7.	8.
too little (scanty)	9.	10.	11.	12.

LESSON 15.4 Disorders of Pregnancy
(continued)

Gestational Diabetes Mellitus (GDM) (LO 15.5, 15.6, and 15.7)

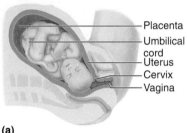

(a)

In some pregnant women, the amount of insulin they can produce decreases and this leads to hyperglycemia. For the mother, gestational diabetes mellitus (**GDM**) increases the risk of preeclampsia and future type 2 diabetes. For the **neonate** (newborn child), it increases the risk of **perinatal** mortality, birth trauma, and **neonatal** hypoglycemia. Later in life, both mother and child are at increased risk for developing type 2 diabetes and obesity.

Hyperemesis Gravidarum (LO 15.5, 15.6, and 15.7)

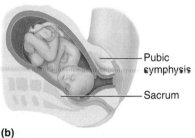

(b)

Eighty percent of pregnant women experience some degree of "morning sickness." It is at its worst between 2 and 12 weeks of pregnancy and resolves in the second trimester. For a few women, nausea is persistent, and vomiting is extreme and can lead to dehydration. This condition is called **hyperemesis gravidarum.** Severe cases may have to be admitted to the hospital for IV fluids.

Teratogenesis (LO 15.5, 15.6, and 15.7)

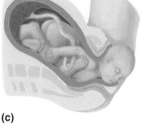

(c)

Teratogenesis is the production of fetal abnormalities—**congenital malformations**—by a chemical agent affecting the mother during the early development of the fetus, while organs and structures are being formed. All medications readily cross the placenta. **Teratogens** include alcohol, isotretinoin (acne medication), valproic acid (an anticonvulsant), and the rubella virus.

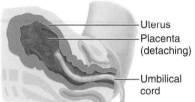

(d)

▲ FIGURE 15.16
The Stages of Childbirth.
(a) First stage: Early dilation. (b) First stage: Late dilation. (c) Second stage: Expulsion of the fetus. (d) Third stage: Expulsion of the placenta.

ABBREVIATION

GDM	gestational diabetes mellitus

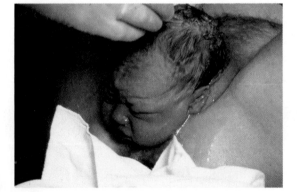

▲ FIGURE 15.17
Delivery of the Head.

Childbirth (LO 15.5 and 15.6)

Labor contractions begin about 30 minutes apart. They have to be intermittent because each contraction shuts down the maternal blood supply to the placenta and to the fetus. Labor pains are due to ischemia of the uterine muscle during contractions.

Labor is divided into three stages *(Figure 15.16),* each of which is usually longer in a **primipara** than in a **multipara.** Another term for pregnant is **gravid,** and a pregnant woman can be called **gravida.** A woman in her first pregnancy is called a **primigravida.**

First Stage—Dilation of the Cervix (LO 15.5 and 15.6)

This is the longest stage of labor. It can be a few minutes in a multipara to more than 1 day in a primipara. **Dilation** is the widening of the cervical canal to the same diameter as that of the baby's head *(Figure 15.16b).* At the same time that dilation occurs, the wall of the cervix becomes thinner--a process called **effacement.** During dilation, the fetal membranes rupture, and the "waters break" as amniotic fluid is released.

Second Stage—Expulsion of the Fetus (LO 15.5 and 15.6)

While the uterus continues to contract, the baby's head generates additional pain as it stretches the cervix and vagina. When the head reaches the vaginal opening and stretches the vulva, the head is said to be **crowning** and the baby can be delivered *(Figure 15.17).* Sometimes, this process can be helped by performing an **episiotomy** and making an incision in the perineum.

After the baby is delivered, blood in the placental vein is drained into the baby, and the umbilical cord is clamped in two places and cut between the two clamps.

Third Stage—Expulsion of the Placenta (LO 15.5 and 15.6)

After the baby is delivered, the uterus continues to contract. It pushes the placenta off the uterine wall and expels it from the vagina *(Figure 15.16d).*

Puerperium (LO 15.5 and 15.6)

The 6 weeks **postpartum** (after the birth) are called the **puerperium.** The uterus shrinks (**involution**) through self-digestion (**autolysis**) of uterine cells by their own enzymes. This generates a vaginal discharge called **lochia** that lasts about 10 days.

478   Chapter 15 The Female Reproductive System

Word	Pronunciation		Elements	Definition
autolysis	awe-**TOL**-ih-sis	P/ R/	auto- *self, same* -lysis *destruction*	Destruction of cells by enzymes within the cells
dilation	die-**LAY**-shun	S/ R/	-ion *process* dilat- *open out*	Stretching or enlarging an opening
effacement	ee-**FACE**-ment	S/ R/	-ment *resulting state* efface- *wipe out*	Thinning of the cervix in relation to labor
episiotomy	eh-piz-ee-**OT**-oh-me	S/ R/CF	-tomy *surgical incision* episi/o- *vulva*	Surgical incision of the vulva
gravid gravida	**GRAV**-id **GRAV**-ih-dah		Latin *pregnant* Latin *pregnant woman*	Pregnant A pregnant woman
hyperemesis	high-per-**EM**-ee-sis	P/ R/	hyper- *excessive* -emesis *vomiting*	Excessive vomiting
labor	**LAY**-bore		Latin *toil, suffering*	Process of expulsion of the fetus
lochia	**LOW**-kee-uh		Greek *relating to childbirth*	Vaginal discharge following childbirth
multipara	mul-**TIP**-ah-ruh	P/ R/	multi- *many* -para *to bring forth*	Woman who has given birth to two or more children
neonate neonatal (adj) (Note: The "e" in the root is dropped because of the following vowel.)	**NEE**-oh-nate **NEE**-oh-**NAY**-tal	P/ R/ S/	neo- *new* -nate *born* -al *pertaining to*	A newborn infant Pertaining to the newborn infant or the newborn period
perinatal	per-ih-**NAY**-tal	S/ P/ R/	-al *pertaining to* peri- *around* -nat- *birth*	Around the time of birth
postpartum	post-**PAR**-tum	P/ R/	post- *after* -partum *childbirth, to bring forth*	After childbirth
primigravida	pree-mih-**GRAV**-ih-dah	P/ R/	primi- *first* -gravida *pregnancy*	A woman in her first pregnancy
primipara	pry-**MIP**-ah-ruh	P/ R/	primi- *first* -para *to bring forth*	Woman giving birth for the first time
puerperium (Note: This term is composed of roots only.)	pyu-er-**PER**-ee-um	R/ R/	puer- *child* -perium *a bringing forth*	Six-week period after birth in which the uterus involutes
teratogen teratogenic (adj) teratogenesis	**TER**-ah-toe-jen **TER**-ah-toe-**JEN**-ik **TER**-ah-toe-**JEN**-eh-sis	S/ R/CF S/ S/	-gen *create, produce* terat/o- *monster, malformed fetus* -ic *pertaining to* -esis *condition*	Agent that produces fetal deformities Capable of producing fetal deformities Process involved in producing fetal deformities

EXERCISES

A. Elements: *Several of these elements you have seen before, and you will certainly see them again in other terms. Learn an element once, and recognize it all the time. Circle the best answer to each question.*

1. The term that contains the prefix meaning *many* is:

   primipara   lochia   multipara

2. The term that contains the suffix meaning *incision* is:

   episiotomy   effacement   dilation

3. The term that contains the root meaning *destruction* is:

   autolysis   involution   effacement

4. The term that contains the root meaning *child* is:

   gravid   multipara   puerperium

- Every newborn *(neonate)* is either:

  o **Premature,** less than 37 weeks gestation;

  o **Full-term,** between 37 and 42 weeks gestation; or

  o **Post-term,** longer than 42 weeks gestation.

C-section	cesarean section
OB	obstetrics
PPH	postpartum hemorrhage
RDS	respiratory distress syndrome

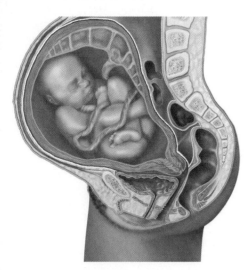

▲ **FIGURE 15.18**
Breech Presentation.

Disorders of Childbirth
(LO 15.5, 15.6, and 15.7)

Fetal distress, due to lack of oxygen, is an uncommon complication of labor, but it is detrimental if not recognized. During labor, there is electronic fetal heart monitoring. Treatment is to give the mother oxygen or increase IV fluids. If distress persists, the baby is delivered as quickly as possible by forceps extraction, vacuum extractor, or **cesarean section (C-section).**

An **abnormal position of the fetus** occurs at the beginning of labor if the baby is not a head-first **(vertex)** presentation facing rearward. Abnormal positions include:

- **Breech:** The buttocks present first *(Figure 15.18).*
- **Face:** The face, instead of the top of the head, presents first.
- **Shoulder:** The shoulder and upper back are trying to exit the uterus first.

If the baby cannot be turned into a vertex presentation, a C-section is usually performed.

In addition, other conditions can occur involving an abnormal placement of the baby's umbilical cord. In **prolapsed umbilical cord,** the cord precedes the baby down the birth canal. Pressure on the cord can cut off the baby's blood supply, which is still being provided through the umbilical arteries.

In **nuchal cord,** the cord is wrapped around the baby's neck during delivery. This occurs in 20% of deliveries.

Premature rupture of the membranes occurs in 10% of normal pregnancies and increases the risk of infection of the uterus and fetus.

Gestational Classification
(LO 15.5, 15.6, and 15.7)

Prematurity occurs in about 8% of newborns. The earlier the baby is born, the more life-threatening problems occur.

Because their lungs are underdeveloped, premature babies can develop **respiratory distress syndrome (RDS),** also called **hyaline membrane disease.** Their lungs are not mature enough to produce **surfactant,** a mixture of lipids and proteins that keeps the alveoli from collapsing. As a result, this prevents the respiratory exchange of oxygen and carbon dioxide.

An immature liver can impair the excretion of bilirubin (yellowish bile pigment) *(see Chapter 9),* and premature babies become jaundiced. High levels of bilirubin can produce **kernicterus,** in which deposits of bilirubin in the brain cause brain damage.

Postmaturity is much less common than prematurity. Its etiology is unknown, but the placenta begins to shrink, making it difficult to supply sufficient nutrients to the baby. For the baby, this leads to: hypoglycemia; loss of subcutaneous fat; dry, peeling skin; and, if oxygen is lacking, fetal distress. The baby can pass stools **(meconium)** into the amniotic fluid. In its distress, the baby can take deep gasping breaths and inhale the meconium fluid. This leads to **meconium aspiration syndrome** and respiratory difficulty at birth.

An **abortion** is the expulsion of an embryo or fetus from the uterus before the 20th week of gestation. It can be spontaneous (occurring from natural causes) or induced medically or surgically.

Placental Disorders
(LO 15.5, 15.6, and 15.7)

Placenta abruptio is the separation of the placenta from the uterine wall before delivery of the baby. The baby's oxygen supply is cut off, and fetal distress appears quickly. It is an **obstetric (OB)** emergency, and usually a **C-section** is performed.

Placenta previa is a low-lying placenta between the baby's head and the internal os of the cervix. It can cause severe bleeding during labor, and a C-section may be necessary.

In a **retained placenta,** all or part of the placenta and/or membranes remain behind in the uterus 30 minutes to an hour after the baby has been delivered. The result of a retained placenta is heavy uterine bleeding called **postpartum hemorrhage (PPH).** Manual removal of the retained placenta may be necessary under spinal, epidural, or general anesthesia *(Figure 15.19).*

▼ **FIGURE 15.19**
Placenta (Afterbirth).

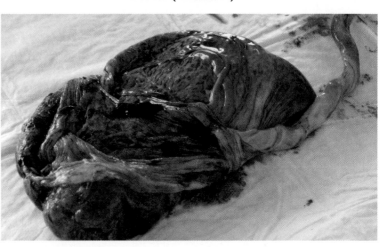

Word	Pronunciation		Elements	Definition
abortion	ah-**BOR**-shun	S/ R/	-ion *action* **abort**- *fail at onset*	Spontaneous or induced expulsion of the embryo or fetus from the uterus at 20 weeks or less
breech	BREECH		Old English *trousers*	Buttocks-first presentation of the fetus at delivery
cesarean section c-section (abbrev)	seh-**ZAH**-ree-an **SEK**-shun		Roman law under the Caesars required that pregnant women who died be cut open and the fetus be extracted	Extraction of the fetus through an incision in the abdomen and uterine wall
kernicterus	ker-**NICK**-ter-us	R/ R/	**kern**- *nucleus* -icterus *jaundice*	Bilirubin staining of the basal nuclei of the brain
meconium	meh-**KOH**-nee-um		Greek *a little poppy*	The first bowel movement of the newborn
nuchal cord	**NYU**-kul KORD		nuchal French *the back (nape) of the neck*	Loop(s) of umbilical cord around the fetal neck
placenta abruptio	plah-**SEN**-tah ab-**RUP**-she-oh		abruptio Latin *to break off*	The premature detachment of the placenta
placenta previa	plah -**SEN**-tah **PREE**-vee-ah	P/ R/	pre- *before, in front of* -via *the way*	Placenta obstructing the fetus during delivery
postmature	post -mah-**TYUR**	P/ R/	post- *after* -mature *ripe, ready*	Infant born after 42 weeks of gestation
postmaturity	post-mah-**TYUR**-ih-tee	S/	-ity *condition, state*	Condition of being postmature
premature (slang term "preemie")	pree -mah-**TYUR**	P/ R/	pre- *before* -mature *ripe, fully developed*	Occurring before the expected time
prematurity (same as *preterm*)	pree-mah-**TYUR**-ih-tee	S/	-ity *condition, state*	Condition of being premature
surfactant	sir-**FAK**-tant		*surface active agent*	A protein and fat compound that creates surface tension to hold the lung alveolar walls apart
vertex	**VER**-teks		Latin *whorl*	Topmost point of the vault of the skull

EXERCISES

A. Patient documentation: *Pick any two terms from the WAD, and use them to create your own patient documentation. You must be able to pronounce, spell, and define every term you use in your sentences as the instructor may ask you to read them aloud in class. Fill in the blanks.*

1. _____

_____

2. _____

_____

B. Meet lesson and chapter objectives *and apply the language of obstetrics to answer the following questions.*

1. What is the result of a retained placenta? _____

2. What is a *spontaneous abortion?* _____

3. What are the other causes of abortion? _____

4. What is another medical term for RDS? _____

5. What is the function of a surfactant? _____

6. What is the medical term for normal presentation of the fetus? _____

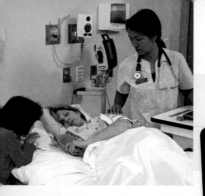

LESSON 15.5

The Female Breast

KEYNOTE

- There is no relation between breast size and the ability to breastfeed.

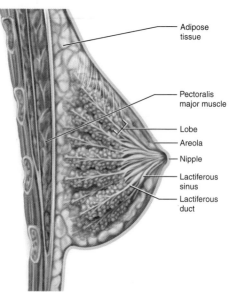

— Adipose tissue

— Pectoralis major muscle

— Lobe
— Areola
— Nipple
— Lactiferous sinus
— Lactiferous duct

▲ **FIGURE 15.20**
Anatomy of the Lactating Breast.

CASE REPORT 15.5

YOU ARE

> . . . a surgical technologist working with Charles Walsh, MD, a surgeon at Fulwood Medical Center.

YOU ARE COMMUNICATING WITH

> . . . Mrs. Victoria Post, a 62-year-old woman who has discovered a lump in her right breast together with some lumps in her right armpit on self-examination. She had not examined her breasts for about 6 months. She began her menopause at age 52. Her mother and a sister died of breast cancer. Physical examination shows a 2-cm firm, painless lesion in the upper outer quadrant of her right breast, and several small, painless lymph nodes in her right axilla. Dr. Walsh has scheduled her for a biopsy of the breast lesion and for DNA testing.

The Breast (LO 15.8)

Anatomy of the Breast (LO 15.8)

The female breasts can be both beautiful and functional. They help to give a woman her distinctive feminine shape, and, after childbirth, they provide natural nourishment for an infant. Each adult female breast has a **body** located over the pectoralis major muscle and an **axillary tail** extending toward the armpit. The **nipple** projects from the breast and contains multiple openings of the main milk ducts. The reddish-brown **areola** surrounds the nipple. The small bumps on its surface are called **areolar glands.** These are sebaceous glands whose secretions prevent chapping and cracking during breastfeeding.

The **nonlactating breast** consists mostly of adipose and connective tissues. It has a system of ducts that branch through the connective tissue and converge on the nipple.

Mammary Gland (LO 15.8)

When the **mammary** gland develops during pregnancy, it is divided into 15 to 20 lobes that contain the secretory **alveoli** which produce milk. The main milk ducts, called **lactiferous ducts** *(Figure 15.20),* drain each lobe immediately before opening onto the nipple .

Lactation (LO 15.8)

In late pregnancy, the secretory alveoli and lactiferous ducts contain **colostrum.** This is the first secretion from the breasts during pregnancy. Colostrum contains more protein but less fat than human milk. It also contains high levels of **immunoglobulins** *(see Chapter 7)* that give the infant protection from infections. Colostrum begins to be replaced by milk 2 or 3 days after the baby's birth, and this replacement is complete by day 5.

The essential stimulus to milk production is the baby's sucking. This stimulates the pituitary gland to produce **prolactin,** which in turn stimulates milk production, and **oxytocin** *(see Chapter 12),* which causes milk to be ejected from the alveoli into the duct system.

After **lactation** completely stops, **involution** of the mammary gland occurs. The epithelial cells of the alveoli are lost through **apoptosis** (programmed cell death), the ducts shrink in size, and adipose and connective tissues return to be the major breast tissues.

S = Suffix   P = Prefix   R = Root   R/CF= Combining Form

Word	Pronunciation	Elements		Definition
apoptosis	AP-op-TOE-sis	P/ R/	apo- *separation from* -ptosis *drooping*	Programmed normal cell death
areola areolar (adj)	ah-**REE**-oh-lah ah-**REE**-oh-lar	S/ R/	Latin *small area* -ar *pertaining to* areol- *areolar*	Circular reddish area surrounding the nipple Pertaining to the areola
colostrum	koh-**LOSS**-trum		Latin *foremilk*	The first breast secretion at the end of pregnancy
involution	in-voh-**LOO**-shun	S/ P/	-ion *action, condition* in- *in*	Decrease in size
involute (verb)	in voh-**LUTE**	R/	-volut- *roll up, shrink*	
lactation (noun)	lak-**TAY**-shun	S/ R/	-ation *action, process of* lact- *milk*	Production of milk
lactate (verb)	**LAK**-tate	S/	-ate *composed of, pertaining to*	To produce milk
lactiferous (adj)	lak-**TIF**-er-us	S/ R/	-ous *pertaining to* -ifer- *to bear, carry*	Pertaining to or yielding milk
mammary	**MAM**-ah-ree	S/ R/	-ary *pertaining to* mamm- *breast*	Pertaining to the lactating breast
nipple	**NIP**-el		Old English *small nose*	Projection from the breast into which the lactiferous ducts open
oxytocin	**OCK**-see-**TOE**-sin	S/ R/ R/	-in *substance* oxy- *oxygen* -toc- *labor*	Pituitary hormone that stimulates the uterus to contract
prolactin	pro-**LAK**-tin	S/ P/ R/	-in *substance* pro- *before* -lact- *milk*	Pituitary hormone that stimulates the production of milk

EXERCISES

A. Review *the Case Report on this spread before answering the questions.*

1. Where did Mrs. Post find the lumps? _____

2. What important fact is in her history? _____

3. Why would Mrs. Post go to the doctor if the lumps in her breast and armpit were not causing her any pain? _____

_____

4. Use an abbreviation to describe where the 2 cm lump was found. _____

5. Use the medical term to describe where the enlarged lymph nodes appeared. _____

B. Spelling *your documentation correctly is a mark of an educated professional. Read the following statements, and insert the correctly spelled term in the blanks.*

1. The circular, reddish area surrounding the nipple is the *(aireola/areola)* _____.

2. After complete cessation of lactation, involution of the *(mamery/mammary)* _____ gland occurs.

3. Programmed cell death is known as *(apotosis/apoptosis)* _____.

4. The first breast secretion at the end of pregnancy is known as *(colestrium/colostrum)* _____.

C. Proofread *the following sentences for error in fact or spelling. Write the corrected sentences on the lines below.*

1. The main milk ducts are called mammary ducts.

_____

2. The term innvolution means to decrease in size.

_____

3. The first secretion from the breasts during pregnancy is called meconium.

_____

- There is some disagreement whether routine mammograms should begin at age 40 or 50 and whether they should be performed annually or every 2 years.

ABBREVIATIONS

BRCA1, breast cancer genes
BRCA2

BSE   breast self-examination

PMS   premenstrual syndrome

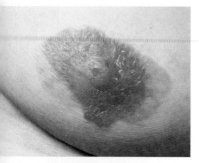

▲ **FIGURE 15.21**
Paget Disease of the Nipple Is Associated with Breast Cancer.

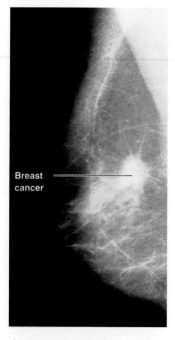

Breast cancer

▲ **FIGURE 15.22**
Mammogram Showing Breast Cancer.

CASE REPORT 15.5 (CONTINUED)

Mrs. Victoria Post's biopsy confirmed that the lump was cancer. DNA testing showed the presence of the BRCA1 gene, which explained the occurrence of breast cancer in her mother and sister. Mrs. Post is to attend a consultation with her surgeon, Dr. Walsh, and her **geneticist,** Ingrid Hughes, MD, PhD, to determine what treatment should be undertaken. For example, because of her high risk of cancer, should she have her left breast, currently cancer-free, removed? With BRCA1, there is also a 20% to 40% risk of ovarian cancer. Therefore, should her ovaries also be removed?

Disorders of the Breast (LO 15.8)

Mastitis, an inflammation of the breast, can occur in association with breastfeeding if the nipple or areola is cracked or traumatized. **Mastalgia** (breast pain) is the most common benign breast disorder. This pain may be associated with breast tenderness or **PMS.**

Paget disease of the nipple presents as a scaling, crusting lesion of the nipple, sometimes with a discharge from the nipple *(Figure 15.21).* It is indicative of an underlying cancer that must be the focus of diagnosis and treatment.

Nipple discharge, particularly if it is bloody and only from one breast, is an indication of an underlying disorder like breast cancer and should be investigated.

Fibroadenomas are confined, small, benign tumors that can be either cystic or solid, and can be multiple. These tumors can be surgically removed.

Fibrocystic breast disease presents as a dense, irregular, cobblestone consistency of the breast, often with intermittent breast discomfort. It occurs in over 60% of all women and is considered by many doctors as a normal condition.

Breast cancer affects one in eight women in their lifetimes. Risk factors include: a family history, particularly if a woman carries either the **BRCA1** or **BRCA2 gene;** the use of postmenopausal estrogen therapy; and an early menarche and late menopause.

Some breast cancers are discovered as a lump by the patient, which is why **monthly breast self-examinations (BSEs)** are important. Another 40% are discovered on routine **mammograms** *(Figure 15.22).* Routine **mammography** reduces breast cancer mortality by 25% to 30%. Breast cancer rarely occurs in males.

Most breast cancers occur in the upper and outer quadrant of the breast. If cancer is suspected, a biopsy should be planned. Currently, it's common to perform a **stereotactic biopsy,** where a needle biopsy is done during mammography. Breast cancer can metastasize to the lymph nodes, lungs, liver, bones, brain, and skin. The surgical treatments available for breast cancer include:

- **Lumpectomy:** the tumor is removed and the surrounding breast tissue is preserved.

- Simple **mastectomy:** the breast with skin and the nipple is removed.

- Modified radical mastectomy: a simple mastectomy with lymph node dissection.

- Radical mastectomy: a modified mastectomy that includes the removal of lymph nodes and the pectoralis major muscle.

Additional radiotherapy and chemotherapy are also used.

Galactorrhea occurs when a woman produces milk when she's not breastfeeding. This can occur in association with hormone therapy, antidepressants, a pituitary gland tumor, and the use of street drugs like cocaine, heroin, and marijuana. In most cases, the milk production ceases with time.

Gynecomastia is an enlargement of the breast that can be unilateral or bilateral. It can occur in both sexes. It is usually associated with either liver disease, marijuana use, or drug therapy involving estrogens, calcium channel blockers, and **antineoplastic** drugs. Gynecomastia remits or disappears after the drug is withdrawn. Occasionally, cosmetic surgery is needed.

Word	Pronunciation		Elements	Definition
antineoplastic	AN-tee-nee-oh-**PLAS**-tik	S/ P/ R/CF R/	-tic *pertaining to* anti- *against* -ne/o- *new* -plas- *growth*	Pertaining to the prevention of the growth and spread of cancer cells
fibroadenoma	FIE-broh-ad-en-**OH**-muh	S/ R/CF R/	-oma *tumor* fibr/o- *fiber* -aden- *gland*	Benign tumor containing much fibrous tissue
fibrocystic disease	fie-broh-**SIS**-tik diz-**EEZ**	S/ R/CF R/	-ic *pertaining to* fibr/o- *fiber* -cyst- *cyst*	Benign breast disease with multiple tiny lumps and cysts
galactorrhea	gah-**LAK**-toe-**REE**-ah	R/ R/CF	-rrhea *flow* galact/o- *milk*	Abnormal flow of milk from the breasts
gene genetics geneticist (Note: 2 suffixes)	JEEN jeh-**NET**-iks jeh-**NET**-ih-sist	 S/ R/ S/	Greek *origin, birth* -ics *knowledge* genet- *origin* -ist *specialist*	Functional segment of DNA molecule Science of the inheritance of characteristics A specialist in genetics
gynecomastia	GUY-nih-koh-**MAS**-tee-ah	S/ R/CF R/	-ia *condition* gynec/o- *female* -mast- *breast*	Enlargement of the breast
lumpectomy	lump-**ECK**-toe-me	S/ R/	-ectomy *surgical excision* lump- *piece*	Removal of a lesion with preservation of surrounding tissue
mammogram mammography	**MAM**-oh-gram mah-**MOG**-rah-fee	S/ R/CF S/	-gram *a record* mamm/o- *breast* -graphy *process of recording*	The record produced by x-ray imaging of the breast Process of x-ray examination of the breast
mastalgia	mass-**TAL**-jee-uh	S/ R/	-algia *pain* mast- *breast*	Pain in the breast
mastectomy	mass-**TECK**-toe-me	S/ R/	-ectomy *surgical excision* mast- *breast*	Surgical excision of the breast
mastitis	mass-**TIE**-tis	S/ R/	-itis *inflammation* mast- *breast*	Inflammation of the breast
Paget disease	**PAJ**-et diz-**EEZ**		Sir James Paget, 1814–1899, English surgeon	Scaling, crusting lesion of the nipple, often associated with an underlying cancer of the breast
stereotactic	**STER**-ee-oh-**TAK**-tic	S/ R/ R/CF	-ic *pertaining to* -tact- *orderly arrangement* stere/o- *three-dimensional*	A precise three-dimensional method to locate a lesion

EXERCISES

A. Review *the Case Report on this spread before answering the questions.*

1. Which diagnostic test confirmed the diagnosis of cancer for Mrs. Post? _____

2. What explains the occurrence of breast cancer in Mrs. Post's mother and sister? _____

3. What type of testing is used for genes? _____

4. What are some options for Mrs. Post's treatment plan? _____

B. Suffixes *always provide a big clue to the meaning of a medical term. Review all the terms in the WAD above, and then answer the following questions. All of these questions can be answered by analyzing the suffix in each term.*

Which of the terms in this WAD means?

1. a condition of enlargement of the breast? _____

2. a glandular tumor? _____

3. process of an x-ray examination of the breast? _____

4. knowledge of the inheritance of characteristics? _____

5. an inflammation of the breast? _____

6. breast pain? _____

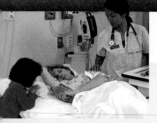

CHAPTER 15 REVIEW FEMALE REPRODUCTIVE SYSTEM

CHALLENGE YOUR KNOWLEDGE

A. Language of gynecology: *Understanding the terminology for the anatomy and physiology of the genitalia and reproductive organs is an important introduction to the female reproductive system. Identify each of the following terms based on its root or combining form and its meaning, and then give the meaning of the medical term. Fill in the chart.*

Medical Term	Root/CF	Meaning of Root/CF	Meaning of Term
progesterone	1.	2.	3.
dyspareunia	4.	5.	6.
gonorrhea	7.	8.	9.
endometrial	10.	11.	12.
hysterectomy	13.	14.	15.
gynecologic	16.	17.	18.
menarche	19.	20.	21.
amenorrhea	22.	23.	24.
colpopexy	25.	26.	27.
menstruation	28.	29.	30.

Use any one of the terms above in a sentence of your choice that could be patient documentation:

_____

_____

B. Build *the following medical terms using the definitions as clues. Write the correct elements on the line, and the meaning of each element under the line. Fill in the blanks.*

1. thinning of cervix in labor _____ / _____ / _____

2. self-digestion _____ / _____ / _____

3. giving birth for the first time _____ / _____ / _____

4. after childbirth _____ / _____ / _____

5. 6-week period after birth _____ / _____ / _____

6. surgical incision to enlarge the opening of the vulva _____ / _____ / _____

7. newborn infant _____ / _____ / _____

8. occurring before the expected time _____ / _____ / _____

C. Prefixes: *The prefix is given in the first column. Identify the meaning of the prefix, give an example of a medical term containing this prefix (the term does not have to be from this chapter), and give the meaning of the term in the last column. Fill in the chart.*

Prefix	Meaning of Prefix	Medical Term Containing This Prefix	Meaning of This Term
a	1.	2.	3.
ab	4.	5.	6.
contra	7.	8.	9.
dys	10.	11.	12.
peri	13.	14.	15.
poly	16.	17.	18.
pre	19.	20.	21.
pro	22.	23.	24.
re	25.	26.	27.
retro	28.	29.	30.
syn	31.	32.	33.

D. Word attack. *This exercise teaches you to think logically about analyzing a medical term.*

Which term means too little *of something?*

    a. polyhydramnios

    b. fibroadenoma

    c. endometriosis

    d. multipara

    e. oligohydramnios

Read the question and the possible answers; then read them again.

The words in the question—*too little*—are describing the quantity of something. *Words* that describe are adjectives, but *elements* that describe how big, how little, the color of something, where something is located, and the like, are usually prefixes.

Here is where your knowledge of elements is important. Slash each term into elements. Start by analyzing just the prefixes.

1. Does every term in this question have a prefix? _____ If not, which terms do not have prefixes?

_____

Analyze the *prefix only* in each of the remaining terms.

2. Which term has the prefix that means *too little?* _____

3. Therefore, the answer is _____.

4. Besides *too little,* what is another meaning for the prefix in the correct answer? _____.

Note: Remember that another way of saying "too little" would be to say "deficient" *(hypo),* so if there had been an answer choice beginning with the element *hypo,* it could have been the correct answer.

Elements can have similar meanings, but they are not interchangeable terms.

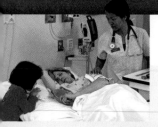

E. Language of obstetrics: *Pregnancy has its own associated set of obstetric terms. Apply your knowledge of obstetric terms to answering the following questions. Write the correct elements on the line, and the identity (P, R, CF, or S) of the element below the line. Remember: Some terms may not contain every element.*

1. disorder in which a fertilized egg continues its development in the fallopian tube instead of the uterus:

   _____ / _____ / _____

2. woman giving birth for the first time:

   _____ / _____ / _____

3. excessive vomiting:

   _____ / _____ / _____

4. removal of amniotic fluid for diagnostic purposes:

   _____ / _____ / _____

5. from conception to birth:

   _____ / _____ / _____

6. first 2 weeks of the developing embryo:

   _____ / _____ / _____

7. too much amniotic fluid:

   _____ / _____ / _____

8. hypertension, edema, and proteinuria during pregnancy:

   _____ / _____ / _____

9. birth occurring before 37 weeks of gestation:

   _____ / _____ / _____

10. destruction of cells by enzymes within the cells:

   _____ / _____ / _____

F. Recall and review: *How well do you remember these word elements from previous chapters? Try to answer without looking back to check. Write your explanation on the lines provided.*

Element	Type of Element	Meaning of Element
1. metro	_____	_____
2. pareun	_____	_____
3. oma	_____	_____
4. syn	_____	_____
5. dys	_____	_____

G. Roots/combining forms *are the core foundation of every term. Circle just the roots or combining forms in the following terms, and give their meanings on the lines provided.*

1. blastocyst: _____

2. gestation: _____

3. ectopic: _____

4. oligohydramnios: _____

5. teratogenic: _____

6. neonatal: _____

7. episiotomy: _____

8. amniocentesis: _____

9. estrogen: _____

10. apoptosis: _____

11. fibrocystic: _____

12. gynecologist: _____

13. mastectomy: _____

14. postpartum: _____

15. cystocele: _____

H. Elements: *Knowing the meanings of word elements is your best tool for building and analyzing medical terms. Choose from among the following word elements, and insert the correct element on the blank to build the medical term.*

1. pertaining to many cysts: _____ cystic

(pick one: mono   poly   cyano   endo)

2. one who studies female diseases: _____ logist

(pick one: neuro   dermato   cardio   gyneco)

3. term synonymous with *menstruation:* _____

(pick one: gynecology   gynecologic   menses   menstrual)

4. inflammation of the uterine tube: _____itis

(pick one: recto   salping   metro   cyst)

5. hormone produced by the ovary: _____ gen

(pick one: menstru   estro   ovari   proges)

6. surgical excision of the vulva: _____ ectomy

(pick one: vulv   hystero   myo   vestibul)

7. pain during sexual intercourse: _____ pareunia

(pick one: dys   a   trans   mal)

8. inner lining of the uterus: _____ metrium

(pick one: endo   myo   peri   pre)

9. surgical fixation of the vagina: _____ pexy

(pick one: vagino   colpo   vestibul   hystero)

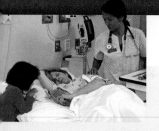

I. Elements: *The following medical terms all have the same prefix, but the rest of their elements make them entirely different terms. Deconstruct each medical term into its basic elements, write their meanings, and then use each term in a sentence of your own making. Fill in the chart, and create the sentences.*

Medical Term	Meaning of Prefix	Meaning of Root/CF	Meaning of Suffix	Meaning of Term
dysplasia	1.	2.	3.	4.
dysmenorrhea	5.	6.	7.	8.
dysplastic	9.	10.	11.	12.
dysfunctional	13.	14.	15.	16.
dyspareunia	17.	18.	19.	20.

Sentences:

1. _____

_____

2. _____

_____

3. _____

_____

4. _____

_____

5. _____

_____

J. Latin and Greek terms *cannot be further deconstructed into prefix, root, or suffix. You must know them for what they are. Test your knowledge of these terms with this exercise. Match the meaning in column 1 with the correct medical term in column 2. There are more answers than you need.*

_____ **1.** smaller

_____ **2.** partition or wall

_____ **3.** lip

_____ **4.** greater

_____ **5.** tampon

_____ **6.** month

_____ **7.** egg

_____ **8.** sheath

_____ **9.** membrane

_____ **10.** come together

A. menses

B. ovary

C. vagina

D. coitus

E. minora

F. hymen

G. majora

H. antrum

I. labium

J. diaphragm

K. plug

L. oocyte

K. Spelling demons: *Every chapter contains spelling demons. Challenge your ability to spell all these terms correctly. Circle the best choice.*

1. choirionic   khorionic   chorionic
2. pre-eclampsia   preeclampsia   preclampsia
3. oligohydramnios   oligohydromios   oligohydrammios
4. puerperpium   puerperium   purperpium
5. cesarian   cesarrian   cesarean
6. obstrician   obstetrican   obstetrician
7. apotosis   apoptossis   apoptosis
8. galactorrhea   galactorhea   galactorea
9. hyperemessis   hyperemmesis   hyperemesis
10. gynecomastia   gyncomastia   gynecomasstia

Write the other terms from this chapter that you found the most difficult to spell and give their definitions.

Term: _____ Definition: _____

_____

Term: _____ Definition: _____

_____

L. Abbreviations: *The following abbreviations have appeared in this chapter. Write out the words each abbreviation stands for, and give a brief definition for it. Refer to your dictionary and/or the Glossary for help. Fill in the blanks.*

1. *LPN* means _____.

    Definition:_____

2. *STD* means _____.

    Definition:_____

3. *HSV* means _____.

    Definition:_____

4. *GYN* means _____.

    Definition:_____

5. *IVF* means _____.

    Definition:_____

6. *c/o* means _____.

    Definition:_____

7. *AIDS* means _____.

    Definition:_____

8. *PCOS* means _____.

    Definition:_____

9. *D & C* means _____.

    Definition:_____

10. *IUD* means _____.

    Definition:_____

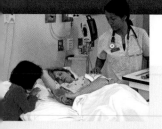

M. Deconstruct terms: *One element in each of the following medical terms has been bolded. First slash the term to isolate the elements. Identify the bolded element as a prefix, root, combining form, or suffix under the line, and write the meaning of the element on the line. Then write another term in which this same element appears. The first one is done for you. Fill in the blanks*

1. ***dysp****areunia*   Meaning: <u>difficult,   painful</u>

   Name another term in which this same element appears: *dyspnea*

2. *gono****rrhea***   Meaning: _____

   Name another term in which this same element appears: _____

3. ***gyneco****logy*   Meaning: _____

   Name another term in which this same element appears: _____

4. *ovul****ation***   Meaning: _____

   Name another term in which this same element appears: _____

5. *recto****cele***   Meaning: _____

   Name another term in which this same element appears: _____

6. *hyster****ectomy***   Meaning: _____

   Name another term in which this same element appears: _____

7. ***salping****itis*   Meaning: _____

   Name another term in which this same element appears: _____

N. Spelling demons: *This chapter contains some very difficult spelling demons. Challenge your ability to spell all these terms correctly. Circle the best choice, and then fill in the blanks.*

1. dyspareuria   dyspareunia   dyspariunia

2. clamidia   clammydia   chlamydia

3. chancre   cankcre   cranchre

4. gonnorhea   gonorrea   gonorrhea

5. trichomonosis   trichomoniasis   trichomonis

6. syphillis   syphilis   syphylis

7. dismenorhea   dysmenorhea   dysmenorrhea

8. liomyoma   leomyoma   leiomyoma

9. menorrhagia   mennoragia   menorhagia

10. diaphragm   diaphram   diaphramm

11. Write a definition for any two terms in the previous list:

Term: _____

Definition: _____

Term: _____

Definition: _____

12. Use any one term in a sentence that is *not* a definition: _____

_____

_____

13. Which term is the most difficult for you to spell correctly?

Term: _____

Definition: _____

O. Abbreviations *must be used carefully to convey the correct information. Circle the best choice to complete the sentence.*

1. This is the patient's first (OB/PGY/RDS).

2. The patient has developed (OR/POC/GDM) in her last trimester.

3. The emergency C-section will be scheduled for the first available (OR/OB/OA).

4. Order 3 units of blood for the patient having the (POC/RDS/PPH).

5. (GDM/RDS/BSE) can save a life.

P. Definitions: *The following medical terms do not deconstruct into elements, so there is no clue as to their meaning. You must know them for what they are. Define the following terms on the lines below.*

1. chorion: _____

_____

2. vertex: _____

_____

3. embryo: _____

_____

4. fetus: _____

_____

5. lochia: _____

_____

6. breech: _____

_____

7. placenta: _____

_____

8. meconium: _____

_____

9. gravida: _____

_____

10. areola: _____

_____

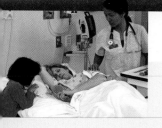

Q. Partner exercise: *On a separate piece of paper, write a multiple-choice question using terms from this chapter. You must have five possible answers. Give your question to your partner, and you answer his or her question. Check your spelling of the terms before submitting your question. Each person should correct the question his or her partner answered. Return all papers to the instructor.*

1. Your question for your partner:

_____

_____

a. _____

b. _____

c. _____

d. _____

e. _____

2. Your partner's question for you:

_____

_____

a. _____

b. _____

c. _____

d. _____

e. _____

R. Dictate *the following sentences to your class partner. Have your partner write them on a separate piece of paper. After he or she has written the sentences, have your partner spell the medical terms for you.* (**Note:** *For the answer to be correct, every word has to be spelled correctly.) If either of you is having difficulties with the pronunciations, check the term on the Student Online Learning Center (*www.mhhe.com/AllanEss2e*). Be prepared to define any of these terms if the instructor should ask!*

1. Some means of contraception are diaphragms, spermicidal foams and gels, intrautcrine devices, and oral contraceptives.

2. Tubal ligation is performed with laparoscopy.

3. An alternative to dilation and curettage is endometrial ablation, in which a laser removes or destroys the lining of the uterus and prevents or reduces menstruation.

Write any misspelled or mispronounced terms on the lines below:

_____

_____

_____

_____

_____

_____

S. Prefixes: *Some of the same prefixes continue to appear throughout these chapters and always have the same meaning. Compare the meanings of medical terms from this chapter with those of medical terms that are from previous chapters and have the same prefix. Each set of elements and two terms requires the meaning for the element (listed first) and the definitions of the two terms below it.*

Element/Term

1. hyper _____

   hyperemesis _____

   hypertension _____

2. neo _____

   neonatal _____

   neoplasm _____

3. oligo _____

   oligohydramnios _____

   oliguria _____

4. poly _____

   polycystic _____

   polyphagia _____

5. pre _____

   preterm _____

   prepatellar _____

6. auto _____

   autolysis _____

   autologous _____

7. post _____

   postpartum _____

   postprandial _____

8. pro _____

   prolactin _____

   prognosis _____

9. anti _____

   antineoplastic _____

   anticoagulant _____

10. peri _____

    perinatal _____

    pericardium _____

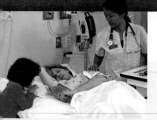

T. Translate *the following sentences from medical language to layperson's language and from layperson's language to medical language.*

Remember to check your spelling, and you should be able to pronounce everything you write. You may be called on to read your sentences in class.

1. From medical language to layperson's language:

"For the neonate, it increases the risk of perinatal mortality, birth trauma, and neonatal hypoglycemia."

_____

2. From layperson's language to medical language:

"The signs of this condition are a sudden, abnormal increase in blood pressure after the 20th week of pregnancy, with swelling of the face, hands, and feet and protein in the urine."

_____

_____

U. Surgical suffixes: *Each of the following terms is an "ectomy," that is, the surgical removal of some body part. What is the doctor removing in each procedure? Fill in the first chart.*

Medical Term	Meaning of Medical Term (What Is Being Removed?)
hysterectomy	1.
salpingectomy	2.
myomectomy	3.
vestibulectomy	4.
cystectomy	5.

Keeping in mind the roots and terms from previous chapters, complete the second chart:

Medical Term	Meaning of Medical Term (What Is Being Removed?)
vasectomy	6.
gastrectomy	7.
pancreatectomy	8.
nephrectomy	9.
laryngectomy	10.
pneumonectomy	11.
cholecystectomy	12.
menisectomy	13.

The principle is the same: Know one suffix, and it is your clue to a dozen different terms. Your knowledge of the roots will help you with the specifics of each term.

V. Short answer: *If you understand the questions below and the terminology well enough, you can explain the concepts to someone else, as you will often have to do on the job. Write your explanation on the lines provided.*

1. Explain how the difference of one word element changes the meanings of these words: *conception* *contraception*

_____

_____

2. A new patient's chart says she is *gravida 4 para 3*. What does that mean? _____

_____

_____

W. Chapter challenge: *Circle the correct answer.*

1. When does the embryo cease being called an embryo and start being called a fetus?

   a. after delivery
   b. after the eighth week
   c. after the third trimester
   d. just before delivery
   e. after the first month

2. Fine, soft hair on the fetal body is called:

   a. lochia
   b. meconium
   c. lanugo
   d. kernicterus
   e. vernix caseosa

3. What is a vertex presentation?

   a. Head presents first, facing rearward
   b. Shoulder and upper back present first
   c. Fetus presents face first
   d. Head presents first, facing downward
   e. Buttocks present first

4. Identify the pair of incorrect spellings:

   a. galactorrhea/gynecomastia
   b. antineoplastic/excisional
   c. fibroadenoma/mammogram
   d. mammography/stereotactic
   e. falopian/corionic

5. The letter "H" in the abbreviation *PPH* stands for:

   a. hemorrhage
   b. hyperemesis
   c. hypoglycemia
   d. hyaline
   e. hysterecomy

6. When the head of the fetus reaches the vaginal opening, the condition is termed:

   a. crowning
   b. effacement
   c. apoptosis
   d. autolysis
   e. involution

7. Previous salpingitis, PID, or endometriosis can sometimes be a cause of:

   a. mastalgia
   b. mastitis
   c. cervical cancer
   d. ectopic pregnancy
   e. eclampsia

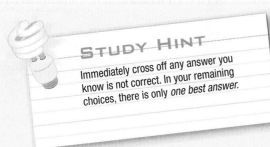

STUDY HINT

Immediately cross off any answer you know is not correct. In your remaining choices, there is only *one best answer*.

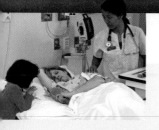

X. Terminology challenge: *Autolysis is a new term you learned in this chapter. It is composed of two elements you have met before in previous chapters. Recall other terms you have already learned that have those elements. Fill in the blanks.*

1. Slash the term *autolysis,* and write the meaning of each element below the line.

_____ / _____ / _____

Other terms with the same elements:

2. *auto:* _____

_____

3. *lysis:* _____

_____

Brain teaser: Why is the term *autolysis* like the term *apoptosis?*

4. _____

Y. Case Report challenge: *Now that you are more comfortable with the terms in this chapter, you can apply that knowledge and briefly answer the questions about the Case Report. If you read the report thoroughly and underline all the medical terminology, this will make it easier to answer the questions.*

CASE REPORT 15.4

YOU ARE

. . . an obstetric assistant employed by Garry Joiner, MD, an obstetrician at Fulwood Medical Center.

YOU ARE COMMUNICATING WITH

Mrs. Gloria Maggay, a 29-year-old housekeeper. Her last menstrual period was 8 weeks ago, and she has a positive home pregnancy test. This is her first pregnancy. She has breast tenderness and mild nausea. For the past 2 days, she has had some cramping, lower right abdominal pain, and this morning had vaginal spotting. Her vital signs are T 99°F, P 80, R 14, BP 130/70.

While you are waiting for Dr. Joiner to come and examine her, Mrs. Maggay complains of feeling faint and has a sharp, severe pain in her lower abdomen on the right side. Her pulse rate has increased to 92. You need to recognize what is happening.

Mrs. Gloria Maggay's symptoms are those of an ectopic pregnancy. The sudden increase in the pain and the rise in pulse rate can indicate that the tube has ruptured and is hemorrhaging into the abdominal cavity. The obstetrician should see Mrs. Maggay immediately and take her to the operating room for laparoscopic surgery to stop the bleeding and evacuate the products of conception.

1. List all of Mrs. Maggay's symptoms:

_____

_____

2. There are abbreviations that could be substituted for medical terms in the Case Report. Write them here:

_____

_____

3. What body quadrant has the "sharp, severe pain"? Use the abbreviation:

_____

_____

4. Mrs. Maggay is "hemorrhaging into the abdominal cavity"—what does this mean?

_____

_____

5. Name one other body cavity: _____

Name one organ located in this cavity: _____

6. What "tube" has ruptured? _____

7. In this case, what happened when the tube ruptured?

_____

_____

8. Define *ectopic pregnancy:*

_____

_____

9. Why, then, has the tube ruptured?

_____

_____

10. What type of instrument will be used in Mrs. Maggay's surgery?

_____

_____

11. What medical term can be applied to Mrs. Maggay since this is her first pregnancy?

_____

_____

12. In Vital Signs, what do the following abbreviations stand for?

T _____

P _____

R _____

BP _____

Word Parts and Abbreviations

Note: For easy identification, the word parts in this appendix appear in the same colors as in the Word Analysis and Definition boxes: suffix, prefix, root, root/combining form. Any term that is used in the text in both root and combining form is shown only in this appendix as a combining form.

Word Part	Definition
a-	not, without
a-	variant of ad
ab-	away from
abdomin/o	abdomen
ability	competence
ablat	take away
-able	capable
abort	fail at onset, expel nonviable fetus
abras	scrape off
absorpt	to swallow, take in
ac-	toward
-ac	pertaining to
-acea	condition, remedy
acid/o	acid, low pH
acin	grape
acous	hearing
acr/o	peak, topmost, extremity, highest point
acromi/o	acromion
act	to do, perform, performance
activ	movement
acu	needle
acu-	sharp
acumin	to sharpen
ad-	to, toward, into
adapt	to adjust
-ade	process
aden/o	gland
adenoid	adenoid
adip	fat
adjust	alter
adjuv	give help
adolesc	beginning of adulthood
adren/o	adrenal gland

Word Part	Definition
aer/o	air, gas
affer	move toward the center
ag-	to
-age	pertaining to
agglutin	sticking together, clumping
-ago	disease
agon	to fight
-agon	to fight
agor/a	marketplace
-agra	severe pain
-al	pertaining to
alanine	an amino acid, protein synthesized in muscle
albicans	white
albino/o	white
albumin	albumin
ald/o	organic compound
-ale	pertaining to
alges	sensation of pain
-algia	pain, painful condition
aliment	nourishment
-alis	pertaining to
alkal	base
all/o	strange, other
allo-	strange, other
alopec-	baldness, mange
alpha-	first letter in the Greek alphabet
alveol	alveolus, air sac
-aly	condition
ambly-	dull
ambulat	to walk, walking
amin/o	nitrogen containing
-amine	nitrogen-containing substance
ammon	ammonia

WORD PART	DEFINITION
amni/o	amnion, fetal membrane
amnios	amnion
amph-	around
ampull	bottle-shaped
amput	to prune, cut off
amyl	starch
an-	not, lack of, without
-an	pertaining to
an/o	anus
ana-	away from, excessive
anabol	build up
analysis	process to study whole in terms of its parts
analyst	one who separates
anastom	provide a mouth
-ance	condition, state of
-ancy	state of
andr/o	male, masculine
aneurysm	dilation
angi/o	blood vessel, lymph vessel
angina	sore throat, chest pain radiating to throat
ankyl	stiff
-ant	forming, pertaining to
ant-	against
ante-	before, forward, in front of
anter	before, front part
anthrac	coal
anti-	against
aort	aorta
apo-	different from, separation from
appendic	appendix
apse	clasp
aqu-	water
-ar	pertaining to
arachn	cobweb, spider
-arche	beginning
areol	areolar
aria	air
-arian	one who is

WORD PART	DEFINITION
-aris	pertaining to
aroma	smell, sweet herb
array	place in order
arter	artery
arteri/o	artery
arteriosus	like an artery
arthr/o	joint
articul	joint
-ary	pertaining to
asbest	asbestos
ascit	fluid in the belly
-ase	enzyme
aspartate	an amino acid
aspergill	aspergillus
aspirat	to breathe on
assay	evaluate
assist	aid, help
asthm	asthma
astr/o	star
-ata	action, place, use
-ate	composed of, pertaining to
-ated	pertaining to a condition
atel	incomplete
ather/o	porrldge, gruel, fatty substance
athet	without position, uncontrolled
-atic	pertaining to
-ation	a process
-ative	pertaining to, quality of
-ator	agent, instrument, person or thing that does something
-atory	pertaining to
atri/o	entrance, atrium
-atric	treatment
attent	awareness
attenu	to weaken
audi/o	hearing
audit	hearing
aur-	ear
auscult	listen to

S = Suffix   P = Prefix   R = Root   R/CF = Combining Form

Word Part	Definition
auto-	self, same
avail	useful
axill	armpit, axilla
ayur-	life
azot	nitrogen
-back	back, toward the starting point
bacteri/o	bacteria
balan	glans penis
bar	pressure
bari	weight
bas/o	base, opposite of acid
basal	deepest part
basil	base, support
be	life
behav	mental or motor activity
beta	second letter of Greek alphabet
bi-	two, twice, double
bi/o	life
-bil	able
bil/i	bile
-blast	germ cell, immature cell
blast/o	germ cell, immature cell
blephar/o	eyelid
body	body, mass, substance
bov	cattle
brachi/o	arm
brachii	of the arm
brachy-	short
brady-	slow
bride	rubbish, rubble
bronch/i	bronchus
bronch/o	bronchus
brucell	pathologist David Bruce
buccinat	cheek
bulb/o	bulb
burs	bursa
calc/i	calcium
calcan	calcaneous
calcul	stone, little stone

Word Part	Definition
callos	thickening
calor	heat
canal	duct or channel
cancer	cancer
candid	*Candida*
capill	hairlike, capillary
capit	head
capn	carbon dioxide
caps	box, cover, shell
capsul	box
carb/o	carbon
carboxy	group of organic compounds
carcin/o	cancer
card	heart
cardi/o	heart
care	be responsible for
carotene	yellow-red pigment
carotid	large neck artery
carp/o	bones of the wrist
cartilag	cartilage
cata-	down
catabol	break down
catechol	tyrosine-containing
catheter	insert, catheter
caud	tail
cav	hollow space
cava	cave
cavern	cave
cec	cecum
-cele	cave, hernia, swelling
celi	abdomen
cellul	cell, small cell
cent-	hundred
-centesis	to puncture
centr/o	central
ceph	head
cephal/o	head
-cephalus	head
cephaly	condition of the head

503

Word Part	Definition
ceps	head
cept	to receive
cerebell	little brain, cerebellum
cerebr/o	brain
cerumin	cerumen
cervic	neck
cess	going forward
chancr	chancre
chem/o	chemical
chemic	chemical
-chete	hair
-chezia	pass a stool
chir/o	hand
chlor	green
chol/e	bile
cholangi	bile duct
cholecyst	gallbladder
choledoch/o	common bile duct
chondr/o	cartilage, rib, granule
chorion	chorion, membrane
chrom/o	color
chromat	color
chron/o	time
chym/o	chyme
-cidal	pertaining to killing
cide	to kill
cili	hairlike structure
circulat	circular route
circum-	around
cirrh	yellow
cis	to cut
cit/i	cell
-clast	break, break down
claudic	limp
claustr/o-	confined space
clav	clavicle
clave	lock
clavicul	clavicle
-cle	small

Word Part	Definition
clitor	clitoris
clon	cutting used for propagation, tumult
-clonus	violent action
co-	with, together
coagul/o	clot, clump
coarct	press together, narrow
cobal	cobalt
cocc	round bacterium
coccus	berry, spherical bacterium
cochle	cochlear
code	information system
cognit	thinking
coit	sexual intercourse
col-	with, together
col	colon
coll	collect, glue
coll/a	glue
colon/o	colon
coloniz	form a colony
colp/o	vagina
com	take care of
com-	with, together
comat	coma
combin	combine
comminut	break into pieces
commodat	adjust
compat	tolerate
compet	strive together
complex	woven together
compli	fulfill
compress	press together
compuls	drive, compel
con-	with, together
concav	arched, hollow
concept	become pregnant
concuss	shake or jar violently
condyl	knuckle
confus	bewildered
congest	accumulation of fluid

S = Suffix   P = Prefix   **R = Root**   **R/CF = Combining Form**

Word Part	Definition
coni	dust
coniz	cone
conjunctiv	conjunctiva
connect	join together
conscious	awareness
constip	press together
constrict	to narrow
contagi/o	transmissible by contact
contaminat/o	to corrupt, make unclean
contin	hold together
contra-	against
contract	draw together, pull together
contus	bruise
convalesc	recover
cor	heart
cori	skin
corne/o	cornea
coron	crown, coronary
corpor/e	body
corpus	body
cortic/o	cortex, cortisone
cortis	cortisone
cost	rib
crani/o	cranium, skull
crease	groove
creat	flesh
creatin	creatine
crete	to separate
cretin	cretin
crimin	distinguish
crine	secrete
crista	cresl
-crit	to separate
cry/o	cold
crypt-	hidden
cub	cube
cubit	elbow
cubitus	lying down
cune/i	wedge

Word Part	Definition
cur	cleanse, cure
curat	to care for
curett	to cleanse
cursor	run
cusp	point
cutan/e	skin
cyan/o	dark blue
-cyst	cyst, bladder
cyst/o	bladder, sac, cyst
cysteine	an amino acid
cyt/o	cell
-cyte	cell
cyte	cell
dacry/o	tears, lacrimal duct
dai	day
de-	without, out of, removal, from
defec	clear out waste
defici	failure, lacking, inadequate
degenerat	deteriorate
deglutit	to swallow
del	visible
deliri	confusion, disorientation
delt	triangle
delus	deceive
dem	the people
demi-	half
dendr/o	treelike
dent	tooth
depend	rely on
depress	press down
derm/a	skin
-derma	skin
dermat/o	skin
dermis	skin
-desis	bind together, fixation of bone or joint
di-	two
dia-	complete
diabet	diabetes
diagnost	decision

Word Part	Definition
dialectic	argument
dialy	separate
diaphor	sweat
diaphragm/a	diaphragm
diastol	diastole, relaxation
dict	consent, surrender
didym/o	testis
didymis	testis
diet	a way of life
different	not identical
digest	to break down food
digit	finger or toe
dilat	open up, expand, widen
dips	thirst
dis-	apart, away from
discipl	understand
disciplin	disciple, instruction
dist	away from the center
-dium	appearance
diuret	increase urine output
diverticul	byroad
dorm	sleep
dors	back
dorsi	of the back
drome	running
drop	liquid globule
duce	to lead
ducer	to lead, leader
duct	to lead, lead
ductus	leading
duoden	twelve, duodenum
dur	dura
dura	hard
dwarf	miniature
dynam/o	power
-dynia	pain
dys-	bad, difficult, painful
e-	out of, from
-eal	pertaining to

Word Part	Definition
ease	normal function, freedom from pain
ec-	out, outside
ech/o	sound wave
echin	hedgehog
eclamps	shining forth
eco-	environment
-ectasis	dilation
-ectomy	excision, surgical excision
ectop	on the outside, displaced
eczem/a	eczema
-ed	pertaining to
edema	edema, swelling
-ee	person who is the object of an action
efface	wipe out
effer	move out from the center
effus	pour out
ejacul	shoot out
ejaculat	shoot out
elasma	plate
elect	choice
electr/o	electric, electricity
elimin	throw away, expel
-elle	small
-em	condition
em-	in, into
-ema	quality of, quantity of
emac/i	make thin
embol	plug
embryon	embryo, fertilized egg
emesis	vomiting
-emesis	to vomit, vomiting
emet	to vomit
emia	a blood condition
-emia	a blood condition
-emic	pertaining to a blood condition
emic	pertaining to a blood condition
emmetr-	measure
emuls	suspend in a liquid
en-	in

S = Suffix   P = Prefix   **R = Root   R/CF = Combining Form**

WORD PART	DEFINITION
-ence	forming, quality of, state of
enceph	brain
encephal/o	brain
encephaly	condition of the brain
-ency	condition, state of, quality of
end-	inside, within
endo-	inside, within
-ent	end result, pertaining to
enter/o	intestine
entery	condition of the intestine
enur	urinate
environ	surroundings
-eon	one who does
eosin/o	dawn
ependym	lining membrane
epi-	above, upon, over
epilept	seizure
epiphys/i	growth
episi/o	vulva
equi-	equal
equin	horse
equip	to fit out
-er	agent, one who does
erect	straight, to set up
erg/o	work
-ergy	process of working
-ery	process of
erysi-	red
erythemat	redness
erythr/o	red
-escent	process
-esis	condition
eso-	inward
esophag/e	esophagus
essent	existence
esthes	sensation, perception
esthet	sensation, perception
estr/o	woman
ethm	sieve

WORD PART	DEFINITION
eti/o	cause
-etic	pertaining to
-etics	pertaining to
-ette	little
eu-	good, normal
ex-	away from, out, out of
exacerbat	increase, aggravate
examin	test, examine
excis	cut out
excret	separate, discharge
exo-	outside, outward
expect	await
expir	breathe out
extra-	out of, outside
faci	face
factor	maker
farct	area of dead tissue
fasc/i	fascia
febr	fever
fec	feces
feed	to give food, nourish
femor	femur
fer	to bear, to carry
ferrit	iron
fertil	able to conceive
fertiliz	to make fruitful
fet/o	fetus
fibr/o	fiber, fibrous
fibrill	small fiber
fibrin/o	fibrin
fibul	fibula
-fication	remove
fida	split
field	definite area
filar	roundworm
filtr	strain through
fiss	split
fistul	tube, pipe
flammat	flame

S = Suffix   P = Prefix   R = Root   R/Cf = Combining Form

Word Part	Definition
flat	flatus
flatul	excessive gas
flavin	yellow
flex	bend
fluid	flowing
fluo-	fluorine
fluor/o	flux, flow
flux	flow
foc	center, focus
follicul	follicle
foramin	opening, foramen
fore-	in front
-form	appearance of, resembling
format	to form
fract	break
fraction	small amount
free	free
frequ	repeated, often
front	front, forehead
fructos	fruit sugar
function	perform
fund/o	fundus
fung/i	fungus
fusion	to pour
galact/o	milk
gall	bile
gastr/o	stomach
gastrin	stomach hormone
gastrocnem	calf of leg
gemin	twin, double
gen/o	produce, create
-gen	create, produce, form
gen-	birth
-gene	production, give birth
gener	create, produce
genesis	origin, creation, production
-genesis	creation, origin, formation, source
genet	origin
-genic	creation, producing

Word Part	Definition
genit	bring forth, birth, primary male or female sex organ
genitor	offspring
ger	old age
geront/o	old age
gest	gestation, pregnancy, produce
gestat	gestation, pregnancy, to bear
gigant	giant
gingiv	gums
gland	gland
glauc	lens opacity, grey
gli/o	glue, supportive tissue of nervous system
-glia	glue, supportive tissue of nervous system
globin/o	protein
globul	globular, protein
glomerul/o	glomerulus
gloss/o	tongue
glott	mouth of windpipe
glottis	mouth of windpipe
gluc/o	glucose, sugar
glut	buttocks
glutin	glue, stick
glyc/o	glycogen, glucose, sugar
glycer	glycerol, sweet
gnath	jaw
gnose	use knowledge
gnosis	knowledge
gomph	bolt, nail
gon/o	seed
gonad/o	gonads, testes, or ovaries
gong	daily practice
-grade	going
graft	splice, transplant
-graft	tissue for transplant
graine	head pain
-gram	a record, recording
grand-	big
grand	big

Word Part	Definition
granul/o	granule, small grain
-graph	to record, write
-grapher	one who records
-graphy	process of recording
gravida	pregnant
gravis	serious
gru	to move
guan	dung
gurgit	flood
gynec/o	woman, female
habilitat	restore
hale	breathe
halit	breath
hallucin	imagination
hallux	big toe
hem/o	blood
hemangi/o	blood vessel
hemat/o	blood
heme	red iron-containing pigment
hemi-	half
hepar	liver
hepat/o	liver
herb/i	plant
herni/o	hernia, rupture
herp	blister
hetero-	different
hiat	opening
hist	derived from histidine
hist/o	tissue
holist	entire, whole
hom/i	man
home/o	the same
homo-	same, alike
hormon	chemical messenger, hormone
human	human being
humor	fluid
hyal	glass
hydr/o	water
hyp-	below

Word Part	Definition
hyper-	above, beyond, excess, excessive
hypn/o	sleep
hypo-	below, deficient, smaller, low, under
hyster/o	uterus
-ia	condition
-iac	pertaining to
-ial	pertaining to
-ian	one who does, specialist
-ias	condition
-iasis	abnormal condition
iatr	medical treatment, physician
-iatric	relating to medicine, medical knowledge
iatrics	medical knowledge
-iatrist	practitioner, one who treats
-iatry	treatment, field of medicine
-ible	can do, able to
-ic	pertaining to
-ica	pertaining to
-ical	pertaining to
-ician	expert
-ics	knowledge
ict	seizure
icterus	jaundice
-id	having a particular quality, pertaining to
-ide	having a particular quality
idi/o	unknown, personal
ifer	to bear, carry
-ify	to become
-il	a thing
-ile	pertaining to
ile/o	ileum
ili/o	ilium (hip bone)
im	in, not
imag	likeness
immun/o	immune, immune response, immunity
immune	protected from
immuniz	make immune
impair	worsen
impede	obstruct

Word Part	Definition
-imus	most
-in	substance, chemical compound
in-	not, into, in
incis	cut into
incub	sit on, lie on, hatch
index	to declare
-ine	pertaining to
infant	infant
infect	internal invasion, infection
infer	below, beneath
infest	invade, attack
inflammat	set on fire
inflat	blow up
infra-	below, beneath
-ing	quality of, doing
ingest	carry in
inguin	groin
inhal	breathe in
inhibit	repress
inject	force in
ino	sinew
insect/i	insect
insert	put together
inspir	breathe in
insul	island
integr	whole
integument	covering of the body
inter-	between
interstiti	space between tissues
intestin	gut, intestine
intra-	inside, within
intrins	on the inside
intus-	within
iod	violet, iodine
-ion	action, condition
-ior	pertaining to
-iosum	pertaining to
-ious	pertaining to
irrig	to water

Word Part	Definition
-is	belonging to, pertaining to
isch	to block
ischi	ischium
-ism	condition, process
-ismus	take action
iso-	equal
-ist	agent, specialist
-istic	pertaining to
-isy	inflammation
-ites	associated with
-ition	process
-itis	inflammation, infection
-ity	condition, state
-ium	structure
-ius	pertaining to
-ive	nature of, quality of, pertaining to
-iz	subject to
-ization	process of inserting or creating
-ize	action, affect in a specific way, policy
-ized	affected in a specific way
-izer	affects in a particular way, line of action
jejun	jejunum
jugul	throat
junct	joining together
juxta-	beside, near, close to
kal	potassium
kary/o	nucleus
kel/o	tumor
kerat	keratin, hard protein
kerat/o	cornea
kern	nucleus
ket/o	ketone
keton	ketone
ketone	organic compound
kin	motion
kinase	enzyme
kinesi/o	movement
kinet	motion
-kinin	move in

Word Part	Definition
klept/o	to steal
kyph/o	bent, humpback
labi	lip
labyrinth	inner ear
lacer	to tear
lacrim	tears, tear duct
lact	milk
lactat	secrete milk
lapar/o	abdomen in general
lapse	clasp, fall together
-lapse	fall together, slide
laryng/o	larynx
lash	end of whip
lat	to take
lateral	at the side
latiss	wide
-le	small
lei/o	smooth
-lemma	covering
-lepsy	seizure
lept	thin, small
-let	small
leuk/o	white
lex	word
librium	balance
ligament	ligament
ligat	tie up, tie off
lign	line
-ling	small
lingu	tongue
lip/o	fat
lipid	fat
lith/o	stone
liv	life, live
load	to carry
lob	lobe
locat	a place
log	to study
-logist	one who studies, specialist

Word Part	Definition
logous	relation
-logy	study of
logy	study of
longev	long life
lord/o	curve, swayback
lubric	make slippery
lucid	bright, clear
lumb	lower back, loin
lump	piece
lun	moon
lupus	wolf
-lus	small
lute	yellow
luxat	dislocate
ly	break down, separate
-ly	every
lymph/o	lymph, lymphatic system
lymphaden/o	lymph node
lymphangi/o	lymphatic vessels
lys/o	decompose, dissolve
lysis	destruction
-lysis	destruction, dissolve, separation
lyt	dissolve, destroy
-lyte	soluble
-lytic	relating to destruction
lyze	destruct, dissolve
macro-	large
macul	spot
magnet	magnet
mak	makes
-maker	one who makes
mal-	bad, difficult
mal	bad, difficult, inadequate
-malacia	abnormal softness
malign	harmful, bad
malleol	small hammer, malleolus
mamm/o	breast
man	frenzy, madness
man/o	pressure

Word Part	Definition
mandibul	mandible
-mania	frenzy, madness
manic	affected by frenzy
manipul	handful, use of hands
marker	sign
mast	breast
mastic	chew
mastoid	mastoid process
mater	mother
matern	mother
matur(e)	ripe, ready, fully developed
maxilla	maxilla
medi	middle
media	middle
mediastin/o	mediastinum
medic	medicine
medulla	middle
mega-	enormous
-megaly	enlargement
mei	lessening
mela	black
melan/o	melanin, black pigment
mellit	sweetened with honey
membran/o	cover, skin
men/o	menses, monthly, month
mening/o	meninges, membranes
menisc	crescent, meniscus
menstr/u	menses, occurring monthly
ment	mind, chin
-ment	action, state, resulting state
mere	part
mero-	partial
meso-	middle
meta-	after, beyond, subsequent to
metabol	change
metacarp	bones of the hand
metatars	bones of the feet
-meter	measure, instrument to measure
metr/o	uterus

Word Part	Definition
-metric	pertaining to measurement
-metrist	skilled in measurement
-metry	process of measuring
mi-	derived from *hemi,* half
micr/o	small
micro-	small
mictur	pass urine
mid-	middle
mileusis	lathe
milli-	one-thousandth
miner	mines
mineral/o	inorganic material
miss	send
mit	thread
mito-	thread
mitr	having two points
mitt	send
mod	nature, form, method
molec	mass
mollusc	soft
mon	single
monas	single unit
monil	type of fungus
mono-	one, single
morbid	disease
morph/o	shape
mort	death
mot	move
motiv	move
muc/o	mucus, mucous membrane
mucosa	lining of a cavity
multi-	many
mune	in service
muscul/o	muscle
mut	silent
muta	genetic change
mutil	to maim
my/o	muscle
myc/o	fungus

Word Part	Definition
myel/o	spinal cord, bone marrow
myelin	in the spinal cord, myelin
myo-	to blink
myop	to blink
myos	muscle
myring/o	tympanic membrane, eardrum
myx-	mucus
narc/o	stupor
nas	nose
nat	born, birth
nate	born, birth
natr/i	sodium
natur/o	nature
ne/o	new
nebul	cloud
necr/o	death
neo-	new
nephr/o	kidney
nerv	nerve
-ness	quality, state
neur/o	nerve, nervous tissue
neutr/o	neutral
nici	lethal
nitr/o	nitrogen
noct-	night
noia	to think
nom	law
non-	no, not
nor-	normal
norm-	normal
nos/o	disease
nucle/o	nucleus
nucleol	small nucleus
nutri	nourish
nutrit	nourishment
o/o	egg
oblong	elongated
obsess	besieged by thoughts
obstetr	pregnancy and childbirth

Word Part	Definition
occipit	back of head
occulta	hidden
ocul/o	eye
-ode	way, road, path
odont	tooth
odyn/o	pain
-oid	resembling
-ol	alcohol, chemical, substance
-ola	small
-ole	small
olfact	smell
oligo-	scanty, too little
om/o	body, tumor
-oma	tumor, mass
onc/o	tumor
-one	chemical substance, hormone
onych/o	nail
ophthalm/o	eye
ophthalmos	eye
-opia	sight
opportun	take advantage of
-opsis	vision
-opsy	to view
opt/o	vision
optic	eye
-or	a doer, one who does, that which does something
or/o	mouth
orbit	orbit
orchi/o	testicle
ordin	arrange
orex	appetite
organ	organ, tool, instrument
orth/o	straight
orthot	correct
-orum	function of
-ory	having the function of
os	mouth
-osa	full of, like

S = Suffix   P = Prefix   R = Root   R/Cf = Combining Form

Word Part	Definition
-ose	full of
-osis	abnormal condition
osmo	push
osmol	concentration
oss/e	bone
oste/o	bone
-osus	condition
ot/o	ear
-otomy	incision
-ous	pertaining to
ov/i	egg
ovari	ovary
ovul	ovum, egg
ox	oxygen
-oxia	oxygen condition
oxid	oxidize
oxy	oxygen
pace	step
palat	palate
palliat	reduce suffering
palm	palm
palpat	touch, stroke
palpit	throb
pan-	all
pancreat	pancreas
panto-	entire
papill/o	pimple
par-	abnormal, beside
para	to bring forth
para-	adjacent to, alongside, beside, abnormal
paresis	weakness
parasit	parasite
pareun	lying beside, sexual intercourse
pariet	wall
paroxysm	irritate; sudden, sharp attack
particul	little piece
partum	childbirth, to bring forth
pat	lie open

Word Part	Definition
patell	patella
patent	lie open
-path	disease
path/o	disease
pathet	suffering
-pathic	pertaining to a disease
pathy	disease, emotion
-pathy	disease
paus	cessation
pause	cessation
pector	chest
ped	child, foot
pedicul	louse
pelas	skin
pelv	pelvis
pen	penis
-penia	deficient, deficiency
peps	digestion
pepsin/o	pepsin
pept	digest
per-	through, intense
perforat	bore through
perfus	to pour
peri-	around
perine	perineum
peripher	external boundary, outer part, outer edge
periton/e	stretch over, peritoneum
perium	a bringing forth
perm/e	pass through
pes	foot
pesti	pest
petit	small
petit-	small
-pexy	fixation, surgical fixation
phaco-	lens
phag/o	to eat
phage	to eat
-phage	to eat

Word Part	Definition
-phagia	swallowing, eating
phagia	swallowing
phalang/e	phalanx, finger, toe
pharmac/o	drug
pharyng/o	pharynx
pharynx	pharynx, throat
phenol	benzene derivative
phenyl	chemical group
pheo-	gray
pher/o	to carry
-pheresis	removal
-phil	attraction
-phile	attraction
-philia	attraction
phim	muzzle
phleb/o	vein
phob	fear
-phobia	fear
phon/o	sound, voice
phor	bear, carry
phosphat	phosphorus
phot/o	light
phren	mind
phylac	protect
phylaxis	protection
-phyll	leaf
physema	blowing
physi/o	body
physis	growth
phyt/o	plant
pia	delicate
pituit	pituitary
pituitar	pituitary
plak	plate, plaque
plant	insert, plant
planus	flat surface
plas	molding, formation, growth
-plasia	formation
-plasm	something formed

Word Part	Definition
plasm/o	to form
-plasty	formation, repair, surgical repair
plate	flat
pleg	paralysis
plete	filled
pleur	pleura
plexy	stroke
-pnea	breathe
pneum/o	air, lung
pneumat	structure filled with air
pneumon	air, lung
pod	foot
-poiesis	to make
-polet	the making
-poietin	the maker
poikilo-	irregular
point	to pierce
pol	pole
polio	gray matter
pollut	unclean
poly-	excessive, many, much
polyp	polyp
poplit/e	ham, back of knee
por/o	opening
post-	after
poster	back part
pract	efficient, practical
prand/i	breakfast
pre-	before, in front of
precis	accurate
pregn	with child, pregnant
presby	old man
press	press close, press down, squeeze
prevent	prevent
primi-	first
pro-	before, in front, projecting forward
proct/o	anus and rectum
product	lead forth
prolifer	bear offspring

515

S = Suffix   P = Prefix   R = Root   R/Cf = Combining Form

Word Part	Definition
pronat	bend down
prosta	prostate
prosthet	artificial part
prot/e	first
protein	protein
proto-	first
provision	provide
proxim	nearest to the center
prurit	itch
pseudo-	false
psych/o	mind, soul
psyche	mind, soul
pteryg	wing
ptosis	drooping, falling
-ptosis	drooping
ptysis	spit
pub	pubis
puer	child
pulmon/o	lung
puls	to drive
pump	pump
punct	puncture
pupill-	pupil
pur	pus
purific	make pure
purul	pus
py/o	pus
pyel/o	renal pelvis
pylor	gate, pylorus
pyr/o	fire, heat
pyrex	fever
pyrid	heat
qi	vital force
quadrant	quadrant
quadri-	four
radi/o	radius, x-ray, radiation
radic	root
re-	again, back, backward
recept	receive

Word Part	Definition
rect/o	rectum
reflex	bend back
refract	bend
regul	to rule, control
remiss	send back, give up
ren	kidney
replic	reply
rescein	resin
resect/o	cut off
resid/u	left over, what is left over
resist	to withstand
respire/a	to breathe
restor	renew
resuscit	revive from apparent death
reticul	fine net, network
retin/o	retina
retinacul	hold back
retro-	backward
rhabd/o	rod shaped, striated
rheumat	a flow, rheumatism
rhin/o	nose
rhythm	rhythm
rib/o	like a rib
ribo	a sugar, pentose
ribo-	from ribose, a sugar
rigid	stiff
rose	rose
rotat	rotate
-rrhagia	excessive flow, discharge
-rrhaphy	suture
rrhea	flow, discharge
-rrhoid	flow
rrhyth	rhythm
rrhythm	rhythm
-rubin	rust colored
rumin	throat
sacchar	sugar
sacr/o	sacrum
sagitt	arrow

Word Part	Definition
saliv	saliva
salping/o	fallopian tube, uterine tube
salpinx	trumpet
san	sound, healthy
sanit	health
sapon	soap
sarc/o	flesh, muscle, sarcoma
satur	to fill
scapul	scapula
schiz/o	to split, cleave
scintill	spark
scler/o	hardness, white of eye
scoli/o	crooked
scope	instrument for viewing
-scope	instrument for viewing, instrument to examine
-scopy	to examine, to view
scorb	scurvy
scrot	scrotum
seb/o	sebum
sebac/e	wax
sebum	wax
secret	secrete, produce, separate
sect	cut off
sedat	to calm
sedent	sitting
segment	section
seiz	to grab
self	me, own individual
semi-	half
semin/i	semen
seminat	scatter seed
sen	old age
senesc	growing old
senil	senile
sens	feel
sensitiv	feeling
sensor/i	sensation, sensory
separat	move apart

Word Part	Definition
seps	decay, infection
sept/o	septum, partition
ser/o	serum
serum	serum
sib	relative
-side	glycoside
sigm	Greek letter "S"
silic	silicon, glass
simi	ape, monkey
simul	imitate
sin/o	sinus
sinus	sinus
sipid	flavor
-sis	abnormal condition, process
sit/u	place
skelet	skeleton
smear	spread
soc	partner
soci/o	society, social
soma	body
somat/o	body
-some	body
somn/o	sleep
son/o	sound
sorbit	fruit of a tree
sorpt	swallow
spad	tear or cut
spasm	spasm, sudden involuntary tightening
spast	tight
specif	species
sperm/i	sperm
spermat/o	sperm
sphen	wedge
spher/o	sphere
sphygm/o	pulse
spin/a	spine
spin/o	spine, spinal cord
spir/o	to breathe
spirat	breathe

S = Suffix   P = Prefix   **R = Root**   **R/Cf = Combining Form**

WORD PART	DEFINITION	WORD PART	DEFINITION
spirit/u	spirit	strict	narrow
spiro-	spiral, coil	study	inquiry
splen/o	spleen	su/i	self
spongios	sponge	sub-	below, under, underneath
spor	spore	suct	suck
stable	steady	suffic/i	enough
stag	standing place	sulf	sulfur
stalsis	constrict, constriction	super	above, excessive
staphyl/o	bunch of grapes	super-	above, excessive
-stasis	stop, stand still, control	supinat	bend backward
stasis	stagnate, to stand still	supplement	supply to remedy a deficiency
stat	stationary	suppress	pressed under, push under
-static	stopped, standing still	supra-	above
-statin	inhibit	surfact	surface
stax	fall in drops	surg	operate
steat	fat	suscept	to take up
stein	stone	-sylated	linked
sten/o	narrow, contract	sym-	together
ster	solid, steroid	symptomat	collection of symptoms
stere/o	three-dimensional	syn-	together
steril	sterile, make sterile	syndesm	bind together
stern	chest, breastbone	synov	synovial membrane
-steroid	steroid	syring/o	tube, pipe
-sterol	steroid	system	the body as a whole
-sterone	steroid	systol/e	contraction, systole
steth/o	chest	tachy-	rapid
sthen	strength	tact	orderly arrangement
stigmat	focus	tag	touch
stimul	excite, strengthen	tain	hold
stin	partition	talip	ankle bone
stip	press	tamin	touch
stiti	space	tampon	plug
stoma	mouth	tangent	touch
-stomy	new opening	tars	ankle
stone	stone, pebble	tax	coordination
storm	crisis	tempor/o	time, temple
strab	squint	ten/o	tendon
strat	layer	tendin	tendon
strept/o	twisted	tens	pressure

Word Part	Definition
-tensin	tense, taut
terat/o	monster, malformed fetus
term	limit, end
test/o	testis, testicle
testicul	testicle, testis
tetra-	four
thalam	thalamus
thalamus	thalamus
thalass	sea
thel	breast, nipple
then	motion
thenar	palm
therap/o	healing, treatment
therapeut	healing, treatment
-therapist	one who treats
therapy	treatment
-therapy	treatment
therm/o	heat
thesis	arrange, place, organize
thet	arrange, place, organize
thi	sulfur
thora	chest
thorac/o	chest
thorax	chest
thromb/o	blood clot, clot
thym	thymus gland
thyr/o	thyroid
tibi	tibia
-tic	pertaining to
-tion	process, being
-tiz	pertaining to
toc	labor, birth
toler	endure
tom/o	cut, slice, layer
-tome	instrument to cut
-tomy	surgical incision
ton/o	pressure, tension
tonsil	tonsil
tonsill/o	tonsil

Word Part	Definition
tope	part, location
topic	local
-tous	pertaining to
tox	poison
-toxic	able to kill
toxic/o	poison
trache/o	trachea, windpipe
tract	draw, pull
tranquil	calm
trans-	across, through
traumat	wound, injury
tresia	a hole
tri-	three
trich/o	hair
-tripsy	crushing
-tripter	crusher
trochle	pulley
trop	turn, turning
troph	development, nourishment
trophy	development, nourishment
-tropic	a turning, change
-tropin	nourishing, stimulation
tryps	friction
tub	tube
tubercul	swelling, nodule, tuberculosis
tubul	small tube
tussis	cough
tympan/o	eardrum, tympanic membrane
-type	model, particular kind
typh	typhus
ulcer	a sore
-ule	little, small
ulent	abounding in
uln	ulnar
ultra-	higher, beyond
-um	tissue, structure
umbilic	navel, umbilicus
un	one
un-	not

WORD PART	DEFINITION	WORD PART	DEFINITION
uni-	one	virus	poison
ur/o	urine, urinary system	viscer	internal organs
-ure	process, result of	viscos	viscous, sticky
uresis	to urinate	visu	sight
uret	ureter, urine, urination	vita	life
ureter/o	ureter	voc	voice
urethr/o	urethra	vol	volume
-uria	urine	volunt	willing
uria urin	urine	volut	shrink, roll up
-us	pertaining to	-volut	rolled up
uter/o	uterus	vuls	tear, pull
uve	uvea	vulv/o	vulva
uvul	uvula	whip	to swing
vaccin	vaccine, giving a vaccine	xanth	yellow
vag	vagus nerve	xeno-	foreign
vagin	sheath, vagina	-xis	condition
valgus	turn out	-yl	substance
valv	valve	zea-	to live
varic/o	varicosity; dilated, tortuous vein	-zoa	animal
vas/o	blood vessel, duct	zyg	zygote
vascul	blood vessel	zygomat	cheekbone
ved	knowledge	zyme	fermenting, enzyme, transform
veget	plants		
vegetat	growth		
ven/a	vein		
ven/o	vein		
ventil	wind		
ventr	belly		
ventricul	ventricle		
vers	turn		
-version	change		
vert	to turn		
vertebr	vertebra		
vesic	sac containing fluid		
vestibul/o	vestibule, entrance		
via	the way		
violet	bluish purple		
viril	masculine		

Abbreviations

ABBREVIATION	DEFINITION
µg	microgram; one-millionth of a gram
∧	increase/ above
∨	decrease/ below
1°	primary
2°	secondary
Ab	antibody
ABGs	arterial blood gases
ABO	agents of biologic origin
ABO	a blood group system
AC	acromioclavicular
ACL	anterior cruciate ligament
ACLS	advanced cardiac life support
ACTH	adrenocorticotropic hormone
AD	right ear
ADD	attention deficit disorder
ADH	antidiuretic hormone
ADHD	attention deficit hyperactivity disorder
ADL	activity of daily living
AED	automatic external defibrillator
Afib	atrial fibrillation
Ag	antigen
AIDS	acquired immunodeficiency syndrome
AKA	above-knee amputation
ALL	acute lymphocytic leukemia
ALS	amyotrophic lateral sclerosis
AMI	acute myocardial infarction
AMS	altered mental state
ANS	autonomic nervous system
AOM	acute otitis media
AP	anteroposterior
ARDS	adult respiratory distress syndrome
ARF	acute respiratory failure
ARF	acute renal failure

ABBREVIATION	DEFINITION
AROM	active range of motion
AS	left ear
ASD	atrial septal defect
ASD	autism spectrum disorder
ASHD	arteriosclerotic heart disease
AU	both ears
AV	atrioventricular
AVM	arteriovenous malformation
BBB	blood brain barrier
BD	brain death
BEP	benign enlargement of the prostate
BKA	below-knee amputation
BM	bowel movement
BMD	bone mineral density
BMR	basal metabolic rate
BOM	bilateral otitis media
BP	blood pressure
BPD	borderline personality disorder
BPH	benign prostatic hyperplasia
BPPV	benign paroxysmal positional vertigo
BRCA1	genetic mutation responsible for breast and ovarian cancer (**br**east **ca**ncer 1)
BRCA2	genetic mutation responsible for breast cancer (**br**east **ca**ncer 2)
BSE	bovine spongiform encephalopathy
BSE	breast self-examination
C1	first cervical vertebra
C5	fifth cervical vertebra or nerve
C7	seventh cervical vertebra
CA	cancer
CABG	coronary artery bypass graft
CAD	coronary artery disease
CAO	chronic airway obstruction

Abbreviation	Definition
CAPD	continuous ambulatory peritoneal dialysis
CBC	complete blood count
CBT	cognitive-behavioral therapy
CD	conduct disorder
CDC	Centers for Disease Control and Prevention
CF	cystic fibrosis
CHD	congenital heart disease
CHES	certified health education specialist
CHF	congestive heart failure
CJD	Creutzfeldt-Jakob disease
CKD	chronic kidney disease
CMA	certified medical assistant
CMV	cytomegalovirus
CNA	certified nurse assistant
CNS	central nervous system
c/o	complains of
CO_2	carbon dioxide
COPD	chronic obstructive pulmonary disease
COT	certified occupational therapist
COTA	certified occupational therapist assistant
CP	cerebral palsy
CPAP	continuous positive airway pressure
CPR	cardiopulmonary resuscitation
CPT	cognitive processing therapy
CRF	chronic renal failure
CRP	C-reactive protein
C-section	cesarean section
CSF	cerebrospinal fluid
CT	computed tomography
CVA	cerebrovascular accident
CVP	central venous pressure
CVS	cardiovascular system
CVT	cardiovascular technologist
CXR	chest x-ray
D & C	dilation and curettage
DASH	dietary approaches to stop hypertension
DEXA	dual-energy x-ray absorptiometry
DI	diabetes insipidus

Abbreviation	Definition
DIC	disseminated intravascular coagulation
DID	dissociative identity disorder
DIFF	differential white blood cell count
DJD	degenerative joint disease
DKA	diabetic ketoacidosis
dL	deciliter; one-tenth of a liter
DM	diabetes mellitus
DMD	Duchenne muscular dystrophy
DNA	deoxyribonucleic acid
DNR	do not resuscitate
DO	Doctor of Osteopathy
DRE	digital rectal examination
DSM-IV	*Diagnostic and Statistical Manual of Mental Disorders,* Fourth Edition
DVT	deep vein thrombosis
EBV	Epstein-Barr virus
ECG	electrocardiogram
ECT	electroconvulsive therapy
ED	erectile dysfunction
ED	emergency department
EEG	electroencephalogram
EKG	electrocardiogram
EMT	emergency medical technician
EMT-P	emergency medical technician–paramedic
EPCA-2	early prostate cancer antigen–2
ER	emergency room
ESR	erythrocyte sedimentation rate
ESRD	end-stage renal disease
ESWL	extracorporeal shock wave lithotripsy
FAS	fetal alcohol syndrome
FDA	U.S. Food and Drug Administration
FEV1	forced expiratory volume in 1 second
FSH	follicle-stimulating hormone
FTT	failure to thrive
FUS	focused ultrasound surgery
FVC	forced vital capacity
Fx	fracture
g	gram

ABBREVIATION	DEFINITION
GAD	generalized anxiety disorder
GDM	gestational diabetes mellitus
GERD	gastroesophageal reflux disease
GFR	glomerular filtration rate
GH	growth hormone, somatotrophin
GI	gastrointestinal
GI	glycemic index
GL	glycemic load
GTT	glucose tolerance test
GYN	gynecology
HAV	hepatitis A virus
Hb	hemoglobin
Hb A1c	glycosylated hemoglobin A one-C
HBOT	hyperbaric oxygen therapy
HBV	hepatitis B virus
HCG	human chorionic gonadotropin
HCl	hydrochloric acid
Hct	hematocrit
HCV	hepatitis C virus
HDL	high-density lipoprotein
HDN	hemolytic disease of the newborn
Hgb	hemoglobin
HIPAA	Health Insurance Portability and Accountability Act
HIV	human immunodeficiency virus
HMD	hyaline membrane disease
HPI	history of present illness
HPV	human papilloma virus
HRT	hormone replacement therapy
HSV	herpes simplex virus
HSV-1	herpes simplex virus, type 1
HTN	hypertension
HUS	hemolytic uremic syndrome
IBS	irritable bowel syndrome
ICD	implantable cardioverter/defibrillator
IDDM	insulin-dependent diabetes mellitus
Ig	immunoglobulin
IgA	immunoglobulin A
IgD	immunoglobulin D

ABBREVIATION	DEFINITION
IgE	immunoglobulin E
IgG	immunoglobulin G
IgM	immunoglobulin M
IM	intramuscular
INR	international normalized ratio
ITP	idiopathic (immunologic) thrombocytopenic purpura
IU	international unit(s)
IUD	intrauterine device
IV	intravenous
IVC	inferior vena cava
IVF	in vitro fertilization
IVP	intravenous pyelogram
JRA	juvenile rheumatoid arthritis
KUB	x-ray of abdomen to show kidneys, ureters, and bladder
LASER	light amplification by stimulated emission of radiation
LCC-ST	certified surgical technologist
LD	learning disability
LDL	low-density lipoprotein
LFT	liver function test
LH	luteinizing hormone
LLQ	left lower quadrant
LOC	loss of consciousness
LPN	licensed practical nurse
LUQ	left upper quadrant
LVN	licensed vocational nurse
mcg	microgram; one-millionth of a gram
MCP	metacarpophalangeal
MCS	minimally conscious state
MD	Doctor of Medicine
mg	milligram
MI	myocardial infarction
mL	milliliter
mm³	cubic millimeter
MOAB	monoclonal antibody
MODY	mature onset diabetes of the young
MONA	morphine, oxygen, nitroglycerine, and aspirin

Abbreviation	Definition
MPD	multiple personality disorder
MRA	magnetic resonance angiography
MRI	magnetic resonance imaging
mRNA	messenger RNA
MRSA	methicillin-resistant *Staphylococcus aureus*
MS	multiple sclerosis
NCI	National Cancer Institute
NIDDM	non-insulin-dependent diabetes mellitus
NIH	National Institutes of Health
NKA	no known allergies
NO	nitric oxide
NRDS	neonatal respiratory distress syndrome
NSAID	nonsteroidal anti-inflammatory drug
O_2	oxygen
OA	osteoarthritis
OA	obstetric assistant
OB	obstetrics
OCD	obsessive compulsive disorder
OD	Doctor of Osteopathy
OD	right eye
ODD	oppositional defiant disorder
OGTT	oral glucose tolerance test
OME	otitis media with effusion
OS	left eye
OSHA	Occupational Safety and Health Administration
OT	ophthalmic technician
OT	oxytocin
OT	occupational therapy
OTC	over the counter
OU	both eyes
P	pulse rate
PA	posteroanterior
PA	pernicious anemia
PaO_2	partial pressure of arterial oxygen
Pap	Papanicolaou (Pap test, Pap smear)
PAT	paroxysmal atrial tachycardia
PCL	posterior cruciate ligament
PCOS	polycystic ovarian syndrome

Abbreviation	Definition
PDA	patent ductus arteriosus
PDD-NOS	pervasive developmental disorder, not otherwise specified
PDT	postural drainage therapy
PE tube	pressure equalization tube
PEEP	positive end-expiratory pressure
PEFR	peak expiratory flow rate
PERRLA	pupils equal, round, reactive to light, and accommodation
PET	positron emission tomography
PFTs	pulmonary function tests
PGY	pregnancy
pH	hydrogen ion concentration
PhD	Doctor of Philosophy
PID	pelvic inflammatory disease
PIP	proximal interphalangeal
PKD	polycystic kidney disease
PMDD	premenstrual dysphoric disorder
PMNL	polymorphonuclear leukocyte
PMS	premenstrual syndrome
PNB	pulseless, nonbreather
PNS	peripheral nervous system
PO	by mouth
POC	products of conception
polio	poliomyelitis
PPH	postpartum hemorrhage
PPS	postpolio syndrome
p.r.n, PRN	when necessary
PSA	prostate-specific antigen
PT	physiotherapy
PT	prothrombin time
PT	physical therapy, physical therapist
PTA	physical therapy assistant
PTCA	percutaneous transluminal coronary angioplasty
PTH	parathyroid hormone
PTSD	posttraumatic stress disorder
PVC	premature ventricular contractions
PVD	peripheral vascular disease
PVS	persistent vegetative state

ABBREVIATION	DEFINITION
q.4.h.	every 4 hours
q.i.d.	four times each day
R	respiration rate
RA	rheumatoid arthritis
RBC	red blood cell
RDA	recommended dietary allowance
RDS	respiratory distress syndrome
Rh	Rhesus
Rho-GAM	Rhesus immune globulin
RICE	rest, ice, compression, and elevation
RLQ	right lower quadrant
RN	registered nurse
RNA	ribonucleic acid
ROM	range of motion
RU-486	mifepristone
RUQ	right upper quadrant
SA	sinoatrial
SAD	seasonal affective disorder
SARS	severe acute respiratory syndrome
SBS	shaken baby syndrome
SC	subcutaneous
SCI	spinal cord injury
SET	self-examination of the testes
SFD	small for date
SG	specific gravity
SGA	small for gestational age
SI	sacroiliac
SIDS	sudden infant death syndrome
SLE	systemic lupus erythematosus
SOB	short(ness) of breath
SP	standard precautions
SSRI	selective serotonin reuptake inhibitor
STAT	immediately
STD	sexually transmitted disease
SVC	superior vena cava
T	temperature
T1	first thoracic vertebra or nerve

ABBREVIATION	DEFINITION
T3	triiodothyronine
T4	tetraiodothyronine (thyroxine)
TB	tuberculosis
TBI	traumatic brain injury
TENS	transcutaneous electrical nerve stimulation
THR	total hip replacement
TIA	transient ischemic attack
t.i.d.	(Latin *ter in die*) three times a day
TMJ	temporomandibular joint
TNM	**t**umor-**n**ode-**m**etastasis staging system for cancer
TOF	tetralogy of Fallot
tPA	tissue plasminogen activator
TSH	thyroid-stimulating hormone
TTM	trichotillomania
TTN	transient tachypnea of the newborn
TTP	thrombotic thrombocytopenic purpura
TURP	transurethral resection of the prostate
UA	urinalysis
UP	universal precautions
URI	upper respiratory infection
USDA	U.S. Department of Agriculture
UTI	urinary tract infection
UV	ultraviolet
VEP	visual evoked potential
Vfib	ventricular fibrillation
VS	vital signs
VSD	ventricular septal defect
V-tach	ventricular tachycardia
vWD	von Willebrand disease
vWF	von Willebrand factor
WAD	Word Analysis and Definition (box)
WBC	white blood cell; white blood (cell) count
WNL	within normal limits
WNV	West Nile virus

Diagnostic and Therapeutic Procedures

A compilation of the diagnostic and therapeutic procedural terms used in this book.

A

abdominoplasty Esthetic operation on the abdominal wall (tummy tuck).

ablation Removal of tissue to destroy its function.

activated partial thromboplastin time (APTT) Blood test used to monitor the dose of heparin, an anticoagulant.

adenoidectomy Surgical removal of the adenoid tissue.

alignment Process of bringing the ends of a fractured bone at the break back opposite each other so that they fit together as they did in the original bone.

ambulatory Surgery or any other care provided without an overnight stay in a medical facility.

ambulatory blood pressure monitor Device that provides a record of blood pressure readings over a 24-hour period as patients go about their daily activities.

amniocentesis Removal of amniotic fluid for diagnostic purposes.

amputation Process of removing a limb, part of a limb, a breast, or other projecting part.

anastomosis Surgically made union between two tubular structures.

angiogram Radiographic image of arteries or veins after injection of contrast material.

angiography The process of obtaining an angiogram.

angioplasty Reopening of a blood vessel by surgery.

anoscopy Examination of the anus and lower rectum with a rigid instrument.

Apgar score Evaluation of a newborn's status.

appendectomy Surgical removal of the appendix.

arterial blood gases The measurement of the levels of oxygen and carbon dioxide in the blood—a good indicator of respiratory function.

arteriography X-ray visualization of an artery after injection of contrast material.

arthrocentesis Aspiration of fluid from a joint; used to establish a diagnosis by laboratory examination of the fluid, drain off infected fluid, or insert medication such as local corticosteroids.

arthrodesis Fixation or stiffening of a joint by surgery.

arthrography X-ray of a joint after injection of a contrast medium into the joint to make the inside details of the joint visible.

arthroplasty Replacement of a joint with a prosthesis.

arthroscopy Procedure performed using an arthroscope to examine the internal compartments of a joint or perform a surgical procedure such as debridement, removal of damaged tissue, or repair of torn ligaments.

aspiration Removal by suction of fluid or gas from a body cavity.

atherectomy Surgical removal of atheroma from a blood vessel.

audiometer Electronic device that generates sounds in different frequencies and intensities to test for hearing loss.

auscultation Diagnostic method of listening to body sounds with a stethoscope.

autograft Graft removed from the patient's own skin.

automatic external defibrillator (AED) Device that sends an electric shock to the heart to stop the heart and allow a normal contraction rhythm to resume.

B

bariatric surgery Surgical treatment of obesity.

barium meal Ingestion of barium sulfate to study the distal esophagus, stomach, and duodenum on x-ray.

barium swallow Ingestion of barium sulfate, a contrast material, to show details of the pharynx and esophagus on x-ray.

biopsy Removal of tissue from a living person for laboratory examination.

blepharoplasty Correction of defects in the eyelids.

bone marrow aspiration or biopsy Use of a needle to remove bone marrow cells.

bone mineral density (BMD) Screening test for osteoporosis using a dual-energy x-ray absorptiometry (DEXA) scan.

brace Appliance to support a part of the body in its correct position.

brachytherapy Radiation therapy in which the source of irradiation is implanted in the tissue to be treated.

bronchoscopy Examination of the interior of the tracheobronchial tree with an endoscope.

C

cannula Tube inserted into a blood vessel or cavity as a channel for fluid or gas.

cardiac catheterization Procedure that detects patterns of pressures and blood flows in the heart. A thin tube is guided into the heart under x-ray guidance after being inserted into a vein or artery.

cardiac stress testing Exercise tolerance test that raises the heart rate and monitors the effect on cardiac function.

cardiopulmonary resuscitation Attempt to restore cardiac and pulmonary function.

cardioversion Restoration of a normal heart rhythm by electrical shock. Also called *defibrillation.*

catheterization Introduction of a catheter.

cerebral angiography Injection of a radiopaque dye into the blood vessels of the neck and brain to detect blood vessels that are partially or completely blocked, aneurysms, or arteriovenous malformations.

cerebral arteriography Procedure used to determine the site of bleeding in hemorrhagic strokes, enabling surgery to be performed to stop the bleed or to clip off the aneurysm.

chest x-ray Radiograph image of the chest that can be taken in anteroposterior (AP), posteroanterior (PA), lateral, and sometimes oblique and lateral decubitus positions.

cholangiography Use of a contrast medium to radiographically visualize the bile ducts.

cholecystectomy Surgical removal of the gallbladder.

cholelithotomy Surgical removal of a gallstone(s).

circumcision Removal of part or all of the prepuce of the penis.

clean-catch, midstream urine specimen Sample collected after the external urethral meatus is cleaned. The first part of the urine stream is not collected, and the sterile collecting vessel is introduced into the urinary stream to collect the last part.

clot-busting drugs Drugs injected within a few hours of an MI or thrombotic stroke to dissolve the thrombus. Also called *thrombolytic drugs.*

colonoscopy Examination of the inside of the colon by endoscopy.

colostomy Artificial opening from the colon to the outside of the body.

colpopexy Surgical fixation of a relaxed and prolapsed vagina to the anterior abdominal wall.

computed tomography (CT) Scan in which images of sections of the body are generated by a computer synthesis of x-rays obtained in many different directions in a given plane.

conization Surgical excision of a cone-shaped piece of tissue, e.g., from the outer lining of the cervix.

constant positive airway pressure (CPAP) Attempt to keep alveoli open by maintaining a positive pressure in the airways. A mask is fitted over the nose and mouth and attached to a ventilator.

continuous ambulatory peritoneal dialysis (CAPD) Dialysis performed by the patient at home through an implanted peritoneal catheter, usually 4 times a day, 7 days a week.

continuous cycling peritoneal dialysis Use of a machine to automatically infuse dialysis solution into and out of the abdominal cavity through a peritoneal catheter during sleep.

coronary angiogram Injection of a contrast dye during cardiac catheterization to identify coronary artery blockages.

coronary artery bypass surgery (CABG) Procedure in which healthy blood vessels harvested as a graft from the leg, chest, or arm are used to bypass (detour) the blood around blocked coronary arteries.

cryosurgery Use of liquid nitrogen or argon gas in a probe to freeze and kill abnormal tissue.

curette Scoop-shaped instrument for scraping or removing new growths (or earwax).

cystoscopy Insertion of a pencil-thin, flexible, tubelike telescope through the urethra into the bladder to examine directly the lining of the bladder and to take a biopsy if needed.

cystourethrogram X-ray image during voiding to show the structure and function of the bladder and urethra.

D

debridement Removal of injured or necrotic tissue.

defibrillation Restoration of uncontrolled twitching of cardiac muscle fibers to a normal rhythm.

dermabrasion Removal of upper layers of the skin using a high-powered rotating brush.

dialysis Artificial method of removing waste materials and excess fluid from blood.

digital rectal examination (DRE) Palpation of the rectum and prostate gland with an index finger.

dilation and curettage (D&C) Dilation of the cervix so that a thin instrument can be inserted to scrape away the lining of the uterus and take tissue samples.

dipstick Plastic strip bearing paper squares of reagent—the most cost-effective method of screening urine. After the stick is dipped in the urine specimen, the color change in each segment of the dipstick is compared to a color chart on the container. Dipsticks can screen for pH, specific gravity, protein, blood, glucose, ketones, bilirubin, nitrite, and leukocyte esterase.

Doppler ultrasound Diagnostic instrument that sends an ultrasonic beam into the body.

E

early morning urine collection Process used to determine the ability of the kidneys to concentrate urine following overnight dehydration.

echocardiography Ultrasound recording of heart function.

echoencephalography Use of ultrasound in the diagnosis of intracranial lesions.

electrocardiogram Record of the electrical signals of the heart.

electrocardiography Interpretation of electrocardiograms.

electroconvulsive therapy (ECT) Passage of electric current through the brain to produce convulsions and treat persistent depression.

electroencephalography Recording of the electrical activity of the brain.

electromyography Recording of electrical activity in muscle.

endarterectomy Surgical removal of plaque from an artery.

endometrial ablation Use of a heat-generating tool or a laser to remove or destroy the lining of the uterus and prevent or reduce menstruation.

endoscope An instrument for the examination of the interior of a hollow or tubular organ.

endoscopy Use of an endoscope to examine the interior of a tubular or hollow organ and perform a biopsy, remove polyps (polypectomy), and coagulate bleeding lesions.

enema Injection of fluid into the rectum and lower bowel.

enteroscopy Examination of the lining of the digestive tract.

episiotomy Surgical incision in the perineum to dilate the opening of the vagina.

evoked responses Use of stimuli for vision, sound, and touch to activate specific areas of the brain and measure their responses with EEG. This provides information about how that specific area of the brain is functioning.

excision Surgical removal of part or all of a structure or organ.

excisional biopsy Removal of a tumor with a surrounding margin of normal tissue.

external fixation Method of maintaining the alignment of a fractured bone by immobilizing the bone through the use of plaster casts, splints, traction, and external fixators such as steel rods and pins.

extracorporeal shock wave lithotripsy (ESWL) Process in which a machine called a *lithotripter* produces shock waves that crumble renal or ureteral stones into small pieces that can pass down the ureter.

F

fasciectomy Surgical removal of fascia.

fecal occult blood test Diagnostic procedure that detects the presence of blood not visible to the naked eye. Trade name: *Hemoccult* test.

fistulectomy Surgical excision of a fistula.

fistulotomy Surgical enlargement or opening up of a fistula.

flexible endoscopy Use of a flexible, slim fiber-optic instrument that transmits light and sends back images to the observer.

forceps extraction Assisted delivery of a baby by an instrument that grasps the head of the baby.

fundoscopy Examination of the retina with an ophthalmoscope.

G

gastroscopy Endoscopic examination of the inside of the stomach.

gavage To feed by a stomach tube.

gingivectomy Surgical removal of diseased gum tissue.

H

heart transplant Surgery in which the heart of a recently deceased person (donor) is transplanted to the recipient after the recipient's diseased heart has been removed.

Hemoccult test Trade name for *fecal occult blood test.*

hemodialysis Process that filters blood through an artificial kidney machine (dialyzer).

hemorrhoidectomy Surgical removal of hemorrhoids.

herniorrhaphy Surgical repair of a hernia.

heterograft Graft from a nonhuman species. Also called *xenograft.*

Holter monitor Continuous ECG recorded on a tape cassette for at least 24 hours as a person works, plays, and rests.

homocysteine Amino acid in the blood. Elevated levels are related to a higher risk of CAD, stroke, and peripheral vascular disease.

homograft Skin graft from another person or a cadaver. Also called *allograft.*

hysterectomy Surgical removal of the uterus.

I

ileostomy Artificial opening from the ileum to the outside of the body.

implantable cardioverter/defibrillator (ICD) Implanted device that senses abnormal rhythms and gives the heart a small electrical shock to return the rhythm to normal.

incision Cut or surgical wound.

internal fixation Use of tissue-compatible materials such as stainless steel and titanium to stabilize fractured bony parts, enabling the patient to return to function more quickly and reducing the incidence of nonunion and malunion (improper healing). The types of internal fixation are wires used as sutures to "sew" the bone fragments together; plates that extend along both or all fragments of bone and are held in place by screws; rods inserted through the medullary cavity of both fragments to align the bones; and screws that can be used on their own as well as with plates.

intradermal injection Introduction of a short, thin needle into the epidermis, thus raising a small wheal. This site is used for allergy and tuberculosis (TB) testing.

intramuscular (IM) injection Use of a long needle that penetrates the epidermis, dermis, and hypodermis to reach into the muscles underneath. Some antibiotics and immunizations are given by this route.

intrauterine insemination Insertion of sperm directly into the uterus via a special catheter to initiate pregnancy.

intravenous pyelogram (IVP) Procedure in which a contrast material containing iodine is injected intravenously and its progress through the urinary tract is then recorded on a series of rapid radiological images.

intubation Insertion of a tube into a canal, hollow organ, or cavity, e.g., into the trachea for anesthesia or control of ventilation.

in vitro fertilization (IVF) Process of combining sperm and egg in a laboratory dish and placing the resulting embryos inside the uterus.

Ishihara color system Test for color vision defects.

J

Jaeger reading card Chart containing type in different sizes of print for testing near vision.

K

keratomileusis Procedure that cuts and shapes the cornea.

keratotomy Incision through the cornea.

kidney transplant Surgery in which the kidney of a donor is transplanted to a recipient; provides a better quality of life than kidney dialysis, if a suitable donor can be found.

KUB X-ray of the abdomen to show **k**idneys, **u**reters, and **b**ladder.

L

laparoscopy Examination of the contents of the abdomen using an endoscope, which can also be used to perform surgery and take samples for biopsy.

laryngoscopy Use of a hollow tube with a light and camera to visualize or operate on the larynx.

laser surgery Use of a concentrated, intense narrow beam of electromagnetic radiation for surgery. (*laser:* **l**ight **a**mplification by **s**imulated **e**mission of **r**adiation)

lipectomy Surgical removal of fatty tissue.

lipid profile Group of blood tests that helps determine the risk of CAD and comprises total cholesterol; high-density lipoprotein (HDL), or "good cholesterol"; low-density lipoprotein (LDL), or "bad cholesterol"; and triglycerides.

liposuction Surgical removal of fatty tissue using suction.

lobectomy Surgical removal of a lobe of a structure, for example, a lobe of a lung.

lumbar puncture Use of a hollow needle to remove CSF so that it can be examined in the laboratory. Also called *spinal tap.*

lumpectomy Removal of a lesion with preservation of surrounding tissue.

lymphadenectomy Surgical removal of a lymph gland(s).

lymphangiogram Radiographic images of lymph vessels and nodes following injection of contrast material.

M

magnetic resonance angiography (MRA) Method of visualizing vessels that contain flowing structures by producing a contrast between them and stationary structures.

magnetic resonance imaging (MRI) Diagnostic technique that creates detailed images of structures and tissues in various planes without exposing patients to radiation as in conventional radiography or computed tomography.

mammogram Record produced by x-ray imaging of the breast.

mammoplasty Surgical reshaping of the breasts.

mastectomy Surgical excision of the breast.

mechanical ventilation Process by which gases are moved into and out of the lungs via a ventilator that is set to meet the respiratory requirements of the patient.

mediastinoscopy Examination of the mediastinum using an endoscope inserted through an incision in the suprasternal notch.

myomectomy Surgical removal of a uterine myoma (fibroid).

myringotomy Incision through the tympanic membrane; e.g., for the placement of pressure equalization (PE) tubes to allow an effusion to drain.

N

nebulizer Device used to deliver liquid medicine in a fine mist.

nephrectomy Surgical removal of a kidney.

nephrolithotomy Incision into the kidney for removal of a stone.

nephroscopy Examination of the pelvis of the kidney.

nerve conduction studies Studies that measure the speed at which motor or sensory nerves conduct impulses.

nuclear imaging of the heart Use of an injection of a radioactive substance in association with a cardiac stress test to assess cardiac function.

O

ophthalmoscopy Examination of the retina using an ophthalmoscope.

orchiopexy Surgical fixation of a testis in the scrotum.

ostomy Artificial opening into a tubular structure, for example, ileostomy and colostomy.

otoscopy Examination of the ear using an otoscope.

P

pacemaker Device that regulates cardiac electrical activity. The device generates electronic signals carried along thin, insulated wires to the heart muscle.

palpation Examination with the fingers and hands.

panendoscopy Visual examination of the inside of the esophagus, stomach, and upper duodenum using a flexible fiber-optic endoscope.

Pap test Examination of cells taken from the cervix.

parathyroidectomy Surgical removal of the parathyroid glands.

peak flow meter Instrument used to record the greatest flow of air that can be sustained for 10 milliseconds on forced expiration, the peak expiratory flow rate (PEFR). It is of value in following the course of asthma and in postoperative care to monitor the return of lung function after anesthesia.

percutaneous nephrolithotomy Insertion of a nephroscope through the skin to locate and remove a renal pelvic or ureteral stone.

percutaneous transluminal coronary angioplasty (PTCA) Procedure in which a balloon-tipped catheter is guided to the site of the blockage and inflated to expand the artery from the inside by compressing the plaque against the walls of the artery.

percutaneous transthoracic needle aspiration Insertion of a needle with a cutting chamber through an intercostal space to hook a specimen of parietal pleura for laboratory examination.

peritoneal dialysis Procedure in which a dialysis solution is infused into and drained out of the abdominal cavity through a small, flexible, implanted catheter.

phlebotomy Process of taking blood from a vein.

photocoagulation Use of a laser beam to form a clot or destroy abnormal capillaries. In the eye, this slows the pace of the visual loss in macular degeneration

phototherapy Treatment using light rays.

pneumonectomy Surgical removal of a lung.

polypectomy Excision or removal of a polyp.

polysomnography Test to monitor brain waves, muscle tension, eye movement, and oxygen levels in the blood as the patient sleeps.

positive end expiratory pressure (PEEP) Technique in ventilation to keep the alveoli from collapsing in adult and neonatal respiratory distress syndromes.

positron emission tomography (PET) Scan that shows the uptake and distribution of substances such as sugar in tissues to locate abnormal, often malignant, structures.

postural drainage therapy (PDT) Treatment that involves positioning and tilting the patient so that gravity promotes drainage of secretions from lung segments. Chest percussion (tapping) on the chest wall can help loosen, mobilize, and drain the retained secretions.

proctoscopy Examination of the inside of the anus and rectum by endoscopy.

prostatectomy Surgical removal of part or all of the prostate.

prosthesis Manufactured substitute for a missing part of the body.

prothrombin time (PT) Test used to monitor the dose of Coumadin, an anticoagulant. It is reported as an *international normalized ratio (INR)* instead of in seconds.

pulmonary rehabilitation Therapeutic restoration of lung function that includes education, breathing exercises and retraining, exercises for the upper and lower extremities, and psychosocial support.

pulse oximeter Sensor placed on the finger to measure the oxygen saturation of the blood.

pyelogram X-ray image of the renal pelvis and ureters.

Q

quadrantectomy Surgical excision of a quadrant of the breast.

R

radical hysterectomy Surgical removal of the fallopian tubes and ovaries as well as the uterus.

radical mastectomy Complete surgical removal of all breast tissue, the pectoralis major muscle, and associated lymph nodes.

radical prostatectomy Complete surgical removal of the prostate and surrounding tissues.

random urine collection Process in which a sample is taken with no precautions regarding contamination. It is often used for collecting samples for drug testing. "Pee into a cup."

reduction Procedure in which the distal segment of a fractured bone is pulled back into alignment with the proximal segment. Anesthesia may be used.

rehabilitation Therapeutic restoration of an ability to function as before after disease, illness, or injury.

renal angiogram X-ray with contrast material used to assess blood flow to the kidneys.

resection Removal of a specific part of an organ or structure.

retrograde pyelogram Injection of contrast material through a urinary catheter into the ureters to locate stones and other obstructions.

rhinoplasty Surgical procedure to alter the size or shape of the nose.

Rinne test Test for a conductive hearing loss.

S

salpingectomy Surgical removal of a fallopian tube.

sclerotherapy Injection of a solution into a vein to thrombose it.

segmentectomy Surgical excision of a segment of a tissue or organ.

sigmoidoscopy Endoscopic examination of the sigmoid colon.

Snellen letter chart Test for acuity of distant vision.

sphygmomanometer Instrument for measuring arterial blood pressure.

spinal tap Placement of a needle through an intervertebral space into the subarachnoid space to withdraw CSF.

spirometer Device used to measure the volume of air that a patient moves in and out of the respiratory system.

splenectomy Surgical removal of the spleen.

staging Process of determining the extent of the distribution of a neoplasm. The TNM (tumor-node-metastasis) staging system can be used.

stent placement Procedure in which a wire mesh tube, or stent, is placed inside the vessel to reduce the likelihood that an occluded artery will close up again. Some stents (drug-eluting stents) are covered with a special medication to help keep the artery open.

sterilization Process of making sterile.

stethoscope Instrument for listening to cardiac, respiratory, and other sounds.

stoma Artificial opening.

subcutaneous (SC) injection Injection in which a needle pierces the epidermis and dermis to reach the hypodermis (subcutaneous) layer. This site is used for insulin injections and for some immunizations.

suprapubic transabdominal needle aspiration of the bladder Procedure used with newborns and small infants to obtain a pure sample of urine.

suture Process or material that brings together the edges of a wound to enhance tissue healing. Also, a form of fibrous joint to unite two bones.

T

thoracentesis Insertion of a needle through an intercostal space to remove fluid from a pleural effusion for laboratory study or to relieve pressure. Also called *pleural tap*.

thoracoscopy Examination of the pleural cavity with an endoscope.

thoracotomy Incision through the chest wall.

thymectomy Surgical removal of the thymus gland.

thyroidectomy Surgical removal of the thyroid gland.

tomography Radiographic image of a selected slice of tissue.

tonometry Measurement of intraocular pressure.

tonsillectomy Surgical removal of the tonsils.

tracheal aspiration Procedure in which a soft catheter is passed in the trachea to allow brushings and washings to remove cells and secretions from the trachea and main bronchi for diagnostic study.

tracheostomy Insertion of a tube into the windpipe to assist breathing.

tracheotomy The process of making an incision into the trachea.

traction Gentle but continuous application of a pulling force that can align a fracture, reduce muscle spasm, and relieve pain.

transdermal application Administration of some medications through the skin by an adhesive transdermal patch that is applied to the skin. The medication diffuses across the epidermis and enters the blood vessels in the dermis. Contraceptive hormones, analgesics, and antinausea/seasickness medications are examples.

transthoracic Going through the chest wall.

tubal ligation Surgery, using laparoscopy, in which both fallopian tubes are cut, a segment is removed, and the ends are tied off and cauterized shut.

24-hour urine collection Process that determines the amount of protein being excreted daily and estimates the kidneys' filtration ability.

tympanostomy Surgically created new opening in the tympanic membrane to allow fluid to drain from the middle ear.

U

ultrasonography Delineation of deep structures using sound waves.

ureteroscopy Examination of the ureter. A small flexible ureteroscope is passed through the urethra and bladder into the ureter. Devices can be passed through the endoscope to remove or fragment stones.

urinalysis (U/A) Examination of urine to separate it into its elements and define their kind and/or quantity. A routine urinalysis in the laboratory can include tests for color, clarity, pH, specific gravity, protein, glucose, ketones, and leukocyte esterase (indicator of infection).

urinalysis (microscopic) Analysis of the solids deposited by centrifuging a specimen of urine. It can reveal RBCs, WBCs, and renal tubular epithelial cells stuck together to form casts (cylindrical molds of cells) in nephrotic syndrome.

urine culture Culture taken from a clean-catch urine specimen. It is the definitive test for a urinary tract infection.

V

vasectomy Excision of a segment of the ductus deferens to interrupt the flow of sperm.

vasovasostomy Microsurgical procedure to suture back together the cut ends of the ductus deferens to restore the flow of sperm. Also called *vasectomy reversal*.

venogram Radiograph of veins after injection of radiopaque contrast material.

vestibulectomy Surgical excision of the vulva.

voiding cystourethrogram (VCUG) Imaging in which a contrast material is inserted into the bladder through a catheter and X-rays are taken during voiding.

W

Weber test Test for sensorineural hearing loss.

X

xenograft Graft from a nonhuman species. Also called *heterograft*.

Pharmacology

A compilation of pharmacologic terms used in this book.

A

acetaminophen Analgesic (reduces response to pain) and antipyretic (reduces fever).

adrenaline (1) Hormone produced by the adrenal medulla that boosts the supply of oxygen and glucose to the brain and increases heart rate and output. (2) Drug used to treat cardiac arrest and dysrhythmias and relieve bronchospasm in asthma. Also called *epinephrine*.

allergen Substance producing a hypersensitivity (allergic) reaction. Examples are animal fur and dander, penicillins, and foods such as eggs, milk, and wheat.

analgesic Substance that reduces or relieves the response to pain without producing loss of consciousness. Examples are aspirin and other NSAIDs, acetaminophen, and codeine.

androgen Hormone that promotes masculine characteristics. An example is testosterone.

anesthetic Agent that causes absence of feeling or sensation. Examples of local anesthetics are lidocaine and novocaine; examples of general anesthetics are nitrous oxide, thiopental, and ketamine.

antacid Agent that neutralizes the acidity of stomach contents. Examples are aluminum hydroxide, magnesium hydroxide, and calcium carbonate.

antibiotic Substance that has the capacity to inhibit the growth of or destroy bacteria and other microorganisms. Examples are penicillin, erythromycin, cefotaxime, and flucloxacillin.

anticoagulant Substance that prevents clotting. Examples are heparin and Coumadin (warfarin).

antidiabetic drugs Medications used to treat diabetes. Those given orally include metformin, acarbose, and thiazolidinediones, such as troglitazone. Insulin is given by injection or inhaled.

antidiuretic Agent that decreases urine production. Examples are vasopressin, amiloride, and chlorpropamide.

antiepileptic Agent capable of preventing or arresting epilepsy. Examples are phenobarbitol, phenytoin, and valproate.

antihistamine Agent used to treat allergic symptoms because of its action antagonistic to histamine. Examples are benadryl, diphenhydramine, and cimetidine.

anti-inflammatory Agent that reduces inflammation by acting on the body's responses, without affecting the causative agent. Examples are corticosteroids and aspirin.

antimicrobial Agent used to destroy or prevent multiplication of organisms. (See antibiotic.)

antineoplastic Agent that prevents the growth and spread of cancer cells. Examples are methotrexate, fluorouracil, and cyclophosphamide.

antipruritic Medication against itching. Examples are calamine lotion, hydrocortisone cream applied topically, and diphenhydramine (Benadryl) taken orally.

antipyretic Agent that reduces fever. Examples are aspirin and acetaminophen.

antiseptic Agent that reduces the number of microorganisms in different situations. Examples are alcohol, chlorhexidine, and providone-iodine.

atropine Agent used to dilate the pupils.

B

beta blocker Agent used in the treatment of a variety of cardiovascular diseases. Examples are propanalol and acebutolol.

bronchodilator Agent that relaxes the smooth muscles of the bronchioles. Examples are theophylline; beta-2 agonists, such as salbutamol and terbutaline; and anticholinergics, such as ipratropium bromide.

C

calcium channel blocker Agent that decreases the force of contraction of the myocardium, dilates coronary arteries, and reduces blood pressure. Examples are amlodipine and verapamil.

chemotherapy Treatment using chemical agents, usually in relation to neoplastic disease. Examples are platinum compounds such as cisplatin or paraplatin.

coagulant Substance that causes clotting. Thrombin and fibrin glue are used surgically to treat bleeding.

contraceptive Agent that prevents conception. Examples are condoms, diaphragms, and birth control pills using a mixture of estrogen and progesterone.

corticosteroids Hormones produced by the adrenal cortex. Examples are cortisol and aldosterone.

cortisol One of the glucocorticoids produced by the adrenal cortex; has anti-inflammatory effects. Also called *hydrocortisone*.

D

decongestant An agent that reduces the swelling and fluid in the nose and sinuses. Examples are pseudoephedrine and phenylephrine.

depressant Substance that diminishes activity, sensation, or tone, particularly in relation to the nervous system. Examples are alcohol, barbiturates, and benzodiazepines.

disease-modifying drug Agent that has partial success in slowing down the accumulation of disabilities in a specific disease process. Examples in multiple sclerosis (MS) include interferons and mitoxantrone.

disinfectant Agent used to destroy pathogenic and other microorganisms on nonliving surfaces. Examples are alcohol, hydrogen peroxide, and hypochlorites.

diuretic Agent that increases urine output. Examples are furosemide, hydrochlorthiazide, spironolactone, and mannitol.

dopamine Chemical neurotransmitter in some specific areas of the brain.

E

epinephrine (1) Hormone produced by the adrenal medulla that boosts the supply of oxygen and glucose to the brain and increases heart rate and output. (2) Drug used to treat cardiac arrest and dysrhythmias and relieve bronchospasm in asthma. Also called *adrenaline*.

estrogen Generic term for hormones that stimulate female secondary sex characteristics.

F

fluorescein Dye that produces a vivid green color under a blue light; used to diagnose corneal abrasions and foreign bodies in the eye.

H

histamine Compound liberated in tissues as a result of injury or an immune response.

hydrocortisone Potent glucocorticoid with anti-inflammatory properties. Also called *cortisol.*

I

immunization Treatment with an agent designed to protect susceptible people from a communicable disease, such as agents that protect against the childhood diseases of measles, rubella, and pertussis.

insulin Hormone produced by the islet cells of the pancreas that promotes glucose use. Injectable insulin preparations are classified by their speed of action.

M

melatonin Hormone formed and secreted by the pineal gland during darkness. Serotonin is a precursor. It assists in the control of daily body rhythms, stimulates the immune system, and is an antioxidant.

morphine Derivative of opium used as an analgesic or sedative.

mucolytic Agent that attempts to break up mucus to allow it to be cleared more effectively from the airways. Examples are guaifenesin (common in over-the-counter cough medications), potassium iodide, and *N*-acetylcysteine (taken through a nebulizer).

N

narcotic Drug derived from opium. Examples are heroin, morphine, codeine, and demerol.

neurotransmitter Chemical that crosses a synapse to stimulate or inhibit another neuron or the cell of a muscle or gland. Examples are norepinephrine, serotonin, and dopamine.

O

opiate Drug derived from opium. Examples are morphine, codeine, heroin, and demerol.

oxygen Gas given by nasal cannula or by mask and intubation to relieve hypoxia. Patients with severe, chronic COPD can be attached to a portable cylinder of oxygen.

P

pharmacist Person licensed by the state to prepare and dispense drugs.

pharmacology Science of the preparation, uses, and effects of drugs.

pharmacy Facility licensed to prepare and dispense drugs.

placebo Inert, medicinally inactive compound with no intrinsic therapeutic value.

progesterone Hormone used to correct abnormalities of menstruation, and as a contraceptive.

psychoactive Agent able to alter mood, behavior, and/or cognition. Examples include narcotics, stimulants, antidepressants, and hallucinogens.

S

saline Salt solution, usually sodium chloride.

somatotropin Hormone of the anterior pituitary gland that stimulates the growth of body tissues. Also called *growth hormone (GH).*

spermicide Agent that destroys sperm. Examples are nonoxynol-9 and benzalkonium chloride.

sterilization Elimination of all microorganisms by high-pressure steam (autoclave), dry heat (oven), or radiation.

steroid Large family of chemical substances found in many drugs, hormones, and body components.

stimulant Agent that excites or strengthens. Examples include caffeine, nicotine, and cocaine.

surfactant Protein and fat compound that creates surface tension to hold the lung alveolar walls apart.

T

teratogen Agent that produces fetal abnormalities—congenital malformations—while organs and structures are being formed. (All medications readily cross the placenta.) Examples include alcohol, isoretinoin (acne medication), valproic acid (anticonvulsant), and the rubella virus.

testosterone The major androgen that promotes development of male sex characteristics.

thrombolytic Agent injected within a few hours of a myocardial infarction (MI) or stroke to dissolve the thrombus causing the arterial blockage. Examples are streptokinase and tissue plasminogen activator (tPA). Also called *clot-busting drug.*

thyroxine Thyroid hormone T4, tetraiodothyronine.

topical Medication applied to the skin to obtain a local effect. Examples are ointments, creams, gels, lotions, patches, and sprays.

toxin Poisonous substance formed by a living cell or organism. Examples are venom from bee stings, snake bites, and jellyfish stings.

V

vaccine Agent used to generate immunity and composed of the antigenic components of a killed or attenuated microorganism or its inactivated toxins. See *immunization.*

vitamin Essential organic substance necessary in small amounts for normal cell function.

W

warfarin Anticoagulant; also used as rat poison. Trade name: *Coumadin.*

A

abdomen (**AB**-doh-men) Part of the trunk between the thorax and the pelvis.

abdominal (ab-**DOM**-in-al) Pertaining to the abdomen.

abdominopelvic (ab-**DOM**-ih-no-**PEL**-vik) Pertaining to the abdomen and pelvis.

abdominoplasty (ab-**DOM**-ih-noh-plas-tee) Surgical removal of excess subcutaneous fat from the abdominal wall (tummy tuck).

abduction (ab-**DUCK**-shun) Action of moving away from the midline.

abductor (ab-**DUCK**-tor) Muscle that moves the thigh away from the midline.

ablation (ab-**LAY**-shun) Removal of tissue to destroy its function.

abortion (ah-**BOR**-shun) Spontaneous or induced expulsion of the fetus from the uterus at 20 weeks or less.

abrasion (ah-**BRAY**-shun) Area of skin or mucous membrane that has been scraped off.

abruptio (ab-**RUP**-she-oh) Placenta abruptio is the premature detachment of the placenta.

absorption (ab-**SORP**-shun) Uptake of nutrients and water by cells in the GI tract.

accommodate (ah-**KOM**-oh-date) To adapt to meet a need.

accommodation (ah-kom-oh-**DAY**-shun) The act of adjusting something to make it fit the needs; for example, the lens of the eye adjusts itself.

accomodative (ah-kom-oh-**DAY**-tiv) Pertaining to accommodation.

acetabulum (ass-eh-**TAB**-you-lum) The cup-shaped cavity of the hip bone that receives the head of the femur to form the hip joint.

acetaminophen (ah-seat-ah-**MIN**-oh-fen) Medication that is an analgesic and an antipyretic.

acetone (**ASS**-eh-tone) Ketone that is found in blood, urine, and breath when diabetes mellitus is out of control.

Achilles tendon (ah-**KILL**-eeze) A tendon formed from gastrocnemius and soleus muscles and inserted into the calcaneus bone. Also called *calcaneal tendon.*

achondroplasia (a-kon-droh-**PLAY**-zee-ah) Condition with abnormal conversion of cartilage into bone, leading to dwarfism.

acne (**AK**-nee) Inflammatory disease of sebaceous glands and hair follicles.

acquired immunodeficiency syndrome (**AIDS**) (ah-**KWIRED IM**-you-noh-dee-**FISH**-en-see **SIN**-drohm) Infection with the HIV virus.

acromegaly (ak-roe-**MEG**-ah-lee) Enlargement of the head, face, hands, and feet due to excess growth hormone in an adult.

acromioclavicular (**AC**) (ah-**CROW**-mee-oh-klah-**VICK**-you-lar) The joint between the acromion and the clavicle.

acromion (ah-**CROW**-mee-on) Lateral end of the scapula, extending over the shoulder joint.

activities of daily living (**ADLs**) (ak-**TIV**-ih-tees of **DAY**-lee **LIV**-ing) Daily routines for mobility, personal care, bathing, dressing, eating, and moving.

acute (ah-**KYUT**) Disease of sudden onset.

adapt (a-**DAPT**) To adjust to different conditions.

adaptation (ad-ap-**TAY**-shun) Change in the function or structure of an organ to meet new conditions.

addict (**ADD**-ikt) One who cannot live without a substance or practice.

addiction (ah-**DIK**-shun) Habitual psychologic and physiologic dependence on a substance or practice.

Addison disease (**ADD**-ih-son diz-**EEZ**) An autoimmune disease leading to decreased production of adrenocortical steroids.

adduction (ah-**DUCK**-shun) Action of moving toward the midline.

adductor (ah-**DUCK**-tor) Muscle that moves the thigh toward the midline.

adenocarcinoma (**ADD**-eh-noh-kar-sih-**NOH**-mah) A cancer arising from glandular epithelial cells.

adenoid (**ADD**-eh-noyd) Single mass of lymphoid tissue in the midline at the back of the throat.

adenoidectomy (**ADD**-eh-noy-**DEK**-toh-me) Surgical removal of the adenoid tissue.

adipose (**ADD**-ih-pose) Containing fat.

adolescence (ad-oh-**LESS**-ence) Stage that begins with puberty and ends with physical maturity.

adolescent (ad-oh-**LESS**-ent) Pertaining to adolescence or a person in that stage.

adrenal gland (ah-**DREE**-nal GLAND) The suprarenal gland on the upper pole of each kidney.

adrenaline (ah-**DREN**-ah-lin) One of the catecholamines. Also called *epinephrine.*

adrenocortical (ah-**DREE**-noh-**KOR**-tih-kal) Pertaining to the cortex of the adrenal gland.

adrenocorticotropic (ah-**DREE**-noh-**KOR**-tih-koh-**TROH**-pik) Hormone of the anterior pituitary that stimulates the cortex of the adrenal gland to produce its own hormones.

afferent (**AFF**-eh-rent) Moving toward a center; for example, nerve fibers conducting impulses to the spinal cord and brain.

aged (**A**-jid) Having lived to an advanced age.

agenesis (a-**JEN**-eh-sis) Failure to develop any organ or any part.

agglutinate (ah-**GLUE**-tin-ate) Stick together to form clumps.

agglutination (ah-glue-tih-**NAY**-shun) Process by which cells or other particles adhere to each other to form clumps.

aging (**A**-jing) The process of human maturation and decline.

agranulocyte (a-**GRAN**-you-loh-site) A white blood cell without any granules in its cytoplasm.

aldosterone (al-**DOS**-ter-own) Mineralocorticoid hormone of the adrenal cortex.

alignment (a-**LINE**-ment) Having a structure in its correct position relative to other structures.

alimentary (al-ih-**MEN**-tar-ee) Pertaining to the digestive tract.

alimentary canal (al-ih-**MEN**-tar-ee kah-**NAL**) Digestive tract.

allergen (**AL**-er-jen) Substance producing a hypersensitivity (allergic) reaction.

allergenic (al-er-**JEN**-ik) Pertaining to the capacity to produce an allergic reaction.

allergic (ah-**LER**-jik) Pertaining to or suffering from an allergy.

allergy (**AL**-er-jee) Hypersensitivity to an allergen.

alloimmune (**AL**-oh-im-**YUNE**) Immune reaction directed against foreign tissue.

alopecia (al-oh-**PEE**-shah) Partial or complete loss of hair, naturally or from medication.

alveolus (al-**VEE**-oh-lus) Terminal element of the respiratory tract where gas exchange occurs. Plural *alveoli*.

Alzheimer disease (**AWLZ**-high-mer **DIZ**-eez) Common form of dementia.

amblyopia (am-blee-**OH**-pee-ah) Failure or incomplete development of the pathways of vision to the brain.

ambulatory (am-byu-**LAY**-tor-ee) Surgery or any other care provided without an overnight stay in a medical facility.

amenorrhea (a-men-oh-**REE**-ah) Absence or abnormal cessation of menstrual flow.

amino acid (ah-**ME**-no **ASS**-id) The basic building block for protein.

ammonia (ah-**MOAN**-ih-ah) Toxic breakdown product of amino acids (proteins).

amniocentesis (**AM**-nee-oh-sen-**TEE**-sis) Removal of amniotic fluid for diagnostic purposes.

amnion (**AM**-nee-on) Membrane around the fetus that contains amniotic fluid.

amniotic (am-nee-**OT**-ic) Pertaining to the amnion.

ampulla (am-**PULL**-ah) Dilated portion of a canal or duct.

amputation (am-pyu-**TAY**-shun) Process of removing a limb, a part of a limb, a breast, or some other projecting part.

amputee (**AM**-pyu-tee) A person with an amputation.

amylase (**AM**-il-aze) One of a group of enzymes that breaks down starch.

amyotrophic (a-my-oh-**TROH**-fik) Pertaining to muscular atrophy.

anabolism (an-**AB**-oh-lizm) The buildup of complex substances in the cell from simpler ones as a part of metabolism.

anal (**A**-nal) Pertaining to the anus.

analgesia (an-al-**JEE**-zee-ah) State in which pain is reduced.

analgesic (an-al-**JEE**-zic) Substance that produces analgesia.

anaphylactic (**AN**-ah-fih-**LAK**-tik) Pertaining to anaphylaxis.

anaphylaxis (**AN**-ah-fih-**LAK**-sis) Immediate severe allergic response.

anastomosis (ah-**NAS**-toh-**MOH**-sis) A surgically made union between two tubular structures. Plural *anastomoses*.

androgen (**AN**-droh-jen) Hormone that promotes masculine characteristics.

anemia (ah-**NEE**-me-ah) Decreased number of red blood cells.

anemic (ah-**NEE**-mik) Pertaining to or suffering from anemia.

anencephaly (**AN**-en-**SEF**-ah-lee) Born without cerebral hemispheres.

anesthesia (an-es-**THEE**-zee-ah) Complete loss of sensation.

anesthesiologist (**AN**-es-thee-zee-**OL**-oh-jist) Medical specialist in anesthesia.

anesthesiology (**AN**-es-thee-zee-**OL**-oh-jee) Medical specialty related to anesthesia.

anesthetic (an-es-**THET**-ik) Agent that causes absence of feeling or sensation.

aneurysm (**AN**-yur-izm) Circumscribed dilation of an artery or cardiac chamber.

angiogram (**AN**-jee-oh-gram) Radiograph obtained after injection of radiopaque contrast material into blood vessels.

angiography (an-jee-**OG**-rah-fee) Radiography of vessels after injection of contrast material.

angioplasty (**AN**-jee-oh-**PLAS**-tee) Recanalization of a blood vessel by surgery.

anomaly (ah-**NOM**-ah-lee) Structural abnormality present at birth.

anorectal junction (**A**-no-**RECK**-tal **JUNK**-shun) Junction between the anus and the rectum.

anorexia (an-oh-**RECK**-see-ah) Without an appetite; *or* having an aversion to food.

anoxia (an-**OCK**-see-ah) Without oxygen.

anoxic (an-**OCK**-sik) Pertaining to or suffering from a lack of oxygen.

antacid (ant-**ASS**-id) Agent that neutralizes the acidity of stomach contents.

antagonist (an-**TAG**-oh-nist) An opposing structure, agent, disease, or process.

antagonistic (an-**TAG**-oh-nist-ik) Having an opposite function.

antecubital (an-teh-**KYU**-bit-al) In front of the elbow.

anterior (an-**TEER**-ee-or) Front surface of body; situated in front.

anteversion (an-teh-**VER**-shun) Forward displacement or tilting of a structure.

anthracosis (an-thra-**KOH**-sis) Lung disease caused by the inhalation of coal dust.

anthrax (**AN**-thraks) A severe, malignant infectious disease.

antibiotic (**AN**-tih-bye-**OT**-ik) A substance that has the capacity to inhibit growth of and destroy bacteria and other microorganisms.

antibody (**AN**-tee-body) Protein produced in response to an antigen. Plural *antibodies*.

anticoagulant (**AN**-tee-koh-**AG**-you-lant) Substance that prevents clotting.

antidiuretic (**AN**-tih-die-you-**RET**-ik) An agent that decreases urine production.

antidiuretic hormone (ADH) (**AN**-tih-die-you-**RET**-ik **HOR**-mohn) Posterior pituitary hormone that decreases urine output by acting on the kidney. Also called *vasopressin*.

antiepileptic (**AN**-tee-epih-**LEP**-tik) A pharmacologic agent capable of preventing or arresting epilepsy.

antigen (**AN**-tee-jen) Substance capable of triggering an immune response.

antihistamine (an-tee-**HIS**-tah-meen) Drug used to treat allergic symptoms because of its action antagonistic to histamine.

antimicrobial (**AN**-tee-my-**KROH**-bee-al) Agent to destroy or prevent multiplication of organisms.

antineoplastic (**AN**-tee-nee-oh-**PLAS**-tik) Pertaining to the prevention of the growth and spread of cancer cells.

antipruritic (**AN**-tee-pru-**RIT**-ik) Medication against itching.

antipyretic (**AN**-tee-pie-**RET**-ik) Agent that reduces fever.

antisepsis (an-tih-**SEP**-sis) Inhibiting the growth of infectious agents.

antiseptic (an-tee-**SEP**-tik) An agent or substance capable of affecting antisepsis.

antiserum (an-tee-**SEER**-um) Serum taken from another human or animal that has antibodies to a disease. Also called *immune serum*.

antrum (**AN**-trum) A closed cavity.

anuria (an-**YOU**-ree-ah) Absence of urine production.

anus (**A**-nus) Terminal opening of the digestive tract through which feces are discharged.

anxiety (ang-**ZI**-eh-tee) Distress and dread caused by fear.

aorta (a-**OR**-tuh) Main trunk of the systemic arterial system.

aortic (a-**OR**-tik) Pertaining to the aorta.

apex (**A**-peks) Tip or end; for example, of the cone-shaped heart.

Apgar score (**AP**-gar SKOR) Evaluation of a newborn's status.

aphthous (**AF**-thus) Painful small oral ulcers (canker sores).

apnea (**AP**-nee-ah) Absence of spontaneous respiration.

apoptosis (**AP**-op-**TOE**-sis) Programmed normal cell death.

appendicitis (ah-pen-dih-**SIGH**-tis) Inflammation of the appendix.

appendix (ah-**PEN**-dicks) Small blind projection from the pouch of the cecum.

aqueous humor (**ACHE**-we-us **HEW**-mor) Watery liquid in the anterior and posterior chambers of the eye.

arachnoid mater (ah-**RACK**-noyd **MAY**-ter) Weblike middle layer of the three meninges.

areola (ah-**REE**-oh-luh) Circular reddish area surrounding the nipple.

areolar (ah-**REE**-oh-lar) Pertaining to the areola.

arrhythmia (a-**RITH**-me-ah) Condition when the heart rhythm is abnormal.

arteriography (ar-teer-ee-**OG**-rah-fee) X-ray visualization of an artery after injection of contrast material.

arteriole (ar-**TIER**-ee-ole) Small terminal artery leading into the capillary network.

arteriosclerosis (ar-**TIER**-ee-oh-skler-**OH**-sis) Hardening of the arteries.

arteriosclerotic (ar-**TIER**-ee-oh-skler-**OT**-ik) Pertaining to or suffering from arteriosclerosis.

artery (**AR**-ter-ee) Thick-walled blood vessel carrying blood away from the heart.

arthritis (ar-**THRI**-tis) Inflammation of a joint or joints.

arthrocentesis (**AR**-throw-sen-**TEE**-sis) Withdrawal of fluid from a joint through a needle.

arthrodesis (ar-**THROW**-dee-sis) Fixation or stiffening of a joint by surgery.

arthrography (ar-**THROG**-rah-fee) X-ray of a joint taken after the injection of a contrast medium into the joint.

arthroplasty (**AR**-throw-plas-tee) Surgery to restore, as far as possible, the function of a joint.

arthroscope (**AR**-thro-skope) Endoscope used to examine the interior of a joint.

arthroscopy (ar-**THROS**-koh-pee) Visual examination of the interior of a joint.

articulate (ar-**TIK**-you-late) Two separate bones have formed a joint.

articulation (ar-tik-you-**LAY**-shun) A joint.

asbestosis (as-bes-**TOE**-sis) Lung disease caused by the inhalation of asbestos particles.

ascites (ah-**SIGH**-teez) Accumulation of fluid in the abdominal cavity.

asepsis (a-**SEP**-sis) Absence of living pathogenic organisms.

Asperger syndrome (**AHS**-per-ger **SIN**-drohm) Developmental disorder of children.

aspiration (**AS**-pih-**RAY**-shun) Removal by suction of fluid or gas from a body cavity.

asthma (**AZ**-mah) Episodes of breathing difficulty due to narrowed or obstructed airways.

asthmatic (az-**MAT**-ik) Suffering from or pertaining to asthma.

astigmatism (ah-**STIG**-mah-tism) Inability to focus light rays that enter the eye in different planes.

asymptomatic (**A**-simp-toe-**MAT**-ik) Without any symptoms experienced by the patient.

asystole (a-**SIS**-toe-lee) Absence of contractions of the heart.

ataxia (a-**TAK**-see-ah) Inability to coordinate muscle activity, leading to jerky movements.

ataxic (a-**TAK**-sik) Pertaining to or suffering from ataxia.

atelectasis (at-el-**ECK**-tah-sis) Collapse of part of a lung.

atherectomy (ath-er-**EK**-toe-me) Surgical removal of atheroma.

atheroma (ath-er-**ROE**-mah) Lipid deposit in the lining of an artery.

atherosclerosis (**ATH**-er-oh-skler-**OH**-sis) Atheroma in arteries.

athetoid (**ATH**-eh-toyd) Resembling or suffering from athetosis.

athetosis (ath-eh-**TOE**-sis) Slow, writhing involuntary movements.

atonic (a-**TOHN**-ik) Without normal muscular tone.

atopic (ay-**TOP**-ik) Pertaining to an allergy.

atopy (**AT**-oh-pee) State of hypersensitivity to an allergen—allergic.

atresia (a-**TREE**-zee-ah) Congenital absence of a normal opening or lumen.

atrial (**A**-tree-al) Pertaining to the atrium.

atrioventricular (AV) (**A**-tree-oh-ven-**TRICK**-you-lar) Pertaining to both the atrium and the ventricle.

atrium (**A**-tree-um) Chamber where blood enters the heart on both right and left sides. Plural *atria*.

atrophy (**AT**-roh-fee) Wasting or diminished volume of a tissue or organ.

atropine (**AT**-ro-peen) Pharmacologic agent used to dilate pupils.

attenuate (ah-**TEN**-you-ate) Weaken the ability of an organism to produce disease.

audiologist (aw-dee-**OL**-oh-jist) Specialist in evaluation of hearing function.

audiology (aw-dee-**OL**-oh-jee) Study of hearing disorders.

audiometer (aw-dee-**OM**-ee-ter) Instrument to measure hearing.

audiometric (**AW**-dee-oh-**MET**-rik) Pertaining to the measurement of hearing.

auditory (**AW**-dih-tor-ee) Pertaining to the sense or the organs of hearing.

aura (**AWE**-rah) Sensory experience preceding an epileptic seizure or a migraine headache.

auricle (**AW**-ri-kul) The shell-like external ear.

auscultation (aws-kul-**TAY**-shun) Diagnostic method of listening to body sounds with a stethoscope.

autism (**AWE**-tizm) Developmental disorder of children.

autoantibody (awe-toe-**AN**-tee-bod-ee) Antibody produced in response to an antigen from the host's own tissue.

autograft (**AWE**-toe-graft) A graft using tissue taken from the same individual who is receiving the graft.

autoimmune (awe-toe-im-**YUNE**) Immune reaction directed against a person's own tissue.

autologous (awe-**TOL**-oh-gus) Blood transfusion with the same person as donor and recipient.

autolysis (awe-**TOL**-ih-sis) Destruction of cells by enzymes within the cells.

autonomic (awe-toh-**NOM**-ik) Self-governing visceral motor division of the peripheral nervous system.

autopsy (**AWE**-top-see) Examination of the body and organs of a dead person to determine the cause of death.

avascular (a-**VAS**-cue-lar) Without a blood supply.

avulsion (a-**VUL**-shun) Forcible separation or tearing away, often of a tendon from bone.

axilla (**AK**-sill-ah) Medical name for the armpit. Plural *axillae*.

axillary (**AK**-sill-air-ee) Pertaining to the armpit.

axon (**ACK**-son) Single process of a nerve cell carrying nervous impulses away from the cell body.

azotemia (azo-**TEE**-me-ah) Excess nitrogenous waste products in the blood.

B

bacterial (bak-**TEER**-ee-al) Pertaining to bacteria.

bacterium (bak-**TEER**-ee-um) A unicellular (single-cell), simple, microscopic organism. Plural *bacteria*.

balanitis (bal-ah-**NIE**-tis) Inflammation of the glans and prepuce of the penis.

bariatric (bar-ee-**AT**-rik) Treatment of obesity.

basilar (**BAS**-ih-lar) Pertaining to the base of a structure.

basophil (**BAY**-so-fill) A basophil's granules attract basic blue stain in the laboratory.

Bell palsy (BELL **PAWL**-zee) Paresis, or paralysis, of one side of the face.

biceps brachii (**BYE**-sepz **BRAY**-key-eye) A muscle of the arm that has two heads or points of origin on the scapula.

bicuspid (by-**KUSS**-pid) Having two points. A bicuspid heart valve has two flaps; a bicuspid (premolar) tooth has two points.

bifid (**BI**-fid) Separated into two parts.

bilateral (by-**LAT**-er-al) On two sides; for example, in both ears.

bile (BILE) Fluid secreted by the liver into the duodenum.

bile acids (BILE **AH**-sids) Steroids synthesized from cholesterol.

biliary (**BILL**-ee-air-ree) Pertaining to bile or the biliary tract.

bilirubin (bill-ee-**RU**-bin) Bile pigment formed in the liver from hemoglobin.

binge eating (BINJ **EE**-ting) Eating with periods of excessive intake.

biopsy (**BI**-op-see) Removing tissue from a living person for laboratory examination.

bipolar disorder (bi-**POH**-lar dis-**OR**-der) A mood disorder with alternating episodes of depression and mania.

bladder (**BLAD**-er) Hollow sac that holds fluid, for example, urine or bile.

blastocyst (**BLAS**-toe-sist) First 2 weeks of the developing embryo.

blepharitis (blef-ah-**RYE**-tis) Inflammation of the eyelid.

blepharoplasty (**BLEF**-ah-roh-**PLAS**-tee) Surgical repair of the eyelid.

blepharoptosis (**BLEF**-ah-**ROP**-toe-sis) Drooping of the upper eyelid.

blood-brain barrier (BBB) (BLUD BRAYN **BAIR**-ee-er) A selective mechanism that protects the brain from toxins and infections.

bolus (**BOH**-lus) Single mass of a substance.

botulism (**BOT**-you-lizm) Food poisoning caused by the neurotoxin produced by *Clostridium botulinum*.

bovine spongiform encephalopathy (**BO**-vine **SPON**-jee-form en-sef-ah-**LOP**-ah-thee) Disease of cattle that can be transmitted to humans, causing Creutzfeldt-Jakob disease. Also called *mad cow disease*.

bowel (**BOUGH**-el) Another name for *intestine*.

brace (BRACE) Appliance to support a part of the body in its correct position.

brachial (**BRAY**-kee-al) Pertaining to the arm.

brachialis (**BRAY**-kee-al-is) Muscle that lies underneath the biceps and is the strongest flexor of the forearm.

brachioradialis (**BRAY**-kee-oh-**RAY**-dee-al-is) Muscle that helps flex the forearm.

brachytherapy (brah-kee-**THAIR**-ah pee) Radiation therapy in which the source of radiation is implanted in the tissue to be treated.

bradycardia (brad-ee-**KAR**-dee-ah) Slow heart rate (below 60 beats per minute).

bradypnea (brad-ip-**NEE**-ah) Slow breathing.

brainstem (**BRAYN**-stem) Comprises the thalamus, pineal gland, pons, fourth ventricle, and medulla oblongata.

breech (BREECH) Buttocks-first presentation of the fetus at delivery.

bronchiectasis (brong-key-**ECK**-tah-sis) Chronic dilation of the bronchi following inflammatory disease and obstruction.

bronchiole (**BRONG**-key-ole) Increasingly smaller subdivisions of bronchi.

bronchiolitis (brong-key-oh-**LYE**-tis) Inflammation of the small bronchioles.

bronchitis (bron-**KI**-tis) Inflammation of the bronchi.

bronchoconstriction (**BRONG**-koh-kon-**STRIK**-shun) Reduction in the diameter of a bronchus.

bronchodilator (**BRONG**-koh-die-**LAY**-tor) Agent that increases the diameter of a bronchus.

bronchogenic (**BRONG**-koh-**JEN**-ik) Arising from a bronchus.

bronchopneumonia (**BRONG**-koh-new-**MOH**-nee-ah) Acute inflammation of the walls of smaller bronchioles with spread to lung parenchyma.

bronchoscope (**BRONG**-koh-skope) Endoscope used for bronchoscopy.

bronchoscopy (brong-**KOS**-koh-pee) Examination of the interior of the tracheobronchial tree with an endoscope.

bronchus (**BRONG**-kuss) One of two subdivisions of the trachea. Plural *bronchi*.

bulbourethral (**BUL**-boh-you-**REE**-thral) Pertaining to the bulbous penis and urethra.

bulimia (byu-**LEEM**-ee-ah) Episodic bouts of excessive eating with compensatory throwing up.

bulla (**BULL**-ah) Bubble-like dilated structure. Plural *bullae*.

bundle of His (**BUN**-del of HISS) Pathway for electrical signals to be transmitted to the ventricles.

bunion (**BUN**-yun) A swelling at the base of the big toe.

bursa (**BURR**-sah) A closed sac containing synovial fluid.

bursitis (burr-**SIGH**-tis) Inflammation of a bursa.

C

cadaver (kah-**DAV**-er) A dead body or corpse.

calcaneal (kal-**KAY**-knee-al) Pertaining to the calcaneus.

calcaneus (kal-**KAY**-knee-us) Bone of the tarsus that forms the heel.

calcitonin (kal-sih-**TONE**-in) Thyroid hormone that moves calcium from blood to bones.

calculus (**KAL**-kyu-lus) Small stone. Plural *calculi.*

calyx (**KAY**-licks) Funnel-shaped structure. Plural *calyces.*

cancer (**KAN**-ser) General term for a malignant neoplasm.

Candida (**KAN**-did-ah) A yeastlike fungus.

Candida albicans (**KAN**-did-ah **AL**-bih-kanz) The most common form of *Candida.*

candidiasis (can-dih-**DIE**-ah-sis) Infection with the yeastlike fungus *Candida.* Also called *thrush.*

canker (**KANG**-ker) Nonmedical term for an aphthous ulcer. Also called *mouth ulcer.*

cannula (**KAN**-you-lah) Tube inserted into a blood vessel or cavity as a channel for fluid.

capillary (**KAP**-ih-lair-ee) Minute blood vessel between the arterial and venous systems.

capsular (**KAP**-syu-lar) Pertaining to a capsule.

capsule (**KAP**-syul) Fibrous tissue layer surrounding a joint or other structure.

carbohydrate (kar-boh-**HIGH**-drate) Group of organic food compounds that includes sugars, starch, glycogen, and cellulose.

carbuncle (**KAR**-bunk-ul) Infection of many furuncles in a small area, often on the back of the neck.

carcinogen (kar-**SIN**-oh-jen) Cancer-producing agent.

carcinogenesis (kar-**SIN**-oh-**JEN**-eh-sis) Origin and development of cancer.

carcinoma (kar-sih-**NOH**-mah) A malignant and invasive epithelial tumor.

carcinoma in situ (kar-sih-**NOH**-mah in **SIGH**-too) Carcinoma that has not invaded surrounding tissues.

cardiac (**KAR**-dee-ak) Pertaining to the heart.

cardiogenic (**KAR**-dee-oh-**JEN**-ik) Of cardiac origin.

cardiologist (**KAR**-dee-**OL**-oh-jist) A medical specialist in the diagnosis and treatment of disorders of the heart (cardiology).

cardiology (**KAR**-dee-**OL**-oh-jee) Medical specialty of diseases of the heart.

cardiomegaly (**KAR**-dee-oh-**MEG**-ah-lee) Enlargement of the heart.

cardiomyopathy (**KAR**-dee-oh-my-**OP**-ah-thee) Disease of the heart muscle, the myocardium.

cardiopulmonary resuscitation (**KAR**-dee-oh-**PUL**-moh-nary ree-sus-ih-**TAY**-shun) The attempt to restore cardiac and pulmonary function.

cardiovascular (**KAR**-dee-oh-**VAS**-kyu-lar) Pertaining to the heart and blood vessels.

cardioversion (**KAR**-dee-oh-**VER**-shun) Restoration of a normal heart rhythm by electric shock. Also called *defibrillation.*

caries (**KARE**-eez) Bacterial destruction of teeth.

carotid (kah-**ROT**-id) Main artery of the neck.

carotid endarterectomy (kah-**ROT**-id **END**-ar-ter-**EK**-toe-me) Surgical removal of diseased lining from the carotid artery to leave a smooth lining and restore blood flow.

carpal (**KAR**-pal) Pertaining to the wrist.

carpus (**KAR**-pus) Collective term for the eight carpal bones of the wrist.

cartilage (**KAR**-tih-lage) Nonvascular, firm connective tissue found mostly in joints.

catabolism (kah-**TAB**-oh-lizm) Breakdown of complex substances into simpler ones as a part of metabolism.

cataplexy (**KAT**-ah-plek-see) Sudden loss of muscle tone with brief paralysis.

cataract (**KAT**-ah-ract) Complete or partial opacity of the lens.

catecholamine (kat-eh-**COAL**-ah-meen) Major element in the stress response; includes epinephrine and norepinephrine.

catheter (**KATH**-eh-ter) Hollow tube to allow passage of fluid into or out of a body cavity, organ, or vessel.

catheterization (**KATH**-eh-ter-ih-**ZAY**-shun) Introduction of a catheter.

catheterize (**KATH**-eh-teh-**RIZE**) To introduce a catheter.

caudal (**KAW**-dal) Pertaining to or nearer to the tailbone.

cautery (**KAW**-ter-ee) Agent or device used to burn or scar a tissue.

cavernosa (kav-er-**NOH**-sah) Resembling a cave.

cavity (**KAV**-ih-tee) Hollow space or body compartment. Plural *cavities.*

cecal (**SEE**-kal) Pertaining to the cecum.

cecum (**SEE**-kum) Blind pouch that is the first part of the large intestine.

celiac (**SEE**-lee-ack) Relating to the abdominal cavity.

celiac disease (**SEE**-lee-ak **DIZ**-eez) Disease caused by sensitivity to gluten.

cell (**SELL**) The smallest unit of the body capable of independent existence.

cellular (**SELL**-you-lar) Pertaining to a cell.

cellulitis (**SELL**-you-**LIE**-tis) Infection of subcutaneous connective tissue.

cephalic (seh-**FAL**-ik) Pertaining to or nearer to the head.

cerebellum (ser-eh-**BELL**-um) The most posterior area of the brain, located between the midbrain and the cerebral hemispheres.

cerebral (**SER**-ee-bral) Pertaining to the cerebral hemispheres or the brain.

cerebrospinal (**SER**-ee-broh-**SPY**-nal) Pertaining to the brain and spinal cord.

cerebrospinal fluid (CSF) (**SER**-ee-broh-**SPY**-nal **FLU**-id) Fluid formed in the ventricles of the brain that surrounds the brain and spinal cord.

cerebrum (**SER**-ee-brum) Cerebral hemispheres.

cerumen (seh-**ROO**-men) Waxy secretion of the ceruminous glands of the external ear.

ceruminous (seh-**ROO**-mih-nus) Pertaining to cerumen.

cervical (**SER**-vih-kal) Pertaining to the cervix or to the neck region.

cervix (**SER**-viks) The lower part of the uterus.

cesarean section (seh-**ZAH**-ree-an **SEK**-shun) Extraction of the fetus through an incision in the abdomen and uterine wall. Also called *C-section.*

chancre (**SHAN**-ker) Primary lesion of syphilis.

chemotherapy (**KEY**-moh-**THAIR**-ah-pee) Treatment using chemical agents.

chiasm (**KYE**-asm) X-shaped crossing of the two optic nerves at the base of the brain. Alternative term *chiasma.*

chickenpox (**CHICK**-en-pocks) Acute, contagious viral disease. Also called *varicella.*

chiropractic (kye-roh-**PRAK**-tik) Diagnosis, treatment, and prevention of mechanical disorders of the musculoskeletal system.

chiropractor (kye-roh-**PRAK**-tor) Practitioner of chiropractic.

chlamydia (klah-**MID**-ee-ah) An STD caused by an infection with *Chlamydia,* a species of bacteria.

cholangiography (**KOH**-lan-jee-**OG**-rah-fee) Use of a contrast medium to radiographically visualize the bile ducts.

cholecystectomy (**KOH**-leh-sis-**TECK**-toe-me) Surgical removal of the gallbladder.

cholecystitis (**KOH**-leh-sis-**TIE**-tis) Inflammation of the gallbladder.

choledocholithiasis (**KOH**-leh-**DOH**-koh-li-**THIGH**-ah-sis) Presence of a gallstone in the common bile duct.

cholelithiasis (**KOH**-leh-lih-**THIGH**-ah-sis) Condition of having bile stones (gallstones).

cholelithotomy (**KOH**-leh-lih-**THOT**-oh-me) Surgical removal of a gallstone(s).

cholesteatoma (**KOH**-less-tee-ah-**TOE**-mah) Yellow, waxy tumor arising in the middle ear.

cholesterol (koh-**LESS**-ter-ol) Formed in liver cells; is the most abundant steroid in tissues and circulates in the plasma attached to proteins of different densities.

chorea (kor-**EE**-ah) Involuntary, irregular spasms of limb and facial muscles.

choreic (kor-**EE**-ik) Pertaining to or suffering from chorea.

chorion (**KOH**-ree-on) The fetal membrane that forms the placenta.

chorionic (koh-ree-**ON**-ick) Pertaining to the chorion.

chorionic villus (koh-ree-**ON**-ik **VILL**-us) Vascular process of the embryonic chorion to form the placenta.

choroid (**KOR**-oid) Region of the retina and uvea.

chromosome (**KROH**-moh-sohm) Body in the nucleus that contains DNA and genes.

chronic (**KRON**-ik) A persistent, long-term disease.

chyle (**KYLE**) A milky fluid that results from the digestion and absorption of fats in the small intestine.

chyme (**KYME**) Semifluid, partially digested food passed from the stomach into the duodenum.

cilium (**SILL**-ee-um) Hairlike motile projection from the surface of a cell. Plural *cilia.*

circulation (**SER**-kyu-**LAY**-shun) Continuous movement of blood through the heart and blood vessels.

circumcision (ser-kum-**SIZH**-un) To remove part or all of the prepuce.

circumduct (ser-kum-**DUCKT**) To move an extremity in a circular motion.

circumduction (ser-kum-**DUCK**-shun) Movement of an extremity in a circular motion.

cirrhosis (sir-**ROE**-sis) Extensive fibrotic liver disease.

claudication (klaw-dih-**KAY**-shun) Intermittent leg pain and limping.

clavicle (**KLAV**-ih-kul) Curved bone that forms the anterior part of the pectoral girdle.

clavicular (klah-**VICK**-you-lar) Pertaining to the clavicle.

cleft lip (KLEFT LIP) Congenital defect of the upper lip.

cleft palate (KLEFT **PAL**-ate) Congenital defect of the palate.

clitoris (**KLIT**-oh-ris) Erectile organ of the vulva.

clonic (**KLON**-ik) State of rapid successions of muscular contractions and relaxations.

closed fracture (KLOSD **FRAK**-chur) A bone is broken but the skin over it is intact.

Clostridium botulinum (klos-**TRID**-ee-um bot-you-**LIE**-num) Bacterium that causes food poisoning.

clot (KLOT) The mass of fibrin and cells that is produced in a wound.

coagulant (koh-**AG**-you-lant) Substance that causes clotting.

coagulate (koh-**AG**-you-late) Form a clot.

coagulation (koh-ag-you-**LAY**-shun) The process of blood clotting.

coagulopathy (koh-ag-you-**LOP**-ah-thee) Disorder of blood clotting. Plural *coagulopathies.*

coarctation (koh-ark-**TAY**-shun) Constriction, stenosis, particularly of the aorta.

coccyx (**KOK**-sicks) Small tailbone at the lower end of the vertebral column.

cochlea (**KOK**-lee-ah) An intricate combination of passages; used to describe the inner ear.

cochlear (**KOK**-lee-ar) Pertaining to the cochlea.

cognition (kog-**NIH**-shun) Process of acquiring knowledge through thinking, learning, and memory.

cognitive-behavioral therapy (CBT) (**KOG**-nih-tiv be-**HAYV**-yur-al **THAIR**-ah-pee) Psychotherapy that emphasizes thoughts and attitudes in one's behavior.

coitus (**KOH**-it-us) Sexual intercourse.

colic (**KOL**-ik) Spasmodic, crampy pains in the abdomen.

colitis (koh-**LIE**-tis) Inflammation of the colon.

collagen (**KOLL**-ah-jen) Major protein of connective tissue, cartilage, and bone.

collateral (koh-**LAT**-er-al) Situated at the side, often to bypass an obstruction.

Colles fracture (**KOL**-ez **FRAK**-chur) Fracture of the distal radius at the wrist.

colloid (**COLL**-oyd) Liquid containing suspended particles.

colon (**KOH**-lon) The large intestine, extending from the cecum to the rectum.

colostomy (koh-**LOSS**-toe-me) Artificial opening from the colon to the outside of the body.

colostrum (koh-**LOSS**-trum) The first breast secretion at the end of pregnancy.

colpopexy (**KOL**-poh-peck-see) Surgical fixation of the vagina.

coma (**KOH**-mah) State of deep unconsciousness.

comatose (**KOH**-mah-toes) In a state of coma.

comedo (**KOM**-ee-doh) A whitehead or blackhead caused by too much sebum and too many keratin cells blocking the hair follicle. Plural *comedones.*

comminuted fracture (**KOM**-ih-nyu-ted **FRAK**-chur) A fracture in which the bone is broken into small pieces.

competent (**KOM**-peh-tent) Capable of performing a task or function.

complement (**KOM**-pleh-ment) Group of proteins in the serum that finish off the work of antibodies to destroy bacteria and other cells.

complete fracture (kom-**PLEET FRAK**-chur) A bone is fractured into two separate pieces.

compliance (kom-**PLY**-ance) Measure of the capacity of a chamber or hollow viscus (e.g., the lungs) to expand; *or* consistency and accuracy with which a patient follows a treatment regimen.

compression (kom-**PRESH**-un) Squeeze together to increase density and/or decrease a dimension of a structure.

compression fracture (kom-**PRESH**-un **FRAK**-chur) Fracture of a vertebra causing loss of height of the vertebra.

compulsion (kom-**PULL**-shun) Uncontrollable impulses to perform an act repetitively.

compulsive (kom-**PULL**-siv) Possessing uncontrollable impulses to perform an act repetitively.

conception (kon-**SEP**-shun) Fertilization of the egg by sperm to form a zygote.

concha (**KON**-kah) Shell-shaped bone on the medial wall of the nasal cavity. Plural *conchae.*

concussion (kon-**KUSH**-un) Mild brain injury.

condom (**KON**-dom) A sheath or cover for the penis or vagina to prevent conception and infection.

conductive hearing loss (kon-**DUK**-tiv) Hearing loss caused by lesions in the outer ear or middle ear.

condyle (**KON**-dile) Large, smooth, rounded expansion of the end of a bone where it forms a joint with another bone.

confusion (kon-**FEW**-zhun) Mental state in which environmental stimuli are not processed appropriately.

congenital (kon-**JEN**-ih-tal) Present at birth, either inherited or due to an event during gestation up to the moment of birth.

conization (koh-ni-**ZAY**-shun) Surgical excision of a cone-shaped piece of tissue.

conjunctiva (kon-junk-**TIE**-vah) Inner lining of the eyelids.

conjunctival (kon-junk-**TIE**-val) Pertaining to the conjunctiva.

conjunctivitis (kon-junk-tih-**VI**-tis) Inflammation of the conjunctiva.

connective tissue (koh-**NECK**-tiv **TISH**-you) The supporting tissue of the body.

consciousness (**KON**-shus-ness) The state of being aware of and responsive to the environment.

constipation (kon-stih-**PAY**-shun) Hard, infrequent bowel movements.

constrict (kon-**STRIKT**) To become or make narrow.

constriction (kon-**STRIK**-shun) A narrowed portion of a structure.

contagious (kon-**TAY**-jus) Infection can be transmitted from person to person or from a person to a surface to a person.

contaminate (kon-**TAM**-in-ate) To cause the presence of an infectious agent to be on any surface or in any substance.

contamination (**KON**-tam-ih-**NAY**-shun) Presence of an infectious agent on a surface or in substances.

contraception (kon-trah-**SEP**-shun) Prevention of pregnancy.

contraceptive (kon-trah-**SEP**-tiv) An agent that prevents conception.

contract (kon-**TRAKT**) Draw together or shorten.

contracture (kon-**TRAK**-chur) Muscle shortening due to spasm or fibrosis.

contrecoup (**KON**-treh-koo) Injury to the brain at a point directly opposite the point of original contact.

contusion (kon-**TOO**-zhun) Hemorrhage into a tissue (bruising), including the brain.

convulsion (kon-**VUL**-shun) Alternative name for seizure.

cor pulmonale (**KOR** pul-moh-**NAH**-lee) Right-sided heart failure arising from chronic lung disease.

cornea (**KOR**-nee-ah) The central, transparent part of the outer coat of the eye covering the iris and pupil.

corneal (**KOR**-nee-al) Pertaining to the cornea.

coronal (**KOR**-oh-nal) Pertaining to the vertical plane dividing the body into anterior and posterior portions.

coronal plane (**KOR**-oh-nal **PLAIN**) Vertical plane dividing the body into anterior and posterior portions.

coronary circulation (**KOR**-oh-nair-ee **SER**-kyu-**LAY**-shun) Blood vessels supplying the heart.

corpus (**KOR**-pus) Major part of a structure. Plural *corpora.*

corpus albicans (**KOR**-pus **AL**-bih-kanz) An atrophied corpus luteum.

corpus callosum (**KOR**-pus kah-**LOW**-sum) Bridge of nerve fibers connecting the two cerebral hemispheres.

corpus luteum (**KOR**-pus **LOO**-teh-um) Yellow structure formed at the site of a ruptured ovarian follicle.

corpuscle (**KOR**-pus-ul) A blood cell.

cortex (**KOR**-teks) Outer portion of an organ, such as bone; gray covering of cerebral hemispheres. Plural *cortices.*

cortical (**KOR**-tih-cal) Pertaining to a cortex.

corticosteroid (**KOR**-tih-koh-**STEHR**-oyd) A hormone produced by the adrenal cortex.

corticotropin (**KOR**-tih-koh-**TROH**-pin) Pituitary hormone that stimulates the cortex of the adrenal gland to secrete corticosteroids.

cortisol (**KOR**-tih-sol) One of the glucocorticoids produced by the adrenal cortex; has anti-inflammatory effects. Also called *hydrocortisone.*

coryza (koh-**RYE**-zah) Viral inflammation of the mucous membrane of the nose. Also called *acute rhinitis.*

coup (**KOO**) Injury to the brain occurring directly under the skull at the point of contact.

coxa (**COCK**-sah) Hipbone. Plural *coxae.*

cranial (**KRAY**-nee-al) Pertaining to the cranium.

craniofacial (**KRAY**-nee-oh-**FAY**-shal) Pertaining to both the face and the cranium.

cranium (**KRAY**-nee-um) The skull.

cretin (**KREH**-tin) A person with severe congenital hypothyroidism.

cretinism (**KREH**-tin-izm) Condition of severe congenital hypothyroidism.

Creutzfeldt-Jakob disease (**KROITS**-felt **YAK**-op **DIZ**-eez) Progressive incurable neurologic disease caused by infectious prions.

cricoid (**CRY**-koyd) Ring-shaped cartilage in the larynx.

crista ampullaris (**KRIS**-tah am-**PULL**-air-is) Mound of hair cells and gelatinous material in the ampulla of a semicircular canal.

Crohn disease (**KRONE** diz-**EEZ**) Narrowing and thickening of terminal small bowel. Also called *regional enteritis.*

croup (**KROOP**) Infection of the upper airways in children, characterized by a barking cough. Also called *laryngotracheobronchitis.*

cruciate (**KRU**-she-ate) Shaped like a cross.

cryosurgery (cry-oh-**SUR**-jer-ee) Use of liquid nitrogen or argon gas in a probe to freeze and kill abnormal tissue.

cryptorchism (krip-**TOR**-kizm) Failure of one or both testes to descend into the scrotum.

curettage (kyu-reh-**TAHZH**) Scraping the interior of a cavity.

curette (kyu-**RET**) Scoop-shaped instrument for scraping the interior of a cavity or removing new growths.

Cushing syndrome (**KUSH**-ing **SIN**-drohm) Hypersecretion of cortisol (hydrocortisone) by the adrenal cortex.

cutaneous (kyu-**TAY**-nee-us) Pertaining to the skin.

cuticle (**KEW**-tih-cul) Nonliving epidermis at the base of the fingernails and toenails.

cyanosis (sigh-ah-**NO**-sis) Blue discoloration of the skin, lips, and nail beds due to low levels of oxygen in the blood.

cyanotic (sigh-ah-**NOT**-ik) Pertaining to or marked by cyanosis.

cyst (SIST) An abnormal, fluid-containing sac.

cystic (**SIS**-tik) Relating to a cyst.

cystic fibrosis (CF) (**SIS**-tik fie-**BROH**-sis) Genetic disease in which excessive viscid mucus obstructs passages, including bronchi.

cystitis (sis-**TIE**-tis) Inflammation of the urinary bladder.

cystocele (**SIS**-toh-seal) Hernia of the bladder into the vagina.

cystoscope (**SIS**-toh-skope) An endoscope inserted to view the inside of the bladder.

cystoscopy (sis-**TOS**-koh-pee) Using a cystoscope to examine the inside of the urinary bladder.

cystourethrogram (sis-toh-you-**REETH**-roe-gram) X-ray image during voiding to show the structure and function of the bladder and urethra.

cytologist (**SIGH**-tol-oh-jist) Specialist in the structure, chemistry, and pathology of the cell.

cytology (**SIGH**-tol-oh-jee) Study of the cell.

cytoplasm (**SIGH**-toh-plazm) Clear, gelatinous substance that forms the substance of a cell except for the nucleus.

cytotoxic (sigh-toh-**TOX**-ik) Destructive to cells.

D

dandruff (**DAN**-druff) Scales in hair from shedding of the epidermis.

death (DETH) Total and permanent cessation of all vital functions.

debridement (day-**BREED**-mon) The removal of injured or necrotic tissue.

decongestant (dee-con-**JESS**-tant) Agent that reduces the swelling and fluid in the nose and sinuses.

decubitus ulcer (de-**KYU**-bit-us **UL**-ser) Sore caused by lying down for long periods of time.

defecation (def-eh-**KAY**-shun) Evacuation of feces from the rectum and anus.

defect (**DEE**-fect) An absence, malformation, or imperfection.

defective (dee-**FEK**-tiv) Imperfect.

defibrillation (de-fib-rih-**LAY**-shun) Restoration of uncontrolled twitching of cardiac muscle fibers to normal rhythm.

defibrillator (de-fib-rih-**LAY**-tor) Instrument for defibrillation.

deformity (de-**FOR**-mih-tee) A permanent structural deviation from the normal.

degenerative (dee-**JEN**-er-a-tiv) Relating to the deterioration of a structure.

deglutition (dee-glue-**TISH**-un) The act of swallowing.

dehydration (dee-high-**DRAY**-shun) Process of losing body water.

delirium (de-**LIR**-ee-um) Acute altered state of consciousness with agitation and disorientation; condition is reversible.

deltoid (**DEL**-toyd) Large, fan-shaped muscle connecting the scapula and clavicle to the humerus.

delusion (dee-**LOO**-shun) Fixed, unyielding false belief held despite strong evidence to the contrary.

dementia (dee-**MEN**-she-ah) Chronic, progressive, irreversible loss of intellectual and mental functions.

demyelination (dee-**MY**-eh-lin-**A**-shun) Process of losing the myelin sheath of a nerve fiber.

dendrite (**DEN**-dright) Branched extension of the nerve cell body that receives nervous stimuli.

dental (**DEN**-tal) Pertaining to the teeth.

dentine (**DEN**-tin) Dense, ivory-like substance located under the enamel in a tooth. (Also spelled *dentin.*)

dentist (**DEN**-tist) Legally qualified specialist in dentistry.

dentistry (**DEN**-tis-tree) Evaluation, diagnosis, prevention, and treatment of conditions of the oral cavity and associated structures.

deoxyribonucleic acid (DNA) (dee-**OCK**-see-**RYE**-boh-noo-**KLEE**-ik **ASS**-id) Source of hereditary characteristics found in chromosomes.

dependent (dee-**PEN**-dent) Having to rely on someone else.

depressant (de-**PRESS**-ant) Substance that diminishes activity, sensation, or tone.

depression (de-**PRESS**-shun) Mental disorder with feelings of deep sadness and despair.

dermabrasion (der-mah-**BRAY**-shun) Removal of upper layers of skin by rotary brush.

dermal (**DER**-mal) Pertaining to the skin.

dermatitis (der-mah-**TYE**-tis) Inflammation of the skin.

dermatologic (der-mah-toh-**LOJ**-ik) Pertaining to the skin and dermatology.

dermatologist (der-mah-**TOL**-oh-jist) Medical specialist in diseases of the skin.

dermatology (der-mah-**TOL**-oh-jee) Medical specialty concerned with disorders of the skin.

dermatomyositis (**DER**-mah-toe-**MY**-oh-site-is) Inflammation of the skin and muscles.

dermis (**DER**-miss) Connective tissue layer of the skin beneath the epidermis.

detoxification (dee-**TOKS**-ih-fih-**KAY**-shun) Remove poison from a tissue or substance.

diabetes insipidus (dye-ah-**BEE**-teez in-**SIP**-ih-dus) Excretion of large amounts of dilute urine as a result of inadequate ADH production.

diabetes mellitus (dye-ah-**BEE**-teez **MEL**-ih-tus) Metabolic syndrome caused by absolute or relative insulin deficiency and/or insulin ineffectiveness.

diabetic (dye-ah-**BET**-ik) Pertaining to or suffering from diabetes.

diagnose (die-ag-**NOSE**) To make a diagnosis.

diagnosis (die-ag-**NO**-sis) The determination of the cause of a disease. Plural *diagnoses.*

diagnostic (die-ag-N**OS**-tik) Pertaining to or establishing a diagnosis.

dialysis (die-**AL**-ih-sis) An artificial method of filtration to remove excess waste materials and water from the body.

diaphoresis (**DIE**-ah-foh-**REE**-sis) Sweat or perspiration.

diaphoretic (**DIE**-ah-foh-**RET**-ic) Pertaining to sweat or perspiration.

diaphragm (**DIE**-ah-fram) A ring and dome-shaped material inserted into the vagina to prevent pregnancy; *or* the muscular sheet separating the abdominal and thoracic cavities.

diaphragmatic (**DIE**-ah-frag-**MAT**-ik) Pertaining to the diaphragm.

diaphysis (die-**AF**-ih-sis) The shaft of a long bone.

diarrhea (die-ah-**REE**-ah) Abnormally frequent and loose stools.

diastasis (die-**ASS**-tah-sis) Separation of normally joined parts.

diastole (die-**AS**-toe-lee) Dilation of heart cavities, during which they fill with blood.

diastolic (die-as-**TOL**-ik) Pertaining to diastole.

differential (dif-er-**EN**-shal) A differential white blood cell count lists percentages of the different leukocytes in a blood sample.

diffuse (di-**FUSE**) To disseminate or spread out.

diffusion (di-**FYU**-zhun) The means by which small particles move between tissues.

digestion (die-**JEST**-shun) Breakdown of food into elements suitable for cell metabolism.

digestive (die-**JEST**-iv) Pertaining to digestion.

digital (**DIJ**-ih-tal) Pertaining to a finger or toe.

dilate (**DIE**-late) To perform or undergo dilation.

dilation (die-**LAY**-shun) Stretching or enlarging an opening or a structure.

diphtheria (dif-**THEER**-ee-ah) Disease with a thick, membranous (leathery) coating of the pharynx.

diplegia (die-**PLEE**-jee-ah) Paralysis of all four limbs, with the two legs affected most severely.

disability (dis-ah-**BILL**-ih-tee) Diminished capacity to perform certain activities or functions.

discipline (**DIS**-ih-plin) Training for proper conduct or action.

disease (**DIZ**-eez) A disorder of body functions, systems, or organs.

disinfectant (dis-in-**FEK**-tant) Agent that disinfects.

disinfection (dis-in-**FEK**-shun) Process of destruction of microorganisms by chemical agents.

dislocation (dis-low-**KAY**-shun) Completely out of joint.

displaced fracture (dis-**PLAYSD FRAK**-chur) A fracture in which the fragments are separated and are not in alignment.

disseminate (dih-**SEM**-in-ate) Widely scattered throughout the body or an organ.

dissociative identity disorder (di-**SO**-see-ah-tiv eye-**DEN**-tih-tee dis-**OR**-der) Part of an individual's personality is separated from the rest, leading to multiple personalities.

distal (**DISS**-tal) Situated away from the center of the body.

diuresis (die-you-**REE**-sis) Excretion of large volumes of urine.

diuretic (die-you-**RET**-ik) Agent that increases urine output.

diverticulitis (**DIE**-ver-tick-you-**LIE**-tis) Inflammation of the diverticula.

diverticulosis (**DIE**-ver-tick-you-**LOW**-sis) Presence of a number of small pouches in the wall of the large intestine.

diverticulum (die-ver-**TICK**-you-lum) A pouchlike opening or sac from a tubular structure (e.g., gut). Plural *diverticula.*

dopamine (**DOH**-pah-meen) Neurotransmitter in specific small areas of the brain.

Doppler (**DOP**-ler) Diagnostic instrument that sends an ultrasonic beam into the body.

Doppler ultrasonography (**DOP**-ler **UL**-trah-soh-**NOG**-rah-fee) Detects direction, velocity, and turbulence of blood flow; used in workup of stroke patients.

dormant (**DOOR**-mant) Inactive.

dorsal (**DOOR**-sal) Pertaining to the back or situated behind.

dorsum (**DOOR**-sum) Upper, posterior, or back surface.

Down syndrome (**DOWN SIN**-drome) A syndrome with variable abnormalities associated with three chromosomes 21.

Duchenne muscular dystrophy (**DOO**-shen **MUSS**-kyu-lar **DISS**-troh-fee) Symmetrical weakness and wasting of pelvic, shoulder, and proximal limb muscles.

ductus arteriosus (**DUK**-tus ar-**TEER**-ih-**OH**-sus) Fetal vessel that connects the descending aorta with the left pulmonary artery.

ductus deferens (**DUK**-tus **DEH**-fuh-renz) Tube that receives sperm from the epididymis. Also known as *vas deferens.*

duodenal (du-oh-**DEE**-nal) Pertaining to the duodenum.

duodenum (du-oh-**DEE**-num) The first part of the small intestine; approximately 12 finger-breadths (9 to 10 inches) in length.

dura mater (**DYU**-rah **MAY**-ter) Hard, fibrous outer layer of the meninges.

dysentery (**DIS**-en-tare-ee) Disease with diarrhea, bowel spasms, fever, and dehydration.

dysfunctional (dis-**FUNK**-shun-al) Difficulty in functioning.

dyslexia (dis-**LEK**-see-ah) Impaired reading and writing ability below the person's level of intelligence.

dyslexic (dis-**LEK**-sik) Pertaining to or suffering from dyslexia.

dysmenorrhea (dis-men-oh-**REE**-ah) Painful and difficult menstruation.

dyspareunia (dis-pah-**RUE**-nee-ah) Pain during sexual intercourse.

dyspepsia (dis-**PEP**-see-ah) "Upset stomach," epigastric pain, nausea, and gas.

dysphagia (dis-**FAY**-jee-ah) Difficulty in swallowing.

dysphoria (dis-**FOR**-ee-ah) Psychiatric mood disorder.

dysplasia (dis-**PLAY**-zee-ah) Abnormal tissue formation.

dysplastic (dis-**PLAS**-tik) Pertaining to or showing abnormal tissue formation.

dyspnea (disp-**NEE**-ah) Difficulty breathing.

dyspneic (disp-**NEE**-ik) Pertaining to or suffering from difficulty in breathing.

dysrhythmia (dis-**RITH**-me-ah) An abnormal heart rhythm.

dysuria (dis-**YOU**-ree-ah) Difficulty or pain with urination.

E

echocardiography (**EK**-oh-kar-dee-**OG**-rah-fee) Ultrasound recording of heart function.

echoencephalography (**EK**-oh-en-sef-ah-**LOG**-rah-fee) Use of ultrasound in the diagnosis of intracranial lesions.

eclampsia (ek-**LAMP**-see-uh) Convulsions in a patient with preeclampsia.

ectopic (ek-**TOP**-ik) Out of place, not in a normal position.

eczema (**EK**-zeh-mah) Inflammatory skin disease, often with a serous discharge.

eczematous (**EK**-zem-ah-tus) Pertaining to or marked by eczema.

edema (ee-**DEE**-mah) Excessive accumulation of fluid in cells and tissues.

edematous (ee-**DEM**-ah-tus) Pertaining to or marked by edema.

effacement (ee-**FACE**-ment) Thinning of the cervix in relation to labor.

efferent (**EFF**-eh-rent) Moving away from a center; for example, conducting nerve impulses away from the brain or spinal cord.

effusion (eh-**FYU**-shun) Collection of fluid that has escaped from blood vessels into a cavity or tissues.

ejaculate (ee-**JACK**-you-late) To expel suddenly; *or* the semen expelled in ejaculation.

ejaculation (ee-**JACK**-you-**LAY**-shun) Process of expelling semen suddenly.

ejaculatory (ee-**JACK**-you-**LAY**-tor-ee) Pertaining to ejaculation.

elective (e-**LEK**-tiv) Surgery or a procedure that is not urgent or vital.

electrocardiogram (ECG or EKG) (ee-**LEK**-troh-**KAR**-dee-oh-gram) Record of the electrical signals of the heart.

electrocardiograph (ee-**LEK**-troh-**KAR**-dee-oh-graf) Machine that makes the electrocardiogram.

electrocardiography (ee-**LEK**-troh-kar-dee-**OG**-rah-fee) Interpretation of electrocardiograms.

electroconvulsive therapy (ECT) (ee-**LEK**-troh-kon-**VUL**-siv **THAIR**-ah-pee) Passage of electric current through the brain to produce convulsions and treat persistent depression.

electrode (ee-**LEK**-trode) A device for conducting electricity.

electroencephalogram (EEG) (ee-**LEK**-troh-en-**SEF**-ah-low-gram) Record of the electrical activity of the brain.

electroencephalograph (ee-**LEK**-troh-en-**SEF**-ah-low-graf) Device used to record the electrical activity of the brain.

electroencephalography (ee-**LEK**-troh-en-**SEF**-ah-**LOG**-rah-fee) The process of recording the electrical activity of the brain.

electrolyte (ee-**LEK**-troh-lite) Substance that, when dissolved in a suitable medium, forms electrically charged particles.

electromyogram (ee-**LEK**-troh-**MY**-oh-gram) Recording of electric currents associated with muscle action.

electromyography (ee-**LEK**-troh-my-**OG**-rah-fee) Recording of electrical activity in muscle.

electroneurodiagnostic (ee-**LEK**-troh-**NYUR**-oh-die-ag-**NOS**-tik) Pertaining to the use of electricity in the diagnosis of a neurologic disorder.

elimination (e-lim-ih-**NAY**-shun) Removal of waste material from the digestive tract.

emaciated (ee-may-see-**AY**-ted) Pertaining to or suffering from emaciation.

emaciation (ee-may-see-**AY**-shun) Abnormal thinness.

embolus (**EM**-boh-lus) Detached piece of thrombus, a mass of bacteria, quantity of air, or foreign body that blocks a blood vessel.

embryo (**EM**-bree-oh) Developing organism from conception until the end of the second month.

embryology (em-bree-**OL**-oh-jee) Science of the origin and early development of an organism.

embryonic (em-bree-**ON**-ic) Pertaining to the embryo.

emesis (**EM**-eh-sis) Vomit.

emmetropia (emm-eh-**TROH**-pee-ah) Normal refractive condition of the eye.

empathy (**EM**-pah-thee) Ability to place yourself into the feelings, emotions, and reactions of another person.

emphysema (em-fih-**SEE**-mah) Dilation of respiratory bronchioles and alveoli.

empyema (**EM**-pie-**EE**-mah) Pus in a body cavity, particularly in the pleural cavity.

emulsify (ee-**MUL**-sih-fye) Break up into very small droplets to suspend in a solution (emulsion).

emulsion (ee-**MUL**-shun) The system that contains small droplets suspended in a liquid.

enamel (ee-**NAM**-el) Hard substance covering a tooth.

encephalitis (en-**SEF**-ah-**LIE**-tis) Inflammation of brain cells and tissues.

encephalocele (en-**SEF**-ah-loh-seal) Congenital defect of the cranium with herniation of brain tissue.

encephalomyelitis (en-**SEF**-ah-loh-**MY**-eh-lie-tis) Inflammation of the brain and spinal cord.

encephalopathy (en-sef-ah-**LOP**-ah-thee) Any disorder of the brain.

encopresis (en-koh-**PREE**-sis) Repeated soiling with feces.

endarterectomy (**END**-ar-ter-**EK**-toe-me) Surgical removal of plaque from an artery.

endemic (en-**DEM**-ik) Pertaining to a disease always present in a community.

endocardial (**EN**-doh-kar-**DEE**-al) Pertaining to the endocardium.

endocarditis (**EN**-doh-kar-**DIE**-tis) Inflammation of the lining of the heart.

endocardium (**EN**-doh-kar-**DEE**-um) The inside lining of the heart.

endocrine (**EN**-doh-krin) A gland that produces an internal or hormonal substance.

endocrinologist (**EN**-doh-krih-**NOL**-oh-jist) A medical specialist in endocrinology.

endocrinology (**EN**-doh-krih-**NOL**-oh-jee) Medical specialty concerned with the production and effects of hormones.

endometrial (en-doh-**ME**-tree-al) Pertaining to the inner lining of the uterus.

endometriosis (**EN**-doh-me-tree-**OH**-sis) Endometrial tissue outside the uterus.

endometrium (en-doh-**ME**-tree-um) Inner lining of the uterus.

endoscope (**EN**-doh-skope) Instrument to examine the inside of a tubular or hollow organ.

endoscopy (en-**DOS**-koh-pee) The use of an endoscope.

endotracheal (en-doh-**TRAY**-kee-al) Pertaining to being inside the trachea.

enema (**EN**-eh-mah) An injection of fluid into the rectum.

enteric (en-**TEHR**-ik) Pertaining to the intestine.

enteroscope (**EN**-ter-oh-**SKOPE**) Slender, tubular instrument with light source and camera to visualize the digestive tract.

enteroscopy (en-ter-**OSS**-koh-pee) The examination of the lining of the digestive tract.

enuresis (en-you-**REE**-sis) Bedwetting; urinary incontinence.

enzyme (**EN**-zime) Protein that induces changes in other substances.

eosinophil (ee-oh-**SIN**-oh-fill) An eosinophil's granules attract a rosy-red color on staining.

epicardial (**EP**-ih-kar-**DEE**-al) Pertaining to the epicardium.

epicardium (**EP**-ih-kar-**DEE**-um) The outer layer of the heart wall.

epicondyle (**EP**-ih-**KON**-dile) Projection above the condyle for attachment of a ligament or tendon.

epidemic (ep-ih-**DEM**-ik) Pertaining to an outbreak in a community of a disease or a health-related behavior.

epidermal (ep-ih-**DER**-mal) Pertaining to the epidermis.

epidermis (ep-ih-**DER**-miss) Top layer of the skin.

epididymis (**EP**-ih-**DID**-ih-miss) Coiled tube attached to the testis.

epididymitis (**EP**-ih-did-ih-**MY**-tis) Inflammation of the epididymis.

epididymoorchitis (**EP**-ih-**DID**-ih-moh-or-**KIE**-tis) Inflammation of the epididymis and testicle. Also called *orchitis.*

epidural (ep-ih-**DYU**-ral) Above the dura.

epidural space (ep-ih-**DYU**-ral SPASE) Space between the dura mater and the wall of the vertebral canal.

epigastric (ep-ih-**GAS**-trik) Pertaining to the abdominal region above the stomach.

epigastrium (ep-ih-**GAS**-tri-um) The abdominal region above the stomach.

epiglottis (ep-ih-**GLOT**-is) Leaf-shaped plate of cartilage that shuts off the larynx during swallowing.

epiglottitis (ep-ih-**GLOT**-eye-tis) Inflammation of the epiglottis.

epilepsy (**EP**-ih-**LEP**-see) Chronic brain disorder due to paroxysmal excessive neuronal discharges.

epileptic (**EP**-ih-**LEP**-tik) Pertaining to or suffering from epilepsy.

epinephrine (ep-ih-**NEF**-rin) Main catecholamine produced by the adrenal medulla. Also called *adrenaline.*

epiphysial (eh-**PIF**-ih-see-al) Pertaining to an epiphysis.

epiphysial plate (eh-**PIF**-ih-see-al PLATE) Layer of cartilage between the epiphysis and the metaphysis where bone growth occurs.

epiphysis (eh-**PIF**-ih-sis) Expanded area at the proximal and distal ends of a long bone to provide increased surface area for attachment of ligaments and tendons.

episiotomy (eh-piz-ee-**OT**-oh-me) Surgical incision of the vulva.

epispadias (ep-ih-**SPAY**-dee-as) Condition in which the urethral opening is on the dorsum of the penis.

epistaxis (ep-ih-**STAK**-sis) Nosebleed.

epithelium (ep-ih-**THEE**-lee-um) Tissue that covers surfaces or lines cavities.

equilibrium (ee-kwi-**LIB**-ree-um) Being evenly balanced.

erectile (ee-**REK**-tile) Capable of erection or being distended with blood.

erection (ee-**REK**-shun) Distended and rigid state of an organ.

erosion (ee-**ROE**-zhun) Form a shallow ulcer in the lining of a structure.

erythroblast (eh-**RITH**-ro-blast) Precursor to a red blood cell.

erythroblastosis (eh-**RITH**-roh-blast-oh-sis) Condition of many immature red cells in blood.

erythrocyte (eh-**RITH**-roh-site) A red blood cell.

erythropoiesis (eh-**RITH**-roh-poy-**EE**-sis) The formation of red blood cells.

erythropoietin (eh-**RITH**-roh-**POY**-ee-tin) Protein secreted by the kidney that stimulates red blood cell production.

eschar (**ESS**-kar) The burnt, dead tissue lying on top of third-degree burns.

Escherichia coli (esh-eh-**RIK**-ee-ah **KOH**-lie) Organism in the intestine; releases an exotoxin that can cause diarrhea.

esophageal (ee-**SOF**-ah-**JEE**-al) Pertaining to the esophagus.

esophagitis (ee-**SOF**-ah-**JI**-tis) Inflammation of the lining of the esophagus.

esophagus (ee-**SOF**-ah-gus) Tube linking the pharynx to the stomach.

esotropia (es-oh-**TROH**-pee-ah) Turning the eye inward toward the nose.

estrogen (**ES**-troh-jen) Generic term for hormones that stimulate female secondary sex characteristics.

ethmoid (**ETH**-moyd) Bone that forms the back of the nose and encloses numerous air cells.

etiology (ee-tee-**OL**-oh-jee) The study of the causes of a disease.

eupnea (yoop-**NEE**-ah) Normal breathing.

eustachian tube (you-**STAY**-shun TYUB) Tube that connects the middle ear to the nasopharynx. Also called *auditory tube.*

euthyroid (you-**THIGH**-royd) Normal thyroid function.

eversion (ee-**VER**-shun) Turning outward.

evert (ee-**VERT**) To turn outward.

evolve (ee-**VOLV**) To develop gradually.

exacerbation (ek-zas-er-**BAY**-shun) Period when there is an increase in the severity of a disease.

exanthem (ek-**ZAN**-them) Skin eruption or rash occurring as the outward sign of a viral or bacterial disease.

excision (ek-**SIZH**-un) Surgical removal of part or all of a structure.

excoriate (eks-**KOR**-ee-ate) To scratch.

excoriation (eks-**KOR**-ee-**AY**-shun) Scratch mark.

excrete (eks-**KREET**) To pass waste products of metabolism out of the body.

excretion (eks-**KREE**-shun) Removal of waste products of metabolism out of the body.

exhale (**EKS**-hail) Breathe out.

exocrine (**EK**-soh-krin) A gland that secretes substances outwardly through excretory ducts.

exophthalmos (ek-sof-**THAL**-mos) Protrusion of the eyeball.

exotropia (ek-soh-**TROH**-pee-ah) Turning the eye outward away from the nose.

expectorate (ek-**SPEK**-toh-rate) Cough up and spit out mucus from the respiratory tract.

expiration (**EKS**-pih-**RAY**-shun) Breathe out.

extension (eks-**TEN**-shun) Straighten a joint to increase its angle.

extracorporeal (**EKS**-tra-kor-**POH**-ree-al) Outside the body.

extravasate (eks-**TRAV**-ah-sate) To ooze out from a vessel into the tissues.

extrinsic (eks-**TRIN**-sik) Any muscle located entirely on the outside of the structure under consideration; for example, the eye.

F

facies (**FASH**-eez) Facial features and expressions.

fallopian tubes (fah-**LOW**-pee-an) Uterine tubes connected to the fundus of the uterus.

Fallot (fah-**LOW**) First described the tetralogy of congenital heart defects.

fascia (**FASH**-ee-ah) Sheet of fibrous connective tissue.

fasciectomy (fash-ee-**EK**-toe-me) Surgical removal of fascia.

fasciitis (fash-ee-**EYE**-tis) Inflammation of fascia.

fasciotomy (fash-ee-**OT**-oh-me) An incision through a band of fascia, usually to relieve pressure on underlying structures.

febrile (**FEB**-ril or **FEB**-rile) Pertaining to or suffering from fever.

fecal (**FEE**-kal) Pertaining to feces.

feces (**FEE**-sees) Undigested, waste material discharged from the bowel.

femoral (**FEM**-oh-ral) Pertaining to the femur.

femur (**FEE**-mur) The thigh bone.

fertilization (**FER**-til-eye-**ZAY**-shun) Union of a male sperm and a female egg.

fertilize (**FER**-til-ize) Penetration of the egg by sperm.

fetal (**FEE**-tal) Pertaining to the fetus.

fetalis (fee-**TAH**-lis) Erythroblastosis fetalis is a hemolytic disease of the newborn.

fetus (**FEE**-tus) Human organism from the end of the eighth week after conception to birth.

fever (**FEE**-ver) Increased body temperature that is a physiologic response to disease.

fibrillation (fi-brih-**LAY**-shun) Uncontrolled quivering or twitching of the heart muscle.

fibrin (**FIE**-brin) Stringy protein fiber that is a component of a blood clot.

fibrinogen (fie-**BRIN**-oh-jen) Precursor of fibrin in blood-clotting process.

fibroadenoma (**FIE**-broh-ad-en-**OH**-muh) Benign tumor containing much fibrous tissue.

fibroblast (**FIE**-broh-blast) Cell that forms collagen fibers.

fibrocystic disease (fie-broh-**SIS**-tik **DIZ**-eez) Benign breast disease with multiple tiny lumps and cysts.

fibroid (**FIE**-broyd) Uterine tumor resembling fibrous tissue.

fibromyalgia (fie-broh-my-**AL**-jee-ah) Pain in the muscle fibers.

fibromyoma (**FIE**-broh-my-**OH**-mah) Benign neoplasm derived from smooth muscle and containing fibrous tissue.

fibrosis (fie-**BROH**-sis) Repair of dead tissue cells by formation of fibrous tissue.

fibrotic (fie-**BROT**-ik) Pertaining to or affected by fibrosis.

fibula (**FIB**-you-lah) The smaller of the two bones of the lower leg.

fibular (**FIB**-you-lar) Pertaining to the fibula.

filter (**FIL**-ter) Porous substance used to separate liquids or gases from particulate matter; *or* to subject a substance to the action of a filter.

filtrate (**FIL**-trate) That which has passed through a filter.

filtration (fil-**TRAY**-shun) Process of passing liquid through a filter.

fimbria (**FIM**-bree-ah) A fringelike structure on the surface of a cell or microorganism. Plural *fimbriae*.

fissure (**FISH**-ur) Deep furrow or cleft. Plural *fissures*.

fistula (**FIS**-tyu-lah) Abnormal passage. Plural *fistulae* or *fistulas*.

flank (**FLANK**) Side of the body between pelvis and ribs.

flatulence (**FLAT**-you-lence) Excessive amount of gas in the stomach and intestines.

flatus (**FLAY**-tus) Gas or air expelled through the anus.

flex (**FLEKS**) To bend a joint so that the two parts come together.

flexion (**FLEK**-shun) Bend a joint to decrease its angle.

flexor (**FLEK**-sor) Muscle or tendon that flexes a joint.

flexure (**FLEK**-shur) A bend in a structure.

flora (**FLO**-rah) Microorganisms covering the exterior and interior surfaces of a healthy animal.

fluorescein (flor-**ESS**-ee-in) Dye that produces a vivid green color under a blue light to diagnose corneal abrasions and foreign bodies.

follicle (**FOLL**-ih-kull) Spherical mass of cells containing a cavity; *or* a small cul-de-sac, such as a hair follicle.

follicular (fo-**LIK**-you-lar) Pertaining to a follicle.

foramen (fo-**RAY**-men) An opening through a structure. Plural *foramina*.

forceps extraction (**FOR**-seps ek-**STRAK**-shun) Assisted delivery of the baby by an instrument that grasps the head of the baby.

foreskin (**FOR**-skin) Skin that covers the glans penis.

fornix (**FOR**-niks) Arch-shaped, blind-ended part of the vagina behind and around the cervix. Plural *fornices*.

fovea centralis (**FOH**-vee-ah sen-**TRAH**-lis) Small pit in the center of the macula that has the highest visual acuity.

frenulum (**FREN**-you-lum) Fold of mucous membrane between the glans and the prepuce.

frontal (**FRON**-tal) Vertical plane dividing the body into anterior and posterior portions.

function (**FUNK**-shun) The ability of an organ or tissue to perform its special work.

fundoscopic (fun-doh-**SKOP**-ik) Pertaining to fundoscopy.

fundoscopy (fun-**DOS**-koh-pee) Examination of the fundus (retina) of the eye.

fundus (**FUN**-dus) Part farthest from the opening of a hollow organ.

fungicide (**FUN**-jee-side) Agent to destroy fungi.

fungus (**FUN**-gus) General term used to describe yeasts and molds. Plural *fungi*.

G

galactorrhea (gah-**LAK**-toe-**REE**-ah) Abnormal flow of milk from the breasts.

gallbladder (**GAWL**-blad-er) Receptacle on the inferior surface of the liver for storing bile.

gallstone (**GAWL**-stone) Hard mass of cholesterol, calcium, and bilirubin that can be formed in the gallbladder and bile duct.

ganglion (**GANG**-lee-on) Collection of nerve cells outside the brain and spinal cord; *or* a fluid-filled cyst. Plural *ganglia*.

gastric (**GAS**-trik) Pertaining to the stomach.

gastrin (**GAS**-trin) Hormone secreted in the stomach that stimulates secretion of HCl and increases gastric motility.

gastritis (gas-**TRY**-tis) Inflammation of the lining of the stomach.

gastrocnemius (gas-trok-**NEE**-me-us) Major muscle in back of the lower leg (the calf).

gastroenteritis (**GAS**-troh-en-ter-**I**-tis) Inflammation of the stomach and intestines.

gastroenterologist (GAS-troh-en-ter-OL-oh-jist) Medical specialist in gastroenterology.

gastroenterology (GAS-troh-en-ter-OL-oh-gee) Medical specialty of the stomach and intestines.

gastroesophageal (GAS-troh-ee-sof-ah-JEE-al) Pertaining to the stomach and esophagus.

gastrointestinal (GI) (GAS-troh-in-TESS-tin-al) Pertaining to the stomach and intestines.

gastroscope (GAS-troh-skope) Endoscope for examining the inside of the stomach.

gastroscopy (gas-TROS-koh-pee) Endoscopic examination of the stomach.

gavage (guh-VAHZH) To feed by a stomach tube.

gene (JEEN) Functional segment of DNA molecule.

geneticist (jeh-NET-ih-sist) A specialist in genetics.

genetics (jeh-NET-iks) Science of the inheritance of characteristics.

genital (JEN-ih-tal) Relating to reproduction or to the male or female sex organs.

genitalia (JEN-ih-TAY-lee-ah) External and internal organs of reproduction.

geriatrician (jer-ee-ah-TRISH-an) Medical specialist in in the process and problems of aging.

geriatrics (jer-ee-AT-riks) Medical specialty that deals with the problems of aging.

gerontologist (jer-on-TOL-oh-jist) Medical specialist in the process and general problems of aging.

gerontology (jer-on-TOL-oh-jee) Study of the process and problems of aging.

gestation (jes-TAY-shun) From conception to birth.

gestational (jes-TAY-shun-al) Pertaining to gestation.

gigantism (JI-gan-tizm) Abnormal height and size of the entire body.

gingiva (JIN-jih-vah) Tissue surrounding the teeth and covering the jaw.

gingival (JIN-jih-val) Pertaining to the gingiva.

gingivectomy (jin-jih-VEC-toe-me) Surgical removal of diseased gum tissue.

gingivitis (jin-jih-VI-tis) Inflammation of the gums.

glans (GLANZ) Head of the penis or clitoris.

glaucoma (glau-KOH-mah) Increased intraocular pressure.

glia (GLEE-ah) Connective tissue that holds a structure together.

glial (GLEE-al) Pertaining to glia or neuroglia.

glioma (gli-OH-mah) Tumor of a glial cell.

glomerulonephritis (glo-MER-you-low-nef-RYE-tis) Infection of the glomeruli of the kidney.

glomerulus (glo-MER-you-lus) Plexus of capillaries; part of a nephron. Plural *glomeruli.*

glossopharyngeal (GLOSS-oh-fah-RIN-jee-al) Ninth (IX) cranial nerve, supplying the tongue and pharynx.

glottis (GLOT-is) Vocal apparatus of the larynx.

glucagon (GLU-kah-gon) Pancreatic hormone that supports blood glucose levels.

glucocorticoid (glu-co-KOR-tih-koyd) Hormone of the adrenal cortex that helps regulate glucose metabolism.

gluconeogenesis (GLU-koh-nee-oh-JEN-eh-sis) Formation of glucose from noncarbohydrate sources.

glucose (GLU-kose) The final product of carbohydrate digestion and the main sugar in the blood.

gluteal (GLU-tee-al) Pertaining to the buttocks.

gluten (GLU-ten) Insoluble protein found in wheat, barley, and oats.

gluteus (GLU-tee-us) Refers to one of three muscles in the buttocks.

glycogen (GLYE-koh-gen) The body's principal carbohydrate reserve, stored in the liver and skeletal muscle.

glycogenolysis (GLYE koh-jen-oh-LYE-sis) Conversion of glycogen to glucose.

glycosuria (GLYE-koh-SYU-ree-ah) Presence of glucose in urine.

glycosylated hemoglobin (Hb A1c) (GLYE-koh-sih-lay-ted HE-moh-GLOW-bin) Hemoglobin A fraction linked to glucose; used as an index of glucose control.

goiter (GOY-ter) Enlargement of the thyroid gland.

gomphosis (gom-FOE-sis) Joint formed by a peg and socket. Plural *gomphoses.*

gonad (GO-nad) Testis or ovary. Plural *gonads.*

gonadotropin (GO-nad-oh-TROH-pin) Any hormone that stimulates gonad function.

gonorrhea (gon-oh-REE-ah) Specific contagious sexually transmitted infection.

grade (GRAYD) In cancer pathology, a classification of the rate of growth of cancer cells.

graft (GRAFT) Transplantation of living tissue.

grand mal (GRAHN MAL) Old name for generalized tonic-clonic seizure.

granulation (gran-you-LAY-shun) New fibrous tissue formed during wound healing.

granulocyte (GRAN-you-loh-site) A white blood cell that contains multiple small granules in its cytoplasm.

granulosa cell (gran-you-LOW-sah SELL) Cell lining the ovarian follicle.

Graves disease (GRAVZ diz-EEZ) Hyperthyroidism with toxic goiter.

gravid (GRAV-id) Pregnant.

gravida (GRAV-ih-dah) A pregnant woman.

gray matter (GRAY MATT-er) Regions of the brain and spinal cord occupied by cell bodies and dendrites.

greenstick fracture (GREEN-stik FRAK-chur) A fracture in which one side of the bone is partially broken and the other side is bent. Occurs mostly in children.

groin (GROYN) Crease where the thigh joins the abdomen.

Guillain-Barré syndrome (GEE-yan bah-RAY SIN-drom) Disorder in which the body makes antibodies against myelin, disrupting nerve conduction.

gynecologic (GUY-nih-koh-LOJ-ik) Pertaining to gynecology.

gynecologist (guy-nih-KOL-oh-jist) Specialist in gynecology.

gynecology (guy-nih-KOL-oh-jee) Medical specialty of diseases of the female.

gynecomastia (GUY-nih-koh-MAS-tee-ah) Enlargement of the breast.

gyrus (JI-rus) Rounded elevation on the surface of the cerebral hemispheres. Plural *gyri.*

H

hairline fracture (**HAIR**-line **FRAK**-chur) A fracture without separation of the fragments.

halitosis (hal-ih-**TOE**-sis) Bad odor of the breath.

hallucination (hah-loo-sih-**NAY**-shun) Perception of an object or event when there is no such thing present.

hallux valgus (**HAL**-uks **VAL**-gus) Deviation of the big toe toward the lateral side of the foot.

Hashimoto disease (hah-shee-**MOH**-toe diz-**EEZ**) Autoimmune disease of the thyroid gland. Also called *Hashimoto thyroiditis*.

Haversian canals (hah-**VER**-shan ka-**NALS**) Vascular canals in bone. Also called *central canals*.

Heberden node (**HEH**-ber-den NOHD) Bony lump on the terminal phalanx of the fingers in osteoarthritis.

hemangioma (he-**MAN**-jee-oh-mah) Abnormal mass of proliferating blood vessels.

hematemesis (he-mah-**TEM**-eh-sis) Vomiting of red blood.

hematocrit (Hct) (**HE**-mat-oh-krit) Percentage of red blood cells in the blood.

hematologist (he-mah-**TOL**-oh-jist) Specialist in hematology.

hematology (he-mah-**TOL**-oh-jee) Medical specialty of disorders of the blood.

hematoma (he-mah-**TOE**-mah) Collection of blood that has escaped from the blood vessels into surrounding tissues. Also called *bruise*.

hematuria (he-mah-**TYU**-ree-ah) Blood in the urine.

heme (HEEM) The iron-based component of hemoglobin that carries oxygen.

hemiparesis (**HEM**-ee-pah-**REE**-sis) Weakness of one side of the body.

hemiplegia (hem-ee-**PLEE**-jee-ah) Paralysis of one side of the body.

hemiplegic (hem-ee-**PLEE**-jik) Pertaining to or suffering from hemiplegia.

Hemoccult test (**HEEM**-o-kult TEST) Trade name for a fecal occult blood test.

hemodialysis (**HE**-moh-die-**AL**-ih-sis) An artificial method of filtration to remove excess waste materials and water directly from the blood.

hemodynamics (**HE**-moh-die-**NAM**-iks) The science of the flow of blood through the circulation.

hemoglobin (**HE**-moh-**GLOW**-bin) Red-pigmented protein that is the main component of red blood cells.

hemoglobinopathy (**HE**-moh-**GLOW**-bih-**NOP**-ah-thee) Disease caused by the presence of an abnormal hemoglobin in the red blood cells.

hemolysis (he-**MOL**-ih-sis) Destruction of red blood cells so that hemoglobin is liberated.

hemolytic (he-moh-**LIT**-ik) Pertaining to the process of destruction of red blood cells.

hemophilia (he-moh-**FILL**-ee-ah) An inherited disease from a deficiency of clotting factor VIII.

hemoptysis (he-**MOP**-tih-sis) Bloody sputum.

hemorrhage (**HEM**-oh-raj) To bleed profusely.

hemorrhoid (**HEM**-oh-royd) Dilated rectal vein producing painful anal swelling. Plural *hemorrhoids*.

hemorrhoidectomy (**HEM**-oh-royd-**ECK**-toh-me) Surgical removal of hemorrhoids.

hemostasis (he-moh-**STAY**-sis) Control of or stopping bleeding.

hemothorax (he-moh-**THOR**-ax) Blood in the pleural cavity.

heparin (**HEP**-ah-rin) An anticoagulant secreted particularly by liver cells.

hepatic (hep-**AT**-ik) Pertaining to the liver.

hepatitis (hep-ah-**TIE**-tis) Inflammation of the liver.

hernia (**HER**-nee-ah) Protrusion of a structure through the tissue that normally contains it.

herniate (**HER**-nee-ate) To protrude.

herniation (**HER**-nee-ay-shun) Protrusion of an anatomical structure from its normal location.

herniorrhaphy (**HER**-nee-**OR**-ah-fee) Repair of a hernia.

herpes simplex virus (HSV) (**HER**-peez **SIM**-pleks **VIE**-rus) Manifests with painful, watery blisters on the skin and mucous membranes.

herpes zoster (**HER**-pees **ZOS**-ter) Painful eruption of vesicles that follows a nerve root on one side of the body. Also called *shingles*.

heterograft (**HET**-er-oh-graft) A graft using tissue taken from another species. Also called *xenograft*.

hiatal (high-**AY**-tal) Pertaining to a hernia.

hiatus (high-**AY**-tus) An opening through a structure.

hilum (**HIGH**-lum) The site where the nerves and blood vessels enter and leave an organ. Plural *hila*.

histamine (**HISS**-tah-mean) Compound liberated in tissues as a result of injury or an allergic response.

histologist (his-**TOL**-oh-jist) Specialist in histology.

histology (his-**TOL**-oh-jee) Study of the structure and function of cells, tissues, and organs.

Hodgkin lymphoma (**HOJ**-kin lim-**FOH**-mah) Marked by chronic enlargement of lymph nodes spreading to other nodes in an orderly way.

holistic (ho-**LIS**-tik) Pertaining to the care of the whole person in physical, mental, emotional, and spiritual dimensions.

homeostasis (hoh-mee-oh-**STAY**-sis) Maintaining the stability of a system or the body's internal environment.

homograft (**HOH**-moh-graft) Skin graft from another person or a cadaver.

hordeolum (hor-**DEE**-oh-lum) Abscess in an eyelash follicle. Also called *stye*.

hormonal (hor-**MOHN**-al) Pertaining to a hormone.

hormone (**HOR**-mohn) Chemical formed in one tissue or organ and carried by the blood to stimulate or inhibit a function of another tissue or organ.

Horner syndrome (**HOR**-ner **SIN**-drome) Disorder of the sympathetic nerves to the face and eye.

hospice (**HOS**-pis) Provides care to the dying and their families.

human immunodeficiency virus (HIV) (**HYU**-man **IM**-you-noh-dee-**FISH**-en-see **VIE**-rus) Etiologic agent of acquired immunodeficiency syndrome (AIDS).

human papilloma virus (HPV) (**HYU**-man pap-ih-**LOW**-mah **VIE**-rus) Causes warts on the skin and genitalia and can increase the risk for cervical cancer.

humerus (**HYU**-mer-us) Single bone of the upper arm.

humoral immunity (**HYU**-mor-al ihm-**YOU**-nih-tee) Defense mechanism arising from antibodies in the blood.

Huntington disease (**HUN**-ting-ton diz-**EEZ**) Progressive inherited, degenerative, incurable neurologic disease. Also called *Huntington chorea*.

hyaline (**HIGH**-ah-line) Cartilage that looks like frosted glass and contains fine collagen fibers.

hyaline membrane disease (**HIGH**-ah-line **MEM**-brain **DIZ**-eez) Respiratory distress syndrome of the newborn.

hydrocele (**HIGH**-droh-seal) Collection of fluid in the space of the tunica vaginalis.

hydrocephalus (high-droh-**SEF**-ah-lus) Excess CSF in the cerebral ventricles; may cause enlarged head.

hydrochloric acid (HCl) (high-droh-**KLOR**-ic **ASS**-id) The acid of gastric juice.

hydrocortisone (high-droh-**KOR**-tih-sohn) Potent glucocorticoid with anti-inflammatory properties. Also called *cortisol.*

hydronephrosis (**HIGH**-droh-neh-**FROH**-sis) Dilation of the pelvis and calyces of a kidney.

hydronephrotic (**HIGH**-droh-neh-**FROT**-ik) Pertaining to or suffering from hydronephrosis.

hymen (**HIGH**-men) Thin membrane partly occluding the vaginal orifice.

hyperactivity (**HIGH**-per-ac-**TIV**-ih-tee) Excessive restlessness and movement.

hypercalcemia (**HIGH**-per-cal-**SEE**-me-ah) Excessive level of calcium in the blood.

hypercapnia (**HIGH**-per-**KAP**-nee-ah) Abnormal increase of carbon dioxide in the arterial bloodstream.

hyperemesis (high-per-**EM**-eh-sis) Excessive vomiting.

hyperflexion (high-per-**FLEK**-shun) Flexion of a limb or part beyond the normal limits.

hyperglycemia (**HIGH**-per-gly-**SEE**-me-ah) High level of glucose (sugar) in blood.

hyperglycemic (**HIGH**-per-gly-**SEE**-mik) Pertaining to or having hyperglycemia.

hyperimmune globulin (**HIGH**-per-im-**YUNE GLOB**-youlin) Immunoglobulin prepared from serum of people with a high antibody titer to a specific antigen.

hyperkalemia (**HIGH**-per-kah-**LEE**-me-ah) High level of potassium in the blood.

hypernatremia (**HIGH**-per-nah-**TREE**-me-ah) High level of sodium in the blood.

hyperopia (high-per-**OH**-pee-ah) Able to see distant objects but unable to see close objects.

hyperosmolar (**HIGH**-per-os-**MOH**-lar) Marked hyperglycemia without ketoacidosis.

hyperparathyroidism (**HIGH**-per-para-**THIGH**-royd-izm) Excessive production of parathyroid hormone.

hyperplasia (**HIGH**-per-**PLAY**-zee-ah) Increase in the number of cells in a tissue or organ.

hyperpnea (high-perp-**NEE**-ah) Deeper and more rapid breathing than normal.

hyperpyrexia (**HIGH**-per-pie-**REK**-see-ah) Extremely high body temperature or fever.

hypersecretion (**HIGH**-per-seh-**KREE**-shun) Excessive secretion (of mucus or enzymes or waste products).

hypersensitivity (**HIGH**-per-sen-sih-**TIV**-ih-tee) Exaggerated abnormal reaction to an allergen.

hypersplenism (high-per-**SPLEN**-izm) Condition in which the spleen removes blood components at an excessive rate.

hypertension (**HIGH**-per-**TEN**-shun) Persistent high arterial blood pressure.

hypertensive (**HIGH**-per-**TEN**-siv) Pertaining to or suffering from high blood pressure.

hyperthyroidism (high-per-**THIGH**-royd-izm) Excessive production of thyroid hormones.

hypertrophy (high-**PER**-troh-fee) Increase in size, but not in number, of an individual tissue element.

hypochondriac (high-poh-**KON**-dree-ack) A person who exaggerates the significance of symptoms.

hypochromic (high-poh-**CROW**-mik) Pale in color, as in RBCs when hemoglobin is deficient.

hypodermic (high-poh-**DER**-mik) Pertaining to the hypodermis.

hypodermis (high-poh-**DER**-miss) Tissue layer of skin below the dermis.

hypogastric (high-poh-**GAS**-trik) Abdominal region below the stomach.

hypoglossal (high-poh-**GLOSS**-al) Twelfth (XII) cranial nerve, supplying muscles of the tongue.

hypoglycemia (**HIGH**-poh-gly-**SEE**-me-ah) Low level of glucose (sugar) in the blood.

hypoglycemic (**HIGH**-poh-gly-**SEE**-mik) Pertaining to or suffering from low blood sugar.

hypogonadism (**HIGH**-poh-**GOH**-nad-izm) Deficient gonad production of sperm or eggs or hormones.

hypokalemia (**HIGH**-poh-kah-**LEE**-me-ah) Low level of potassium in the blood.

hyponatremia (**HIGH**-poh-nah-**TREE**-me-ah) Low level of sodium in the blood.

hypoparathyroidism (**HIGH**-poh-par-ah-**THIGH**-royd-izm) Deficient production of parathyroid hormone.

hypophysis (high-**POF**-ih-sis) Another name for *pituitary gland.*

hypopituitarism (**HIGH**-poh-pih-**TYU**-ih-tah-rizm) Condition of one or more deficient pituitary hormones.

hypospadias (high-poh-**SPAY**-dee-as) Urethral opening more proximal than normal on the ventral surface of the penis.

hypotension (**HIGH**-poh-**TEN**-shun) Persistent low arterial blood pressure.

hypotensive (**HIGH**-poh-**TEN**-siv) Pertaining to or suffering from low blood pressure.

hypothalamic (high-poh-thah-**LAM**-ik) Pertaining to the hypothalamus.

hypothalamus (high-poh-**THAL**-ah-muss) An area of gray matter lying below the thalamus.

hypothenar eminence (high-poh-**THAY**-nar **EM**-in-nens) The fleshy mass at the base of the little finger.

hypothermia (high-poh-**THER**-me-ah) Very low core body temperature.

hypothyroidism (high-poh-**THIGH**-royd-izm) Deficient production of thyroid hormones.

hypovolemic (**HIGH**-poh-vo-**LEE**-mick) Decreased blood volume in the body.

hypoxia (high-**POCK**-see-ah) Below-normal levels of oxygen in tissues, gases, or blood.

hypoxic (high-**POCK**-sik) Deficient in oxygen.

hysterectomy (his-ter-**EK**-toe-me) Surgical removal of the uterus.

I

ictal (**ICK**-tal) Pertaining to, or a condition caused by, a stroke or epilepsy.

idiopathic (**ID**-ih-oh-**PATH**-ik) Pertaining to a disease of unknown etiology.

ileocecal (**ILL**-ee-oh-**SEE**-cal) Pertaining to the junction of the ileum and cecum.

ileocecal sphincter (**ILL**-ee-oh-**SEE**-cal **SFINK**-ter) A band of muscle that encircles the junction of the ileum and cecum.

ileoscopy (ill-ee-**OS**-koh-pee) Endoscopic examination of the ileum.

ileostomy (ill-ee-**OS**-toe-me) Artificial opening from the ileum to the outside of the body.

ileum (**ILL**-ee-um) Third portion of the small intestine.

iliac (**ILL**-ee-ack) A structure related to the ilium (pelvic bone).

ilium (**ILL**-ee-um) Large wing-shaped bone at the upper and posterior part of the pelvis. Plural *ilia*.

immune (im-**YUNE**) Protected from an infectious disease.

immune serum (im-**YUNE SEER**-um) Serum taken from another human or animal that has antibodies to a disease. Also called *antiserum*.

immunity (im-**YOU**-nih-tee) State of being protected.

immunization (**IM**-you-nih-**ZAY**-shun) Administration of an agent to provide immunity.

immunize (**IM**-you-nize) To make resistant to an infectious disease.

immunodeficiency (**IM**-you-noh-dee-**FISH**-en-see) Failure of the immune system.

immunoglobulin (**IM**-you-noh-**GLOB**-you-lin) Specific protein evoked by an antigen. All antibodies are immunoglobulins.

immunologist (im-you-**NOL**-oh-jist) Medical specialist in immunology.

immunology (im-you-**NOL**-oh-jee) The science and practice of immunity and allergy.

immunosuppression (**IM**-you-noh-suh-**PRESH**-un) Failure of the immune system caused by an outside agent.

impacted (im-**PAK**-ted) Immovably wedged, as with earwax blocking the external canal.

impacted fracture (im-**PAK**-ted **FRAK**-chur) A fracture in which one bone fragment is driven into the other.

impairment (im-**PAIR**-ment) The state of being worse, weaker, or damaged.

impetigo (im-peh-**TIE**-go) Infection of the skin producing thick, yellow crusts.

implant (im-**PLANT**) To insert material into tissues; *or* the material inserted into tissues.

implantable (im-**PLAN**-tah-bul) A device that can be inserted into tissues.

implantation (im-plan-**TAY**-shun) Attachment of a fertilized egg to the endometrium.

impotence (**IM**-poh-tence) Inability to achieve an erection.

impulsive (im-**PUL**-siv) Inability to resist performing inappropriate actions.

in situ (IN **SIGH**-tyu) In the correct place.

in utero (in **YOU**-ter-oh) Within the womb; not yet born.

in vitro fertilization (IVF) (IN **VEE**-troh **FER**-til-ih-**ZAY**-shun) Process of combining sperm and egg in a laboratory dish and placing the resulting embryos inside the uterus.

inattention (**IN**-ah-**TEN**-shun) Lack of concentration and direction.

incision (in-**SIZH**-un) A cut or surgical wound.

incompetence (in-**KOM**-peh-tense) Failure of valves to close completely.

incomplete fracture (in-kom-**PLEET FRAK**-chur) A fracture that does not extend across the bone, as in a hairline fracture.

incontinence (in-**KON**-tin-ence) Inability to prevent discharge of urine or feces.

incontinent (in-**KON**-tin-ent) Denoting incontinence.

incubation (in-kyu-**BAY**-shun) Process to develp an infection.

incus (**IN**-cuss) Middle one of the three ossicles in the middle ear; shaped like an anvil.

independence (in-dee-**PEN**-dense) The state of being able to think and act for oneself.

independent (in-dee-**PEN**-dent) Pertaining to the ability to think and act for oneself.

indigestion (in-dee-**JESS**-chun) Symptoms resulting from difficulty in digesting food.

infancy (**IN**-fan-see) The first year of life.

infant (**IN**-fant) Child in the first year of life.

infarct (in-**FARKT**) Area of cell death resulting from blockage of its blood supply.

infarction (in-**FARK**-shun) Sudden blockage of an artery.

infect (in-**FEKT**) To invade an organism by a microorganism.

infection (in-**FEK**-shun) Invasion of the body by disease-producing microorganisms.

infectious (in-**FEK**-shus) Capable of being transmitted to a person; *or* a disease caused by the action of a microorganism.

inferior (in-**FEE**-ree-or) Situated below.

infertility (in-fer-**TIL**-ih-tee) Failure to conceive.

infestation (in-fes-**TAY**-shun) Act of being invaded on the skin by a troublesome other species, such as a parasite.

inflammation (in-flah-**MAY**-shun) A complex of cell and chemical reactions in response to an injury or a chemical or biologic agent.

inflammatory (in-**FLAM**-ah-tor-ee) Causing or affected by inflammation.

influenza (in-flew-**EN**-zah) An acute, viral infection of upper and lower respiratory tracts.

infusion (in-**FYU**-zhun) Introduction intravenously of a substance other than blood.

ingestion (in-**JEST**-shun) Intake of food, either by mouth or through a nasogastric tube.

inguinal (**ING**-gwin-ahl) Pertaining to the groin.

inhale (**IN**-hail) Breathe in.

insanity (in-**SAN**-ih-tee) Nonmedical term for a person unable to be responsible for his or her actions.

insecticide (in-**SEK**-tih-side) Agent to destroy insects.

inseminate (in-**SEM**-ih-nate) To introduce semen into the vagina.

insemination (in-sem-ih-**NAY**-shun) The introduction of semen into the vagina.

insertion (in-**SIR**-shun) The insertion of a muscle is the attachment of a muscle to a more movable part of the skeleton, as distinct from the origin.

inspiration (in-spih-**RAY**-shun) Breathe in.

instability (in-stah-**BIL**-ih-tee) Abnormal tendency of a joint to partially or fully dislocate.

insufficiency (in-suh-**FISH**-en-see) Lack of completeness of function; for example, for a heart valve to fail to close properly.

insulin (**IN**-syu-lin) A hormone produced by the islet cells of the pancreas.

integument (in-**TEG**-you-ment) Organ system that covers the body, the skin being the main organ within the system.

integumentary (in-**TEG**-you-**MENT**-ah-ree) Pertaining to the covering of the body.

interatrial (**IN**-ter-**AY**-tree-al) Between the atria of the heart.

intercostal (**IN**-ter-**KOS**-tal) The space between two ribs.

intermittent (**IN**-ter-**MIT**-ent) Alternately ceasing and beginning again.

interosseous (in-ter-**OSS**-ee-us) A structure between bones; for example, muscles.

interphalangeal (**IN**-ter-fay-**LAN**-jee-al) Finger or toe joint between two phalanges.

interstitial (in-ter-**STISH**-al) Pertaining to spaces between cells in a tissue or organ.

interventricular (**IN**-ter-ven-**TRIK**-you-lar) Between the ventricles of the heart.

intervertebral (**IN**-ter-**VER**-teh-bral) The space between two vertebrae.

intestinal (in-**TESS**-tin-al) Pertaining to the intestine.

intestine (in-**TESS**-tin) The digestive tube from stomach to anus.

intolerance (in-**TOL**-er-ance) Inability of the small intestine to digest and dispose of a particular dietary substance.

intracellular (in-trah-**SELL**-you-lar) Within the cell.

intracranial (in-trah-**KRAY**-nee-al) Within the cranium (skull).

intradermal (in-trah-**DER**-mal) Within the epidermis.

intramuscular (in-trah-**MUSS**-kew-lar) Within the muscle.

intraocular (in-trah-**OCK**-you-lar) Pertaining to the inside of the eye.

intrathecal (**IN**-trah-**THEE**-kal) Within the subarachnoid or subdural space.

intrauterine (**IN**-trah-**YOU**-ter-ine) Inside the uterine cavity.

intravenous (**IN**-trah-**VEE**-nus) Through a vein.

intrinsic (in-**TRIN**-sik) Any muscle located entirely within (inside) the structure under consideration; for example, muscles inside the vocal cords or the eye.

intrinsic factor (in-**TRIN**-sik **FAK**-tor) Makes the absorption of vitamin B_{12} happen.

intubation (**IN**-tyu-**BAY**-shun) Insertion of a tube into the trachea.

intussusception (**IN**-tuss-sus-**SEP**-shun) The slipping of one part of bowel inside another to cause obstruction.

inversion (in-**VER**-shun) Turning inward.

invert (in-**VERT**) Turn inward.

involuntary (in-**VOL**-un-tah-ree) Not under control of the will.

involute (in-voh-**LUTE**) Regressive changes in a tissue.

involution (in-voh-**LOO**-shun) Decrease in size.

iodine (**EYE**-oh-dine or **EYE**-oh-deen) Chemical element, the lack of which causes thyroid disease.

iris (**EYE**-ris) Colored portion of the eye with the pupil in its center.

irrigation (ih-rih-**GAY**-shun) Use of water to remove wax out of the external ear canal.

ischemia (is-**KEY**-me-ah) Lack of blood supply to tissue.

ischemic (is-**KEY**-mik) Pertaining to or affected by the lack of blood supply to tissue.

ischial (**IS**-key-al) Pertaining to the ischium.

ischium (**IS**-key-um) Lower and posterior part of the hip bone. Plural *ischia*.

Ishihara color system (ish-ee-**HAR**-ah) Test for color vision defects.

islet cells (**EYE**-let SELLS) Hormone-secreting cells of the pancreas.

islets of Langerhans (**EYE**-lets of **LAHNG**-er-hahnz) Areas of pancreatic cells that produce insulin and glucagon.

isotope (**I**-so-tope) Radioactive element used in diagnostic procedures.

J

Jaeger reading cards (**YA**-ger) Type of different sizes for testing near vision.

jaundice (**JAWN**-dis) Yellow staining of tissues with bile pigments, including bilirubin.

jejunal (je-**JEW**-nal) Pertaining to the jejeunum.

jejunum (je-**JEW**-num) Segment of small intestine between the duodenum and the ileum.

K

Kaposi sarcoma (kah-**POH**-see sar-**KOH**-mah) A skin cancer seen in AIDS patients.

keloid (**KEY**-loyd) Raised, irregular, lumpy scar due to excess collagen fiber production during healing of a wound.

keratin (**KER**-ah-tin) Protein found in the skin, nails, and hair.

keratomileusis (ker-ah-**TOE**-mill-oo-sis) Cuts and shapes the cornea.

keratotomy (ker-ah-**TOT**-oh-mee) Incision in the cornea.

kernicterus (ker-**NICK**-ter-us) Bilirubin staining of the basal nuclei of the brain.

ketoacidosis (**KEY**-toe-ass-ih-**DOE**-sis) Excessive production of ketones, making the blood acid.

ketone (**KEY**-tone) Chemical formed in uncontrolled diabetes or in starvation.

ketosis (key-**TOE**-sis) Excess production of ketones.

kidney (**KID**-nee) Organ of excretion.

kyphosis (ki-**FOH**-sis) A normal posterior curve of the thoracic spine that can be exaggerated in disease.

kyphotic (ki-**FOT**-ik) Pertaining to or suffering from kyphosis.

L

labium (**LAY**-bee-um) Fold of the vulva. Plural *labia*.

labor (**LAY**-bore) Process of expulsion of the fetus.

labyrinth (**LAB**-ih-rinth) The inner ear.

labyrinthitis (**LAB**-ih-rin-**THI**-tis) Inflammation of the inner ear.

laceration (lass-eh-**RAY**-shun) A tear of the skin.

lacrimal (**LAK**-rim-al) Pertaining to tears; *or* bone that forms the medial wall of the orbit.

lactase (**LAK**-tase) Enzyme that breaks down lactose (milk sugar) to glucose and galactose.

lactate (**LAK**-tate) To produce milk.

lactation (lak-**TAY**-shun) Production of milk.

lacteal (**LAK**-tee-al) A lymphatic vessel carrying chyle away from the intestine.

lactiferous (lak-**TIF**-er-us) Pertaining to or yielding milk.

lactose (**LAK**-toes) The disaccharide found in cow's milk.

lanugo (la-**NYU**-go) Fine, soft hair on the fetal body.

laparoscope (**LAP**-ah-roh-skope) Instrument (endoscope) used for viewing the abdominal contents.

laparoscopic (**LAP**-ah-roh-**SKOP**-ik) Pertaining to laparoscopy.

laparoscopy (lap-ah-**ROS**-koh-pee) Examination of the contents of the abdomen using an endoscope.

laryngeal (lah-**RIN**-jee-al) Pertaining to the larynx.

laryngitis (lah-rin-**JEYE**-tis) Inflammation of the larynx.

laryngopharynx (lah-**RIN**-go-**FAH**-rinks) Region of the pharynx below the epiglottis that includes the larynx.

laryngoscope (lah-**RING**-oh-skope) Hollow tube with a light and camera used to visualize or operate on the larynx.

laryngotracheobronchitis (lah-**RING**-oh-**TRAY**-kee-oh-brong-**KIE**-tis) Inflammation of the larynx, trachea, and bronchi. Also called *croup.*

larynx (**LAH**-rinks) Organ of voice production.

laser surgery (**LAY**-zer **SUR**-jer-ee) Use of a concentrated, intense narrow beam of electromagnetic radiation for surgery.

lateral (**LAT**-er-al) Situated at the side of a structure.

latissimus dorsi (lah-**TISS**-ih-muss **DOOR**-sigh) The widest (broadest) muscle in the back.

leiomyoma (**LIE**-oh-my-**OH**-mah) Benign tumor derived from smooth muscle.

lens (LENZ) Transparent refractive structure behind the iris.

lentigo (len-**TIE**-go) Age spot; small, flat, brown-black spot in the skin of older people. Plural *lentigines.*

leptin (**LEP**-tin) Hormone secreted by adipose tissue.

lesion (**LEE**-zhun) Pathologic change or injury in a tissue.

leukemia (loo-**KEE**-mee-ah) Disease when the blood is taken over by white blood cells and their precursors.

leukemic (loo-**KEE**-mik) Pertaining to or affected by leukemia.

leukocyte (**LOO**-koh-site) Another term for a white blood cell. Alternative spelling *leucocyte.*

leukocytosis (**LOO**-koh-sigh-**TOE**-sis) An excessive number of white blood cells.

leukopenia (loo-koh-**PEE**-nee-ah) A deficient number of white blood cells.

libido (lih-**BEE**-doh) Sexual desire.

life expectancy (LIFE eck-**SPEK**-tan-see) Statistical determination of the number of years an individual is expected to live.

life span (LIFE SPAN) The age that a person reaches.

ligament (**LIG**-ah-ment) Band of fibrous tissue connecting two structures.

limbic (**LIM**-bic) Array of nerve fibers surrounding the thalamus.

linear fracture (**LIN**-ee-ar **FRAK**-chur) A fracture running parallel to the length of the bone.

lipase (**LIE**-paze) Enzyme that breaks down fat.

lipectomy (lip-**ECK**-toe-me) Surgical removal of adipose tissue.

lipid (**LIP**-id) General term for all types of fatty compounds; for example, cholesterol, triglycerides, and fatty acids.

lipoprotein (**LIP**-oh-pro-teen) Bonding of molecules of fat and protein.

liposuction (**LIP**-oh-suck-shun) Surgical removal of adipose tissue using suction.

lithotripsy (**LITH**-oh-trip-see) Crushing stones by sound waves.

lithotripter (**LITH**-oh-trip-ter) Machine that generates sound waves.

liver (**LIV**-er) Body's largest organ, located in the right upper quadrant of the abdomen.

lobar (**LOW**-bar) Pertaining to a lobe.

lobe (LOBE) Subdivision of an organ or other part.

lobectomy (low-**BECK**-toe-me) Surgical removal of a lobe.

lochia (**LOW**-kee-uh) Vaginal discharge following childbirth.

longevity (lon-**JEV**-ih-tee) Duration of life beyond the normal expectation.

lordosis (lore-**DOH**-sis) A normal forward curvature of the lumbar spine that can be exaggerated in disease.

lordotic (lore-**DOT**-ik) Pertaining to or suffering from lordosis.

louse (LOWSE) Parasitic insect. Plural *lice.*

lumbar (**LUM**-bar) Region in the back and sides between the ribs and pelvis.

lumen (**LOO**-men) The interior space of a tubelike structure.

lumpectomy (lump-**ECK**-toe-me) Removal of a lesion with preservation of surrounding tissue.

luteal (**LOO**-teh-al) Pertaining to a corpus luteum.

lutein (**LOO**-tee-in) Yellow pigment.

luteum (**LOO**-tee-um) Corpus luteum is the yellow (lutein) body formed after an ovarian follicle ruptures.

lymph (LIMF) A clear fluid collected from body tissues and transported by lymph vessels to the venous circulation.

lymphadenectomy (lim-**FAD**-eh-**NECK**-toe-me) Surgical excision of a lymph node(s).

lymphadenitis (lim-**FAD**-eh-neye-tis) Inflammation of a lymph node(s).

lymphadenopathy (lim-**FAD**-eh-**NOP**-ah-thee) Any disease process affecting a lymph node.

lymphangiogram (lim-**FAN**-jee-oh-gram) Radiographic images of lymph vessels and nodes following injection of contrast material.

lymphatic (lim-**FAT**-ik) Pertaining to lymph or the lymphatic system.

lymphedema (**LIMF**-eh-dee-mah) Tissue swelling due to lymphatic obstruction.

lymphocyte (**LIM**-foh-site) Small white blood cell with a large nucleus.

lymphoid (**LIM**-foyd) Resembling lymphatic tissue.

lymphoma (lim-**FOH**-mah) Any neoplasm of lymphatic tissue.

M

macrocyte (**MACK**-roh-site) Large red blood cell.

macrocytic (mack-roh-**SIT**-ik) Pertaining to a macrocyte.

macrophage (**MACK**-roh-fayj) Large white blood cell that removes bacteria, foreign particles, and dead cells.

macula lutea (**MACK**-you-lah **LOO**-tee-ah) Yellowish spot on the back of the retina; contains the fovea centralis.

macule (**MACK**-yul) Small, flat spot or patch on the skin.

majus (**MAY**-jus) Bigger or greater; for example, labium majus. Plural *majora*.

malabsorption (mal-ab-**SORP**-shun) Inadequate gastrointestinal absorption of nutrients.

malformation (**MAL**-for-**MAY**-shun) Failure of proper or normal development.

malfunction (mal-**FUNK**-shun) Inadequate or abnormal function.

malignancy (mah-**LIG**-nan-see) State of being malignant.

malignant (mah-**LIG**-nant) Tumor that invades surrounding tissues and metastasizes to distant organs.

malleus (**MAL**-ee-us) Outer (lateral) one of the three ossicles in the middle ear; shaped like a hammer.

malnutrition (mal-nyu-**TRISH**-un) Inadequate nutrition from poor diet or inadequate absorption of nutrients.

malunion (mal-**YOU**-nee-un) The two bony ends of a fracture fail to heal together in the correct position.

mammary (**MAM**-ah-ree) Relating to the lactating breast.

mammogram (**MAM**-oh-gram) The record produced by x-ray imaging of the breast.

mammography (mah-**MOG**-rah-fee) The process of x-ray examination of the breast.

mammoplasty (**MAM**-oh-plas-tee) Surgical reshaping of the breast.

mandible (**MAN**-di-bel) Lower jawbone.

mandibular (man-**DIB**-you-lar) Pertaining to the mandible.

mania (**MAY**-nee-ah) Mood disorder with hyperactivity, irritability, and rapid speech.

manic (**MAN**-ik) Pertaining to or suffering from mania.

marrow (**MAH**-roe) Fatty, blood-forming tissue in the cavities of long bones.

mastalgia (mass-**TAL**-jee-uh) Pain in the breast.

mastectomy (mass-**TECK**-toe-me) Surgical excision of the breast.

masticate (**MASS**-tih-kate) To chew.

mastication (mass-tih-**KAY**-shun) The process of chewing.

mastitis (mass-**TIE**-tis) Inflammation of the breast.

mastoid (**MASS**-toyd) Small bony protrusion immediately behind the ear.

maternal (mah-**TER**-nal) Pertaining to or derived from the mother.

matrix (**MAY**-triks) Substance that surrounds and protects cells, is manufactured by the cells, and holds them together.

maturation (mat-you-**RAY**-shun) Process to achieve full development.

mature (mah-**TYUR**) Fully developed.

maxilla (mak-**SILL**-ah) Upper jawbone, containing right and left maxillary sinuses.

maxillary (mak-**SILL**-ah-ree) Pertaining to the maxilla.

maximus (**MAKS**-ih-mus) The gluteus maximus muscle is the largest muscle in the body, covering a large part of each buttock.

meatal (me-**AY**-tal) Pertaining to a meatus.

meatus (me-**AY**-tus) The external opening of a passage.

meconium (meh-**KOH**-nee-um) The first bowel movement of the newborn.

medial (**ME**-dee-al) Nearer to the middle of the body.

mediastinal (**ME**-dee-ass-**TIE**-nal) Pertaining to the mediastinum.

mediastinoscopy (**ME**-dee-ass-tih-**NOS**-koh-pee) Examination of the mediastinum using an endoscope.

mediastinum (**ME**-dee-ass-**TIE**-num) Area between the lungs containing the heart, aorta, venae cavae, esophagus, and trachea.

medius (**ME**-dee-us) The gluteus medius muscle is partly covered by the gluteus maximus.

medulla (meh-**DULL**-ah) Central portion of a structure surrounded by cortex.

medulla oblongata (meh-**DULL**-ah ob-lon-**GAH**-tah) Most posterior subdivision of the brainstem; continuation of the spinal cord.

medullary (meh-**DULL**-ah-ree) Pertaining to a medulla.

meiosis (my-**OH**-sis) Two rapid cell divisions, resulting in half the number of chromosomes.

melanin (**MEL**-ah-nin) Black pigment found in the skin, hair, and retina.

melanoma (mel-ah-**NO**-mah) Malignant neoplasm formed from cells that produce melanin.

melatonin (mel-ah-**TONE**-in) Hormone formed by the pineal gland.

melena (mel-**EN**-ah) The passage of black, tarry stools.

membrane (**MEM**-brain) Thin layer of tissue covering a structure or cavity.

membranous (**MEM**-brah-nus) Pertaining to a membrane.

menarche (meh-**NAR**-key) First menstrual period.

Ménière disease (men-**YEAR DIZ**-eez) Disorder of the inner ear with acute attacks of tinnitus, vertigo, and hearing loss.

meninges (meh-**NIN**-jeez) Three-layered covering of the brain and spinal cord.

meningitis (men-in-**JIE**-tis) Inflammation of the meninges.

meningocele (meh-**NING**-oh-seal) Protrusion of the meninges from the spinal cord or brain through a defect in the vertebral column or cranium.

meningococcal (meh-nin-goh-**KOK**-al) Pertaining to the *meningococcus* bacterium.

meningomyelocele (meh-nin-goh-**MY**-el-oh-seal) Protrusion of the spinal cord and meninges through a defect in the vertebral arch of one or more vertebrae.

meniscectomy (men-ih-**SEK**-toh-me) Excision (cutting out) of all or part of a meniscus.

meniscus (meh-**NISS**-kuss) Disc of cartilage between the bones of a joint; for example, in the knee joint. Plural *menisci*.

menopausal (**MEN**-oh-paws-al) Pertaining to the menopause.

menopause (**MEN**-oh-paws) Permanent ending of menstrual periods.

menorrhagia (men-oh-**RAY**-jee-ah) Excessive menstrual bleeding.

menses (**MEN**-seez) Monthly uterine bleeding.

menstrual (**MEN**-stru-al) Pertaining to menstruation.

menstruate (**MEN**-stru-ate) The act of menstruation.

menstruation (men-stru-**AY**-shun) Synonym of *menses.*

mesentery (**MESS**-en-ter-ree) A double layer of peritoneum enclosing the abdominal viscera.

metabolic (met-ah-**BOL**-ik) Pertaining to metabolism.

metabolic acidosis (met-ah-**BOL**-ik ass-ih-**DOE**-sis) Decreased pH in the blood and body tissues as a result of an upset in metabolism.

metabolism (meh-**TAB**-oh-lizm) The constantly changing physical and chemical processes occurring in the cell that are the sum of anabolism and catabolism.

metacarpal (**MET**-ah-**KAR**-pal) The five bones between the carpus and the fingers.

metacarpophalangeal (**MET**-ah-**KAR**-poh-fay-**LAN**-jee-al) The articulations (joints) between the metacarpal bones and the phalanges.

metastasis (meh-**TAS**-tah-sis) Spread of a disease from one part of the body to another. Plural *metastases.*

metastasize (meh-**TAS**-tah-size) To spread to distant parts.

metastatic (meh-tah-**STAT**-ik) Pertaining to the character of cells that can metastasize.

metatarsal (**MET**-ah-**TAR**-sal) Pertaining to the metatarsus.

metatarsus (**MET**-ah-**TAR**-sus) The five parallel bones of the foot between the tarsus and the phalanges.

metrorrhagia (**MEH**-troh-**RAY**-jee-ah) Irregular uterine bleeding between menses.

microbe (**MY**-krohb) Short for *microorganism.*

microcephalic (**MY**-kroh-**SEF**-ah-lik) Pertaining to or suffering from a small head.

microcephaly (**MY**-kroh-**SEF**-ah-lee) An abnormally small head.

microcyte (**MY**-kroh-site) Small red blood cell.

microcytic (my-kroh-**SIT**-ik) Pertaining to a small cell.

microorganism (**MY**-kroh-**OR**-gan-izm) Any organism too small to be seen by the naked eye.

microscope (**MY**-kroh-skope) Instrument for viewing something small that cannot be seen in detail by the naked eye.

microscopic (**MY**-kroh-**SKOP**-ik) Visible only with the aid of a microscope.

micturate (**MIK**-choo-rate) Pass urine.

micturition (mik-choo-**RISH**-un) Act of passing urine.

migraine (**MY**-grain) Paroxysmal severe headache confined to one side of the head.

mineral (**MIN**-er-al) Inorganic compound usually found in the earth's crust.

mineralocorticoid (**MIN**-er-al-oh-**KOR**-tih-koyd) Hormone of the adrenal cortex that influences sodium and potassium metabolism.

minimus (**MIN**-ih-mus) The gluteus minimus is the smallest of the gluteal muscles and lies under the gluteus medius.

minus (**MY**-nus) Smaller or lesser; for example, labium minus. Plural *minora.*

mitochondrion (my-toe-**KON**-dree-on) Organelle that generates, stores, and releases energy for cell activities. Plural *mitochondria.*

mitosis (my-**TOE**-sis) Cell division that creates two identical cells, each with 46 chromosomes.

mitral (**MY**-tral) Shaped like the headdress of a Catholic bishop.

modify (**MOD**-ih-fie) Change the form or qualities of something.

molar (**MO**-lar) One of six teeth in each jaw that grind food.

mole (MOLE) Benign localized area of melanin-producing cells.

molecule (**MOLL**-eh-kyul) Very small particle.

molluscum contagiosum (moh-**LUS**-kum kon-**TAY**-jee-oh-sum) STD caused by a virus.

monocyte (**MON**-oh-site) Large white blood cell with a single nucleus.

mononeuropathy (**MON**-oh-nyu-**ROP**-ah-thee) Disorder affecting a single nerve.

mononucleosis (**MON**-oh-nyu-klee-**OH**-sis) Presence of large numbers of specific, diagnostic mononuclear leukocytes.

monoplegia (**MON**-oh-**PLEE**-jee-ah) Paralysis of one limb.

monoplegic (**MON**-oh-**PLEE**-jik) Pertaining to or suffering from monoplegia.

mons pubis (MONZ **PYU**-bis) Fleshy pad with pubic hair, overlying the pubic bone.

morbidity (mor-**BID**-ih-tee) The frequency of the appearance of a disease.

morphine (**MOR**-feen) Derivative of opium used as an analgesic or sedative.

mortality (mor-**TAL**-ih-tee) Death rate.

motile (**MOH**-til) Capable of spontaneous movement.

motility (moh-**TILL**-ih-tee) The ability for spontaneous movement.

motor (**MOH**-tor) Structures of the nervous system that send impulses out to cause muscles to contract or glands to secrete.

mouth (MOWTH) External opening of a cavity or canal.

mucin (**MYU**-sin) Protein element of mucus.

mucocutaneous (**MYU**-koh-kyu-**TAY**-nee-us) Junction of skin and mucous membrane; for example, the lips.

mucolytic (**MYU**-koh-**LIT**-ik) Agent capable of dissolving or liquefying mucus.

mucosa (myu-**KOH**-sah) Lining of a tubular structure that secretes mucus. Another name for *mucous membrane.*

mucous (**MYU**-kus) Pertaining to mucus or the mucosa.

mucus (**MYU**-kus) Sticky secretion of cells in mucous membranes.

multipara (mul-**TIP**-ah-ruh) Woman who has given birth to two or more children.

murmur (**MUR**-mur) Abnormal heart sound heard with a stethoscope when a valve closes or opens abnormally.

muscle (**MUSS**-el) A tissue consisting of contractile cells.

musculoskeletal (**MUSS**-kyu-loh-**SKEL**-eh-tal) Pertaining to the muscles and the bony skeleton.

mutation (myu-**TAY**-shun) Change in the chemistry of a gene.

mute (MYUT) Unable or unwilling to speak.

mutism (**MYU**-tizm) Absence of speech.

myasthenia gravis (my-as-**THEE**-nee-ah **GRA**-vis) Disorder of fluctuating muscle weakness.

myelin (**MY**-eh-lin) Material of the sheath around the axon of a nerve.

myelitis (**MY**-eh-**LIE**-tis) Inflammation of the spinal cord.

myelocele (**MY**-eh-low-seal) Protrusion of the spinal cord through a defect in the vertebral arch.

myelomeningocele (**MY**-eh-low-meh-**NING**-oh-seal) Protrusion of the spinal cord and meninges through a defect in the vertebral arch of one or more vertebrae.

myocardial (my-oh-**KAR**-dee-al) Pertaining to heart muscle.

myocarditis (**MY**-oh-kar-**DIE**-tis) Inflammation of the heart muscle.

myocardium (**MY**-oh-**KAR**-dee-um) All the heart muscle.

myoma (my-**OH**-mah) Benign tumor of muscle.

myomectomy (my-oh-**MEK**-toe-me) Surgical removal of a myoma (fibroid).

myometrium (my-oh-**MEE**-tree-um) Muscle wall of the uterus.

myopia (my-**OH**-pee-ah) Able to see close objects but unable to see distant objects.

myringotomy (mir-in-**GOT**-oh-me) Incision in the tympanic membrane.

myxedema (miks-eh-**DEE**-muh) Nonpitting, waxy edema of the skin in hypothyroidism.

N

narcolepsy (**NAR**-koh-lep-see) Involuntary falling asleep.

narcotic (nar-**KOT**-ik) Drug derived from opium or any drug with effects similar to those of opium derivatives.

naris (**NAH**-ris) Nostril. Plural *nares*.

nasal (**NAY**-zal) Pertaining to the nose.

nasogastric (**NAY**-zoh-**GAS**-trik) Pertaining to the nose and stomach.

nasolacrimal duct (**NAY**-zoh-**LAK**-rim-al DUKT) Passage from the lacrimal sac to the nose.

nasopharyngeal (**NAY**-zoh-fah-**RIN**-jee-al) Pertaining to the nasopharynx.

nasopharynx (**NAY**-zoh-**FAH**-rinks) Region of the pharynx at the back of the nose and above the soft palate.

natal (**NAY**-tal) Pertaining to birth.

nebulizer (**NEB**-you-liz-er) Device used to deliver liquid medicine in a fine mist.

necrosis (neh-**KROH**-sis) Pathologic death of cells or tissue.

necrotic (neh-**KROT**-ik) Pertaining to or affected by necrosis.

necrotizing fasciitis (neh-kroh-**TIZE**-ing fash-ee-**EYE**-tis) Inflammation of fascia producing death of the tissue.

neonatal (**NEE**-oh-**NAY**-tal) Pertaining to the newborn infant or the newborn period.

neonate (**NEE**-oh-nate) A newborn infant.

neonatologist (**NEE**-oh-nay-**TOL**-oh-jist) Medical specialist in disorders of the newborn.

nephrectomy (nef-**REK**-toe-me) Surgical removal of a kidney.

nephritis (nef-**RY**-tis) Inflammation of the kidney.

nephroblastoma (**NEF**-roh-blas-**TOE**-mah) Cancerous kidney tumor of childhood. Also known as *Wilms tumor*.

nephrolithiasis (**NEF**-roe-lih-**THIGH**-ah-sis) Presence of a kidney stone.

nephrolithotomy (**NEF**-roe-lih-**THOT**-oh-me) Incision for removal of a stone.

nephrologist (nef-**ROL**-oh-jist) Medical specialist in disorders of the kidney.

nephrology (nef-**ROL**-oh-jee) Medical specialty of diseases of the kidney.

nephron (**NEF**-ron) Filtration unit of the kidney; glomerulus + renal tubule.

nephropathy (nef-**ROP**-ah-thee) Any disease of the kidney.

nephroscope (**NEF**-roe-skope) Endoscope to view the inside of the kidney.

nephroscopy (nef-**ROS**-koh-pee) To examine the kidney.

nephrosis (nef-**ROH**-sis) Same as *nephrotic syndrome*.

nephrotic syndrome (nef-**ROT**-ik **SIN**-drome) Glomerular disease with marked loss of protein. Also called *nephrosis*.

nerve (NERV) A cord of nerve fibers bound together by connective tissue.

nervous (**NER**-vus) Pertaining to a nerve or the nervous system; *or* easily excited or agitated.

nervous system (**NER**-vus **SIS**-tem) The whole, integrated nerve apparatus.

neural (**NYU**-ral) Pertaining to nervous tissue.

neuralgia (nyu-**RAL**-jee-ah) Pain in the distribution of a nerve.

neuroglia (nyu-roh-**GLEE**-ah) Connective tissue holding nervous tissue together.

neurohypophysis (**NYU**-roh-high-**POF**-ih-sis) Posterior lobe of the pituitary gland.

neurologic (**NYU**-roh-**LOJ**-ik) Pertaining to the nervous sytem.

neurologist (nyu-**ROL**-oh-jist) Medical specialist in disorders of the nervous system.

neurology (nyu-**ROL**-oh-jee) Medical specialty of disorders of the nervous system.

neuromuscular (**NYU**-roh-**MUSS**-kyu-lar) A junction where a nerve supplies muscle tissue.

neuron (**NYU**-ron) Technical term for a nerve cell; consists of the cell body with its dendrites and axons.

neuropathy (nyu-**ROP**-ah-thee) Any disorder affecting the nervous system.

neurosurgeon (**NYU**-roh-**SUR**-jun) One who operates on the nervous system.

neurosurgery (**NYU**-roh-**SUR**-jer-ee) Operating on the nervous system.

neurotoxin (**NYU**-roh-tock-sin) Agent that poisons the nervous system.

neurotransmitter (**NYU**-roh-trans-**MIT**-er) Chemical agent that relays messages from one nerve cell to the next.

neutropenia (**NEW**-troh-**PEE**-nee-ah) A deficiency of neutrophils.

neutrophil (**NEW**-troh-fill) A neutrophil's granules take up (purple) stain equally, whether the stain is acid or alkaline.

neutrophilia (**NEW**-troh-**FILL**-ee-ah) An increase in neutrophils.

nevus (**NEE**-vus) Congenital lesion of the skin. Plural *nevi*.

nipple (**NIP**-el) Projection from the breast into which the lactiferous ducts open.

nitrite (**NI**-trite) Chemical formed in urine by *E. coli* and other microorganisms.

nitrogenous (ni-**TROJ**-en-us) Containing or generating nitrogen.

nocturia (nok-**TYU**-ree-ah) Excessive urination at night.

node (NOHD) A circumscribed mass of tissue.

nonunion (non-**YOU**-nee-un) Total failure of healing of a fracture.

norepinephrine (**NOR**-ep-ih-**NEFF**-rin) Catecholamine hormone of the adrenal gland that is a parasympathetic neurotransmitter. Also called *noradrenaline*.

nosocomial (noh-soh-**KOH**-mee-al) Acquired while in the hospital.

nuchal cord (**NYU**-kul KORD) Loop(s) of umbilical cord around the fetal neck.

nuclear (**NYU**-klee-ar) Pertaining to a nucleus.

nucleolus (nyu-**KLEE**-oh-lus) Small mass within the nucleus.

nucleus (**NYU**-klee-us) Functional center of a cell or structure.

nutrient (**NYU**-tree-ent) A substance in food required for normal physiologic function.

nutrition (nyu-**TRISH**-un) The study of food and liquid requirements for normal function of the human body.

O

obesity (oh-**BEE**-sih-tee) Excessive amount of fat in the body.

oblique fracture (ob-**LEEK FRAK**-chur) A diagonal fracture across the long axis of the bone.

obsession (ob-**SESH**-un) Persistent, recurrent, uncontrollable thoughts or impulses.

obsessive (ob-**SES**-iv) Possessing persistent, recurrent, uncontrollable thoughts or impulses.

obstetrician (ob-steh-**TRISH**-un) Medical specialist in obstetrics.

obstetrics (OB) (ob-**STET**-ricks) Medical specialty for the care of women during pregnancy and the postpartum period.

occipital (ock-**SIP**-it-al) The back of the skull.

occipital lobe (ock-**SIP**-it-al LOBE) Posterior area of the cerebral hemispheres.

occlude (oh-**KLUDE**) To close, plug, or completely obstruct.

occlusion (oh-**KLU**-zhun) A complete obstruction.

occult (oh-**KULT**) Not visible on the surface, hidden.

occult blood (oh-**KULT** BLUD) Blood that cannot be seen in the stool but is positive on a fecal occult blood test.

ocular (**OCK**-you-lar) Pertaining to the eye.

olfaction (ol-**FAK**-shun) Sense of smell.

olfactory (ol-**FAK**-toh-ree) Related to the sense of smell.

oligohydramnios (**OL**-ih-goh-high-**DRAM**-nee-os) Too little amniotic fluid.

oliguria (ol-ih-**GYUR**-ee-ah) Scanty production of urine.

omentum (oh-**MEN**-tum) Membrane that encloses the bowels.

onychomycosis (oh-nih-koh-my-**KOH**-sis) Condition of a fungus infection in a nail.

oocyte (**OH**-oh-site) Female egg cell.

oogenesis (oh-oh-**JEN**-eh-sis) Development of a female egg cell.

open fracture (**OH**-pen FRAK-chur) The skin over the fracture is broken.

ophthalmia neonatorum (off-**THAL**-me-ah ne-oh-nay-**TOR**-um) Conjunctivitis of the newborn.

ophthalmic (off-**THAL**-mick) Pertaining to the eye.

ophthalmologist (off-thal-**MALL**-oh-jist) Medical specialist in ophthalmology.

ophthalmology (off-thal-**MALL**-oh-jee) Diagnosis and treatment of diseases of the eye.

ophthalmoscope (off-**THAL**-moh-skope) Instrument for viewing the retina.

ophthalmoscopic (**OFF**-thal-**MOS**-koh-pik) Pertaining to the use of an ophthalmoscope.

ophthalmoscopy (**OFF**-thal-**MOS**-koh-pee) The process of viewing the retina.

opiate (**OH**-pee-ate) A drug derived from opium.

opportunistic (**OP**-or-tyu-**NIS**-tik) An organism or a disease in a host with lowered resistance.

opportunistic infection (**OP**-or-tyu-**NIS**-tik in-**FEK**-shun) An infection that causes disease when the immune system is compromised for other reasons.

optic (**OP**-tick) The eye or vision; *or* second (II) cranial nerve, which carries visual information.

optical (**OP**-tih-kal) Pertaining to the eye or vision.

optometrist (op-**TOM**-eh-trist) Someone skilled in the measurement of vision but who cannot treat eye diseases or prescribe medication.

optometry (op-**TOM**-eh-tree) The profession of the measurement of vision.

oral (**OR**-al) Pertaining to the mouth.

orbit (**OR**-bit) The bony socket that holds the eyeball.

orbital (**OR**-bit-al) Pertaining to the orbit.

orchiectomy (or-key-**ECK**-toe-me) Removal of one or both testes.

orchiopexy (**OR**-key-oh-**PEK**-see) Surgical fixation of a testis in the scrotum.

orchitis (or-**KIE**-tis) Inflammation of the testis. Also called *epididymoorchitis*.

organ (**OR**-gan) Structure with specific functions in a body system.

organelle (**OR**-gah-nell) Part of a cell having specialized function(s).

organism (**OR**-gan-izm) Any whole, living individual animal or plant.

orifice (**OR**-ih-fis) Any opening or aperture.

origin (**OR**-ih-gin) Fixed source of a muscle at its attachment to bone.

oropharyngeal (**OR**-oh-fah-**RIN**-jee-al) Pertaining to the oropharynx.

oropharynx (**OR**-oh-fah-rinks) Region at the back of the mouth between the soft palate and the tip of the epiglottis.

orthopedic (or-tho-**PEE**-dik) Pertaining to the correction and cure of deformities and diseases of the musculoskeletal system; originally, most of the deformities treated were in children. Also spelled *orthopaedic*.

orthopedist (or-tho-**PEE**-dist) Specialist in orthopedics.

orthopnea (or-**THOP**-nee-ah) Difficulty in breathing when lying flat.

orthopneic (or-**THOP**-nee-ik) Pertaining to or affected by orthopnea.

orthotic (or-**THOT**-ik) Orthopedic appliance to correct an abnormality.

orthotist (or-**THOT**-ist) Maker and fitter of orthopedic appliances.

os (OSS) Opening into a canal; for example, the cervix.

ossicle (**OSS**-ih-kel) A small bone, particularly relating to the three bones in the middle ear.

osteoarthritis (**OSS**-tee-oh-ar-**THRI**-tis) Chronic inflammatory disease of the joints, with pain and loss of function.

osteoblast (**OSS**-tee-oh-blast) Bone-forming cell.

osteocyte (**OSS**-tee-oh-site) A bone-maintaining cell.

osteogenesis imperfecta (**OSS**-tee-oh-**JEN**-eh-sis im-per-**FEK**-tah) Inherited condition when bone formation is incomplete, leading to fragile, easily broken bones.

osteogenic sarcoma (**OSS**-tee-oh-**JEN**-ik sar-**KOH**-mah) Malignant tumor originating in bone-producing cells.

osteomalacia (**OSS**-tee-oh-mah-**LAY**-she-ah) Soft, flexible bones lacking in calcium (rickets).

osteomyelitis (**OSS**-tee-oh-my-eh-**LIE**-tis) Inflammation of bone tissue.

osteopath (**OSS**-tee-oh-path) Practitioner of osteopathy.

osteopathy (**OSS**-tee-**OP**-ah-thee) Medical practice based on maintaining the balance of the body.

osteopenia (**OSS**-tee-oh-**PEE**-nee-ah) Decreased calcification of bone.

osteoporosis (**OSS**-tee-oh-poh-**ROE**-sis) Condition in which the bones become more porous, brittle, and fragile and more likely to fracture.

ostomy (**OSS**-toe-me) Artificial opening into a tubular structure.

otitis media (oh-**TIE**-tis **ME**-dee-ah) Inflammation of the middle ear.

otolith (**OH**-toe-lith) A calcium particle in the vestibule of the inner ear.

otologist (oh-**TOL**-oh-jist) Medical specialist in diseases of the ear.

otology (oh-**TOL**-oh-jee) Study of the function and diseases of the ear.

otorhinolaryngologist (**OH**-toe-**RHINO**-lah-rin-**GOL**-oh-jist) Ear, nose, and throat medical specialist.

otosclerosis (oh-toe-sklair-**OH**-sis) Hardening at the junction of the stapes and oval window that causes loss of hearing.

otoscope (**OH**-toe-skope) Instrument for examining the ear.

otoscopic (oh-toe-**SKOP**-ik) Pertaining to examination with an otoscope.

otoscopy (oh-**TOS**-koh-pee) Examination of the ear.

ovarian (oh-**VAIR**-ee-an) Pertaining to the ovary(ies).

ovary (**OH**-vah-ree) One of the paired female egg-producing glands. Plural *ovaries.*

ovulate (**OV**-you-late) Release the oocyte from a follicle.

ovulation (**OV**-you-**LAY**-shun) Release of an oocyte from a follicle.

ovum (**OH**-vum) Egg. Also called *oocyte.* Plural *ova.*

oxygen (**OCK**-see-jen) The gas essential for life.

oxyhemoglobin (**OCK**-see-he-moh-**GLOW**-bin) Hemoglobin in combination with oxygen.

oxytocin (**OCK**-see-**TOE**-sin) Pituitary hormone that stimulates the uterus to contract.

P

pacemaker (**PACE**-may-ker) Device that regulates cardiac electrical activity.

palate (**PAL**-ate) Roof of the mouth.

palatine (**PAL**-ah-tine) Bone that forms the hard palate and parts of the nose and orbits.

palliative care (**PAL**-ee-ah-tiv **KAIR**) To relieve symptoms and pain without curing.

pallor (**PAL**-or) Paleness of the skin.

palm (PAHLM) Flat or anterior surface of the hand.

palmar (**PAHL**-mar) Pertaining to the palm.

palpate (**PAL**-pate) To examine with the fingers and hands.

palpation (pal-**PAY**-shun) Examination with the fingers and hands.

palpitation (pal-pih-**TAY**-shun) Forcible, rapid beat of the heart felt by the patient.

palsy (**PAWL**-zee) Paralysis or paresis from brain damage.

pancreas (**PAN**-kree-as) Lobulated gland, the head of which is tucked into the curve of the duodenum.

pancreatic (**PAN**-kree-**AT**-ik) Pertaining to the pancreas.

pancreatitis (**PAN**-kree-ah-**TIE**-tis) Inflammation of the pancreas.

pancytopenia (**PAN**-site-oh-**PEE**-nee-ah) Deficiency of all types of blood cells.

pandemic (pan-**DEM**-ik) Pertaining to a disease attacking the population of a very large area.

panendoscopy (pan-en-**DOS**-koh-pee) A visual examination of the inside of the esophagus, stomach, and upper duodenum using a flexible fiber-optic endoscope.

panhypopituitarism (pan-**HIGH**-poh-pih-**TYU**-ih-tah-rizm) Deficiency of all the pituitary hormones.

Pap test (PAP TEST) Examination of cells taken from the cervix.

papilla (pah-**PILL**-ah) Any small projection. Plural *papillae.*

papilledema (pah pill eh-**DEE**-mah) Swelling of the optic disc in the retina.

papillomavirus (pap-ih-**LOH**-mah-vi-rus) Virus that causes warts and is associated with cancer.

papule (**PAP**-yul) Small, circumscribed elevation on the skin.

para (**PAH**-rah) Abbreviation for number of deliveries.

paralysis (pah-**RAL**-ih-sis) Loss of voluntary movement.

paralytic (par-ah-**LYT**-ik) Suffering from paralysis.

paralyze (**PAR**-ah-lyze) To make incapable of movement.

paranasal (**PAR**-ah **NAY**-zal) Adjacent to the nose.

paranoia (par-ah-**NOY**-ah) Presence of persecutory delusions.

paranoid (**PAR**-ah-noyd) Having delusions of persecution.

paraphimosis (**PAR**-ah-fih-**MOH**-sis) Condition in which a retracted prepuce cannot be pulled forward to cover the glans.

paraplegia (par-ah-**PLEE**-jee-ah) Paralysis of both lower extremities.

paraplegic (par-ah-**PLEE**-jik) Pertaining to or suffering from paraplegia.

parasite (**PAR**-ah-site) An organism that attaches itself to, lives on or in, and derives its nutrition from another species.

parasitic (par-ah-**SIT**-ik) Pertaining to a parasite.

parasympathetic (par-ah-sim-pah-**THET**-ik) Division of the autonomic nervous system; has opposite effects of the sympathetic division.

parathyroid (par-ah-**THIGH**-royd) Endocrine glands embedded in the back of the thyroid gland.

paraurethral (**PAR**-ah-you-**REE**-thral) Situated around the urethra.

parenchyma (pah-**RENG**-kih-mah) Characteristic functional cells of a gland or organ that are supported by the connective tissue framework.

parenteral (pah-**REN**-ter-al) Giving medication by any means other than the gastrointestinal tract.

paresis (par-**EE**-sis) Partial paralysis (weakness).

paresthesia (par-es-**THEE**-ze-ah) An abnormal sensation; for example, tingling, burning, prickling. Plural *parasthesias.*

parietal (pah-**RYE**-eh-tal) Pertaining to the outer layer of the pericardium and the wall of any body cavity; *or* the two bones forming the sidewalls and roof of the cranium.

parietal lobe (pah-**RYE**-eh-tal LOBE) Area of the brain under the parietal bone.

Parkinson disease (**PAR**-kin-son **DIZ**-eez) Disease of muscular rigidity, tremors, and a masklike facial expression.

paronychia (par-oh-**NICK**-ee-ah) Infection alongside the nail.

parotid (pah-**ROT**-id) Parotid gland is the salivary gland beside the ear.

paroxysmal (par-ock-**SIZ**-mal) Occurring in sharp, spasmodic episodes.

particle (**PAR**-tih-kul) A small piece of matter.

particulate (par-**TIK**-you-late) Relating to a fine particle.

patella (pah-**TELL**-ah) Thin, circular bone in front of the knee joint and embedded in the patellar tendon. Also called *kneecap.* Plural *patellae.*

patellar (pah-**TELL**-ar) Pertaining to the patella.

patent (**PAY**-tent) Open.

patent ductus arteriosus (**PAY**-tent **DUK**-tus ar-**TER**-ee-oh-sus) An open, direct channel between the aorta and the pulmonary artery.

pathogen (**PATH**-oh-jen) A disease-causing microorganism.

pathogenic (path-oh-**JEN**-ik) Causing disease.

pathologic fracture (path-oh-**LOJ**-ik **FRAK**-chur) Fracture occurring at a site already weakened by a disease process, such as cancer.

pathologist (pa-**THOL**-oh-jist) A specialist in pathology.

pathology (pa-**THOL**-oh-jee) Medical specialty dealing with the structural and functional changes of a disease process or the cause, development, and structural changes in disease.

pectoral (**PEK**-tor-al) Pertaining to the chest.

pectoral girdle (**PEK**-tor-al **GIR**-del) Incomplete bony ring that attaches the upper limb to the axial skeleton.

pectoralis (**PEK**-tor-ah-lis) Pertaining to the chest.

pedal (**PEED**-al) Pertaining to the foot.

pediatrician (**PEE**-dee-ah-**TRISH**-an) Medical specialist in pediatrics.

pediatrics (pee-dee-**AT**-riks) Medical specialty of treating children during development from birth through adolescence.

pediculosis (peh-dick-you-**LOH**-sis) An infestation with lice.

peer (PEER) A person at the same level or standing.

pelvic (**PEL**-vik) Pertaining to the pelvis.

pelvis (**PEL**-viss) A basin-shaped ring of bones, ligaments, and muscles at the base of the spine; *or* a basin-shaped cavity, as in the pelvis of the kidney.

penile (**PEE**-nile) Pertaining to the penis.

penis (**PEE**-nis) Conveys urine and semen to the outside.

pepsin (**PEP**-sin) Enzyme produced by the stomach that breaks down protein.

pepsinogen (pep-**SIN**-oh-jen) Converted by HCl in stomach to pepsin.

peptic (**PEP**-tik) Relating to the stomach and duodenum.

percutaneous (**PER**-kyu-**TAY**-nee-us) Passage through the skin.

perforated (**PER**-foh-ray-ted) Punctured with one or more holes.

perforation (per-foh-**RAY**-shun) A hole through the wall of a structure.

perfuse (per-**FYUSE**) To force blood to flow through a lumen or a vascular bed.

perfusion (per-**FYU**-shun) The act of perfusing.

pericardial (per-ih-**KAR**-dee-al) Pertaining to the pericardium.

pericarditis (**PER**-ih-kar-**DIE**-tis) Inflammation of the pericardium, the covering of the heart.

pericardium (per-ih-**KAR**-dee-um) A double layer of membranes surrounding the heart.

perimetrium (per-ih-**ME**-tree-um) The covering of the uterus; part of the peritoneum.

perinatal (per-ih-**NAY**-tal) Around the time of birth.

perineal (**PER**-ih-**NEE**-al) Pertaining to the perineum.

perineum (**PER**-ih-**NEE**-um) Area between the thighs, extending from the coccyx to the pubis.

periodontal (**PER**-ee-oh-**DON**-tal) Around a tooth.

periodontics (**PER**-ee-oh-**DON**-tiks) Branch of dentistry specializing in disorders of tissues around the teeth.

periodontist (**PER**-ee-oh-**DON**-tist) Specialist in periodontics.

periodontitis (**PER**-ee-oh-don-**TIE**-tis) Inflammation of tissues around a tooth.

periorbital (per-ee-**OR**-bit-al) Pertaining to tissues around the orbit.

periosteal (**PER**-ee-**OSS**-tee-al) Pertaining to the periosteum.

periosteum (**PER**-ee-**OSS**-tee-um) Fibrous membrane covering a bone.

peripheral (peh-**RIF**-er-al) Pertaining to the periphery or external boundary.

peripheral vision (peh-**RIF**-er-al **VIZH**-un) Ability to see objects as they come into the outer edges of the visual field.

peristalsis (per-ih-**STAL**-sis) Waves of alternate contraction and relaxation of the muscle wall of a tube; for example, of the intestinal wall to move food along the digestive tract.

peritoneal (**PER**-ih-toe-**NEE**-al) Pertaining to the peritoneum.

peritoneum (**PER**-ih-toe-**NEE**-um) Membrane that lines the abdominal cavity.

peritonitis (**PER**-ih-toe-**NIE**-tis) Inflammation of the peritoneum.

pernicious anemia (per-**NISH**-us ah-**NEE**-me-ah) Chronic anemia due to lack of vitamin B_{12}.

pertussis (per-**TUSS**-is) Infectious disease with a spasmodic, intense cough ending on a whoop (stridor). Also called *whooping cough*.

pes planus (PES **PLAY**-nuss) A flat foot with no plantar arch.

pessary (**PES**-ah-ree) Appliance inserted into the vagina to support the uterus.

petechia (peh-**TEE**-kee-ah) Pinpoint capillary hemorrhagic spot in the skin. Plural *petechiae*.

petit mal (peh-**TEE** MAL) Old name for absence seizures.

phagocyte (**FAG**-oh-site) Blood cell that ingests and destroys foreign particles and cells.

phagocytic (fag-oh-**SIT**-ik) Pertaining to a phagocyte.

phagocytosis (**FAG**-oh-sigh-**TOE**-sis) Process of ingestion and destruction.

phalanx (**FAY**-lanks) A bone of a finger or toe. Plural *phalanges*.

pharmacist (**FAR**-mah-sist) Person licensed by the state to prepare and dispense drugs.

pharmacology (far-mah-**KOLL**-oh-jee) Science of the preparation, uses, and effects of drugs.

pharmacy (**FAR**-mah-see) Facility licensed to prepare and dispense drugs.

pharyngeal (fah-**RIN**-jee-al) Pertaining to the pharynx.

pharyngitis (fah-rin-**JIE**-tis) Inflammation of the pharynx.

pharynx (**FAH**-rinks) Tube from the back of the nose to the larynx.

phimosis (fih-**MOH**-sis) Prepuce cannot be retracted.

phlebitis (fleh-**BIE**-tis) Inflammation of a vein.

phlebotomist (fleh-**BOT**-oh-mist) Person skilled in taking blood from veins.

phlebotomy (fleh-**BOT**-oh-me) Taking blood from a vein.

phlegm (FLEM) Abnormal amounts of mucus expectorated from the respiratory tract.

phobia (**FOH**-bee-ah) Pathologic fear or dread.

photocoagulation (foh-toe-koh-ag-you-**LAY**-shun) Using light (laser beam) to form a clot.

photophobia (foh-toe-**FOH**-bee-ah) Fear of the light because it hurts the eyes.

photophobic (foh-toe-**FOH**-bik) Pertaining to or suffering from photophobia.

photoreceptor (foh-toe-ree-**SEP**-tor) A photoreceptor cell receives light and converts it into electrical impulses.

photosensitive (**FOH**-toe-**SEN**-sih-tiv) Abnormally sensitive to light.

photosensitivity (**FOH**-toe-**SEN**-sih-tiv-ih-tee) Light produces pain in the eye.

phototherapy (**FOH**-toe-**THAIR**-ah-pee) Treatment using light rays.

pia mater (**PEE**-ah **MAY**-ter) Delicate inner layer of the meninges.

pica (**PIE**-kah) Eating substances not considered to be food.

pineal (**PIN**-ee-al) Pertaining to the pineal gland.

pink eye (PINK EYE) Conjunctivitis.

pinna (**PIN**-ah) Another name for *auricle*. Plural *pinnae*.

pitting edema (ee-**DEE**-mah) An indentation made by a finger in an edematous area persists for a long time.

pituitary (pih-**TYU**-ih-tary) Pertaining to the pituitary gland.

placebo (plah-**SEE**-boh) An inert compound with no innate therapeutic value.

placenta (plah-**SEN**-tah) Organ that allows metabolic interchange between the mother and the fetus.

placenta abruptio (plah-**SEN**-tah ab-**RUP**-she-oh) Premature detachment of the placenta.

placenta previa (plah-**SEN**-tah **PREE**-vee-ah) Placenta obstructing the fetus during delivery.

plaque (PLAK) Patch of abnormal tissue.

plasma (**PLAZ**-mah) Fluid, noncellular component of blood.

platelet (**PLAYT**-let) Cell fragment involved in the clotting process. Also called *thrombocyte*.

pleura (**PLUR**-ah) Membrane covering the lungs and lining the ribs in the thoracic cavity. Plural *pleurae*.

pleural (**PLUR**-al) Pertaining to the pleura.

pleurisy (**PLUR**-ih-see) Inflammation of the pleura.

plexus (**PLEK**-sus) A weblike network of joined nerves. Plural *plexuses*.

pneumoconiosis (**NEW**-moh-koh-nee-**OH**-sis) Fibrotic lung disease caused by the inhalation of different dusts.

pneumonectomy (**NEW**-moh-**NECK**-toe-me) Surgical removal of a lung.

pneumonia (new-**MOH**-nee-ah) Inflammation of the lung parenchyma (tissue).

pneumonitis (new-moh-**NYE**-tis) Synonym for pneumonia.

pneumothorax (new-moh-**THOR**-ax) Air in the pleural cavity of the chest.

podiatrist (poh-**DIE**-ah-trist) Practitioner of podiatry.

podiatry (poh-**DIE**-ah-tree) The diagnosis and treatment of disorders and injuries of the foot.

poliomyelitis (**POE**-lee-oh-**MY**-eh-lie-tis) Inflammation of the gray matter of the spinal cord, leading to paralysis of the limbs and muscles of respiration. Abbreviation *polio*.

pollutant (poh-**LOO**-tant) Substance that makes an environment unclean or impure.

pollution (poh-**LOO**-shun) Condition that is unclean, impure, and a danger to health.

polycystic (pol-ee-**SIS**-tik) Composed of many cysts.

polycythemia vera (**POL**-ee-sigh-**THEE**-me-ah VERA) Chronic disease with bone marrow hyperplasia, increase in number of RBCs, and increase in blood volume.

polydipsia (pol-ee-**DIP**-see-ah) Excessive thirst.

polyhydramnios (**POL**-ee-high-**DRAM**-nee-os) Too much amniotic fluid.

polymenorrhea (**POL**-ee-men-oh-**REE**-ah) More than normal frequency of menses.

polymorphonuclear (**POL**-ee-more-foh-**NEW**-klee-ahr) White blood cell with a multilobed nucleus.

polyneuropathy (**POL**-ee-nyu-**ROP**-ah-thee) Disorder affecting many nerves.

polyp (**POL**-ip) Any mass of tissue that projects outward.

polypectomy (pol-ip-**ECK**-toh-mee) Excision or removal of a polyp.

polyphagia (pol-ee-**FAY**-jee-ah) Excessive eating.

polyposis (pol-ih-**POH**-sis) Presence of several polyps.

polysomnography (**POLL**-ee-som-**NOG**-rah-fee) Test to monitor brain waves, muscle tension, eye movement, and oxygen levels in the blood as the patient sleeps.

polyuria (pol-ee-**YOU**-ree-ah) Excessive production of urine.

pons (PONZ) Part of the brainstem.

popliteal (pop-**LIT**-ee-al) Pertaining to the back of the knee.

popliteal fossa (pop-**LIT**-ee-al **FOSS**-ah) The hollow at the back of the knee.

portal vein (**POR**-tal) The vein that carries blood from the intestines to the liver.

postcoital (post-**KOH**-ih-tal) After sexual intercourse.

posterior (pos-**TEER**-ee-or) Pertaining to the back surface of the body; situated behind.

postictal (post-**IK**-tal) Transient neurologic deficit after a seizure.

postmature (post-mah-**TYUR**) Infant born after 42 weeks of gestation.

postmaturity (post-mah-**TYUR**-ih-tee) Condition of being postmature.

postmortem (post-**MOR**-tem) Examination of the body and organs of a dead person to determine the cause of death.

postnatal (post-**NAY**-tal) After the birth.

postpartum (post-**PAR**-tum) After childbirth.

postpolio syndrome (PPS) (post-**POE**-lee-oh **SIN**-drome) Progressive muscle weakness in a person previously affected by polio.

postprandial (post-**PRAN**-dee-al) Following a meal.

posttraumatic (post-traw-**MAT**-ik) Occurring after and caused by trauma.

Pott fracture (POT **FRAK**-shur) Fracture of the lower end of the fibula, often with fracture of the tibial malleolus.

precancerous (pree-**KAN**-ser-us) Lesion from which cancer can develop.

precipitate labor (pree-**SIP**-ih-tate **LAY**-bore) A very rapid labor and delivery.

precursor (pree-**KUR**-sir) Cell or substance formed earlier in the development of the cell or substance.

preeclampsia (pree-eh-**KLAMP**-see-uh) Hypertension, edema, and proteinuria during pregnancy.

preemie (**PREE**-me) Slang for *premature baby.*

pregnancy (**PREG**-nan-see) State of being pregnant.

pregnant (**PREG**-nant) Having conceived.

prehypertension (pree-**HIGH**-per-**TEN**-shun) Precursor to hypertension.

premature (pree-mah-**TYUR**) Occurring before the expected time; for example, an infant born before 37 weeks of gestation.

prematurity (pree-mah-**TYUR**-ih-tee) Condition of being premature.

premenstrual (pree-**MEN**-stru-al) Pertaining to the time immediately before the menses.

prenatal (pree-**NAY**-tal) Before birth.

prepatellar (pree-pah-**TELL**-ar) In front of the patella.

prepuce (**PREE**-puce) Fold of skin that covers the glans penis. Same as *foreskin.*

presbyopia (prez-bee-**OH**-pee-ah) Difficulty in nearsighted vision occurring in middle and old age.

preterm (**PREE**-term) Baby delivered before 37 weeks of gestation. Also called *premature.*

previa (**PREE**-vee-ah) Anything blocking the fetus during its birth; for example, an abnomally situated placenta, *placenta previa.*

priapism (**PRY**-ah-pizm) Persistent erection of the penis.

primary (**PRY**-mah-ree) The first of a disease or symptom, after which others may occur as complications arise.

primigravida (pry-mih-**GRAV**-ih-dah) First pregnancy.

primipara (pry-**MIP**-ah-ruh) Woman giving birth for the first time.

prion (**PREE**-on) Small infectious protein particle.

proctitis (prok-**TIE**-tis) Inflammation of the lining of the rectum.

proctoscopy (prok-**TOSS**-koh-pee) Examination of the inside of the anus by endoscopy.

progesterone (pro-**JESS**-ter-own) Hormone that prepares the uterus for pregnancy.

progestin (pro-**JESS**-tin) A synthetic form of progesterone.

prognathism (**PROG**-nah-thizm) Condition of a forward-projecting jaw.

prognosis (prog-**NO**-sis) Forecast of the probable future course and outcome of a disease.

prolactin (pro-**LAK**-tin) Pituitary hormone that stimulates the production of milk.

prolapse (pro-**LAPS**) A sinking down of an organ or tissue.

proliferate (pro-**LIF**-eh-rate) To increase in number through reproduction.

pronate (**PRO**-nate) Rotate the forearm so that the surface of the palm faces posteriorly in the anatomical position.

pronation (pro-**NAY**-shun) Process of lying face down or of turning a hand or foot with the volar (palm or sole) surface down.

prone (PRONE) Lying face down, flat on your belly.

prophylactic (pro-fih-**LAK**-tik) The act or the agent that prevents a disease.

prophylaxis (pro-fih-**LAX**-is) Prevention of disease.

prostaglandin (**PROS**-tah-**GLAN**-din) Hormone present in many tissues but first isolated from the prostate gland.

prostate (**PROS**-tate) Organ surrounding the urethra at the base of the male urinary bladder.

prostatectomy (pros-tah-**TEK**-toe-me) Surgical removal of the prostate.

prostatic (pros-**TAT**-ik) Pertaining to the prostate.

prostatitis (pros-tah-**TIE**-tis) Inflammation of the prostate.

prosthesis (**PROS**-thee-sis) Manufactured substitute for a missing part of the body.

prosthetic (pros-**THET**-ik) Pertaining to a prosthesis.

prostrate (pros-**TRAYT**) To lay flat or to be overcome by physical weakness and exhaustion.

prostration (pros-**TRAY**-shun) To be lying flat or to be overcome by physical weakness and exhaustion.

protein (**PRO**-teen) Class of food substances based on amino acids.

proteinuria (pro-tee-**NYU**-ree-ah) Presence of protein in urine.

prothrombin (pro-**THROM**-bin) Protein formed by the liver and converted to thrombin in the blood-clotting mechanism.

provisional diagnosis (pro-**VISH**-un-al die-ag-**NO**-sis) A temporary diagnosis pending further examination or testing.

proximal (**PROK**-sih-mal) Situated nearest the center of the body.

pruritic (proo-**RIT**-ik) Itchy.

pruritus (proo-**RYE**-tus) Itching.

psoriasis (so-**RYE**-ah-sis) Rash characterized by reddish, silver-scaled patches.

psychiatric (sigh-kee-**AH**-trik) Pertaining to psychiatry.

psychiatrist (sigh-**KIGH**-ah-trist) Licensed medical specialist in psychiatry.

psychiatry (sigh-**KIGH**-ah-tree) Diagnosis and treatment of mental disorders.

psychologic (sigh-koh-**LOJ**-ik) Pertaining to psychology.

psychological (sigh-koh-**LOJ**-ik-al) Pertaining to psychology.

psychologist (sigh-**KOL**-oh-jist) One who studies and becomes a specialist in psychology.

psychology (sigh-**KOL**-oh-jee) Study of the behavior of the human mind.

psychopath (**SIGH**-koh-path) Person with antisocial personality disorder.

psychosis (sigh-**KOH**-sis) Disorder causing mental disruption and loss of contact with reality.

psychosocial (**SIGH**-koh-**SOH**-shal) Involving both the mind and various social and community aspects of life.

psychosomatic (**SIGH**-koh-soh-**MAT**-ik) Disorders of the body influenced by the mind.

psychotic (sigh-**KOT**-ik) Pertaining to or affected by psychosis.

ptosis (**TOE**-sis) Sinking down of the upper eyelid or an organ.

pubarche (pyu-**BAR**-key) Development of pubic and axillary hair.

puberty (**PYU**-ber-tee) Process of maturing from child to young adult.

pubic (**PYU**-bik) Pertaining to the pubis.

pubis (**PYU**-bis) Alternative name for *pubic bone.*

puerperium (pyu-er-**PER**-ee-um) Six-week period after birth in which the uterus involutes.

pulmonary (**PULL**-moh-**NAR**-ee) Pertaining to the lungs.

pulmonologist (**PULL**-moh-**NOL**-oh-jist) Specialist in treating disorders of the lungs.

pulmonology (**PULL**-moh-**NOL**-oh-jee) Study of the lungs, or the medical specialty of disorders of the lungs.

pulp (PULP) Dental pulp is the connective tissue in the cavity in the center of the tooth.

pupil (PYU-pill) The opening in the center of the iris that allows light to reach the lens. Plural *pupillae*.

pupillary (PYU-pill-ah-ree) Pertaining to the pupil.

purge (PURJ) Consciously throw up or cause bowel evacuation.

Purkinje fibers (per-KIN-jee fi-BERS) Network of nerve fibers in the myocardium.

purpura (PUR-pyu-rah) Skin hemorrhages that are red initially and then turn purple.

purulent (PURE-you-lent) Showing or containing a lot of pus.

pustule (PUS-tyul) Small protuberance on the skin that contains pus.

pyelitis (pie-eh-LYE-tis) Inflammation of the renal pelvis.

pyelogram (PIE-el-oh-gram) X-ray image of renal pelvis and ureters.

pyelonephritis (PIE-eh-loh-neh-FRY-tis) Inflammation of the kidney and renal pelvis.

pyloric (pie-LOR-ik) Pertaining to the pylorus.

pylorus (pie-LOR-us) Exit area of the stomach.

pyorrhea (pie-oh-REE-ah) Purulent discharge.

pyrexia (pie-REK-see-ah) An abnormally high body temperature or fever.

Q

quadrant (KWAD-rant) One-quarter of a circle; *or* one of four regions of the surface of the abdomen.

quadrantectomy (kwad-ran-TEK-toe-me) Surgical excision of a quadrant of the breast.

quadriceps femoris (KWAD-rih-seps FEM-or-is) An anterior thigh muscle with four heads.

quadriplegia (kwad-rih-PLEE-jee-ah) Paralysis of all four limbs.

quadriplegic (kwad-rih-PLEE-jik) Pertaining to or suffering from quadriplegia.

R

radial (RAY-dee-al) Pertaining to the forearm or to any of the structures (artery, vein, nerve) named after it; *or* diverging in all directions from any given center.

radiation (ray-dee-AY-shun) To spread out.

radiologic (RAY-dee-oh-LOJ-ik) Pertaining to radiology.

radiologist (ray-dee-OL-oh-jist) Medical specialist in the use of x-rays and other imaging techniques.

radiology (ray-dee-OL-oh-jee) Study of medical imaging.

radius (RAY-dee-us) The forearm bone on the thumb side.

rale (RAHL) Crackle heard through a stethoscope when air bubbles through liquid in the lungs. Plural *rales.*

rash (RASH) Skin eruption.

rectocele (RECK-toe-seal) Hernia of the rectum into the vagina.

rectum (RECK-tum) Terminal part of the colon from the sigmoid to the anal canal.

reduction (ree-DUCK-shun) Restore a structure to its normal position.

reflex (REE-fleks) An involuntary response to a stimulus.

reflux (REE-fluks) Backward flow.

refract (ree-FRACT) Make a change in the direction of, or bend, a ray of light.

refraction (ree-FRAK-shun) The bending of light

regenerate (ree-JEN-eh-rate) Reconstitution of a lost part.

regeneration (ree-JEN-eh-RAY-shun) The process of reconstitution.

regulate (reg-you-LATE) To control the way in which a process progresses.

regulation (reg-you-LAY-shun) Control of the way in which a process progresses.

regurgitate (ree-GUR-jih-tate) To flow backward; for example, blood through a heart valve.

regurgitation (ree-gur-jih-TAY-shun) Expel contents of the stomach into the mouth, short of vomiting.

rehabilitation (REE-hah-bill-ih-TAY-shun) Therapeutic restoration of an ability to function as before.

remission (ree-MISH-un) Period when there is a lessening or absence of the symptoms of a disease.

renal (REE-nal) Pertaining to the kidney.

replication (rep-lih-KAY-shun) Reproduction to produce an exact copy.

reproduction (ree-pro-DUK-shun) The process by which organisms produce offspring.

reproductive (ree-pro-DUK-tiv) Pertaining to reproduction.

resection (ree-SEK-shun) Removal of a specific part of an organ or structure.

resectoscope (ree-SEK-toe-skope) Endoscope for transurethral removal of lesions of the prostate.

residual (reh-ZID-you-al) Pertaining to anything left over.

resistance (reh-ZIS-tants) Ability of an organism to withstand the effects of an antagonistic agent.

resistant (reh-ZIS-tant) Able to resist.

respiration (RES-pih-RAY-shun) Process of breathing; fundamental process of life used to exchange oxygen and carbon dioxide.

respirator (RES-pih-RAY-tor) Another name for *ventilator.*

respiratory (RES-pih-rah-tor-ee) Pertaining to respiration.

retention (ree-TEN-shun) Holding back in the body what should normally be discharged (e.g., urine).

retina (RET-ih-nah) Light-sensitive innermost layer of the eyeball.

retinal (RET-ih-nal) Pertaining to the retina.

retinoblastoma (RET-in-oh-blas-TOE-mah) Malignant neoplasm of primitive retinal cells.

retinopathy (ret-ih-NOP-ah-thee) Any disease of the retina.

retrograde (RET-roh-grade) Reversal of a normal flow; for example, back from the bladder into the ureters.

retroversion (reh-troh-VER-shun) Tipping backward of the uterus.

retroverted (REH-troh-vert-ed) Tilted backward.

retrovirus (REH-troh-vie-rus) Virus with an RNA core.

rheumatic (ru-MAT-ik) Pertaining to or affected by rheumatism.

rheumatism (RU-mat-izm) Pain in various parts of the musculoskeletal system.

rheumatoid arthritis (RA) (RU-mah-toyd ar-**THRI**-tis) Disease of connective tissue, with arthritis as a major manifestation.

rhinitis (rye-**NIE**-tis) Inflammation of the nasal mucosa. Also called *coryza*.

rhinoplasty (**RYE**-no-plas-tee) Surgical procedure to change size or shape of the nose.

rhonchus (**RONG**-kuss) Wheezing sound heard on auscultation of the lungs; made by air passing through a constricted lumen. Plural *rhonchi*.

ribonucleic acid (RNA) (**RYE**-boh-nyu-**KLEE**-ik **ASS**-id) Information carrier from DNA in the nucleus to an organelle to produce protein molecules.

ribosome (**RYE**-boh-sohm) Structure in the cell that assembles amino acids into protein.

rickets (**RICK**-ets) Disease due to vitamin D deficiency, producing soft, flexible bones.

rigidity (ri-**JID**-ih-tee) Increased muscle tone at rest.

Rinne test (**RIN**-eh TEST) Test for conductive hearing loss.

root (ROOT) Fundamental or beginning part of a structure.

rooting (rue-**TING**) A neonatal reflex to turn toward the nipple and open the mouth when a nipple is placed on the cheek.

rosacea (roh-**ZAY**-she-ah) Persistent erythematous rash of the central face.

rotator cuff (roh-**TAY**-tor CUFF) Part of the capsule of the shoulder joint.

rumination (**ROO**-min-ay-shun) To bring back food into the mouth to chew over and over.

rupture (**RUP**-tyur) Break or tear of any organ or body part.

S

sacral (**SAY**-kral) Pertaining to or in the neighborhood of the sacrum.

sacroiliac joint (say-kroh-**ILL**-ih-ak JOINT) The joint between the sacrum and the ilium.

sacrum (**SAY**-crum) Segment of the vertebral column that forms part of the pelvis.

sagittal (**SAJ**-ih-tal) Vertical plane through the body dividing it into right and left portions.

saline (**SAY**-leen) Salt solution, usually sodium chloride.

saliva (sa-**LIE**-vah) Secretion in the mouth from salivary glands.

salivary (**SAL**-ih-var-ee) Pertaining to saliva.

salpingectomy (sal-pin-**JEK**-toe-me) Surgical excision of a fallopian tube.

salpingitis (sal-pin-**JIE**-tis) Inflammation of the uterine tube.

saphenous (**SAPH**-ih-nus) Relating to the saphenous vein in the thigh.

sarcoidosis (sar-koy-**DOH**-sis) Granulomatous lesions of the lungs and other organs; cause is unknown.

sarcoma (sar-**KOH**-mah) A malignant tumor originating in connective tissue.

sarcopenia (sar-koh-**PEE**-nee-ah) Progressive loss of muscle mass and strength with aging.

saturated fatty acid (satch-you-**RAY**-ted **FAT**-ee **ASS**-id) Lipid that is incapable of absorbing any more hydrogen.

scab (SKAB) Crust that forms over a wound or sore during healing.

scabies (**SKAY**-bees) Skin disease produced by mites.

scald (SKAWLD) Burn from contact with hot liquid or steam.

scapula (**SKAP**-you-lah) Shoulder blade. Plural *scapulae*.

scapular (**SKAP**-you-lar) Pertaining to the scapula.

scar (SKAR) Fibrotic seam that forms when a wound heals.

schizophrenia (skitz-oh-**FREE**-nee-ah) Disorder of perception, thought, emotion, and behavior.

Schwann cell (SHWANN SELL) Connective tissue cell of the peripheral nervous system that forms a myelin sheath.

sclera (**SKLAIR**-ah) Fibrous outer covering of the eyeball and the white of the eye.

scleral (**SKLAIR**-al) Pertaining to the sclera.

scleritis (sklair-**RI**-tis) Inflammation of the sclera.

scleroderma (sklair-oh-**DERM**-ah) Thickening and hardening of the skin due to new collagen formation.

sclerose (skleh-**ROSE**) To harden or thicken.

sclerosis (skleh-**ROH**-sis) Thickening or hardening of a tissue; in the nervous system, hardening of nervous tissue by fibrous and glial connective tissue.

sclerotherapy (**SKLAIR**-oh-**THAIR**-ah-pee) Injection of a solution into a vein to thrombose it.

scoliosis (skoh-lee-**OH**-sis) An abnormal lateral curvature of the vertebral column.

scoliotic (**SKOH**-lee-**OT**-ik) Pertaining to or suffering from scoliosis.

scrotal (**SKRO**-tal) Pertaining to the scrotum.

scrotum (**SKRO**-tum) Sac containing testes.

seasonal affective disorder (see-**ZON**-al af-**FEK**-tiv dis-**OR**-der) Depression that occurs at the same time every year, often in winter.

sebaceous glands (seh-**BAY**-shus GLANZ) Glands in the dermis that open into hair follicles and secrete an oily fluid called *sebum*.

seborrhea (seb-oh-**REE**-ah) Excessive amount of sebum.

seborrheic (seb-oh-**REE**-ik) Pertaining to seborrhea.

sebum (**SEE**-bum) Waxy secretion of the sebaceous glands.

secondary (**SEK**-ond-ah-ree) Diseases or symptoms following a primary disease or symptom.

secrete (seh-**KREET**) To produce a chemical substance in a cell and release it from the cell.

secretion (seh-**KREE**-shun) The production of a chemical substance in a cell and its release from the cell.

sedation (seh-**DAY**-shun) State of being calmed.

sedative (**SED**-ah-tiv) Agent that calms nervous excitement.

segment (**SEG**-ment) A section of an organ or structure.

segmentectomy (seg-men-**TEK**-toe-me) Surgical excision of a segment of a tissue or organ.

seizure (**SEE**-zhur) Event due to excessive electrical activity in the brain.

self-examination (**SELF**-ek-zam-ih-**NAY**-shun) Conduct an examination of one's own body.

self-mutilation (self-myu-tih-**LAY**-shun) Injury or disfigurement made to one's own body.

semen (**SEE**-men) Penile ejaculate containing sperm and seminal fluid.

semilunar (sem-ee-**LOO**-nar) Appears like a half moon.

seminal vesicle (**SEM**-in-al **VES**-ih-kull) Sac of the ductus deferens that produces seminal fluid.

seminiferous (sem-ih-**NIF**-er-us) Pertaining to carrying semen.

seminiferous tubule (sem-ih-**NIF**-er-us **TU**-byul) Coiled tubes in the testes that produce sperm.

seminoma (sem-ih-**NO**-mah) Neoplasm of germ cells of a testis.

senescence (seh-**NES**-ens) The state of being old.

senescent (seh-**NES**-ent) Growing old.

senile (**SEE**-nile) Characteristic of old age.

senility (seh-**NIL**-ih-tee) Mental disorders occurring in old age.

sensation (sen-**SAY**-shun) The conscious feeling of the effects of a stimulation.

sensorineural hearing loss (**SEN**-sor-ih-**NYUR**-al) Hearing loss caused by lesions of the inner ear or the auditory nerve.

sensory (**SEN**-soh-ree) Having the function of sensation; structures of the nervous system that carry impulses to the brain.

sepsis (**SEP**-sis) Presence of pathogenic organisms or their toxins in blood or tissues.

septicemia (sep-tih-**SEE**-mee-ah) Microorganisms circulating in, and infecting, the blood (blood poisoning).

septum (**SEP**-tum) A thin wall separating two cavities or tissue masses. Plural *septa.*

serotonin (ser-oh-**TOE**-nin) A neurotransmitter in the central and peripheral nervous systems.

serum (**SEER**-um) Fluid remaining after removal of cells and fibrin clot from blood.

shock (SHOCK) Sudden physical or mental collapse or circulatory collapse.

shunt (SHUNT) A bypass or diversion of fluid; for example, blood.

sigmoid (**SIG**-moyd) Sigmoid colon is shaped like an "S."

sigmoidoscopy (sig-moi-**DOS**-koh-pee) Endoscopic examination of the sigmoid colon.

sign (SINE) Physical evidence of a disease process.

silicosis (sil-ih-**KOH**-sis) Fibrotic lung disease from inhaling silica particles.

sinoatrial (SA) node (sigh-noh-**AY**-tree-al NODE) The center of modified cardiac muscle fibers in the wall of the right atrium that acts as the pacemaker for the heart rhythm.

sinus (**SIGH**-nus) Cavity or hollow space in a bone or other tissue.

sinus rhythm (**SIGH**-nus **RITH**-um) The normal (optimal) heart rhythm arising from the sinoatrial node.

sinusitis (sigh-nyu-**SIGH**-tis) Inflammation of the lining of a sinus.

skeletal (**SKEL**-eh-tal) Pertaining to the skeleton.

skeleton (**SKEL**-eh-ton) The bony framework of the body.

Skene glands (SKEEN GLANZ) Paraurethral glands in the anterior wall of the vagina. Also called *paraurethral glands.*

smegma (**SMEG**-mah) Oily material produced by the glans and prepuce.

Snellen letter chart (**SNEL**-en) Test for acuity of distant vision.

snore (SNOR) Noise produced by vibrations in the structures of the nasopharynx.

sociopath (**SOH**-see-oh-path) Person with antisocial personality disorder.

somatic (soh-**MAT**-ik) Relating to the body in general; *or* a division of the periperal nervous system serving the skeletal muscles.

somatostatin (**SOH**-mah-toh-**STAT**-in) Hormone that inhibits release of growth hormone and insulin.

somatotropin (**SOH**-mah-toh-**TROH**-pin) Hormone of the anterior pituitary that stimulates the growth of body tissues. Also called *growth hormone.*

spasm (SPASM) Sudden involuntary contraction of a muscle group.

spasmodic (spaz-**MOD**-ik) Intermittent contractions.

spastic (**SPAZ**-tik) Increased muscle tone on movement.

specific (speh-**SIF**-ik) Relating to a particular entity.

specificity (spes-ih-**FIS**-ih-tee) State of having a fixed relation to a particular entity.

sperm (SPERM) Mature male sex cell. Also called *spermatozoon.*

spermatic (**SPER**-mat-ik) Pertaining to sperm.

spermatid (**SPER**-mat-id) A cell late in the development process of sperm.

spermatocele (**SPER**-mat-oh-seal) Cyst of the epididymis that contains sperm.

spermatogenesis (**SPER**-mat-oh-**JEN**-eh-sis) The process by which male germ cells differentiate into sperm.

spermatozoa (**SPER**-mat-oh-**ZOH**-ah) Sperm (plural of *spermatozoon*).

spermicidal (sper-mih-**SIGH**-dal) Pertaining to the killing of sperm; *or* destructive to sperm.

spermicide (**SPER**-mih-side) Agent that destroys sperm.

sphenoid (**SFEE**-noyd) Wedge-shaped bone at the base of the skull.

sphincter (**SFINK**-ter) Band of muscle that encircles an opening; when it contracts, the opening squeezes closed.

sphygmomanometer (**SFIG**-moh-mah-**NOM**-ih-ter) Instrument for measuring arterial blood pressure.

spina bifida (**SPY**-nah **BIH**-fih-dah) Failure of one or more vertebral arches to close during fetal development.

spina bifida cystica (**SIS**-tik-ah) Meninges and spinal cord protruding through the absent vertebral arch and having the appearance of a cyst.

spina bifida occulta (**OH**-kul-tah) The deformity of the vertebral arch is not apparent from the surface.

spinal (**SPY**-nal) Pertaining to the spine.

spinal tap (**SPY**-nal TAP) Placement of a needle through an intervertebral space into the subarachnoid space to withdraw CSF.

spine (SPINE) The vertebral column; *or* a short bony projection.

spiral fracture (**SPY**-ral **FRAK**-chur) A fracture in the shape of a coil.

spirochete (**SPY**-roh-keet) Spiral-shaped bacterium causing a sexually transmitted disease (syphilis).

spirometer (spy-**ROM**-eh-ter) An instrument used to measure respiratory volumes.

spirometry (spy-**ROM**-eh-tree) Use of a spirometer.

spleen (SPLEEN) Vascular, lymphatic organ in the left upper quadrant of the abdomen.

splenectomy (sple-**NECK**-toe-me) Surgical removal of the spleen.

splenomegaly (sple-noh-**MEG**-ah-lee) Enlarged spleen.

spondylosis (spon-dih-**LOH**-sis) Degenerative osteoarthritis of the spine.

spongiosum (spun-jee-**OH**-sum) Spongelike tissue.

sprain (SPRAIN) A wrench or tear in a ligament.

sputum (**SPYU**-tum) Matter coughed up and spat out by individuals with respiratory disorders.

squamous cell (**SKWAY**-mus SELL) Flat, scalelike epithelial cell.

stage (STAYJ) Definition of the extent and dissemination of a malignant neoplasm.

staging (**STAY**-jing) Process of determination of the extent of the distribution of a neoplasm.

stapes (**STAY**-peas) Inner (medial) one of the three ossicles of the middle ear; shaped like a stirrup.

Staphylococcus (**STAF**-ih-loh-**KOK**-us) Genus of gram-positive bacteria that divide in more than one plane to form clusters. Plural *staphylococci.*

starch (STARCH) Complex carbohydrate made of multiple units of glucose attached together.

stasis (**STAY**-sis) Stagnation in the flow of any body fluid.

status (**STAT**-us) A state or condition.

status epilepticus (**STAT**-us ep-ih-**LEP**-tik-us) Latin phrase for being in a prolonged or recurrent seizure for longer than a specific time frame.

stem cell (STEM SELL) Undifferentiated cell found in a differentiated tissue that can divide to yield the specialized cells in that tissue.

stenosis (steh-**NOH**-sis) Narrowing of a canal or passage.

stent (STENT) Wire-mesh tube used to keep arteries open.

stereopsis (ster-ee-**OP**-sis) Three-dimensional vision.

stereotactic (**STER**-ee-oh-**TAK**-tic) A precise three-dimensional method to locate a lesion.

stereotype (**STER**-ee-oh-tipe) An image held in common by members of a group.

sterile (**STER**-isle) Free from all living organisms and their spores; *or* unable to fertilize or reproduce.

sterility (ster-**RIL**-ih-tee) Inability to reproduce.

sterilization (**STER**-ih-lih-**ZAY**-shun) Process of making sterile.

sterilize (**STER**-ih-lize) To make sterile.

sternum (**STIR**-num) Long, flat bone forming the center of the anterior wall of the chest.

steroid (**STER**-oyd) Large family of chemical substances found in many drugs, hormones, and body components.

stethoscope (**STETH**-oh-skope) Instrument for listening to cardiac and respiratory sounds.

stimulant (**STIM**-you-lant) Agent that excites or strengthens.

stimulation (stim-you-**LAY**-shun) Arousal to increased functional activity.

stimulus (**STIM**-you-lus) Something that excites or strengthens the functional activity of an organ or part. Plural *stimuli.*

stoma (**STOW**-mah) Artificial opening.

strabismus (strah-**BIZ**-mus) Turning of an eye away from its normal position.

strain (STRAIN) Overstretch or tear in a muscle or tendon.

stratum basale (**STRAH**-tum bay-**SAL**-eh) Deepest layer of the epidermis, from which the other cells originate and migrate.

Streptococcus (strep-toe-**KOK**-us) Genus of gram-positive bacteria that grow in chains. Plural *streptococci.*

striated muscle (**STRI**-ay-ted **MUSS**-el) Another term for *skeletal muscle.*

stricture (**STRICK**-shur) Narrowing of a tube.

stridor (**STRY**-door) High-pitched noise made when there is a respiratory obstruction in the larynx or trachea.

stroke (STROHK) Acute clinical event caused by impaired cerebral circulation.

subarachnoid space (sub-ah-**RACK**-noyd SPASE) Space between the pia mater and the arachnoid membrane.

subclavian (sub-**CLAY**-vee-an) Underneath the clavicle.

subcutaneous (sub-kew-**TAY**-nee-us) Below the skin. Also called *hypodermic.*

subdural space (sub-**DYU**-ral SPACE) Space between the arachnoid and dura mater layers of the meninges.

sublingual (sub-**LING**-wal) Underneath the tongue.

subluxation (sub-luck-**SAY**-shun) An incomplete dislocation when some contact between the joint surfaces remains.

submandibular (sub-man-**DIB**-you-lar) Underneath the mandible.

submucosa (sub-mew-**KOH**-sa) Tissue layer underneath the mucosa.

substernal (sub-**STER**-nal) Under (behind) the sternum or breastbone.

suction (**SUK**-shun) Use of a catheter to clear the upper airway or other tubes.

sulcus (**SUL**-cuss) Groove on the surface of the cerebral hemispheres that separates gyri. Plural *sulci.*

superficial (soo-per-**FISH**-al) Situated near the surface.

superior (soo-**PEE**-ree-or) Situated above.

supinate (**SOO**-pih-nate) Rotate the forearm so that the surface of the palm faces anteriorly in the anatomical position.

supination (soo-pih-**NAY**-shun) Process of lying face upward or of turning a hand or foot so that the palm or sole is facing up.

supine (soo-**PINE**) Lying face up, flat on your spine.

suprapubic (**SOO**-prah-pyu-bik) Above the symphysis pubis.

surfactant (sir-**FAK**-tant) A protein and fat compound that creates surface tension to hold the lung alveolar walls apart.

suture (**SOO**-chur) Two bones are joined together by a fibrous band continuous with their periosteum, as in the skull; *or* a stitch to hold the edges of a wound together; *or* to stitch the edges of a wound together. Plural *sutures.*

sympathetic (sim-pah-**THET**-ik) Division of the autonomic nervous system operating at an unconscious level.

sympathy (**SIM**-pah-thee) Appreciation and concern for another person's mental and emotional state.

symphysis (**SIM**-feh-sis) Two bones joined by fibrocartilage. Plural *symphyses.*

symptom (**SIMP**-tum) Departure from the normal experienced by a patient.

symptomatic (simp-toe-**MAT**-ik) Pertaining to the symptoms of a disease.

synapse (**SIN**-aps) Junction between two nerve cells or a nerve fiber and its target cell, where electrical impulses are transmitted between the cells.

syncope (**SIN**-koh-peh) Temporary loss of consciousness and posture due to diminished cerebral blood flow.

syndesmosis (sin-dez-**MOH**-sis) Binding together of two bones with ligaments. Plural *syndesmoses.*

syndrome (**SIN**-drohm) Combination of signs and symptoms associated with a particular disease process.

synovial (sin-**OH**-vee-al) Pertaining to synovial fluid and the synovial membrane.

synthesis (**SIN**-the-sis) The process of building a compound from different elements.

synthetic (sin-**THET**-ik) Built up or put together from simpler compounds.

syphilis (**SIF**-ih-lis) Sexually transmitted disease caused by a spirochete.

syringomyelia (sih-**RING**-oh-my-**EE**-lee-ah) Abnormal longitudinal cavities in the spinal cord cause paresthesias and muscle weakness.

systemic (sis-**TEM**-ik) Relating to the entire organism.

systemic lupus erythematosus (sis-**TEM**-ik **LOO**-pus er-ih-**THEE**-mah-toe-sus) Inflammatory connective tissue disease affecting the whole body.

systole (**SIS**-toe-lee) Contraction of the heart muscle.

systolic (sis-**TOL**-ik) Pertaining to systole.

T

tachycardia (tack-ih-**KAR**-dee-ah) Rapid heart rate (above 100 beats per minute).

tachypnea (tack-ip-**NEE**-ah) Rapid breathing.

talipes (**TAL**-ip-eze) Deformity of the foot involving the talus.

talus (**TAY**-luss) The tarsal bone that articulates with the tibia to form the ankle joint.

tampon (**TAM**-pon) Plug or pack in a cavity to absorb or stop bleeding.

tamponade (tam-poh-**NAID**) Pathologic compression of an organ, such as the heart.

tapeworm (TAPEWORM) Intestinal parasitic worm.

tarsal (**TAR**-sal) Pertaining to the tarsus.

tarsus (**TAR**-sus) The collection of seven bones in the foot that form the ankle and instep; *or* the flat fibrous plate that gives shape to the outer edges of the eyelids.

tartar (**TAR**-tar) Calcified deposit at the gingival margin of the teeth.

Tay-Sachs disease (TAY SAKS **DIZ**-eez) Congenital fatal disorder of fat metabolism.

temperament (**TEM**-per-ah-ment) Predisposition to character or personality.

temporal (**TEM**-pore-al) Bone that forms part of the base and sides of the skull.

temporal lobe (**TEM**-pore-al LOBE) Posterior two-thirds of the cerebral hemispheres.

temporomandibular joint (TMJ) (**TEM**-pore-oh-man-**DIB**-you-lar JOYNT) The joint between the temporal bone and the mandible.

tendinitis (ten-dih-**NYE**-tis) Inflammation of a tendon. Also spelled *tendonitis*.

tendon (**TEN**-dun) Fibrous band that connects muscle to bone.

tenosynovitis (**TEN**-oh-sin-oh-**VIE**-tis) Inflammation of a tendon and its surrounding synovial sheath.

teratogen (**TER**-ah-toe-jen) Agent that produces fetal deformities.

teratogenesis (**TER**-ah-toe-**JEN**-eh-sis) Process involved in producing fetal deformities.

teratogenic (**TER**-ah-toe-**JEN**-ik) Pertaining to or capable of producing fetal deformities.

teratoma (ter-ah-**TOE**-mah) Neoplasm of a testis or ovary containing multiple tissues from other sites in the body.

testicle (**TES**-tih-kul) One of the male reproductive glands. Also called *testis*.

testicular (tes-**TICK**-you-lar) Pertaining to the testicle.

testis (**TES**-tis) A synonym for *testicle*. Plural *testes*.

testosterone (tes-**TOSS**-ter-own) Powerful androgen produced by the testes.

tetany (**TET**-ah-nee) Severe muscle twitches, cramps, and spasms.

tetralogy (te-**TRAL**-oh-jee) A set of four congenital heart defects occurring together.

tetralogy of Fallot (TOF) (te-**TRAL**-oh-jee of fah-**LOW**) Set of four congenital heart defects occurring together.

thalamus (**THAL**-ah-mus) Mass of gray matter underneath the ventricle in each cerebral hemisphere.

thalassemia (thal-ah-**SEE**-mee-ah) Group of inherited blood disorders that produce a hemolytic anemia.

thelarche (thee-**LAR**-key) Onset of breast development.

thenar (**THAY**-nar) The thenar eminence is the fleshy mass at the base of the thumb.

therapeutic (**THAIR**-ah-**PYU**-tik) Pertaining to the treatment of a disease or disorder.

therapy (**THAIR**-ah-pee) Systematic treatment of a disease, dysfunction, or disorder.

thoracentesis (**THOR**-ah-sen-**TEE**-sis) Insertion of a needle into the pleural cavity to withdraw fluid or air. Also called *pleural tap*.

thoracic (**THOR**-ass-ik) Pertaining to the chest (thorax).

thoracic cavity (**THOR**-ass-ik **KAV**-ih-tee) Space within the chest containing the lungs, heart, aorta, venae cavae, esophagus, trachea, and pulmonary vessels.

thoracoscopy (thor-ah-**KOS**-koh-pee) Examination of the pleural cavity with an endoscope.

thoracotomy (thor-ah-**KOT**-oh-me) Incision through the chest wall.

thorax (**THOR**-acks) The part of the trunk between the abdomen and the neck.

thrombin (**THROM**-bin) Enzyme that forms fibrin.

thrombocyte (**THROM**-boh-site) Another name for *platelet*.

thrombocytopenia (**THROM**-boh-site-oh-**PEE**-nee-uh) Deficiency of platelets in circulating blood.

thromboembolism (**THROM**-boh-**EM**-boh-lizm) A piece of detached blood clot (embolus) blocking a distant blood vessel.

thrombolysis (throm-**BOL**-ih-sis) Dissolving of a thrombus (clot).

thrombolytic (throm-boh-**LIT**-ik) Able to dissolve a thrombus.

thrombophlebitis (**THROM**-boh-fleh-**BY**-tis) Inflammation of a vein with clot formation.

thrombosis (throm-**BOH**-sis) Formation of a thrombus.

thrombus (**THROM**-bus) A clot attached to a diseased blood vessel or heart lining. Pleural *thrombi*.

thrush (THRUSH) Infection with *Candida albicans*.

thymectomy (thigh **MEK** toe me) Surgical removal of the thymus gland.

thymoma (thigh-**MOH**-mah) Benign tumor of the thymus.

thymus (**THIGH**-mus) Lymphoid and endocrine gland located in the mediastinum.

thyroid (**THIGH**-royd) Endocrine gland in the neck; *or* a cartilage of the larynx.

thyroid hormone (**THIGH**-royd **HOR**-mohn) Collective term for the two thyroid hormones, T3 and T4.

thyroid storm (**THIGH**-royd STORM) Medical crisis and emergency due to excess thyroid hormones.

thyroidectomy (thigh-royd-**ECK**-toe-me) Surgical removal of the thyroid gland.

thyroiditis (thigh-royd-**EYE**-tis) Inflammation of the thyroid gland.

thyrotoxicosis (**THIGH**-roe-toks-ih-**KOH**-sis) Disorder produced by excessive thyroid hormone production.

thyrotropin (thigh-roe-**TROH**-pin) Hormone from the anterior pituitary gland that stimulates function of the thyroid gland.

thyroxine (thigh-**ROCK**-sin) Thyroid hormone T4, tetraiodothyronine.

tibia (**TIB**-ee-ah) The larger bone of the lower leg.

tibial (**TIB**-ee-al) Pertaining to the tibia.

tic (TIK) Sudden, involuntary, repeated contraction of muscles.

tic douloureux (tik duh-luh-**RUE**) Painful, sudden, spasmodic involuntary contractions of the facial muscles supplied by the trigeminal nerve. Also called *trigeminal neuralgia.*

tinea (**TIN**-ee-ah) General term for a group of related skin infections caused by different species of fungi.

tinnitus (**TIN**-ih-tus) Persistent ringing, whistling, clicking, or booming noise in the ears.

tissue (**TISH**-you) Collection of similar cells.

tomography (toe-**MOG**-rah-fee) Radiographic image of a selected slice of tissue.

tone (TONE) Tension present in resting muscles.

tongue (TUNG) Mobile muscle mass in the mouth; bears the taste buds.

tonic (**TON**-ik) State of muscular contraction.

tonic-clonic (**TON**-ik **KLON**-ik) The body alternates between excessive muscular rigidity (tonic) and jerking muscular contractions (clonic).

tonic-clonic seizure (**TON**-ik **KLON**-ik **SEE**-zhur) Generalized seizure due to epileptic activity in all or most of the brain.

tonometer (toe-**NOM**-eh-ter) Instrument for determining intraocular pressure.

tonometry (toe-**NOM**-eh-tree) The measurement of intraocular pressure.

tonsil (**TON**-sill) Mass of lymphoid tissue on either side of the throat at the back of the tongue.

tonsillectomy (ton-sih-**LEK**-toh-me) Surgical removal of the tonsils.

tonsillitis (ton-sih-**LIE**-tis) Inflammation of the tonsils.

topical (**TOP**-ih-kal) Medication applied to the skin to obtain a local effect.

torsion (**TOR**-shun) The act or result of twisting.

Tourette syndrome (tur-**ET SIN**-drome) Disorder of multiple motor and vocal tics.

toxic (**TOK**-sick) Pertaining to a toxin.

toxicity (toks-**ISS**-ih-tee) The state of being poisonous.

toxin (**TOK**-sin) Poisonous substance formed by a cell or organism.

trachea (**TRAY**-kee-ah) Air tube from the larynx to the bronchi.

trachealis (tray-kee-**AY**-lis) Pertaining to the trachea.

tracheostomy (tray-kee-**OST**-oh-me) Incision into the windpipe into which a tube can be inserted to assist breathing.

tracheotomy (tray-kee-**OT**-oh-me) Incision made into the trachea to create a tracheostomy.

tract (TRACKT) Bundle of nerve fibers with a common origin and destination.

traction (**TRAK**-shun) Pulling or dragging force.

trait (TRAYT) A discrete characteristic that has a known quality.

tranquilizer (**TRANG**-kwih-lie-zer) Agent that calms without sedating or depressing.

transdermal (tranz-**DER**-mal) Going across or through the skin.

transfusion (tranz-**FYU**-zhun) Transfer of blood or a blood component from donor to recipient.

transplant (**TRANZ**-plant) The tissue or organ used; *or* the act of transferring tissue from one person to another.

transplantation (**TRANZ**-plan-**TAY**-shun) The moving of tissue or an organ from one person or place to another.

transthoracic (tranz-thor-**ASS**-ik) Going through the chest wall.

transurethral (**TRANZ**-you-**REE**-thral) Procedure performed through the urethra.

transverse (tranz-**VERS**) Horizontal plane dividing the body into upper and lower portions.

transverse fracture (tranz-**VERS FRAK**-chur) A fracture perpendicular to the long axis of the bone.

tremor (**TREM**-or) Small, shaking, involuntary, repetitive movements of hands, extremities, neck, or jaw.

triceps brachii (**TRY**-sepz **BRAY**-key-eye) Muscle of the arm that has three heads or points of origin.

Trichomonas (trik-oh-**MOH**-nas) A parasite causing an STD.

trichomoniasis (**TRIK**-oh-moh-**NIE**-ah-sis) Infection with *Trichomonas vaginalis.*

tricuspid (try-**KUSS**-pid) Having three points; a tricuspid heart valve has three flaps.

triglyceride (try-**GLISS**-eh-ride) Lipid containing three fatty acids.

trimester (**TRY**-mes-ter) One-third of the length of a full-term pregnancy.

triplegia (try-**PLEE**-jee-ah) Paralysis of three limbs.

triplegic (try-**PLEE**-jik) Pertaining to or suffering from triplegia.

trochanter (troh-**KAN**-ter) One of two bony prominences near the head of the femur.

tropic (**TROH**-pik) Tropic hormones stimulate other endocrine glands to produce hormones.

tuberculosis (too-**BER**-kyu-**LOW**-sis) Infectious disease that can infect any organ or tissue.

tumor (**TOO**-mor) Any abnormal swelling.

tunica (**TYU**-nih-kah) A covering layer in the wall of a blood vessel or other tubular structure.

tunica vaginalis (**TYU**-nih-kah vaj-ih-**NAHL**-iss) The sheath of the testis and epididymis.

tympanic (tim-**PAN**-ik) Pertaining to the tympanic membrane (eardrum) or tympanic cavity.

tympanostomy (tim-pan-**OS**-toe-me) Surgically created new opening in the tympanic membrane to allow fluid to drain from the middle ear.

U

ulna (**UL**-nah) The medial and larger of the bones of the forearm.

ulnar (**UL**-nar) Pertaining to the ulna or to any of the structures (artery, vein, nerve) named after it.

ultrasonography (**UL**-trah-soh-**NOG**-rah-fee) Delineation of deep structures using sound waves.

ultraviolet (ul-trah-**VIE**-oh-let) Light rays at a higher frequency than the violet end of the spectrum.

umbilical (um-**BILL**-ih-kal) Pertaining to the umbilicus or the center of the abdomen.

umbilicus (um-**BILL**-ih-kuss) Pit in the abdomen where the umbilical cord entered the fetus.

unilateral (you-nih-**LAT**-er-al) Pertaining to one side.

urea (you-**REE**-ah) End product of nitrogen metabolism.

uremia (you-**REE**-me-ah) The complex of symptoms arising from renal failure.

ureter (you-**REE**-ter) Tube that connects a kidney to the urinary bladder.

ureteral (you-ree-**TER**-al) Pertaining to the ureter.

ureteroscope (you-**REE**-ter-oh-scope) Endoscope to view the inside of the ureter.

ureteroscopy (you-**REE**-ter-os-koh-pee) To examine the ureter.

urethra (you-**REE**-thra) Canal leading from the bladder to the outside.

urethritis (you-ree-**THRI**-tis) Inflammation of the urethra.

urinalysis (yur-ih-**NAL**-ih-sis) Examination of urine to separate it into its elements and define their kind and/or quantity.

urinary (**YUR**-in-ary) Pertaining to urine.

urinate (**YUR**-in-ate) To pass urine.

urination (yur-ih-**NAY**-shun) The act of passing urine.

urine (**YUR**-in) Fluid and dissolved substances excreted by the kidney.

urological (yur-oh-**LOJ**-ih-kal) Pertaining to urology.

urologist (you-**ROL**-oh-jist) Medical specialist in disorders of the urinary system.

urology (you-**ROL**-oh-jee) Medical specialty of disorders of the urinary system.

urticaria (ur-tee-**KARE**-ee-ah) Rash of itchy wheals (hives).

uterine (**YOU**-ter-ine) Pertaining to the uterus.

uterus (**YOU**-ter-us) Organ in which a fertilized egg develops into a fetus.

uvea (**YOU**-vee-ah) Middle coat of the eyeball—includes the iris, ciliary body, and choroid.

uveitis (you-vee-**EYE**-tis) Inflammation of the uvea.

uvula (**YOU**-vyu-lah) Fleshy projection of the soft palate.

V

vaccinate (**VAK**-sin-ate) To administer a vaccine.

vaccination (vak-sih-**NAY**-shun) Administration of a vaccine.

vaccine (**VAK**-seen) Preparation to generate active immunity.

vagina (vah-**JIE**-nah) Female genital canal extending from the uterus to the vulva.

vaginal (**VAJ**-ih-nal) Pertaining to the vagina.

vaginitis (vah-jih-**NIE**-tis) Inflammation of the vagina.

vaginosis (vah-jih-**NOH**-sis) A disease of the vagina.

vagus (**VAY**-gus) Tenth (X) cranial nerve; supplies many different organs throughout the body.

varicocele (**VAIR**-ih-koh-seal) Varicose veins of the spermatic cord.

varicose (**VAIR**-ih-kos) Characterized by or affected with varices.

varicosities (vair-ih-**KOS**-ih-tees) Collection of varicose veins.

varix (**VAIR**-iks) Dilated, tortuous vein. Plural *varices.*

vasectomy (vah-**SEK**-toe-me) Excision of a segment of the ductus deferens.

vasoconstriction (**VAY**-soh-con-**STRIK**-shun) Reduction in the diameter of a blood vessel.

vasodilation (**VAY**-soh-dih-**LAY**-shun) Increase in the diameter of a blood vessel.

vasovasostomy (**VAY**-soh-vay-**SOS**-toe-me) Reanastomosis of the ductus deferens to restore the flow of sperm. Also called *vasectomy reversal.*

vegetative (**VEJ**-eh-tay-tiv) Functioning unconsciously, as plant life is assumed to do.

vein (**VANE**) Blood vessel carrying blood toward the heart.

vena cava (**VEE**-nah **KAY**-vah) One of the two largest veins in the body. Plural *venae cavae.*

venogram (**VEE**-noh-gram) Radiograph of veins after injection of radiopaque contrast material.

venous (**VEE**-nuss) Pertaining to a vein.

ventilation (ven-tih-**LAY**-shun) Movement of gases into and out of the lungs.

ventilator (**VEN**-tih-lay-tor) Device that breathes for the patient.

ventral (**VEN**-tral) Pertaining to the belly or situated nearer to the surface of the belly.

ventricle (**VEN**-trih-kel) Chamber of the heart (pumps blood) or brain (produces cerebrospinal fluid).

venule (**VEN**-yule or **VEEN**-yule) Small vein leading from the capillary network.

vernix caseosa (**VER**-nicks kay-see-**OH**-sah) Cheesy substance covering the skin of the fetus.

verruca (ver-**ROO**-cah) Wart caused by a virus.

vertebra (**VER**-teh-brah) One of the bones of the spinal column. Plural *vertebrae.*

vertebral (**VER**-teh-bral) Pertaining to a vertebra.

vertex (**VER**-teks) Topmost point of the vault of the skull.

vertigo (**VER**-tih-go) Sensation of spinning or whirling.

vesicle (**VES**-ih-kull) Small sac containing liquid; for example, a blister.

vestibular (ves-**TIB**-you-lar) Pertaining to the vestibule.

vestibule (**VES**-tih-byul) Space at the entrance to a canal.

vestibulectomy (ves-tib-you-**LEK**-toe-me) Surgical excision of the vulva.

villus (**VILL**-us) Thin, hairlike projection, particularly of a mucous membrane lining a cavity. Plural *villi.*

virus (**VIE**-rus) Group of infectious agents that require living cells for growth and reproduction.

viscera (**VISS**-er-ah) Internal organs, particularly in the abdomen.

visceral (**VISS**-er-al) Pertaining to the internal organs.

viscosity (viss-**KOS**-ih-tee) The resistance of a fluid to flow.

viscous (**VISS**-kus) Sticky fluid that is resistant to flow.

viscus (**VISS**-kus) Any single internal organ.

visual acuity (**VIH**-zhoo-al ah-**KYU**-ih-tee) Sharpness and clearness of vision.

vitamin (**VYE**-tah-min) Essential organic substance necessary in small amounts for normal cell function.

vitreous (**VIT**-ree-us) Vitreous humor is a gelatinous liquid in the posterior cavity of the eyeball with the appearance of glass.

vocal (**VOH**-kal) Pertaining to the voice.

void (VOYD) To evacuate urine or feces.

voluntary muscle (**VOL**-un-tare-ee **MUSS**-el) Muscle that is under the control of the will.

vomer (**VOH**-mer) Lower nasal septum.

vulva (**VUL**-vah) Female external genitalia.

vulvar (**VUL**-var) Pertaining to the vulva.

vulvodynia (vul-voh-**DIN**-ee-uh) Chronic vulvar pain.

vulvovaginal (**VUL**-voh-**VAJ**-ih-nal) Pertaining to the vulva and vagina.

vulvovaginitis (**VUL**-voh-vaj-ih-**NIE**-tis) Inflammation of the vulva and vagina.

W

warfarin (**WAR**-fuh-rin) Anticoagulant; also used as rat poison; trade name *Coumadin.*

Weber test (**VA**-ber TEST) Test for sensorineural hearing loss.

wheal (WHEEL) Small, itchy swelling of the skin. Wheals raised by an injection do not itch. Also called *hives.*

whiplash (**HWIP**-lash) Symptoms caused by sudden, uncontrolled extension and flexion of the neck, often in an automobile accident.

white matter (WITE **MATT**-er) Regions of the brain and spinal cord occupied by bundles of axons.

whooping cough (**WHO**-ping KAWF) Infectious disease with spasmodic, intense cough ending on a whoop (stridor). Also called *pertussis.*

Wilms tumor (WILMZ **TOO**-mor) Cancerous kidney tumor of childhood. Also known as *nephroblastoma.*

wound (WOOND) Any injury that interrupts the continuity of skin or a mucous membrane.

X

xenograft (**ZEN**-oh-graft) A graft from another species. Also called *heterograft.*

Y

yeast (YEEST) Microscopic fungus.

Z

zygoma (zye-**GO**-mah) Bone that forms the prominence of the cheek.

zygomatic (zye-go-**MAT**-ik) Pertaining to the zygoma.

zygote (**ZYE**-goat) Cell resulting from the union of the sperm and egg.

Photo Credits

Front Matter

Title Page: © The McGraw-Hill Companies, Inc./Rick Brady, photographer; Page xiii: © C Squared Studios/Getty RF; Page xviii: © Banana Stock RF.

Welcome Chapter

Opener: © The McGraw-Hill Companies, Inc./Rick Brady, photographer; W.1, W2: © The McGraw-Hill Companies, Inc./Rick Brady, photographer; W.3: Corbis RF; W.4: © The McGraw-Hill Companies, Inc./Rick Brady, photographer; W.5: © Vol. 115/PhotoDisc/Getty RF.

Chapter 1

Opener: © The McGraw-Hill Companies, Inc./Rick Brady, photographer.

Chapter 2

Opener: © The McGraw-Hill Companies, Inc./Rick Brady, photographer; 2.1: © The McGraw-Hill Companies, Inc./Joe DeGrandis, photographer; 2.2: © The McGraw-Hill Companies, Inc./Eric Wise, photographer; 2.3, 2.5: © The McGraw-Hill Companies, Inc./Joe DeGrandis, photographer; 2.6: © Francis Leroy, BIOCOSMOS/Photo Researchers, Inc.

Chapter 3

Opener: © The McGraw-Hill Companies, Inc./Rick Brady, photographer; 3.4: © Dr. P. Marazzi/SPL/Photo Researchers, Inc.; 3.5: © BioPhoto Associates/Photo Researchers, Inc.; 3.6: © James Stevenson/Photo Researchers, Inc.; 3.7: © Medical-on-line/Alamy; 3.8: © Kenneth Greer/Visuals Unlimited; 3.9: © Logical Images; 3.10: © SPL/Photo Researchers, Inc.; 3.11: © Dr. P. Marazzi/SPL/Photo Researchers, Inc.; 3.12: © A. M. Siegelman/Visuals Unlimited; 3.13: © Eye of Science/Photo Researchers, Inc.; 3.14: © Farrar, W, E., Woods, M. J., Innes, J. S.: *Infectious Diseases: Text and Color Atlas*, ed. 2. London, Mosby, Europe, 1992; 3.15: © Dr P. Marazzi /SPL/Photo Researchers, Inc.; 3.16: Courtesy Dr. Maureen Mayes; 3.17: © Mediscan/Visuals Unlimited; 3.18: © Medical-on-line/Alamy; 3.20: © Kenneth Greer/Visuals Unlimited; 3.24: © Dr. Harout Tanielian/Photo Researchers, Inc.; 3.25: © Logical Images; 3.26a: © Sheila Terry/Photo Researchers, Inc.; 3.26b: © Dr, P. Marazzi/Photo Researchers, Inc.; 3.26c: © John Radcliffe Hospital/Photo Researchers, Inc.; 3.31: © Ken Geer/Visuals Unlimited.

Chapter 4

Opener: © The McGraw-Hill Companies, Inc./Rick Brady, photographer; 4.2a: © The McGraw-Hill Companies, Inc./Christine Eckel, photographer; 4.4: © Dr. Michael Klein/Peter Arnold, Inc.; 4.5: © The McGraw-Hill Companies, Inc./Joe DeGrandis, photographer; 4.14: © Zephyr/Photo Researchers, Inc.; 4.15: © Dr. P. Marazzi/Science Photo Library; Photo Researchers, Inc.; 4.16: © Ralph Hutchings/Visuals Unlimited; 4.18: © Joshua Alan Manchester/Custom Medical Stock Photo; 4.20: © AJPhoto/Photo Researchers Inc.; 4.23: © Charles McRae, M.D./Visuals Unlimited.

Chapter 5

Opener, 5.3: © The McGraw-Hill Companies, Inc./Rick Brady, photographer; 5.6: © The McGraw-Hill Companies, Inc./Eric Wise, photographer; 5.11: © Courtesy of North Coast Medical; 5.12: © Roger Ressmeyer/Corbis.

Chapter 6

Opener, 6.8: © The McGraw-Hill Companies, Inc./Rick Brady, photographer; 6.10: © Ed Reschke; 6.11: © Pasieka/SPL/Photo Researchers, Inc.; 6.15: © Dr. P. Marazzi/Photo Researchers, Inc.

Chapter 7

Opener: © Vol. 40/PhotoDisc/Getty; 7.1b: © Bill Longcore/Photo Researchers, Inc.; 7.2: © Meckes/Ottawa/Photo Researchers, Inc.; 7.3-7.7: © Ed Reschke; 7.9a: © Medical-on-line/Alamy; 7.9b: © Dr. P. Marazzi/SPL/Photo Researchers, Inc.; 7.15: © The McGraw-Hill Companies, Inc./Dennis Strete, photographer; 7.17: © Peter Arnold, Inc.; 7.18: © Visuals Unlimited.

Chapter 8

Opener: © The McGraw-Hill Companies, Inc./Rick Brady, photographer; 8.7: © Phototake; 8.10, 8.12: © Ralph Hutchings/Visuals Unlimited; 8.13: © Collection CNRI/Phototake; 8.14: © Wellcome Images.

Chapter 9

Opener: © The McGraw-Hill Companies, Inc./Rick Brady, photographer; 9.5: © Photo Network Stock/Grant Heilman Photography Inc.; 9.6: © ISM/Phototake; 9.7: © Medical-on-line/Alamy; 9.8: © Mediscan; 9.14: © CNRI/SPL/Photo Researchers Inc.; 9.18: © SIU Biomedical/Photo Researchers, Inc.; 9.21b: © CNRI/Photo Researchers, Inc.; 9.23: © Susan Leavine/Photo Researchers Inc.; 9.24: © Dr. P. Marazzi/SPL/Photo Researchers, Inc.; 9.25: © Phototake Inc./Alamy.

Chapter 10

Opener: © The McGraw-Hill Companies, Inc./Rick Brady, photographer; 10.8: © Phototake Inc./Alamy; 10.9a: © Wellcome Images; 10.10: © NIH/Phototake; 10.11: © James Cavallini/Photo Researchers, Inc.; 10.12a: © Wellcome Images; 10.12b: © Simon Fraser/Newcastle Hospitals NHS/Science Photo Library; Photo Researchers, Inc. 10.13: © Dr. M.A. Ansary/Custom Medical Stock Photo; 10.14: © NMSB/Custom Medical Stock Photo; 10.15: © Vol. 15 PhotoDisc/Getty.

Chapter 11

Opener: © The McGraw-Hill Companies, Inc./Rick Brady, photographer; 11.1: © The McGraw-Hill Companies, Inc./Joe DeGrandis, photographer; 11.3: © Phototake, Inc./Alamy; 11.4: © Western Ophthalmic Hospital/Photo Researchers Inc.; 11.5: © Mediscan; 11.6: © ISM/Phototake; 11.7: © BioPhoto Associates/Photo Researchers Inc.; 11.8: © Matt Harris Photography/Alamy; 11.14: © Phototake Inc./Alamy; 11.15 © National Eye Institute, National Institutes of Health; 11.16: © Dr. P. Marazzi/Photo Researchers, Inc.; 11.17: National Eye Institute, National Institutes of Health; 11.18: © Volume 58/PhotoDisc/Getty; 11.19: © Paul Parker/Photo Researchers, Inc.; 11.20: © Chris Barry/Phototake; 11.21: National Eye Institute, National Institutes of Health; 11.24: © The McGraw-Hill Companies, Inc./Rick Brady, photographer; p. 356: © The McGraw-Hill Companies, Inc./Rick Brady, photographer; 11.27: © Wellcome Images; 11.29: © ISM/Phototake; 11.31: © Lester V. Bergman/Corbis; 11.32: © ISM/Phototake; 11.33: © Clinica Claros/IMS/Phototake.

Chapter 12

Opener: © The McGraw-Hill Companies, Inc./Rick Brady, photographer; 12.4: Reprinted by permission of publisher from Albert Mendeloff, "Acromegaly, diabetes, hypermetabolism, proteinurs, and heart failure," *American Journal of Medicine*: 20:1, 01-56, p. 135. © by Excerpta Medica, Inc.; 12.7: © Dr. M.A. Ansary/Photo Researchers, Inc.; 12.8: © Dr. P. Marazzi/SPL/Photo Researchers, Inc.; 12.9: © Mediscan; 12.10: © Bettmann/Corbis.

Chapter 13

Opener: © The McGraw-Hill Companies, Inc./Rick Brady, photographer; 13.4: © Medical-on-line/Alamy; 13.8: © Saturn Stills/SPL/Photo Researchers, Inc.

Chapter 14

Opener: © The McGraw-Hill Companies, Inc./Rick Brady, photographer.

Chapter 15

Opener: © The McGraw-Hill Companies, Inc./Rick Brady, photographer; 15.3: © Kenneth Greer/Visuals Unlimited; 15.4: © Biophoto Associates/Photo Researchers, Inc.; 15.6: © The William Boyd Museum, Dept. of Pathology and Laboratory Medicine, The University of British Columbia; 15.7: © Wellcome Photo Library; 15.8: © The William Boyd Museum, Dept. of Pathology and Laboratory Medicine, The University of British Columbia; 15.9: © Parviz M. Pour/Photo Researchers, Inc.; 15.11: © The McGraw-Hill Companies, Inc./Jill Braaten, photographer; 15.15: © BrandX Pictures/Punchstock; 15.17: © Photo Researchers, Inc.; 15.19: © Picture Partners/Photo Researchers, Inc.; 15.21: © Wellcome Photo Library; 15.22: © ALIX/Phanie/Photo Researchers, Inc.

A